Orthopedic
Anesthesia

Orthopedic Anesthesia

Edited by

Denise J. Wedel, M.D.

Associate Professor
Department of Anesthesiology
Mayo Medical School
Chair
Division of Orthopedic Anesthesia
Department of Anesthesiology
Mayo Clinic
Rochester, Minnesota

Churchill Livingstone
New York, Edinburgh, London, Melbourne, Tokyo

Library of Congress Cataloging-in-Publication Data

Orthopedic anesthesia / edited by Denise J. Wedel.
   p. cm.
  Includes bibliographical references and index.
   ISBN 0-443-08873-X
   1. Anesthesia in orthopedics. I. Wedel, Denise J.
   [DNLM: 1. Anesthesia. 2. Orthopedics. WO 200 077]
RD751.078 1993
617.0'673—dc20
DNLM/DLC
for Library of Congress   92-49142
                       CIP

Distributed in the United States by Churchill Livingstone Inc., 650 Avenue of the Americas, New York, NY 10011. Distributed in the United Kingdom by Churchill Livingstone, Robert Stevenson House, 1-3 Baxter's Place, Leith Walk, Edinburgh EH1 3AF, and by associated companies, branches, and representatives throughout the world.

Accurate indications, adverse reactions, and dosage schedules for drugs are provided in this book , but it is possible that they may change. The reader is urged to review the package information data of the manufacturers of the medications mentioned.

The Publishers have made every effort to trace the copyright holders for borrowed material. If they have inadvertently overlooked any, they will be pleased to make the necessary arrangements at the first opportunity.

Acquisitions Editor: *Toni M. Tracy*
Copy Editor: *Bridgett Dickinson*
Production Supervisor: *Jeanine Furino*

Printed in the United States of America

First published in 1993   7 6 5 4 3 2 1

Contributors

David L. Brown, M.D.
Associate Professor, Department of Anesthesiology, Mayo Medical School; Consultant, Department of Anesthesiology, Mayo Clinic, Rochester, Minnesota

William J. Davis, M.D.
Clinical Fellow, Department of Anesthesiology, Mayo Clinic, Rochester, Minnesota

Edward P. Didier, M.D.
Associate Professor, Department of Anesthesiology, Mayo Medical School; Consultant, Division of Orthopedic Anesthesia, Department of Anesthesiology, Mayo Clinic, Rochester, Minnesota

Beth A. Elliott, M.D.
Assistant Professor, Department of Anesthesiology, Mayo Medical School; Consultant, Division of Orthopedic Anesthesia, Department of Anesthesiology, Mayo Clinic, Rochester, Minnesota

Ronald J. Faust, M.D.
Associate Professor, Department of Anesthesiology, Mayo Medical School; Consultant, Department of Anesthesiology, Mayo Clinic, Rochester, Minnesota

Brian A. Hall, M.D.
Instructor, Department of Anesthesiology, Mayo Medical School; Senior Associate Consultant, Department of Anesthesiology, Mayo Clinic, Rochester, Minnesota

Terese T. Horlocker, M.D.
Instructor, Department of Anesthesiology, Mayo Medical School; Consultant, Division of Orthopedic Anesthesia, Department of Anesthesiology, Mayo Clinic, Rochester, Minnesota

Tim J. Lamer, M.D.
Assistant Professor, Department of Anesthesiology, Mayo Medical School; Consultant, Department of Anesthesiology, Mayo Clinic, Jacksonville, Florida

Robert L. Lennon, D.O.
Associate Professor, Department of Anesthesiology, Mayo Medical School; Consultant, Department of Anesthesiology, Mayo Clinic, Rochester, Minnesota

Lance A. Proctor, M.D.
Clinical Fellow, Department of Anesthesiology, Mayo Clinic, Rochester, Minnesota

Steven H. Rose, M.D.
Assistant Professor, Department of Anesthesiology, Mayo Medical School; Consultant, Division of Orthopedic Anesthesia, Department of Anesthesiology, Mayo Clinic, Rochester, Minnesota

Kenneth P. Scott, M.D.
Instructor, Department of Anesthesiology, Mayo Medical School; Senior Associate Consultant, Department of Anesthesiology, Mayo Clinic, Rochester, Minnesota

Denise J. Wedel, M.D.
Associate Professor, Department of Anesthesiology, Mayo Medical School; Chair, Division of Orthopedic Anesthesia, Department of Anesthesiology, Mayo Clinic, Rochester, Minnesota

Peter R. Wilson, M.B.B.S.
Associate Professor, Department of Anesthesiology, Mayo Medical School; Consultant, Division of Pain Services, Department of Anesthesiology, Mayo Clinic, Rochester, Minnesota

Foreword

In the era of rapidly expanding scientific knowledge and medical technology the proliferation of medical textbooks seems to be keeping pace. While it would appear that many such efforts are duplications or redundancies, a textbook focused on orthopedic anesthesia is most appealing and will prove to be of considerable value to the practicing anesthesiologist and orthopedic surgeon alike.

With any surgical specialty, an interdisciplinary management is essential for the optimum welfare of our patients. At Mayo such a philosophy of patient management is integral to our practice. For the orthopedic surgeon no aspect of surgical practice relies more completely on the expertise and cooperation of a colleague than does the care rendered by the orthopedic anesthesiologist.

In my opinion the orthopedic anesthesiologists of Mayo Clinic are eminently qualified to provide the special insight required of this procedure. An immense volume of difficult cases representing a broad spectrum of orthopedic intervention is superbly managed by this group of physicians. In addition to the typical support role under the direction of Dr. Wedel, the orthopedic anesthesiologists have demonstrated a keen and genuine interest in the nuances of orthopedic practice and surgical procedures that goes well beyond what would ordinarily be expected of our colleagues at the "head of the table." Because of this involvement the perception once related to me that "patients come to the Mayo Clinic for their surgery, not their anesthesia," may be less true than might be thought. Today, the orthopedic anesthesiologist is intimately involved not only in the procedure but also in the basic science foundation of the anesthetic being administered and in the postoperative pain management of many complex patients.

From this perspective I have specifically found the topic, organization, and structure of *Orthopedic Anesthesia* both thorough and comprehensive. The organization reflects a detailed knowledge of the topic that arises from experience gained from managing the anesthesia of over 9,000 major orthopedic cases each year. The full spectrum of orthopedic procedures, pediatric, microvascular, tumor, foot, and adult reconstructive surgery of all types, are regularly managed by the Mayo Orthopedic Anesthesia Division. This group is in a singular position therefore to provide practical insight into the care of the orthopedic patients. As importantly, the dynamic and ongoing research effort provides the all-important scientific basis for this clinical practice.

In summary, this comprehensive and definitive text is provided by a highly qualified and dedicated staff of orthopedic anesthesiologists. This group is in a unique position to provide a most comprehensive, useful, and timely contribution to the anesthesia literature. I applaud my colleagues for this outstanding accomplishment.

B.F. Morrey, M.D.
Professor, Department of
Orthopedic Surgery
Mayo Medical School
Chair, Department of
Orthopedic Surgery
Mayo Clinic
Rochester, Minnesota

Preface

Orthopedic anesthesia is a logical outgrowth of the burgeoning subspecialization that has been taking place in the field of anesthesiology. Several factors bind this diverse patient group together. Patients vary in age from infancy to extremely elderly, but the surgical procedures involving bone, muscle, and related soft tissues require similar approaches to monitoring and anesthetic techniques. For example, many orthopedic surgical procedures lend themselves to the use of regional anesthesia. This produces both intraoperative surgical anesthesia as well as postoperative pain relief, and creates a further subspecialty within orthopedic anesthesia. Another seemingly trivial, but vitally important function of the orthopedic anesthesia care provider is patient positioning. Patient positioning, other than during supine surgery, is a common feature in orthopedic cases and requires experience and specific knowledge to produce optimal surgical conditions and avoid potential injuries. Orthopedic procedures are frequently associated with major blood loss and its related risks. The orthopedic anesthesia care provider must be experienced in techniques that decrease these risks, must be able to use intraoperative hypotension and blood salvage techniques, and must be able to manage transfusion-related complications. The orthopedic patient undergoing surgery is also at risk for deep venous thrombosis and potentially fatal pulmonary embolus. These complications require extensive knowledge of the current methods available to prevent their occurrence. Therefore, the pharmacology of presently available anticoagulants and antiplatelet agents that may interact with anesthetic drugs or techniques must be thoroughly understood.

Knowledge of specific orthopedic surgical techniques, including duration, extent, predicted blood loss, and associated complications, is invaluable to the anesthesia care provider working in a team to provide the best possible patient care. Orthopedic surgical patients usually require early mobilization and rehabilitation, both of which can be expedited by appropriate selection of anesthetic techniques and management of postoperative analgesia. This knowledge can only be gained by specialized training and experience.

In *Orthopedic Anesthesia* the authors share their experience as anesthesia care providers in a large orthopedic practice that encompasses all major areas of orthopedics. We believe this information will be helpful to both the specialist and the "generalist," and will encourage anesthesia care providers to approach orthopedic anesthesia with renewed interest and confidence. We also believe that this information will be useful to orthopedic surgeons themselves, by giving insight into the problems and complexities of "just a whiff of gas."

Denise J. Wedel, M.D.

Contents

Introduction

Anesthesiology as a medical subspecialty has evolved rapidly during this century. The impetus for this has been in part the occurrence of two world wars and several other major conflicts. These caused battle casualties that required much greater sophistication in anesthesia care as the severity and complexity of the injuries became more amenable to surgical intervention. The medical complexity of patients requiring anesthesia for surgery in civilian life also increased. This, unlike the wartime situation, has been in part related to the significant increase in an elderly population with multiple medical conditions, which has also fueled the development of anesthesiology as a specialty as surgical techniques evolved. In addition, neonates were beginning to survive previously lethal physiologic and anatomic abnormalities. These groups at the extremes of age all require anesthesia for surgery.

The specialization of anesthesiology has developed over the past two or three decades in response to a number of factors related to anesthesia, surgery, and the developing practices of critical care medicine. The chronic shortage of anesthesia care providers has been addressed by training greater numbers of anesthesiologists. It also became necessary to create additional subspecialty training as it became apparent that it was impossible for any individual to obtain encyclopedic knowledge of all aspects of anesthesia. The development of more sophisticated invasive and noninvasive monitoring and computing equipment has been accelerating. The medical and surgical complexity of the patient population is increasing. This has further encouraged the trend towards subspecialty training.

Medicolegal issues have also had a significant impact on anesthesia practice. Standards of care are difficult to define at best, and issues concerning adequate care become more complicated if a subspecialist is asked to interpret a generalist's actions in a legal setting. The tendency for the surgical community to subspecialize, to the extent of entire hospitals dedicated to a particular specialty such as orthopedics or ophthalmology, has also encouraged development of analogous anesthetic practice.

Applications for some specialized monitoring techniques designed for medical diagnostic procedures have been found in clinical anesthesia. For example, transesophageal echocardiographic monitoring is used in cardiac and neuroanesthesia, specifically for detection of embolic phenomena and measurement of cardiac performance. Somatosensory evoked potential monitoring and motor evoked responses are used to monitor neurologic function during neurosurgery and spinal surgery. Electroencephalography is used in neuro-, cardiac, and vascular anesthesia. These techniques require extensive training and experience to be used effectively.

It is unrealistic to expect all anesthesia practitioners to be equally qualified in these high technology procedures. As previously mentioned, the complexity of medical problems seen in many surgical patients has continuously increased. Premature neonates, elderly patients with multisystem disease processes, and patients with severe life-threatening medical conditions scheduled for elective surgery are now commonplace. A decade ago such individuals were frequently denied surgery because they "could not tolerate the anesthetic." However, advances in monitoring, dissemination of knowledge about the actual risks involved, and improvements in the skills and training of the anesthesia care provider are all responsible for these changes. Subspecialization allows the anesthesia care provider to acquire skills and confidence in one or more specific areas. This encourages complete familiarity in the use and interpretation of specialized monitoring and invasive techniques used for that surgical and patient subset. This background of experience and knowledge also encourages bonds of mutual trust and cooperation between the anesthesiologist and subspecialty surgeon. A further important advantage of subspecialty practice in anesthesia is educational. Anesthesia trainees who work with experienced specialists are exposed to the most current practices and knowledge available. They are able to make the most of the training period by learning from experts in each area. Finally, research is also facilitated by subspecialty practices due to the availability for study of larger numbers of cases with similar problems and unanswered questions.

However, anesthetic subspecialization also has negative aspects. While gaining confidence in a specific area of expertise, the anesthesia care provider may be unable to maintain skills in other areas. This may result in a voluntary limitation of practice and, ultimately, professional dissatisfaction. Furthermore, if the individual is required to occasionally cover other areas (e.g., when on-call) there may be a perceived inadequacy related to diminished confidence in technical skills and knowledge.

While the development of complex monitoring devices in medicine has been pervasive, often little evidence exists to support an improvement in patient outcome related to the use of newly available monitors. Furthermore, monitoring equipment is costly, not only because of the capital cost and maintenance expenses of the equipment but also because the anesthesia care provider trained in its use must recover personal training costs. Finally, subspecialty trained anesthesia care providers can become quite isolated in their practice, resulting in a biased view of anesthesia care being passed on in education and research.

On balance, however, in spite of theoretical disadvantages, anesthesia subspecialization has resulted in many positive benefits to anesthesiology as well as to patients. This subspecialization began initially in the surgical areas with the highest patient risk, such as cardiovascular surgery and neurosurgery, or in areas with unique patient factors, such as pediatric anesthesia. However, as patient complexity increased in all surgical areas, and both invasive and noninvasive monitoring became more widely available and accepted as the standard of care, subspecialization has extended to diverse areas such as ear, nose, and throat, solid organ transplants, and orthopedics.

Denise J. Wedel, M.D.

1

Preoperative Evaluation

Kenneth P. Scott
Brian A. Hall

Preoperative evaluation is an essential component of the anesthetic process. Older patients with concurrent cardiac, pulmonary, renal, and metabolic dysfunction frequently present for elective and emergency orthopedic procedures. Furthermore, there is often a progressive decline in the physical activity and fitness of orthopedic patients secondary to joint or spinal disease. This makes assessment of cardiovascular and pulmonary reserve more difficult, as joint pain, rather than angina or claudication, may be the limiting factor. Pediatric orthopedic patients may have associated congenital abnormalities that might affect anesthetic management. Patients of any age, particularly children, may present with full stomachs after trauma. Therefore, a comprehensive preoperative evaluation of these patients is essential to provide safe, high quality anesthesia care.

The preoperative evaluation is divided into four distinct phases.

1. The patient's current medical records, including appropriate medical consultations, are reviewed.
2. The history of the presenting complaint and relevant previous medical history and surgical procedures are obtained. Particular attention is paid to symptoms or episodes of cardiovascular and pulmonary disease.
3. A physical examination is carried out. This must include assessment of the patient's airway and pulmonary status, as well as an examination to rule out neurologic, cardiovascular, metabolic, and orthopedic disorders. The site of any proposed regional anesthetic block procedure is also examined for anatomic abnormalities and any signs of infection.
4. Pertinent laboratory tests and diagnostic procedures are ordered and reviewed.

Each phase of the evaluation is addressed in this chapter, with particular emphasis on the newer methods available for assessing the risk of cardiac events in the perioperative period. Specific medical or age-related conditions associated with an orthopedic surgical practice, such as scoliosis and osteoarticular disease, are discussed.

The preoperative visit presents the opportunity to inform the patient of goals, risks, and alternatives regarding anesthetic management, and to obtain informed consent. The patient must also be encouraged to ask questions and to address any fears or misperceptions con-

1

cerning the planned surgical procedure and anesthetic. Accurate preoperative assessment can provide a rational basis for the anesthetic plan and facilitates the delivery of high-quality anesthesia care. The goal of the preoperative evaluation is to identify factors that may increase the risk of perioperative morbidity and mortality or conversely minimize their effects.

RECORD REVIEW

A thorough review of the patient's current medical records may reveal conditions having anesthetic implications. Pertinent medical consultations, as well as laboratory and diagnostic studies, should be examined. The availability of cross-matched blood and/or blood products should be determined if appropriate. It is extremely important that all available previous anesthetic records be reviewed. Useful information that can be found on the previous anesthetic records includes ease of previous endotracheal intubation, problems during past exposure to anesthetic agents and techniques, and history of perioperative complications. If the patient is currently hospitalized or has been recently discharged following medical or surgical treatment, the discharge summary and hospital notes will be invaluable in assessing the patient's current medical status.

MEDICAL HISTORY AND PHYSICAL EXAMINATION

Obtaining a thorough patient history is the most important part of the preoperative anesthetic evaluation. Information derived directly from the patient will often be more clinically relevant than results from less efficient and more expensive laboratory tests. The patient's age, medication use, and current general medical condition are important initial questions. The latter should be determined prior to any elective procedure. Questions that aid in assessing the patient's general medical status include the patient's level of exercise tolerance, a history of recent acute illness, and the limits of physical activity during the 2 weeks prior to surgery.

The spectrum of patients for orthopedic procedures is broad, ranging from the pediatric patient presenting for reconstructive limb procedures or trauma surgery to the frail geriatric patient requiring fracture reduction or joint replacement. Specific preoperative questions should address age-related concerns as well as associated problems. For example, while the pediatric patient with orthopedic abnormalities may have concomitant congenital heart disease or craniofacial anomalies affecting airway management, the elderly rheumatoid patient should be questioned regarding ischemic cardiac symptoms and cervical spine abnormalities.

Anesthetic History

As described above, a very relevant portion of the patient history pertains to previous anesthetic exposures. Many orthopedic patients have undergone multiple surgical procedures. Important details relating to previous anesthetics can be derived from the record review and directly from the patient. A history of problems with previous anesthetics in the patient or blood relatives may uncover a variety of problems, including susceptibility to malignant hyperthermia, pseudocholinesterase deficiency or abnormality, and specific drug reactions or allergies. Other preoperative concerns center on patient conditions that may affect airway management, infection control precautions, and intraoperative blood replacement. It is important to ascertain whether the patient has ever received a blood transfusion or experienced a transfusion reaction. The patient should also be questioned concerning the presence of dentures, partial plates, removable prosthetics, or loose teeth. It is much easier to identify a loose tooth or dental appliance preoperatively than to search for it at the time of induction or at the end of the anesthetic. Finally, the patient should be interviewed concerning significant symptoms or history of heartburn, hiatal hernia, or gastroesophageal reflux. The most recent time of oral intake must be ascertained as well as the presence of factors that may delay gastric emptying such as diabetes with associated autonomic dysfunction, obesity, pain, and the use of narcotics.

Medications

A detailed preoperative review of the patient's medication regimen is essential for anesthetic management. Some patients have lengthy "drug lists," which may include nonsteroidal anti-inflammatory agents, anticoagulants, cardiac or antihypertensive medications, bronchodilators, steroids or other immunosuppressants, antidepressants, and antineoplastic agents. Some pharmacologic agents have minimal anesthetic implications, while others may profoundly affect anesthetic management. Specific pharmacologic implications are covered under the relevant organ systems.

Important information concerning the drug history can be ascertained by careful preoperative questioning. The anesthesia care provider should determine whether medications have been taken reliably, the time of ingestion of the last scheduled dose, and the reason the medication was prescribed. If the patient gives a history of an allergic response to a medication, a history of the specific reaction should be obtained. Frequently, careful questioning will reveal that the "allergy" is not a true IgE-mediated response, but some other adverse reaction such as nausea associated with codeine or tachycardia secondary to injection of local anesthetic solution containing epinephrine.

Cardiac Disease

Cardiac disease may profoundly affect the outcome of surgery and anesthesia. Identifying patients at increased risk for cardiac morbidity is a crucial step in the preoperative evaluation. Exercise tolerance is an excellent indicator of cardiopulmonary reserve. Unfortunately, many orthopedic patients may be limited in their activities by their degenerative joint disease. Patients with a cardiomyopathy; ischemic, valvular, or subvalvular heart disease; dysrhythmias; hypertension; or symptoms of congestive heart failure should be identified in the preoperative period so that appropriate diagnostic and laboratory studies can be ordered and reviewed prior to surgery.

Myocardial ischemia occurs when oxygen delivery to the heart is less than myocardial oxygen consumption. Factors that increase myocardial oxygen use include increased heart rate, increases in preload or afterload, and any conditions that results in an increased inotropic state. Factors that decrease oxygen delivery to the myocardium include hypotension, tachycardia, hypoxemia, anemia, increased filling pressures, coronary artery disease, and increased coronary artery vascular tone. Manipulation of these variables to maintain a favorable oxygen supply and demand balance is the goal and challenge of the anesthetic management.

Several risk factors for perioperative cardiac morbidity have been identified.[1] Others have been postulated but conclusive evidence is still lacking. Perioperative cardiac morbidity may be manifested as myocardial ischemia or infarction, congestive heart failure, serious dysrhythmia, and cardiac death. Risk factors associated with increased perioperative cardiac morbidity include angina, previous myocardial infarction, congestive heart failure, and diabetes mellitus. Geriatric patients are at increased risk for adverse perioperative cardiac events because of the increased likelihood of having one of the known risk factors. Advanced age alone is not a specific risk factor, and it is not uncommon to encounter a relatively healthy octogenarian. On the other hand, a much younger patient may have significant heart disease, emphasizing the necessity of reviewing and assessing each patient's cardiac risk factors regardless of age. Specific inquiry should be made as to the presence and severity of these risk factors so that appropriate consultations and diagnostic tests are obtained, the patient's cardiac condition optimized prior to surgery, and preanesthetic preparations taken. Important questions to be asked include the patient's anginal pattern, associated dyspnea, exercise tolerance, palpitations, and history of syncopal episodes.

The risk of perioperative myocardial infarction in cardiac patients undergoing noncardiac surgery has been extensively studied. The risk of perioperative myocardial infarction in the general population ranges from 0 to 0.7 percent. This risk is increased to 1.1 percent in patients with coronary artery disease, to 5 to 8 percent in patients with a previous myocardial infarction, and is even higher if the myocardial infarction is recent (within 3 to 6 months).[2] A newer study has shown a decrease in the risk of perioperative myocardial infarction if aggressive intraoperative hemodynamic monitoring and postoperative intensive care unit (ICU) care are instituted.[3] Those data have yet to be reproduced.

Theories regarding the pathophysiology of myocardial ischemia have recently been reassessed.[4] Recent studies indicate that decreases in regional cardiac blood flow are related to hemodynamic parameters, and that there is a dynamic interaction between the presence of atherosclerotic plaques, thrombus formation, and local vasoreactivity. In a patient with stable angina, the mechanism of ischemia is more likely to fit the traditional theory suggesting that coronary blood flow is unable to increase to meet the increase in oxygen demand of stressed myocardium due to coronary stenosis. However, the threshold for ischemia may change depending on the degree of coronary vasospasm. The prognosis in this type of disease is related to both the degree of the coronary arterial disease and the level of ventricular dysfunction. Ischemic events are related to an imbalance between blood flow and stress level, but are modulated by local vasoreactivity. On the other hand, in the case of unstable angina the ischemic events are related to decreased coronary blood flow due to atherosclerotic plaque rupture and thrombus formation. This process is also modulated by local arterial vasoreactivity, and is associated with a high incidence of acute ischemic events, including myocardial infarctions occurring during the immediate perioperative period despite initial stabilization on medical therapy. Transmural myocardial infarctions are caused by the same mechanism as unstable angina except there is total occlusion of the affected coronary artery.

It is vitally important to continue preoperative cardiac medications, right up to the time of transportation of the patient to the operating room. Preoperative withdrawal of β-blockers, nitrates, and calcium channel blockers has been associated with an increased incidence of perioperative myocardial ischemia and infarction, dysrhythmias, and cardiac death.

It is well known that patients who have survived a previous coronary bypass operation have a lower risk of perioperative cardiac morbidity compared to those patients with coronary artery disease who have not been revascularized. There is now evidence that coronary angioplasty may have a similar protective effect.[5]

One valvular heart lesion that deserves mention because of its relevance to regional blockade is aortic stenosis. This lesion may be associated with an increased perioperative mortality whether a general or regional anesthetic technique is used.[1] Spinal and epidural anesthesia are relatively contraindicated in the presence of moderate to severe aortic stenosis. There may be a profound and irreversible fall in cardiac output, blood pressure, and coronary perfusion if venous return and cardiac filling pressures are reduced by the sympathetic blockade and decreased preload. Preoperative evaluation of suspected valvular lesions is easily accomplished with precordial echocardiography.

Vascular Disease

Hypertension is a common, often symptomless, medical condition, the sequelae of which may affect all organ systems. Medical treatment of this disorder significantly affects anesthetic management. Chronic hypertension may cause occlusive vascular disease affecting all portions of the body, including the heart, brain, and kidneys, and resulting in strokes, ischemic heart disease, and renal failure. Preoperative hypertension or withdrawal from antihypertensive medications is associated with intraoperative blood pres-

sure lability. This may cause an imbalance between myocardial oxygen supply and demand, which is particularly dangerous in patients with coronary artery disease. All antianginal and antihypertensive medications, such as β-blockers, calcium channel blockers, and clonidine, must be continued throughout the perioperative period whenever possible. The oral route is acceptable preoperatively, but parenteral routes may be necessary during the postoperative period. Patients with vascular disease are considered to be at risk for ischemic heart disease. For example, patients with symptomatic carotid artery disease have a 5 percent 1-year mortality rate from myocardial infarction.

Pulmonary Disease

Thorough preoperative evaluation is also required in patients with symptoms of pulmonary disease. Patients with complaints of shortness of breath either at rest or with exertion should be evaluated for problems affecting the upper airway, pulmonary, and cardiac systems. Appropriate diagnostic and laboratory studies are needed to establish a diagnosis and document the extent of dysfunction. A patient with good exercise tolerance probably has adequate respiratory reserve, but in those individuals whose activity is limited by orthopedic problems, laboratory and diagnostic studies may identify patients at increased risk of perioperative pulmonary complications. A history of bronchospasm should be further evaluated to determine whether pulmonary function can be optimized prior to surgery. Cigarette smoking is the leading cause of chronic obstructive airways disease. In addition, it predisposes the patient to increased perioperative pulmonary morbidity.[6] This morbidity includes elevated temperature with purulent sputum production, bronchospasm requiring bronchodilator therapy, pleural effusions or pneumothorax requiring drainage, and segmental pulmonary collapse.

Patients with severe pulmonary disease may benefit from the use of regional anesthesia under many circumstances. However, spinal and epidural anesthesia can precipitate respiratory failure if high levels result in weakness of the accessory respiratory muscles. Supraclavicular brachial plexus and intercostal blocks with a potential for pneumothorax may also cause serious respiratory distress in such patients. In addition, interscalene brachial plexus blocks cause phrenic nerve paralysis and should not be performed bilaterally.

Neurologic Disease

All patients should be questioned preoperatively about any history of neurologic disease. This should be followed by a physical examination for significant neurologic deficits, particularly if a regional anesthetic technique is contemplated or if succinylcholine is to be used to facilitate endotracheal intubation. Important information includes the history of seizure, stroke, paralysis, peripheral nerve or head injury, multiple sclerosis, polio, tremor, or other sensory or motor deficits. In today's medicolegal atmosphere, documentation of pre-existing neurologic deficits is paramount. Patients with a seizure disorder, myasthenia gravis, and Parkinson's disease should have their medication regimen reviewed and optimized. An appropriate workup might include serum drug levels and dosage adjustment.

Renal Disease

A history of chronic renal failure is usually unattainable unless the patient has end-stage disease and is undergoing dialysis. If renal disease is suspected or the patient is 40 years of age or older, a serum creatinine level should be obtained prior to surgery. Further laboratory evaluation with serum electrolyte, urea, and hemoglobin levels and assessment of platelet function are carried out if indicated. If renal impairment exists, appropriate adjustment can be made in the anesthetic plan to allow for abnormal drug metabolism and electrolyte disturbances.

Hepatic Disease

Hepatic dysfunction may occur as the result of a variety of disease processes and carries with it several anesthetic implications. Any patient with a history of jaundice should be further evaluated so that the presence of infection, biliary obstruction, and hepatic dysfunction may be detected prior to surgery. Coagulation and liver enzyme studies should be obtained to evaluate the extent of liver dysfunction. Pharmacokinetics of anesthetic drugs are altered in the presence of liver disease by changes in metabolism, altered volume of distribution, and decreases in substances such as pseudocholinesterase produced by the liver. Changes in drug metabolism as well as alterations in coagulation may influence the choice of anesthetic techniques, particularly if regional anesthesia is being considered.

Endocrine–Metabolic Disease

Several endocrinologic diseases may alter anesthetic care of the orthopedic patient. They include diabetes mellitus; thyroid, parathyroid, or adrenal gland dysfunction; and carcinoid tumors. Questions that can be asked to evaluate these problems pertain to thirst and frequency of urination, palpitations, sweating, flushing, heat or cold intolerance, and muscular cramping.

Hematologic Disease

All patients should be questioned regarding the personal or family history of easy bruising and bleeding. If such a history is uncovered, appropriate laboratory evaluation is indicated. Coagulation abnormalities can be related to primary inherited abnormalities of the coagulation cascade such as hemophilia or von Willebrand's disease, underlying liver or renal disease, acquired idiopathic processes as with certain types of thrombocytopenia, and prescribed or self-administered anticoagulants or antiplatelet medications. Disorders of coagulation can cause major complications during regional anesthesia as well as increase the risk of transfusion due to significant intraoperative bleeding. Efforts to identify and treat these problems preoperatively are an important aspect of the preanesthetic evaluation.

The Preoperative Visit: Beneficial Effects

The anesthetic preoperative visit has been shown to reduce patient apprehension concerning the operative procedure more effectively in most cases than preoperative sedation.[7] The preoperative visit is the anesthesia care provider's opportunity to establish rapport with the patient, to ask pertinent questions regarding the medical and anesthetic history, to examine the patient, and to obtain informed consent for the anesthetic. A much more complete picture of the patient's physical status and general condition can be gained from the preoperative visit than from a record review alone.

A relevant physical examination, in-

cluding auscultation of the heart and lungs, examination of the head and neck, and determination of the individual's physical limitations in anticipation of positioning for anesthetic and surgical procedures is indicated in all patients. Specific physical examination of the patient's neurovascular status as well as specific sites for needle placement if regional anesthesia is considered should also be performed during the preoperative visit. In patients with significant medical problems, a more detailed physical examination should be performed to evaluate the extent of the pathologic process and to determine appropriate preoperative laboratory evaluation and treatment.

LABORATORY TESTS AND DIAGNOSTIC STUDIES

"Routine" Laboratory Evaluation

In the healthy patient undergoing elective or emergency surgery, no "routine" laboratory evaluation is required. Appropriate laboratory testing is chosen based on the history and physical examination.[8]

Cardiac Evaluation

A good history will identify most patients with ischemic heart disease. Advances in cardiology have enabled us to further stratify these patients according to the severity of their disease and the need for further work-up, medical therapy, or surgical intervention. Patients with only one of the cardiac risk factors (angina, previous myocardial infarction, congestive heart failure, or diabetes mellitus) are at low risk for cardiac morbidity and usually do not need additional work-up.

Stress Radionuclide Perfusion Imaging

Stress radionuclide perfusion imaging is a useful tool for estimating the probability of adverse outcome (ischemia, myocardial infarction) in patients with an intermediate number (two or three) of the risk factors for perioperative cardiac morbidity. The classic test of this type is the dipyridamole–thallium study, which is performed with simultaneous electrocardiographic (ECG) monitoring. Patients having all four risk factors, indicating severe symptoms and disease, should probably be evaluated directly with coronary angiography. The most commonly used radionuclide marker for stress perfusion imaging is thallium-201. It has biochemical properties similar to potassium and is highly extracted by the metabolically active myocardial cells. Thallium is distributed throughout the myocardium in a fashion that is dependent on the regional blood flow. Areas of high perfusion have increased uptake of thallium compared with areas of lesser perfusion. After initial uptake into the myocardium the thallium distribution changes continuously as a function of time. There is a dynamic process of washout from areas of high perfusion into the blood stream. Similarly, areas of poor perfusion have both slower uptake and slower washout. "Cold spots" represent regions of decreased perfusion and hence decreased uptake in contrast to those with normal perfusion and uptake. Increased uptake in the lungs suggests left ventricular failure.[9]

Radionuclide imaging is carried out first during exercise or pharmacologically induced stress and repeated approximately 4 hours later.[10] Stress increases coronary artery blood flow in all arteries except those that have significant stenoses. A "steal" phenomenon may exist, but is not necessary to create differential blood flow to various regions of the myocardium. The stress images show areas that are highly perfused during exercise. In the delayed images, the thallium has been washed out of the highly perfused areas and is often increased in the less well-perfused regions, a process known as *redistribution*. Regions of the heart with low perfusion during both stress and delayed phases of imaging represent areas of old myocardial infarction. These are called *fixed defects*. Conversely, areas of delayed redistribution suggest myocardial ischemia and are referred to as *reversible defects*. Such regions of myocardium are at risk for ischemia in the stressful perioperative period.

Stress-induced coronary artery dilation during radionuclide perfusion imaging can be produced by one of two techniques: through exercise or pharmacologically. Dipyridamole and adenosine are the agents used for the latter. Producing differential blood flow through exercise has the advantage of identifying a given heart rate and blood pressure at the time symptoms of ischemia are first noted by the patient or detected by ECG monitoring. It also gives some estimate of the patient's exercise tolerance by noting which portion of the exercise protocol the patient is able to complete. Some individuals may not be able to engage in exercise at all because of severe physical (orthopedic, pulmonary, etc.) limitations. In such cases dipyridamole or adenosine can be used.[11,12] Dipyridamole inhibits adenosine uptake by myocardial cells and therefore dilates coronary arteries. Minimal decreases in systemic blood pressure with a mildly increased heart rate are usually noted during dipyridamole infusion; however, profound hypotension, chest pain, and ECG changes may also be seen. These side effects are usually short-lived and easily reversed by administration of aminophylline. Administration of adenosine causes physiologic effects similar to those produced by dipyridamole but shorter in duration.

Images are obtained immediately following peak exercise or injection of dipyridamole (or adenosine) and approximately 4 hours later. Appearance of left ventricular dilation during initial imaging that resolves prior to delayed imaging may represent severe coronary artery disease.[13] There are two types of images in use at this time. They are planar and single-photon emission computed tomography (SPECT) images. The SPECT images appear to be superior because of an increased specificity for coronary artery disease compared to the planar images.[14] The sensitivity for each technique is comparable, but low (approximately 80 percent). For this reason, the test is not a good screening tool for coronary artery disease in asymptomatic individuals.

The two new radioactive agents are technetium-99 sestamibi and technetium-99 teboroxime.[15] They are attached to either red blood cells or albumin in a fashion similar to that employed in multigated acquisition (MUGA) studies. These isotopes have several advantages over thallium-201, including a higher energy level and a shorter half-life. For this reason they produce higher-resolution images and allow estimation of left ventricular ejection fraction.

SPECIAL CONSIDERATIONS

Pediatric Patients

The preanesthetic visit is an important aspect of the anesthesia care of the pediatric patient. Many children who present for orthopedic surgery have undergone multiple surgical procedures in the past and may have associated fears and concerns that should be addressed. These children and their parents often have clear preferences for premedication, induction techniques, anesthetic management, and postoperative pain techniques. The preoperative visit is important in establishing trust with the parent and child. A history of airway problems, recent upper respiratory infections, susceptibility to malignant hyperthermia, and other anesthetic complications should be specifically sought along with a general review of systems. A brief physical examination should focus on the cardiorespiratory system, intravenous access, and potential sites of needle insertion for proposed regional anesthetic techniques. An accurate preoperative weight is important for calculation of fluid replacement and drug dosages. Consent should be obtained for anticipated anesthetic procedures during the visit, including postoperative pain blocks.

Elderly Patients

Elderly patients frequently present for emergency orthopedic surgery with fractures of the hip or humerus. These patients often have degenerative disease involving several organ systems. In patients presenting with a hip fracture, metabolic, neurologic, and cardiac causes for a fall should be sought. While the emergency nature of these procedures often places pressure on the anesthesia care provider to proceed without a full preanesthetic evaluation, it is imperative to fully examine the elderly patient with special emphasis on the cardiovascular, pulmonary, and renal systems. Often such individuals are taking a number of prescription and over-the-counter medications that may affect the anesthetic management. The patient may be severely dehydrated and incapable of giving an accurate history due to pain or confusion.

As a larger proportion of the population survives into its seventh decade and beyond, more and more elderly patients are presenting for elective orthopedic surgery because of degenerative bone disease. In general, these individuals tolerate the stress of surgery and anesthesia well and require only standard monitoring and postoperative care.[16]

Rheumatoid Arthritis

Rheumatoid arthritis is a chronic inflammatory disease that predominantly affects females. Severity is variable, and all age groups are affected. The onset of adult rheumatoid arthritis most often occurs between the ages of 30 and 50 years. It is a polyarthropathy that may affect any joint, but frequently occurs symmetrically in the hands, wrists, and knees. It may also affect the heart, kidneys, lungs, and eyes.

Patients with rheumatoid arthritis commonly present for joint replacement, surgery involving the neck and back, and arthrodeses. As with any patient presenting for surgery, the preoperative evaluation should begin with a thorough history and physical examination. Since direct or indirect involvement of the airway is a potential problem in rheumatoid patients, meticulous attention should be paid to the evaluation of this area. Range of cervical spine motion should be ascertained, as should the limits of comfort with extension and flexion of the neck. If cervical spine instability is suspected, flexion and extension films of the neck should be obtained. The extent of jaw mobility should also be evaluated as the temporomandibular joint may be involved. History of hoarseness or evidence of recent vocal changes should raise suspicion of rheumatoid involvement of the cricoarytenoid joints, which may require use of a smaller endotracheal tube. Further evaluation by an otolaryngologist should be considered for such patients.

Cardiac involvement may be manifested by aortic regurgitation or other valvular abnormalities, pericardial effusion, coronary arteritis, and cardiac conduction abnormalities. The latter can be easily diagnosed on preoperative ECG. If a heart murmur is detected on physical examination and valvular heart disease is suspected, an echocardiogram may be useful in determining valvular competence. The calculated ejection fraction and evidence of regional wall motion abnormalities indicate ischemic heart disease. Further evaluation by stress radionuclide perfusion imaging may be indicated. If a friction rub is heard on examination, pericardial effusion may also be ruled out by echocardiographic examination.

Pleural effusion is the most common pulmonary manifestation of rheumatoid arthritis. Rheumatoid nodules may appear on the pleural surfaces or in the lung parenchyma and may be confused with tuberculosis or neoplasm. Progressive pulmonary fibrosis is a rare complication associated with this disease. Any patient with a history of progressive cough or dyspnea should be evaluated with chest x-ray and pulmonary function studies to assess for restrictive lung disease. A decreased forced expiration volume in 1 second (FEV_1) and forced vital capacity (FVC) may also be seen in rheumatoid patients with severe costochondral involvement.

The frequent use of aspirin and other nonsteroidal anti-inflammatory drugs in patients with rheumatoid arthritis may result in chronic blood loss through the gastrointestinal tract and mild chronic anemia. If leukopenia is also present, Felty syndrome (the triad of anemia, hepatosplenomegaly, and leukopenia) should be suspected. Patients who have received corticosteroid therapy for a period longer than 2 weeks in the preceding 6 months should receive steroid supplementation during the perioperative period.

Scoliosis

The cardiorespiratory evaluation for the patient presenting for spinal surgery is focused on the pulmonary system. Scoliosis can be divided into two major categories; idiopathic and nonidiopathic (i.e., scoliosis associated with other diseases). The etiology of the spinal curvature in the nonidiopathic group is related to underlying congenital, neuromuscular, or myopathic processes. The congenital category includes patients with meningomyelocele who may have concomitant neurologic deficits. There is a higher incidence of congenital cardiac and genitourinary anomalies in patients with this form of scoliosis. Neuromuscular and myopathic scoliosis may be associated with cerebral palsy, polio, and muscular dystrophy. Since the advent of the polio vaccine, most patients fall into the idiopathic group. Idiopathic scoliosis can be further subdivided into three major types depending on age of onset: infantile, juvenile, and adolescent. The age of onset in the infantile group is 0 to 4 years. There is a male predominance and spontaneous resolution of the disease usually occurs. The juvenile group (ages 4 to 9 at onset) has no gender predominance. The adolescent group is characterized by female predominance and thoracic curvature to the right. The clinical presentation varies widely among patients presenting for corrective surgery.

Scoliosis is graded by a system using a measurement referred to as *Cobb angle*. The greater the angle, the more severe the spinal curvature. In patients with idiopathic scoliosis, the Cobb angle can be correlated with pulmonary dysfunction. Patients with angles less than 50 degrees usually have no respiratory abnormality. If the angle is greater than 100 degrees, the patient may have marked signs and symptoms of respiratory failure. Patients with nonidiopathic scoliosis may have much lower pulmonary reserves because of muscular dysfunction. It may not be possible, however, to obtain accurate pulmonary function testing because of associated developmental problems. In this case, exercise tolerance and the frequency of pulmonary infections can give some assessment of pulmonary reserve. Good pulmonary function testing, when it is obtainable, can predict the patient's postoperative course. If FVC is less than 30 to 40 percent of predicted values, the need for postoperative ventilatory support is likely. Pulmonary function testing should be obtained with and without bronchodilators so that any reversible component of obstructive disease can be identified and treated preoperatively. The classic pulmonary function abnormality is consistent with a restrictive pattern with a decrease in total lung capacity (TLC), FEV_1, and FVC.

The primary gas exchange disorder in these patients is secondary to ventilation/perfusion mismatch. Mild to moderate hypoxia is usually seen on arterial blood gas sampling. The presence of hypercarbia signifies severe disease. Chronic hypoxia may lead to progressive pulmonary arterial hypertension and ultimately cor pulmonale. Signs and symptoms of right-sided heart failure should be sought in the preoperative period so that appropriate monitoring can be instituted. Scoliosis is associated with an increased incidence of mitral valve prolapse and congenital heart disease. Any patient in whom cardiac dysfunction is suspected should undergo ECG and echocardiographic testing and preoperative evaluation by a cardiologist.

The preoperative visit for these patients should include a description of the contemplated anesthetic technique and a discussion of the possibility of a wake-up test. The likelihood of blood transfusion and postoperative ventilatory support should also be discussed, as well as the strategy for postoperative pain control. Other preoperative considerations include assessment of the risk of susceptibility to malignant hyperthermia, documentation of any pre-existing neurologic deficits, and confirmation of adequate blood availability for transfusion during the procedure.

Ankylosing Spondylitis

Ankylosing spondylitis is a nonrheumatoid arthropathy characterized by inflammation of the sacroiliac joints and spine. In 50 percent of patients there is extraspinal joint involvement at some time during the course of the disease. Ankylosing spondylitis is relatively common, affecting 1.6 percent of the population. It was previously held that this disease predominated in males. More recent studies, however, have shown that the disease occurs in both sexes with the same frequency. Signs and symptoms, however, tend to be more severe in men. Ankylosing spondylitis may have extensive extra-articular involvement affecting many organ systems.[17]

Cervical spine involvement is variable, but when present may have a profound impact on airway management. The degree of deformity ranges from minimal involvement to complete ankylosis, usually in flexion. Patients with advanced disease are at increased risk for cervical fractures, often after trivial injury. This emphasizes the necessity for a thorough but gentle airway evaluation. A sudden increase in cervical spine range of motion with or without pain should raise suspicion for cervical spine fracture. Cervical spine films in flexion and extension should be obtained. The temporomandibular joint may also be involved, as may the cricoarytenoids. Hoarseness or changes in phonation should be evaluated by an otolaryngologist.

Cardiac involvement is found in 3.5 percent of patients with a 15-year history of ankylosis spondylitis and is even higher in patients with a longer history. Cardiac complications of this disease may include cardiac conduction abnormalities, aortic valve, and occasionally mitral valve involvement. A preoperative ECG should be obtained to identify conduction delays, heart block, or any acute changes. If a heart murmur is heard on physical examination, an echocardiogram is warranted to detect and quantify any aortic valve or other valvular lesions.

Pulmonary involvement in these patients may include upper lobe pulmonary fibrosis, restrictive lung disease, and on rare occasion, secondary amyloidosis. Preoperative pulmonary evaluation should include, in addition to a careful history and physical examination, a chest x-ray and pulmonary function studies. Restrictive lung disease may occur secondary to thoracic spine involvement as well as pulmonary fibrosis. Neurologic manifestations are not uncommon in patients with ankylosing spondylitis and may include spinal cord compression, peripheral nerve lesions, epilepsy, cauda equina syndrome, and vertebral basilar insufficiency. Any patient with a history suggesting neurologic involvement should be evaluated by a neurologist preoperatively.

In conclusion, the preoperative evaluation of patients is partially driven by cost–benefit concerns, particularly in the choice of laboratory tests. The primary goal of the preanesthetic visit is to identify risk factors so that the patient's condition can be optimized prior to surgery. The most expensive portion of the workup is the laboratory evaluation. The anesthesia care provider must attempt to select appropriate tests that will either influence the anesthetic management of the patient or help predict the risk of perioperative complications.

An increasing number of patients are being admitted on an outpatient or morning-admit basis to contain costs. Many of these patients are seen for their preanesthetic evaluation as they are being prepared for their operative procedure. Preanesthetic clinics provide a less-pressured environment for evaluation of these patients, but are time-consuming and costly for the anesthesia care provider. In such patients the preoperative evaluation should focus on items that will affect the anesthetic management, similar to an assessment done for patients undergoing urgent or emergency operations.

REFERENCES

1. Mangano DT: Perioperative cardiac morbidity. Anesthesiology 72:153, 1990
2. Tarhan S, Moffitt EA, Taylor WF et al: Myocardial infarction after general anesthesia. JAMA 220:1451, 1972
3. Rao TLK, Jacobs KH, El-Etr AA: Reinfarction following anesthesia in patients with myocardial infarction. Anesthesiology 59:499, 1983
4. Vetrovec GW: Changing concepts in the pathophysiology of myocardial ischemia. Am J Cardiol 64:3F, 1989
5. Huber KC, Evans MA, Bresnahan JF et al: Outcome of noncardiac operations in patients with severe coronary artery disease successfully treated preoperatively with coronary angioplasty. Mayo Clin Proc 67:15, 1992
6. Warner MA, Divertie MB, Tinker JH: Preoperative cessation of smoking and pulmonary complications in coronary artery bypass patients. Anesthesiology 60:380, 1984
7. Dripps RD, Eckenhoff JE, Vandam LD: Introduction to Anesthesia. The Principles of Safe Practice. 2nd Ed. WB Saunders, Philadelphia, 1982
8. Narr BJ, Hansen TR, Warner MA: Preoperative laboratory screening in healthy Mayo patients: cost-effective elimination of tests and unchanged outcomes. Mayo Clin Proc 66:155, 1991
9. Villanueva FS, Watson DD, Smith WH et al: Significance of increased lung/heart ratio on dipyridamole thallium-201 scintigraphy. Circulation 80(suppl II):II-210, 1989
10. Hosen K, Berman DS, Maddahi J et al: Late reversibility of tomographic myocardial thallium-201 defects: an accurate marker of myocardial viability. J Am Coll Cardiol 12:1456, 1988
11. Beller GA: Pharmacologic stress imaging. JAMA 265:633, 1991
12. Coyne EP, Belvedere DA, Vande Streek PR et al: Thallium-201 scintigraphy after intravenous infusion of adenosine compared with exercise thallium testing in the diagnosis of coronary artery disease. J Am Coll Cardiol 17:1289, 1991
13. Weiss AT, Berman DS, Lew AS et al: Transient ischemic dilation of the left ventricle on stress thallium-201 scintigraphy: a marker of severe and extensive coronary artery disease. J Am Coll Cardiol 9:752, 1987
14. Iskandrian AS: Single-photon emission computed tomographic thallium imaging with adenosine, dipyridamole, and exercise. Am Heart J 122:279, 1991
15. Berman DS, Hosen K, Maddahi J: The new Tc-99 myocardial perfusion imaging agents: Tc-99 sestamibi and Tc-99 teboroxime. Circulation 84(suppl I):I-7, 1991
16. Hosking MP, Warner MA, Lobdell CM et al: Outcomes of surgery in patients 90 years of age and older. JAMA 261(13):1909, 1989
17. Sinclair JR, Mason RA: Ankylosing spondylitis. The case for awake intubation. Anaesthesia 39:3, 1984

2

Transfusion Medicine

Ronald J. Faust

Fear of acquired immunodeficiency syndrome (AIDS) has had a major impact on transfusion practices in the last decade. Public awareness of the risk of human immunodeficiency virus (HIV) transmission via blood products has pressured physicians to change the way they use blood components. For years blood bank specialists have sought changes in the way clinicians use homologous blood products because of the risk of a much more common transfusion-associated infection, hepatitis. The AIDS epidemic has motivated clinicians to make those changes. Those involved in orthopedic anesthesia are confronted with changing transfusion practices. After reviewing AIDS and other risks, this chapter presents an approach to blood replacement and methods to avoid homologous transfusion.

INFECTIOUS RISKS

Post-transfusion AIDS

It has been estimated that 29,000 patients were transfused with blood infected with HIV virus before screening for the virus became possible in 1985.[1,2] Because of the long latency (up to 7 years) between HIV infection and the devel-

opment of clinical AIDS, many of these patients may die of other diseases before AIDS is diagnosed. Through March 1992, transfusion-associated AIDS cases reported to the Centers for Disease Control totalled 4,833.[3] This was 2 percent of adult AIDS cases and 8 percent of pediatric AIDS cases.

Even homologous blood that has been screened for HIV and is negative for the antibody to this virus is not absolutely safe with regard to transfusion-associated AIDS. In 1988, Ward et al[4] reported 13 recipients of blood components who became infected with HIV after receiving seronegative blood from 7 donors. Blood donation had been obtained during a 6- to 14-week "window" period between infection and development of a detectable anti-HIV antibody level. AIDS transmission by all components that are not heat treated (red blood cells, platelet concentrate, fresh frozen plasma [FFP], cryoprecipitate) was documented in these 13 recipients.[4]

Nevertheless, the actual risk of transfusion-associated AIDS has become extremely low since antibody screening and other measures were introduced. In 1989 and 1991, estimates of the risk of contracting HIV from a single unit ranged between 1 in 61,000 to 1 in 153,000.[5,6] This should be reassuring to patients since this level of risk is lower than the risk of death associated with many other common diseases and even common, nonmedical activities such as driving a car.[7]

Studies of blood donors have shown the highest rates of HIV seropositivity among new male donors and the lowest rates among repeat female donors.[5] Continued and more frequent donation from previously tested donors has been encouraged. Designated donors who direct their blood for a given patient could pose a slightly higher risk because they are more often previously untested, first-time donors.[5,8] Also, some designated donors with risk factors might feel pressured to donate even though they would normally exclude themselves. Fatal graft-versus-host disease has also been reported in recipients of blood from related designated donors.[9] As an alternative, minimal-exposure transfusion has been introduced to decrease homologous blood exposure for certain patients anticipating the need of multiple homologous units.[10] To minimize infectious exposure, one committed donor, usually a parent of the recipient, donates multiple units of blood over a period of weeks. FFP and platelet concentrate can also be obtained from the same donor, limiting infectious risk.

Hepatitis

Transmission of hepatitis was the most common serious risk of transfusion throughout recent decades. Even after testing for hepatitis B virus (HBV) was developed, post-transfusion hepatitis continued to occur in 7 to 12 percent of transfused patients during the late 1970s.[11] The cause was non-A, non-B (NANB) hepatitis, recognized as hepatitis C (HCV) in 1989.[12] During the 1980s the incidence of transfusion-associated NANB declined for a number of reasons. Paid donors were eliminated and surrogate testing was introduced that tested donor blood for antibody to HBV core antigen (anti-HBc) and serum alanine aminotransferase (ALT). While not specific for NANB hepatitis, these two factors had been found to be associated with NANB infection. Further reductions in this infection rate were brought about by the introduction of HCV screening. It is speculated that the incidence of post-transfusion hepatitis is now between 1 and 2 percent, but there are few studies in the literature to actually document this.[13,14] While 10 percent of HBV patients become carriers, as many as 50 percent of patients infected with HCV become chronic carriers (Table 2–1). HCV

Table 2-1.   Viral Agents Causing Hepatitis

Virus	Agent	Percentage of Infected Persons Becoming Carriers	Mean Incubation (wk)
HAV	17-nm RNA	None	4
HBV	42-nm DNA	10	12
Delta virus	Defective RNA core requiring HBsAg coat	25 (?)	Unknown
HCV (NANB)	Single-stranded RNA	50	8
CMV	Member of herpesvirus group	100	3

HAV, hepatis A virus; HBV, hepatitis B virus; HCV, hepatitis C virus; NANB, non-A, non-B viral hepatitis; CMV, cytomegalovirus.

is initially much milder than HBV, with fatigue being the only symptom in most cases and fewer than 4 percent of patients becoming icteric.[15] Before the HCV virus was identified, the disease was diagnosed (as NANB) when elevations of ALT or aspartate aminotransferase (AST) were noted in a previously transfused patient after all other sources of liver disease had been excluded. Estimates are that at least 10 percent of chronic HCV carriers eventually develop cirrhosis and one-fourth of those patients eventually develop severe complications of cirrhosis: bleeding esophageal varices or hepatocellular carcinoma.[16]

Other Infectious Risks

Conceivably, almost any infectious agent can be transmitted by transfusion. Other viruses, spirochetes (syphilis, and potentially, Lyme disease), and bacteria can all cause infections after transfusion (Table 2-2).[17–19] In addition to screening for syphilis, HBV, HCV, HIV-1 and 2, and human T-cell lymphotrophic virus type 1 and 2 (HTLV-1/2), careful history taking before blood donation is used to eliminate potentially infected donors.[20] Those who have recently traveled to areas of endemic disease are temporarily deferred. Veterans of the Vietnam War were deferred to prevent malarial transmission; in 1991, those returning from Operation Desert Storm were deferred after it was learned that a number of them had returned with visceral leishmaniasis due to *Leishmania tropica*. But the goal of a zero-risk blood supply should be considered impossible.[7] Even if it were possible to test for all infectious agents with 100 percent sensitivity, new infectious agents with probably continue to evolve. One can only speculate whether the last unit transfused might have contained a new

Table 2-2.   Transfusion Risks

Infections transmitted by transfusion
  Viruses
    Hepatitis A, B, delta, C
    HIV, type 1 and type 2
    HTLV-I/II
    CMV
    Epstein-Barr virus
  Bacteria
    Staphylococcus spp.
    Yersinia enterocolitica
    Pseudomonas spp.
    Enterobacter spp.
    Klebsiella spp.
    Bacillus spp.
  Spirochetes
    Syphilis
    Lyme disease
  Parasites
    Malaria
    Chagas disease
    Babesiosis
    Toxoplasmosis
    Filariasis
    Kala-azar
    Trypanosomiasis
    Visceral leishmaniasis
Immune-mediated transfusion reactions
  Hemolytic
    Acute
    Delayed
  Febrile
  Transfusion-related acute lung injury
  Mild allergic
  Anaphylaxis
  Post-transfusion purpura
Immunosuppression
  Increased spread of malignancy
  Decreased resistance to infection

infectious agent whose clinical manifestations will not be apparent for years to come.

Anesthesia care providers must also be aware of the risk of transfusion-associated sepsis. Ten percent of transfusion-related deaths reported to the U.S. Food and Drug Administration between 1976 and 1985 were caused by bacterial contamination of the product.[21,22] Sepsis can present as a fever or shock-like symptoms appearing just after the start of a transfusion. Platelets are at special risk of bacterial contamination because they are stored at room temperature for up to 5 days. Yet, transfusion-associated sepsis can be caused by any component as a result of contamination during the blood donation process or from inapparent septicemia in a donor. Although stored at 4°C, bacteria can multiply in red blood cells as well. Multiple bacterial agents have been identified as pathogens, but several reports described deaths caused by *Yersinia enterocolitica*, a gram-negative organism that is able to grow even at temperatures as low as 4°C in the blood bank refrigerator.[23,24]

NONINFECTIOUS RISKS

Hemolytic Transfusion Reactions

The most recent review of transfusion-associated deaths found acute hemolysis to be the most frequent fatal reaction excluding hepatitis and AIDS.[21] Most, but not all, of these reactions were caused by clerical or system errors leading to the transfusion of ABO-incompatible blood.[21,25,26] Most hemolytic reactions occur in anesthetized patients or in the intensive care unit setting. They are preventable. When patient and blood identification practices are scrupulously adhered to, most can be avoided.

Fatal hemolytic reactions also occur when non-ABO antibodies react with red blood cell antigens. Anti-c and other antibodies of the Rh group, anti-K (Kell), anti-Fy^a (Duffy), and anti-Jk^a (Kidd) have been most frequently implicated.[21,27] Any red blood cell antibody/antigen reaction that binds complement is capable of producing hemolysis.

Pathophysiology of the acute hemolytic transfusion reaction stems from the production of hemodynamic alterations leading to renal ischemia and activation of the clotting system causing disseminated intravascular coagulation (DIC).[11,28] The clinical presentation commonly includes fever, chills, chest and lumbar pain, nausea, hypotension, and tachycardia. Hemoglobinuria and generalized oozing are seen later and, in addition to tachycardia and hypotension, might be the only signs of a hemolytic transfusion reaction in an anesthetized patient. Mortality in most large series is above 17 percent, although it is hoped that aggressive therapy will decrease the current risk of death.[27] Therapy is aimed at preventing the renal ischemia. The transfusion should be stopped immediately since the reaction is dose-dependent. Crystalloids and furosemide should be used to increase urine volume. The efficacy of mannitol, alkalinization of the urine, and steroid therapy is controversial. Cardiovascular function should be maintained pharmacologically, if necessary, and the patient's coagulation system should be monitored.

Transfusion-Related Lung Injury

Sazama's review listed acute pulmonary edema as the second most frequent cause of transfusion-associated deaths between 1976 and 1985, after deaths from infectious agents had been excluded.[21] Anaphylaxis was implicated in only 8 of the 31 deaths reported. While volume overload is probably the most frequent cause of pulmonary edema after transfusion, transfusion-related lung injury (TRALI) should also be recognized as a form of noncardiogenic pulmonary edema occasionally seen in transfused patients who are not hypervolemic. The syndrome is probably underdiagnosed and is not widely reported in the literature. Many anesthesia care providers, however, will remember patients who developed pulmonary edema after transfusion when the diagnosis of volume overload was unlikely. The patient usually presents with hypoxemia, bronchospasm, and wheezing, but if a pulmonary artery catheter is inserted, pulmonary artery diastolic pressures and pulmonary artery occlusion pressures are normal. The chest x-ray will usually show bilateral pulmonary infiltrates. The reaction usually is noted 2 to 4 hours after transfusion and is often accompanied by a fever.

Intensive respiratory support is necessary for these patients, who usually respond to 24 to 48 hours of increased inspired oxygen, intubation, mechanical ventilation, and positive end-expiratory pressure, as indicated. The reaction is immunologically mediated between an antibody to a human leukocyte antigen (HLA system) in the donor's plasma and an antigen on the recipient's leukocytes that cause pulmonary injury through complement activation.[29–31] White blood cells are thought to aggregate and become trapped in the pulmonary microcirculation during a TRALI reaction. Special antibody identification studies are necessary to confirm the diagnosis.

Febrile Reactions

Febrile and mild allergic reactions are the most common adverse responses to transfusion. Mediated by leukoagglutinins in the recipient, most febrile reactions present with only fever, chills, and tachycardia developing after transfusion. The reaction is usually self-limited and patients may be treated with antipyretics, but the dilemma is excluding other more serious causes of the fever. Postoperative infections and sepsis must be recognized and differentiated from a post-transfusion

febrile reaction. If a fever starts during a transfusion, the transfusion must be interrupted to confirm that the blood component being administered is not contaminated with bacteria (see discussion of transfusion-associated sepsis, above). Also, a fever is the most frequent sign of acute intravascular hemolysis, and an acute hemolytic transfusion reaction must be ruled out before a transfusion is continued in a patient with a fever or chill.[27]

Mild Allergic Reactions

Allergic reactions are mediated by antibodies to other substances in the transfused blood products. Mild allergic reactions usually consist of an urticarial rash with multiple smooth or slightly elevated patches that are either more erythematous or paler than the surrounding skin. Pruritus is common. These reactions are fairly common (occurring in 1 to 4 percent of transfused patients), but are not part of the symptomatology of hemolytic transfusion reactions. If there are no associated signs of anaphylaxis, the transfusion may be continued when a patient develops an urticarial rash; the pruritus can be treated symptomatically with diphenhydramine.

Anaphylactic Reactions

Although rare, anaphylactic reactions can follow transfusion of blood components in some patients. These present with severe hypotension, tachycardia, flushing, dyspnea, cyanosis, and wheezing. These reactions usually occur in patients who have no IgA immunoglobulins but form antibodies against this class of proteins. They will develop anaphylactic reactions to any component other than washed red blood cells because it contains plasma. Even albumin and plasma protein fraction must be avoided in resuscitation.[32] Methods for preparation of IgA-deficient platelets are also being developed.[33]

Immunosuppressive Effects

Immunosuppressive effects of transfusion have been known since the 1970s. It was initially discovered that renal transplant recipients who had been previously transfused actually had higher allograft survival than those who had not received blood.[34] However, adverse effects of transfusion were noted in cancer patients who received blood; their immune systems seemed to have suppressed resistance to growth of malignant cells. Some studies of patients with cancers originating in a number of organs showed significant differences in survival or recurrence rates when patients who had received transfusions were compared to nontransfused patients.[35] One study even showed a higher survival rate in patients transfused with (packed) red blood cells compared to those receiving whole blood.[36] Immunosuppression is also thought to be related to postoperative infection rates in transfused patients. Studies in 1992 and 1991 showed lower infection rates in autotransfused patients after cancer surgery, when compared to matched control patients who received homologous blood.[37,38] Yet not all studies showed significant differences. Ness et al[39] reported no difference in recurrence rates after radical retropubic prostatectomy when patients receiving autologous blood (collected and stored preoperatively) were compared to a group receiving homologous blood. As Schreimer has emphasized, correlations between transfusion and poor survival do not prove that there is a cause-and-effect relationship. Studies have suggested that transfusion-induced immunosuppression may be mediated through effects on the body's natural

killer cell lymphocytes, low helper/suppressor cell ratios, depression of lymphocyte responses to antigen and mitogen, or a reduction of interleukin-2 production.[37]

INTRAOPERATIVE HOMOLOGOUS BLOOD REPLACEMENT

This section approaches blood replacement as a spectrum extending from minimal to massive blood loss. After discussing commonly used components, crystalloids, and colloids, the limits of anemia and how low the hemoglobin can be allowed to drop when blood loss is not excessive is covered before reviewing replacement for massive blood loss. Figure 2-1 illustrates a replacement scheme with the washout curve for the patient's original blood. The washout curve is adapted from Collins' mathematically derived relationship.[40] It describes the percentage of original blood remaining at various levels of transfusion. When blood loss is less than 20 percent and the patient is not anemic, crystalloids are used to restore volume. Red blood cell products become necessary as blood loss increases. As bleeding continues, transfused blood is lost along with the patient's own blood, and after 1 blood volume replacement (10 U in an adult), only 65 percent of the patient's own blood is replaced. This tends to delay the need for replacement of platelets and coagulation factors. Coagulation components usually are not necessary until at least 1.5 blood volumes have been replaced. Blood exchange approaches 95 percent when approximately 3 blood volumes have been replaced. The curve shifts downward and to the left when volume replaced lags behind the volume lost; less of the patient's original

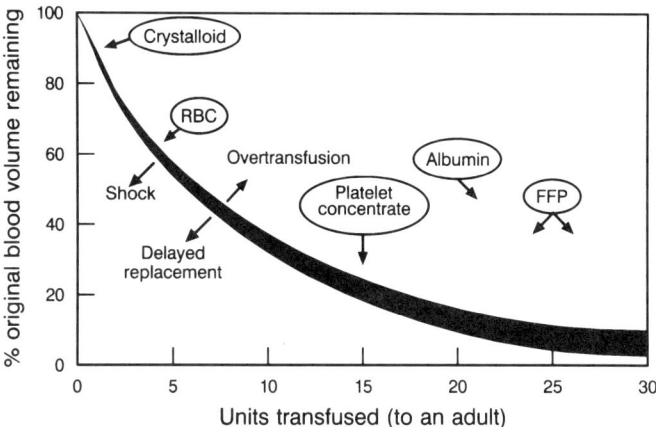

Fig. 2-1. The washout curve depicts the fraction of a 70-kg patient's original blood remaining as the volume transfused increases. Because transfused blood is being shed with the patient's original blood, approximately one-third of the original blood should still be circulating after 1 blood volume (10 U of red blood cells) have been replaced. Red blood cells are not usually indicated for nonanemic adult patients until a 1 to 2 L blood loss has occurred; platelet concentrate and FFP are not necessary until at least 1.5 blood volumes has been transfused. Shock or delayed replacement shifts the curve down and to the left so that washout occurs earlier.

blood remains at a given point in the exchange transfusion.

Components

Although the term *packed red blood cells* can be found extensively in the literature, *red blood cells* is the preferred terminology for the liquid stored red blood cell product. Red blood cells are usually stored in citrate phosphate dextrose adenine (CPDA-1) anticoagulant, or Adsol preservative. When Adsol is used, 100 ml of an additive solution containing adenine, saline, and mannitol is added to the red blood cells after collection in a CPDA-type solution. Shelf life is prolonged to 42 days and viscosity is reduced. While the hematocrit of CPDA-1 red blood cells is approximately 70 percent and that of Adsol red blood cells is 55 percent, the hematocrit of whole blood is usually about 35 percent. Blood stored by freezing is technically called *red blood*

cells deglycerolized. This component is mixed with glycerol for freezing to protect the red blood cells. When the unit is used, it must first be thawed slowly, and the red blood cells then washed with saline to remove the glycerol. Suspended in saline after washing, red blood cells deglycerolized outdate 24 hours after the unit is thawed and entered to wash the cells.

Red blood cells washed can also be prepared in a continuous-flow centrifuge from red blood cells that have not been frozen. Red blood cells washed or deglycerolized are indicated for patients with clinically significant antibodies to IgA proteins. Both products also have been used to avoid febrile reactions in patients with leukoagglutinins, but *leukocyte-reduced red blood cells* also can be prepared by differential centrifugation or filtration through leukocyte depletion filters, which have been shown to be very effective in removing white blood cells.[20]

Platelet concentrate is prepared by

centrifugation of whole blood just after it is collected. Platelet-rich plasma is then separated from the red blood cells and a higher-rpm centrifugation separates platelet concentrate from the rest of the plasma.[41] Each unit of platelet concentrate comes from a single donor and should contain 5.5×10^{10} platelets in approximately 50 ml of plasma. If platelet consumption in the recipient is not excessive, each unit of platelet concentrate should increase an adult's platelet count by approximately 10×10^9/L. Platelet concentrates are stored up 5 days at room temperature, and multiple units are usually pooled just before administration.[42] *Pheresis platelets* are obtained by pheresing a single donor's blood to obtain the equivalent of multiple units of platelet concentrate. Platelets or plasma can be pheresed from a donor using a semicontinuous-flow centrifuge, which returns red blood cells to the donor after separating the desired component. More than 3×10^{11} platelets are collected when they are obtained by pheresis.[43] Although they can be used for any patient needing platelets, pheresis platelets are particularly indicated for patients refractory to platelets from unmatched donors because an HLA-compatible donor can be chosen for pheresis.

Fresh frozen plasma is frozen within 8 hours of collection from a single donor and contains all coagulation factors except platelets. It is particularly useful in patients who require replacement of labile coagulation factors (V and VIII) and volume expansion as well. Stored at temperatures below $-18°C$, it is thawed just before being transfused.

Cryoprecipitate (technically cryoprecipitated antihemophilic factor [AHF]) is prepared by thawing FFP slowly in a refrigerator and recovering and refreezing the precipitate. Each unit comes from a single donor and contains 80 or more factor VIII units and at least 150 mg of fi-

brinogen in 10 to 15 ml of plasma. Each unit of cryoprecipitate or FFP shares the same infectious risks as 1 U of red blood cells; thus the use of heat-treated factor VIII concentrates are increasing as compared to the single-donor components.

Crystalloids and Colloids

In addition to replacing water lost through the skin, lungs, kidneys, and gastrointestinal tract, crystalloids are used intraoperatively to replace lost blood when oxygen carrying capacity is adequate. Lactated Ringer's solution is used most commonly because its composition is closer to normal extracellular fluid than is saline, although little data exist to show its advantages. Five percent dextrose can be used in crystalloid solutions to treat mildly hypoglycemic patients and infants incapable of adequate gluconeogenesis. Adults, however, maintain normal or elevated glucose levels intraoperatively because of catecholamine release caused by the stress of anesthesia and surgery. Elevated glucose levels can increase the risk of neurologic sequelae if neuronal ischemia occurs.[44–46] Thus routine use of 5 percent dextrose in saline or in lactated Ringer's solution is no longer recommended. When crystalloids are used during moderate hemorrhage, usually three times the volume of the estimated blood loss is administered so that intravascular volume will be maintained after the crystalloid solutions equilibrate between the intra- and extravascular spaces.

The importance of colloid administration to replace blood loss and maintain the colloid osmotic pressure (COP) in the vascular system is controversial. While a great deal of research has been done and studies can be found for and against colloid use, the bulk of evidence suggests that colloid therapy for volume replacement does not affect outcome. A number of reviews are available in the literature.[47–49] Although hemodilution resulting in extremely low COP can result in marked peripheral edema, pulmonary edema does not follow as long as hydrostatic pressures (pulmonary artery wedge pressure) and capillary permeability are normal.[47]

Colloid solutions are useful in clinical practice in situations where it is desirous to avoid excessive crystalloids, yet volume is needed and blood transfusion is still unnecessary because oxygen carrying capacity is still adequate. *Hydroxyethyl starch* or serum *albumin* can be used as both are free of infectious risk. While hydroxyethyl starch is slightly less expensive, it has significant effects on the coagulation system and it remains in the reticuloendothelial system for weeks after administration.[50]

Pathophysiology of Anemia

Limits of Hemodilution

Few would question replacing minimal blood loss (<20 percent estimated blood volume) with crystalloids or colloids; 10 percent of blood volume is routinely collected from blood donors with no replacement and rarely a reaction of any type. The decision as to when red blood cell replacement becomes necessary in the face of larger hemorrhage is not simple; the medical judgment to be made requires an understanding of the pathophysiology involved and an assessment of the risks in a particular patient. The era of medicine when patients could be transfused to unnecessarily high hemoglobin levels with no questions asked is now over.

In chronic anemia, compensation mechanisms center around an increase in 2,3-diphosphoglycerate (2,3-DPG) levels in the red blood cell. The 2,3-DPG molecule, a glycolytic intermediate, binds the two β chains of the hemoglobin molecule together, decreasing the affinity of hemoglobin for oxygen so that more oxygen is unloaded in the tissues.[11] Through increases in 2,3-DPG, the oxygen–hemoglobin curve is shifted to the right in chronic anemia; the oxygen tension at which hemoglobin is 50 percent saturated (P_{50}) is higher than the normal 26 mmHg.

By contrast, the compensation for acute anemia is cardiovascular. In essence, the heart increases its work to increase perfusion of critical organ tissues so that oxygen transport may remain adequate. In actuality, a variety of cardiovascular compensation mechanisms have been described and recently reviewed.[51–53] They include

1. Decreased blood viscosity
2. Increased cardiac output
3. Increased stroke volume
4. Increased myocardial oxygen consumption
5. Decreased afterload
6. Increased venous return
7. Increased myocardial blood flow
8. Increased cerebral blood flow
9. Decreased renal, mesenteric, and hepatic blood flow
10. Decreased peripheral resistance
11. Increased heart rate
12. Increased circulating catecholamines, renin, and vasopressin

Decreases in blood viscosity increase oxygen transport independent of other mechanisms as the hemoglobin concentration drops to 10 g%. Although it has been questioned by some, most authors believe oxygen transport is maximal at 10 g%.[54,55] This is primarily based on in vitro studies in which blood flow through glass capillary tubes was measured as hemoglobin concentration was varied (Fig. 2-2). Crowell and Smith[56] found that 27.5 percent was the optimal hematocrit for

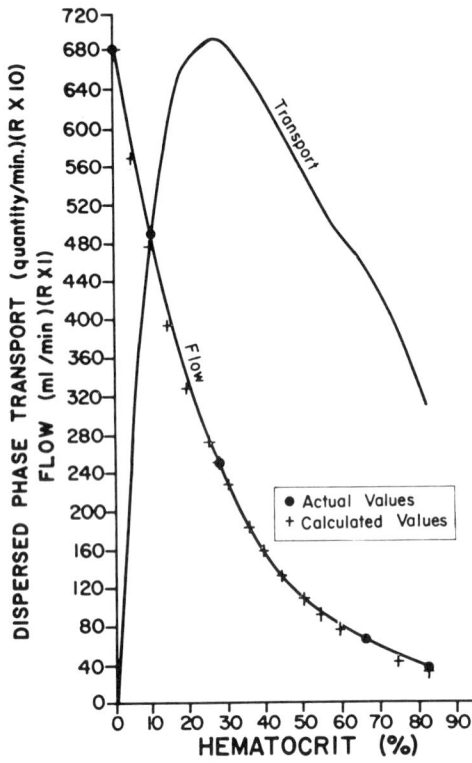

Fig. 2-2. A comparison of the flow of blood and the transport of oxygen through a glass tube at constant pressure as affected by changing the hematocrit. (From Crowell & Smith,[56] with permission.)

blood flowing through 747.4-μ glass tubes. The applicability of the data to blood flow through human capillary beds is questionable.

In normovolemic anemia, cardiac output increases by increasing stroke volume through increased end-diastolic volume.[51] In hypovolemic anemia, increased heart rate is also important. These adjustments take place even under resting conditions at the cost of increased myocardial oxygen consumption, blood flow, and coronary vasodilation, although normal myocardium compensates for this without evidence of ischemia.[57,58] Cerebral blood flow increases during extreme hemodilution, while the cerebral meta-

bolic rate of oxygen ($CMRO_2$) is unaffected.[59,60]

As in most other physiologic systems, the body possesses extraordinary reserves for oxygen transport to tissues. When the hemoglobin is 15 g/dl and saturation is normal (99 percent), the content of arterialized blood is 20 ml/dl. Therefore, a cardiac output of 5 L/min transports 1,000 ml oxygen/min (oxygen delivery [DO_2]), while the total body oxygen consumption of a 70-kg adult is only 250 ml/min (VO_2).[53] Thus, mixed venous blood returns to the heart with an oxygen content of 15 ml/dl, the red blood cells still carrying 75 percent of the oxygen loaded when they last passed through the lungs, 75 percent of that carried to the tissues by arterial blood (Table 2-3).[52] Whole body oxygen extraction (O_2Ex) is normally about 25 percent. Oxygen extraction increases with progressing anemia. Oxygen extraction is the ratio of oxygen consumption to oxygen delivery (VO_2/DO_2). In a hemodiluted pig preparation, Trouwborst tried to define a critical extraction ratio at which oxygen consumption started to decline during stepwise reductions of oxygen delivery. Although he found that the critical extraction ratio averaged 0.57, his data showed a wide variation between animals.[61] His data did show a close correlation between mixed venous oxygen saturation ($S\bar{v}O_2$) and extraction ratio. Mixed venous oxygen saturation can be continuously monitored clinically with an Oximetric pulmonary artery catheter. This might be a way to monitor the effects of extreme hemodilution in patients, but the value of mixed venous oxygen saturation can be affected by other variables in addition to oxygen delivery. This is predicable from the Fick principle (Table 2-3). Changes in metabolic rate, oxygen consumption, arterial oxygen content (CaO_2), and cardiac output (CO) will also affect mixed venous oxygen saturation, and

Table 2-3. Oxygen Transport Definitions and Norms

Symbol	Definition	Normal
PaO_2	Arterial oxygen tension	>80 mmHg
$P\bar{v}O_2$	Mixed venous oxygen tension	35–45 mmHg
P_{50}	Oxygen tension at which hemoglobin is 50% saturated with oxygen	27 mmHg
SaO_2	Percent oxygen saturation of arterial hemoglobin (Hb)	≥95%
$S\bar{v}O_2$	Percent oxygen saturation of mixed venous Hb	70–75%
CaO_2	Arterial oxygen content = $SaO_2/100$ (1.34 × Hg) + (0.003 × PaO_2)	20 ml/dl
$C\bar{v}O_2$	Mixed venous oxygen content = ($S\bar{v}O_2/100$) (1.34 × Hb) + (0.003 × $P\bar{v}O_2$)	15 ml/dl
DO_2	Oxygen delivery = CaO_2 × cardiac output (CO)	1,000 ml/min
$\dot{V}O_2$	Oxygen consumption = CO × arteriovenous oxygen content difference	250 ml/min
$C(a\text{-}\bar{v})O_2$	Arteriovenous oxygen content difference = CaO_2 − $C\bar{v}O_2$	5 ml/dl
O_2Ex	Oxygen extraction = $\dot{V}O_2/DO_2$	25–30%
Fick principle	$$CO = \frac{\dot{V}O_2}{CaO_2 - C\bar{v}O_2}$$ $$C\bar{v}O_2 = CaO_2 - \frac{\dot{V}O_2}{CO}$$	

(Adapted from Robertie & Gravlee,[52] with permission.)

these variables can change in response to numerous other factors.[62] The other problem with reliance on mixed venous oxygen saturation as a monitor for extremes of hemodilution is that it measures only whole body oxygen extraction and not the adequacy of oxygen transport to specific tissues such as the myocardium and central nervous system.

Compensatory mechanisms described at the beginning of this section portray the amazing adaptations healthy mammals can make to extreme anemia, but theoretical, laboratory, and clinical evidence suggest that humans with cardiovascular and cerebrovascular disease have limited ability to compensate for acute anemia below hemoglobin levels of 8 to 10 g%. From a theoretical standpoint, relationships between cardiac output, he-moglobin, and arterial oxygen content (Fig. 2-3) demonstrate the much greater increases in cardiac output necessary to maintain oxygen delivery when hemoglobin concentration is below 10 g% than when it is above 10 g%.[63] Even the viscosity-related advantages from hemodilution are questioned by some.[55] Furthermore, hemodilution is usually studied primarily in anesthetized or, at least, resting subjects in whom all factors that might challenge the cardiovascular system are controlled. A given patient's metabolic requirements may need to increase at any time because of physical activity, pain, fever, or other factors. Reserve oxygen carrying capacity may be crucial at these times to prevent ischemia in myocardial or other critical tissues.

A number of laboratory studies docu-

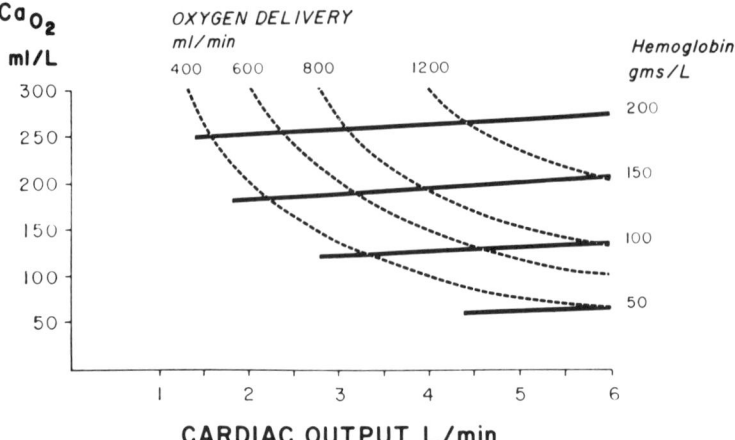

Fig. 2-3. Interrelation of cardiac output, oxygen delivery, and hemoglobin level, computed mathematically. When the hemoglobin level is 100 g/L or less (solid lines), much greater increases in cardiac output are necessary to maintain constant oxygen delivery (broken lines). (From Sullivan,[63] with permission.)

ment the safety of hemodilution but many also demonstrate the increased risk of severe anemia or hemodilution when other pharmacologic or pathologic conditions are present. Crystal et al[64] found impaired myocardial metabolism and a decrease in the ratio of coronary blood flow to endocardial versus epicardial tissues in hemodiluted dogs with coronary stenosis. As in an earlier study from the same laboratory, as hemodilution became more extreme, cardiac failure was demonstrated at higher hemoglobin levels in dogs with coronary stenosis than in the control group.[64,65] Impaired myocardial wall motion has been demonstrated in dogs with critical coronary artery stenosis when hematocrit was reduced from 45 to 15 percent.[66] Estafanous et al[67] showed impaired response to hemodilution (no increase in cardiac output or stroke volume) in a rat preparation in which myocardial depression had been produced pharmacologically. Crystal and Salem[57] studied hemodilution and nitroprusside-induced controlled hypotension in dogs. Decreased blood flow was reported in

certain peripheral tissues, especially the kidney. Adverse hemodynamic effects have been reported from the interactions of β-blockers and hemodilution in some preparations.[68] Plewes and Farhi[69] showed major decreases in oxygen delivery to renal cortex and retina after 90 minutes of hemodilution and controlled hypotension in dogs.

Adverse effects of relatively mild hemodilution also have been demonstrated in a few studies in humans with cardiovascular disease. Weisel et al[70] randomized patients undergoing coronary artery bypass grafting into a group whose hemoglobin level was maintained at 12 ± 1.6 g/dl and a hemodilution group whose hemoglobin level was allowed to drift to a mean 8.9 ± 1.7 g/dl perioperatively. Sensitive indices of myocardial ischemia demonstrated abnormalities in myocardial metabolism postoperatively. Delayed recovery of myocardial lactate and oxygen extraction capabilities were demonstrated in the hemodiluted group. Coronary sinus oxygen tension was found to correlate directly with postoperative hemoglobin level, suggesting a lack of myocardial compensation reserves.[70]

Rao and Montoya[71] hemodiluted cardiopulmonary bypass patients to an average hematocrit of 28 percent and reported that ischemic ST segment changes were most common in those with elevated left ventricular end-diastolic pressures (LVEDP), suggesting that oxygen-carrying capacity reserves were diminished in mildly anemic patients with impaired myocardium. In a small group of total hip arthroplasty patients, Rosberg and Wulff[72] reported that older patients (68 years mean age) were unable to increase cardiac output after hemodilution to 28 percent; old age by itself was suggested as a contraindication to extreme hemodilution by these authors.

The Transfusion Trigger

Most clinicians have now properly abandoned the "magic" 10 g as a *transfusion trigger*, or a preoperative hemoglobin requirement in healthy patients. Its origin has been reviewed by Zauder[73] and its validity appropriately criticized: "The etiology of this requirement is cloaked in tradition, shrouded in obscurity, and unsubstantiated by clinical or experimental evidence." However, the studies reviewed in the previous section suggest there are risks involved when older patients or those with significant cardiovascular, cerebrovascular, or pulmonary disease are hemodiluted below 10 g/dl.[52,70–72] A hemoglobin level of 8 g/dl is reasonable for healthy patients and those with only mild, asymptomatic disease-states. While some patients might be managed with more severe anemia, they should be carefully monitored for any problems that might develop that would compromise their ability to compensate. Neither 10 g/dl nor any hemoglobin level between 10 and 7 g/dl should be regarded as a rigid indication for transfusion; medical judgment must be based on the ability of an individual patient to compensate for the anemia.

Replacement for Massive Blood Loss

Coagulopathy

In both trauma surgery and elective orthopedic surgery and elective orthopedic surgery, bleeding occasionally becomes severe and the anesthesia care provider must be ready to manage a massive transfusion to keep a patient alive. Surgeons and anesthesia care providers have recognized for many decades that some patients developed coagulopathies when transfused massively and that fresh blood was often effective in treating such a coagulopathy. Studies during the Vietnam War showed that massively transfused patients developed a dilutional thrombocytopenia; the severity of the thrombocytopenia correlated with the number of units transfused.[74] Miller[74] reported that a hemorrhagic diathesis was "likely" when the platelet count was approximately 65×10^9/L. His data also showed that 21 percent of patients with platelet counts between 75 and 100×10^9/L developed bleeding problems and that 64 percent of patients with platelet counts between 50 and 75×10^9/L developed coagulopathies.

This knowledge has led many clinicians to use platelet concentrates in all patients transfused massively; however, three more recent massive transfusion studies clearly condemn this practice.[75–77] While a 5- to 7-unit transfusion in an adult meets some physicians' definition of "massive," Miller and others define a massive transfusion as one that is greater than 1.5 times the estimated blood volume of the recipient. His work and subsequent studies showed that significant dilutional thrombocytopenia did not usually occur until patients had received a transfusion large enough to replace 1.5 to 2 blood volumes.[74–76]

Even during transfusions in the range to 15 to 20 U and greater, prophylactic platelet therapy has been shown to be unnecessary. In 1986, Reed et al[75] reported a prospective, randomized, double-blind clinical study on the effectiveness of prophylactic platelets in massively transfused patients. Trauma patients who were expected to require massive transfusion were randomized into two groups. One group was given 6 U of platelet concentrate after transfusion of each 12 U of blood. The other group received only 2 U of FFP and no platelets after every 12 U of blood. The FFP was used as a control to blind clinicians treating each patient; it matched the volume of plasma the patients in the platelet group received with their platelets. The results showed a nearly identical incidence of microvascular bleeding in groups who were or were not given platelet concentrate. Prophylactic platelet therapy was found ineffective in preventing diffuse microvascular bleeding. Very close to 20 percent of massively transfused patients developed nonsurgical bleeding regardless of whether they had received platelets. Although the patients in the platelet group had a slightly higher mean platelet count after receiving platelet therapy, the declining trend in their platelet counts was not altered (Fig. 2-4). Thrombocytopenia was found to develop early in large transfusions with later changes becoming progressively smaller. A patient's initial count before transfusion was an important determinant of how much the subsequent counts would be lowered by dilution. Later, platelet counts were thought to be sustained by splenic release to some extent.

A similar study had previously been performed by Counts et al[76] to determine the effectiveness of prophylactic FFP in massively transfused patients. In this

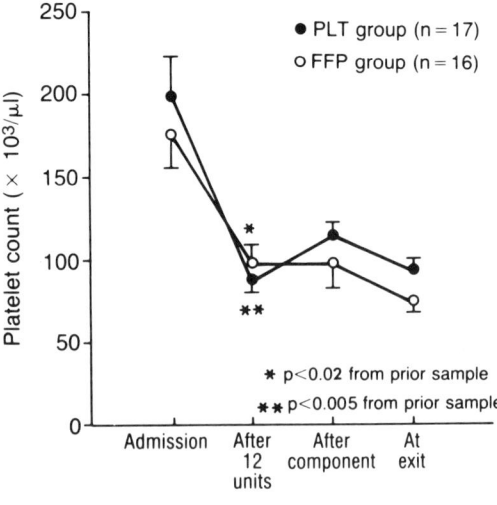

Fig. 2-4. Alterations in group mean platelet counts (± SEM) at four sample time points during massive transfusion in the study by Reed et al.[75] PLT, patients receiving prophylactic platelet component therapy; FFP, patients receiving prophylactic FFP therapy. No significant differences between the two study groups exist. (From Reed et al,[75] with permission.)

study, 27 patients entering the same institution in shock were followed closely with platelet counts and coagulation factor assays. Platelet concentrates, plasma, and cryoprecipitate were given only when there was abnormal microvascular bleeding and laboratory evidence of a platelet or coagulation factor deficiency. Of 27 patients, 8 developed hemostatic abnormalities. Five of these eight patients developed thrombocytopenia, and three patients developed DIC. Platelet therapy alone was effective in reversing the coagulopathies in six of eight bleeding patients. FFP and cryoprecipitate were used only for the patients in whom DIC was diagnosed. Thus, prophylactic FFP was determined to be not indicated in massively transfused patients. Multiple studies have shown that coagulopathies actually develop in only a minority (18 to 30 percent) of massively transfused patients.[75,76,78] Thus, most hemostatic components given prophylactically to massively transfused patients are transfused to patients who would not have developed coagulopathy anyway.[79]

The depletion of both platelets and soluble clotting factors is greatest when shock accompanies severe blood loss.[80] Even in this situation, however, FFP supplementation in normal doses does not effectively restore coagulation activity. FFP and platelet concentrates should be used only in those patients in whom an actual coagulopathy is present and can be attributed to specific clotting factor deficiencies or thrombocytopenia.

In the clinical studies by Reed et al[75] and Counts et al,[76] strict criteria were used to define microvascular bleeding and most of the blood used was modified whole blood. This is blood that has had platelet concentrate removed after which the plasma is returned to the red blood cells. Would the same results hold true if red blood cells were used instead of modified whole blood? Murray et al[77] studied coagulation changes during replacement with red blood cells stored in Adsol preservative, currently the most commonly used anticoagulant/preservative. Twelve patients requiring major elective surgery were studied. Platelet concentrates and FFP were withheld until laboratory studies showed that they were warranted. Platelets were administered in patients with excessive bleeding with platelet counts below $100 \times 10^9/L$. FFP was administered to replace 20 percent of plasma volume in those patients who continued to bleed after platelet therapy. The prothrombin time (PT) and activated partial thromboplastin time (aPTT) increased above control levels prior to replacement of 1 blood volume in 9 of 12 patients. None of these patients developed any observable bleeding tenden-

cies. Four of seven patients who required greater than 1 blood volume developed excessive bleeding with platelet counts less than $100 \times 10^9/L$. Platelets corrected the hemostatic deficiencies in two of the four patients. Two patients who had replacements of between 1.75 and 2 blood volumes continued to bleed until 2 to 4 U of FFP also were given. Since less plasma is contained in Adsol red blood cells, it is reasonable to expect a greater dilution of fibrinogen and soluble clotting factors, which Murray et al demonstrated.[77] Decreases in fibrinogen levels were thought to be a guide to significant declines in other coagulation factor levels. Fibrinogen levels less than 75 mg/dl were associated with a coagulopathy that responded to FFP replacement.

Coagulation Monitoring

In the Murray et al study, the PT and aPTT became elevated prior to 1 blood volume replacement in the absence of clinical bleeding. Abnormalities of these two coagulation profiles do not correlate with clinical bleeding and are not an indication for FFP replacement.[74–77] During a large transfusion, the platelet count, fibrinogen level, and thromboelastography (TEG) are the laboratory parameters most likely to be useful in determining when platelet or clotting factor replacement may be necessary. In addition to the fact that it takes more than 1 hour to get the PT and aPTT done in most institutions, these tests are too sensitive in massively transfused patients. The TEG is a more useful test that is performed on whole blood and can help to differentiate between clotting factor deficiencies and platelet problems.[81] Although thrombocytopenia can be quickly determined with a platelet count, the TEG is the best clinical measure of platelet function in the surgical setting. The bleeding time is difficult to do intraoperatively because it is affected by temperature and technique, and should not be performed on a limb in which intravenous fluids are running. In addition, recent reviews have found the bleeding time of no use as a preoperative screening test.[82] If DIC is suspected, fibrin split products should also be checked.

Metabolic Considerations in Massive Transfusion

Maintenance of patient temperature is critical; in a large transfusion all units must be warmed to avoid hypothermia in the patient. When unwarmed blood is being infused rapidly, the myocardial temperature can quickly drop below core temperature, leading to ventricular fibrillation. Although banked blood is acidotic during storage, prophylactic sodium bicarbonate is not recommended during large transfusions.[74] Blood gas levels should be monitored and the patient treated appropriately; metabolic alkalosis can be a problem after massive transfusion, even when sodium bicarbonate is not used.[83] When citrate anticoagulant in the transfused units accumulates in the patient faster than it can be metabolized by the liver, hypocalcemia can develop. This has been demonstrated at infusion rates above 50 ml/min for whole blood (in a 70-kg adult), but is seldom a problem with slower transfusions.[84] Although prolonged QT intervals can appear on the electrocardiogram, empiric calcium administration is not recommended.[85] In addition to causing arrhythmias, administration of high doses of calcium salts has also been linked to pancreatitis in patients after cardiac surgery.[86]

AUTOTRANSFUSION

Four types of autotransfusion are defined: preoperative donation, normovolemic hemodilution, intraoperative blood salvage, and postoperative blood salvage.[87] All have been used in orthopedic surgery and alone or in combination they have been proved extremely effective in reducing homologous transfusion (Table 2-4).

Preoperative Donation

Utilization of preoperative donation, the simplest form of autotransfusion, lagged behind the popularization of intraoperative blood salvage in the 1980s. A 1987 multi-institutional study reviewed 4,996 surgical patients at 18 tertiary care centers and reported that only 5 percent of eligible patients actually predeposited blood.[131] It was estimated that 68 percent of the patients who required transfusion but did not predonate could have avoided homologous transfusion through preoperative donation. Only 13 percent of those who predeposited subsequently required homologous blood as compared to 36 percent of those who did not predonate ($P <$ 0.01).[131] More recent studies have shown that up to 97 percent of patients scheduled for orthopedic procedures could avoid homologous transfusion through predeposit autologous transfusion.[94,100,109] Participation of orthopedic patients in one predeposit autologous donation program increased from 5 to 73 percent between 1985 and 1989.[98] A 1991 American Association of Blood Banks/Gallup Public Opinion survey found that 93 percent of Americans would prefer to donate their own blood prior to surgery.

Physical requirements for autologous donors have been made much more liberal than those for regular donors, and several large series have shown elderly patients could donate safely before surgery. A 1987 reported showed that 95 percent of transfusion requirements could be supplied by combining predeposit donation and intraoperative blood salvage for elderly patients.[105] In this series 91 percent of the 1,672 donors were older than 50 years and 8.4 percent were between 80 and 91 years of age. Elawad et al[94] collected 130 U of blood preoperatively from 45 patients (aged 60 to 82 years) and were able to supply 100 percent of the perioperative transfusion needs and 97 percent of the total transfusion requirements for these patients.

Mild donor reactions such as fainting, dizziness, or hematomas are a risk of donation; serious reactions such as myocardial infarction or stroke are more of a concern, especially in patients with significant health problems. Greenwalt[132] reported that by 1987 the immediate postdonation reaction rate stood at zero for 1,145 donations from a group between 66 and 78 years old. Other reports relate donor reaction rates of 0.6 to 2.26 percent in donor groups averaging 60 years of age and older.[133–135] McVay et al[135] reported in a large series of 10,200 autologous and 219,307 homologous donors that the incidences of mild (2.26 percent), moderate (0.22 percent), and severe reactions (0.037 percent) were essentially identical between autologous and homologous donors. Mann et al[136] reported a 4 percent donor reaction rate in high risk patients, but Spiess et al[137,138] actually established an autologous donor service specifically for high risk patients. The latter group monitored patients noninvasively during and after donation in their postanesthesia care unit and administered crystalloid or colloid for volume replacement after donation.[137,138]

Preoperative collection in a pediatric patient as young as 16 months of age has been described, and series of pediatric patients as young as 6 years have been reported.[114,119,121,139] Most of these patients were scheduled for scoliosis surgery; preoperative donation alone was enough to supply all transfusion needs for 50 to 63 percent of the patients.[114,119] By combining preoperative donation and intraoperative blood salvage 77 to 88 percent of the pediatric patients were able to supply all their blood requirements.[119,121] Preoperative donation has also been shown to be safe in pregnant patients.[140] Preoperative donation alone has been shown more effective in reducing homologous transfusion than preoperative donation combined with designated donation.[99]

Longer storage periods (42 days for Adsol red blood cells) have facilitated preoperative autologous donation and, for most patients, obviated the need to freeze red blood cells collected for this purpose. In addition to the extra expense imposed by their use, deglycerolized red blood cells must be transfused within 24 hours after thawing, increasing the chance of waste. When blood is donated either weekly or even every 3 to 4 days, 4 to 6 U can often be collected if the patient is maintained on supplemental iron (300 mg ferrous sulfate three times daily); anemia, however, is usually the limiting factor.[101] Plasma volume and composition is known to be back to prephlebotomy steady state within 48 to 72 hours after donation.[141] The mild anemias produced in most patients by this type of a donation program are not adequate to increase endogenous erythropoietin substantially above the normal range.[142,143] Recombinant human erythropoietin has been used to increase hemoglobin levels in the anemia of renal failure; it has also been shown to be effective in increasing the amount of autologous blood that can be collected in donors preoperatively.[144,145] In a randomized, controlled trial in 47 adults scheduled for elective orthopedic procedures, Goodnough et al[145] found more units could be collected from patients treated with erythropoietin. The red blood cell volume donated by patients who received erythropoietin was 41 percent greater than that donated by patients

Table 2-4. Orthopedic Autologous Transfusion Studies

Author(s)	Year Published	Procedure	No. of Patients	Preoperative Deposit	Isovolemic Hemodilution	Intraoperative Blood Salvage	Postoperative Salvage	Patients Using Only Autologous (%)	Transfusion Needs Supplied by Autologous (%)
Ahlberg et al[88]	1977	THA	20		x				50
Bailey & Mahoney[89]	1987	Spinal fusion	52	x				85	
Barbier-Bohm et al[90]	1980	THA	10		x			78	
Bernstein & Rosenberg[91]	1987	Misc. ortho	75	x				71	
Bovill & Norris[92]	1989	Shoulder	72			x		75	
Elawad et al[93]	1991	THA	60	x				100	
Elawad et al[94]	1991	THA	45	x					97
Endresen et al[95]	1991	THA	34			x			76
		THA, revision	14			x			67
Faris et al[96]	1991	THA & TKA	153				x		
Ganon et al[97]	1991	THA & TKA	239				x	87	
Goodnough et al[98]	1990	THA		x				82	
		TKA		x				88	
Goodnough et al[99]	1989	60% orth.	112	x				90	
Goodnough et al[100]	1990	Misc. ortho	276	x				86	
Goodnough et al[101]	1989	Misc. ortho	145	x				87	
Groh et al[102]	1990	TKA	25				x	92	
Haberkern & Dangel[103]	1991	Spinal	30		x	x			75
Hansen[104]	1989	THA & TKA	12	x					54
Haugen & Hill[105]	1987	Misc. ortho	1672	x		x			95
Johnson & Murphy[106]	1990	Lumbar fusion	97	x		x		98	
Kafer et al[107]	1986	Scoliosis	12		x				
Kay & Noble[108]	1990	Misc. ortho	204	x					72
Komatsu[109]	1990	Misc. ortho		x				89	

Study	Year	Procedure	No.					
Kruger & Colbert[110]	1985	Spinal	25		x			
Law & Wiedel[111]	1989	THA, revision	64	x				72
Lehner et al[112]	1981	Spinal	16	x		x		20
Lichtiger et al[113]	1990	Misc. cancer	235			x	73	
MacEwen et al[114]	1990	Scoliosis	118	x		x	63	
MacFarlane et al[115]	1988	THA & TKA	99	x		x	74	
Mann et al[116]	1989	Scoliosis	54		x			54
			41		x	x	90	69
			10					
Martin & Ott[117]	1981	Scoliosis	26			x		83
McMurray et al[118]	1991	THA	49	x				19
		THA, revision	57	x				35
Novak[119]	1988	Scoliosis	82	x		x	77	94
Semkiw et al[120]	1989	THA & TKA	74	x	x	x	83	
Silvergleid[121]	1987	Misc. ortho	180			x	88	
Slagis et al[122]	1991	Bilat. TKA	22		x			54
		THA	50		x			35
		Single TKA	30		x			20
Thomson et al[123]	1987	THA & TKA	159	x		x	71	
Trammell et al[124]	1991	Misc. ortho	96		x			
Turner et al[125]	1990	THA	476	x	x	x	76	58
		THA, revision	1017	x		x	51	
		Spinal	339	x		x	81	
Viviani et al[126]	1978	Spinal	20	x		x	85	
Wasman & Goodnough[127]	1987	Misc. ortho	44	x		x		75
Wilson[128]	1989	THA, revision	98			x		42
Woolson & Watt[129]	1991	THA	143	x		x	92	90
Woolson et al[130]	1987	THA	50	x		x	62	

THA, total hip arthroplasty; TKA, total knee arthroplasty.

given a placebo. The cost of recombinant human erythropoietin might prohibit this therapy's widespread use, but it could make preoperative donation possible in some patients (i.e., those having small body size or chronic anemia) who could not otherwise donate. Even without erythropoietin therapy or frozen blood storage, preoperatively donated autologous blood costs as much as homologous blood, yet its safety can make it a real bargain in the long run. In their report of a large series of 1,832 autologous orthopedic cases, Turner et al[125] documented 22 cases of hepatitis and two cases of HIV-1 exposure in the homologous group. In an amazing display of shortsightedness, the Health Care Financing Administration (HCFA) ruled in 1991 that predeposit autotransfusion was part of a surgical procedure and thus could not be billed separately for Medicare patients. The effectiveness of preoperative donation, when used alone or in combination with other autologous techniques in orthopedic patients, is demonstrated in Table 2-4.

Normovolemic Hemodilution

Acute normovolemic hemodilution is the autotransfusion technique most dependent on the anesthesia care provider's intervention intraoperatively. The patient's red blood cell mass is actively lowered before surgery and blood loss in an effort to reduce intraoperative hemoglobin waste. Volume is replaced with crystalloids or colloids, and the red blood cells are returned to the patient at the end of surgery. It is most often employed during cardiac surgery, where it can be facilitated by large venous cannulae and hypothermia. A number of authors have reported its use in orthopedic surgery as well. Barbier-Bohm et al[90] studied induced hypotension and normovolemic hemodilution and found them both effective in decreasing homologous blood use in patients undergoing total hip arthroplasty. In scoliosis surgery, Martin and Ott,[117] reported that the homologous transfusion requirements could be reduced from a mean of 4,370 ml to 750 ml with extreme hemodilution to a hematocrit of 15 percent. Haberkem and Dangel[103] reported a 75 percent reduction in homologous blood transfusion by combining extreme hemodilution, controlled hypotension, and intraoperative blood salvage in children and adolescents between 3.4 and 19.9 years of age.

Advantages of acute normovolemic hemodilution are that it can be applied to patients who might not be able to donate blood preoperatively and can be used during cancer surgery, where intraoperative blood salvage might be contraindicated. It requires little in the way of special equipment, but it does demand an increase in the intensity of attention from the anesthesia care provider, especially during the period when units are being collected.

When the technique is performed, blood is drawn from an arterial catheter, central line, or large peripheral antecubital vein and collected into anticoagulant bags that are constantly mixed to ensure anticoagulation. The amount of blood to be collected is calculated based on the patient's blood volume (EBV), original hematocrit ($H_{original}$), final hematocrit (H_{final}), and average hematocrit (H_{avg}) according to the formula below:

Volume to be removed

$$= EBV \times \frac{H_{original} - H_{final}}{H_{avg}}$$

The volume collected is measured with a scale during collection. As blood is being withdrawn, volume is replaced with crystalloid or colloid to maintain normovolemia. Three liters of nondextrose-containing crystalloid solutions can be administered for every liter of blood withdrawn. Colloid can be substituted at a lower ratio. Crystalloid is advantageous because its removal at the end of surgery by the kidneys can be facilitated with a diuretic. Peripheral edema is frequently noted, but pulmonary edema is said to be rare.[146] Substitution of colloid decreases the formation of edema during the procedure.

The most serious risks of normovolemic hemodilution involve limitation of oxygen transport to critical tissues such as the myocardium and brain (see Limits of Hemodilution, above). Renal function must be adequate to mobilize the extra load. Although probably reduced as compared to homologous blood, the possibility of a technical error resulting in ABO-incompatible hemolytic transfusion reaction still could exist if blood is not retransfused before the patient leaves the operating room. Protocols for identifying and labeling units must be strictly adhered to. If blood is not reinfused within 6 hours, it must be refrigerated, as bacterial contamination is a risk.

Although the technique has been described in the literature in many types of surgical procedures, there are few, if any, prospective, well-controlled studies proving that acute normovolemic hemodilution actually decreases homologous replacement.[146] In procedures in which blood loss is small and no transfusion is necessary, normovolemic hemodilution could present added risk to a patient. In procedures in which large volumes of blood are lost, the number of units obtained through hemodilution is unlikely to be adequate to prevent homologous replacement.

Intraoperative Blood Salvage

Intraoperative blood salvage is performed by two basic techniques, cell washing and filtration. A number of devices are available that spin cells in a semicontinuous-flow centrifuge in which

Table 2-5. Devices Used for Intraoperative Blood Salvage

Filtration devices for autotransfusion
  Receptal Autotransfusion System (Abbott Laboratories, Abbott Park, IL)
  Solcotrans (Solco Basle, Inc., Rockland, MA)
  Intraop Autotransfusion System (Davol Inc., Cranston, RI)
  O.R. Bloodbanker Autotransfusion System (International Technidyne Corp., Edison, NJ)
  Autovac Intraoperative Autotransfusion System (Boehringer Laboratories, Wynnewood, PA)
Red cell recovery and washing equipment
  Low-flow systems
    Cell Saver 1 and 3 (Haemonetics Corp., Braintree, MA)
    Shiley/Dideco Autotrans BT-795A and BT-795AA (Shiley Co., Irvine, CA)
    Electromedics AT 500 and AT 750 (Electromedics Inc., Englewood, CO)
  Rapid processing systems
    Baylor Rapid Autologous Transfusion System (BRAT) (Cobe Laboratories Inc., Lakewood, CO)
    Cell Saver 4 (Haemonetics Corp., Braintree, MA)
    Shiley Therapeutic Autotransfusion System (STAT) (Shiely/Dideco, Irvine, CA)
    AT-1000 (Electromedics Inc., Englewood, CO)

(Modified from Leach et al,[147] with permission.)

cells are washed with saline before being retransfused. Alternatively, the cells can be simply collected in a filtration device and subsequently washed or directly infused into the patient without washing. Autotransfusion equipment is listed in Table 2-5 and has been described by Leach et al[147] in a recent monograph.

The Red Blood Cell Product

Several authors have looked at the quality of the blood recovered perioperatively.[148–150] Davies et al[149] used a filtration system, a Sorenson Receptal device, for 25 patients undergoing aortic surgery. The plasma hemoglobin level was higher in blood recovered with this filtration system, which does not wash cells, as compared with that recovered from cell wash systems; red blood cell survival was identical in autologous and homologous blood.

McShane et al[150] studied blood scavenged with a Dideco BT 795 autotransfusion machine and compared it to homologous blood. They reported a high hematocrit, which is easily adjustable with this machine, and a more normal pH and electrolyte content in red blood cells washed with this device. 2,3-DPG levels were also documented as higher. In the 1970s, higher 2,3-DPG levels were a promised advantage of autologous transfusion. Because the red blood cells are fresher, their higher 2,3-DPG content improves the efficiency of oxygen unloading in the tissues. However, the clinical significance of improving 2,3-DPG levels in transfused blood has never been proven.

Effects on the Coagulation System

One concern of those using intraoperative blood salvage for autotransfusion is whether these systems can adversely affect coagulation. Activation of the coagulation system in a bleeding patient produces fibrinogen. The fibrinolytic system keeps the clotting system in control by breaking down fibrin after it has been formed. Fibrin degradation products (fibrin split products) are known to inhibit coagulation by interfering with platelet adhesion and aggregation as well as with fibrin polymerization. Since these products should be soluble in blood salvaged from the wound, a theoretical appeal of autotransfusion systems that wash blood is that fibrin split products, thromboplastin, and activated plasmin should be washed out of collected cells before they are reinfused.

The Bentley autotransfusion system of the 1970s was withdrawn from the market because of coagulation problems, although the literature contains little information on this.[139,151] DIC is alleged, but not clearly documented, in humans with this system. Sharp et al[151] reported coagulopathies in 15 percent of patients in whom the Bentley device was used but gave few details. Animal studies did show marked decreases in platelet count, fibrinogen, hematocrit, and serum proteins after the Bentley machine was used.[152,153] Air embolism was also a problem with the Bentley device but has also been reported with early Haemonetics autotransfusion devices.[151]

Lawrence-Brown et al[154] studied blood collected from 10 patients during aortic surgery using heparinized suction and a Sorenson filtration collecting system, which filtered but did not wash red blood cells. They found the D-dimer levels to be elevated in the blood collected, also that D-dimer levels could be effectively eliminated by washing in saline (using a Cobe 2991 cell washer).[154] D-dimers are the smallest unique degradation product resulting from the action of plasmin on fibrin. Their presence is a measure of fibrinolytic activity and could lead to further interference with platelet aggregation and fibrin polymerization. D-dimer levels have been found to be elevated in patients with DIC, pulmonary embolus, and deep venous thrombosis.

Cell washing systems are not without their effects on coagulation, however. Although they remove soluble products, which could induce a coagulopathy, they also remove coagulation factors and platelets, which might do some good if reinfused into the patient. Sharp et al[151] reported a 5.1 percent incidence of coagulopathy in 136 cases in which a Haemonetics system was used. Boldt[155] studied the effects of cell separation and hemofiltration autotransfusion techniques in 40 patients undergoing coronary artery bypass grafting. This group used the Haemonetics Cell Saver 4 machines for their cell-separated group and a Fresenius HF60 hemofilter (Bad Homburg, Germany) for their filtration group. The Cell Saver apparatus produced a product with higher hemoglobin, lower heparin, and lower free hemoglobin levels. Platelet counts were lower; however, the volume was less, and it took longer to process blood with the cell washing device. Five hours post-transfusion, the patients who received washed cells had a higher hemoglobin level and lower PT. Nevertheless, hemoglobin, platelet count, free hemoglobin, antithrombin III, fibrinogen, PT, PTT, and colloid osmotic pressure were all close to normal in both groups.

Thus, while there is a theoretical risk of fibrinolysis and inhibition of the clotting system and possibly DIC from filtration-type autotransfusion systems, cell washing systems also affect coagulation. The product they produce is deficient in coagulation factors and platelets. Although this should not be a problem in an average transfusion, it could lead to coagulopathy in a massive transfusion situation in which the autotransfuser is employed to process more than the equivalent of 1 blood volume.[156] The coagulation system should be monitored during such a transfusion. It should be emphasized that from the standpoint of infectious risk, the empiric use of platelet concentrate and FFP in this type of situation may undo any infectious risk advantages gained from the use of the autotransfusion device.

Infection

Most centers consider the presence of pus or spillage of bowel contents to be contraindications to the use of autotransfusion devices. At least four reports support the belief that in vivo, at least, this is not a problem.[157-160] Schwieger et al[157] cultured the washings from 19 Haemonetics Cell Savers used for cardiopulmonary bypass. This group also followed patients for clinical infection, defined as fever greater than 38.5°C, a productive cough, urinary tract infection, pneumonia diagnosed by chest x-ray, or septic shock. Of the 19 Cell Saver washings, 4 were positive (21 percent); however, none of these patients had clinical infections. Five of the 19 patients (26 percent) did have clinical infections but negative Cell Saver cultures.

Andrews et al[160] reported positive cultures in 100 percent of scavenged blood samples from 18 patients. All but two were skin contaminants with low colony counts, and no patients had positive blood cultures. Davies et al[149] reported 12 positive cultures in autologous blood collected from 35 patients with the Sorenson device. All but 1 of the 12 were skin contaminants. He also noted that these organisms could be cultured from 2 of 25 homologous units. Although sporadic positive blood cultures are widely recognized, sepsis has not been attributed to autotransfusion. Intraoperative blood salvage is routinely employed for cases of subacute bacterial endocarditis in which it is known preoperatively that bacteremia is present.

Bourdreaux et al[158] reported a low incidence of infectious complications in patients autotransfused with blood contaminated with intestinal contents. They reported eight patients in whom this was necessary as a life-saving measure; only one of the eight patients died, and this death was due to a nonrelated cause.[158] In 1943, Griswold and Ortner[159] reported on the use of autotransfusion in 25 patients with abdominal wounds involving intestinal perforations. In the one patient who died of infection, 13 perforations had been found at various intestinal locations. His autotransfusion had been discontinued when the needle became blocked with feces. Glover et al[161] reported 14 patients given blood contaminated by intestinal contents. Six of 14 died, but the significance of the contamination was not clear.

Laboratory work by Boudreaux et al[158] suggests, however, that autotransfusion should only be used in the presence of sepsis or intestinal perforations when it is necessary as a lifesaving measure. Banked blood was injected with *Escherichia coli* to simulate light, moderate, or heavy bacterial contamination. Cultures showed that at least 23 percent of the bacteria were not removed by the cell washing process (Haemonetics Model 15) when 1 L of sterile saline was used for washing at a rate of 175 to 200 ml/min. Increasing the saline volume to 5 or 10 L did not make any difference. Prophylactic antibiotics would be indicated in any patient receiving intraoperative blood salvage in whom there is a possibility of spillage of abdominal contents or evidence of preoperative infection. Autotransfusion is considered indicated only as a life-saving measure in trauma cases once spillage of bowel contents has been noted.

Malignancy

Most centers consider malignancy a contraindication to intraoperative autotransfusion, although cancer surgery frequently requires transfusion of large amounts of homologous blood. Theoretical and clinical evidence suggests, however, that intraoperative autotransfusion could be safely used in these patients. Although Yaw et al[162] showed that cancer cells could be demonstrated in blood salvaged intraoperatively, there is evidence that cancer does not spread through the circulatory system when it metastasizes. Hematogenous spread of cancer during surgery was studied in the 1970s and several authors showed no correlation between cancer spread and the presence of circulating tumor cells during surgical procedures.[163–165] Some authors even found that 5-year survival was better in patients in whom circulating cancer cells were found during surgery.[164,165] Studies have also pointed to immunosuppressive effects of homologous blood, which may increase the risk of metastasis in patients given homologous blood instead of autologous transfusion during surgery for cancer.[35]

Hart et al[166] and Klimberg et al[167] followed 49 patients with transitional cell carcinoma of the bladder who underwent radical cystectomy with autotransfusion. Thirty-three of these patients were followed for at least 1 year, with a mean follow-up time of 24 months. Twenty-five of the 33 patients had no evidence of recurrence. Of the seven patients who did have recurrence, five had only local recurrence and only two patients had evidence of distant metastasis without local recurrence. The authors said recurrence and survival rates were similar to other reports for this type of surgery. Although these authors point out that their follow-up time is brief, and although there was no control group, it would appear that it would be very reasonable to question the generally accepted belief that autotransfusion should not be used during cancer surgery. Randomized, controlled studies should be instituted.

In 1991, Miller et al[168] reported that tumor cells cultured from four different cell lines were not removed by processing with a standard autotransfusion device (Haemonetics Cell Saver), but that they were completely removed when the washed red blood cells were passed through a RC100 leukocyte depletion filter. The ability to use intraoperative blood salvage during surgery for cancer would be a major autotransfusion advance in many centers.

Risks of Intraoperative Blood Salvage/Autologous Transfusion

The efficacy and usefulness of intraoperative blood salvage have been clearly demonstrated in the literature and the practice has become the standard of care in most areas of the country. Large series report few complications; Turner et al,[125] for example, reported no known complications in 1,922 procedures over 8 years. Coagulopathy is the most important risk physicians should keep in mind when caring for patients being autotransfused in the perioperative period. With filtration techniques, fibrin degradation products have been demonstrated and could lead to impaired platelet aggregation and even DIC. Cell washing techniques are not free of risk, however, as they can produce a dilutional coagulopathy because their product contains lower levels of soluble clotting factors than does homologous blood. Also, low levels of heparin are frequently demonstrated and could be a problem where large amounts of autologous blood are processed. Predeposit autotransfusion has a slight risk of transfusion-related sepsis if collected units become contaminated, as do occasional homologous units. Although autologous blood is the only immunologically perfectly compatible blood a person can receive, there is always the remote risk of a clerical error leading to a serious hemolytic reaction.

One case report exists in which hypertension and tachycardia were seen following autotransfusion for pheochromocytoma.[169] Although renal insufficiency is frequently mentioned and renal damage is a theoretical concern when free hemoglobin is present in autotransfused blood, renal insufficiency is relatively frequent after the types of surgery in which autotransfusion is used and it is difficult to prove whether renal problems are from autotransfusion or the surgery it-

Table 2-6. Autotransfusion Risks

Preoperative deposit
    Clerical errors leading to misidentification
    Bacterial contamination
    Hypotension due to hypersensitivity to substances in the blood bags and tubing[171]
    Complications related to the freezing, thawing, and washing process[172]
Normovolemic hemodilution
    Inadequate oxygen delivery to tissues
    Fluid overload
Intraoperative blood salvage
    Effects on coagulation[173]
        Dilutional coagulopathy
        Reinfusion of anticoagulant
    Air embolism
    Bacterial contamination
    Spread of malignancy?
    Transfusion of antibiotic irrigants, microfibrillar collagen, or other substances from the wound[170]
    Salvaged blood syndrome[174,175]
Postoperative salvage
    Effects on coagulation
    Bacterial contamination

self. Microfibrillar collagen hemostat (Avitine) is not removed by cell washing; intraoperative blood salvage should be discontinued in areas of a wound where it has been applied.[170] Air embolism, a problem with the Bentley machine, has been also reported with Haemonetics machines.[151] Modern devices have alarm systems that should prevent reinfusion of air. Spread of cancer or infection by autotransfusion is probably also more a theoretical than an actual concern. Reported risks of autotransfusion are quite remote but are listed in Table 2-6; in practice, few problems have been demonstrated.

Postoperative Blood Salvage

The fourth type of autotransfusion is postoperative blood salvage. It has been employed extensively after cardiovascu-

Table 2-7.   Devices Used for
Postoperative Blood Salvage

Thora-Klex Autotransfusion Kit (Davol, Inc.,
  Cranston, RI)
Pleur-evac Autotransfusion System (Dekna-
  tel, Fall River, MA)
Pleura-Gard Autotransfusion Harvesting Unit
  (Conmed Corp., Utica, NY)
Atrium Blood Recovery System (Atrium Med-
  ical Corp., Hollis, NH)
Richards Solcotrans Orthopedic Autotransfu-
  sion System (Richards Medical Co., Mem-
  phis, TN)
Orthopedic Autovac Autotransfusion System
  (Boehringer Laboratories, Inc., Norristown,
  PA)

(Modified from Leach et al,[147] with permission.)

lar surgical procedures, in which the collection of large amounts of blood postoperatively from chest and mediastinal
drains is predictable. This blood does not
clot because it is defibrinated, primarily
by mechanical factors in the pleural and
pericardial cavities.[176] Since the coagulation process is already activated in the
areas from which the blood drains, the effects of blood salvage postoperatively on
the coagulation system have been closely
questioned. In theory, fibrin degradation
products in the salvaged blood could act
as procoagulants, stimulating the patient's coagulation system adversely after
reinfusion, and possibly even producing
DIC. Numerous clinical studies have
found that postoperative blood salvage
does not lead to adverse effects on the coagulation system in patients after cardiovascular surgery.[176–178] Temporary mild
increases in coagulation profiles such as
the aPTT are sometimes described, but
these return to normal relatively quickly.
Usually relatively inexpensive devices
are used to filter but not wash the red
blood cells collected postoperatively
(Table 2-7). After cardiovascular surgery,
the blood collected from pleural and mediastinal drains typically has a hemoglobin level half that of normal, but platelet

counts in the range of 100×10^9/L.[177] The
plasma hemoglobin level is elevated and
fibrinogen degradation products can be
demonstrated.[178] Bengston et al[179] have
demonstrated increased concentration of
anaphylatoxins (C3A and C5A) in blood
collected from patients after total joint arthroplasty. Activation of the complement
cascade was thought to occur in the collection system or in the wound, but there
were no signs of systemic complement activation in the patients after reinfusion.
Bacterial contamination has been demonstrated in blood collected during intraoperative blood salvage, and the potential
for sepsis with postoperative collection is
also a concern. For this reason, most postoperative blood salvage systems can be
used for only a limited number of hours.
Concerns over whether free hemoglobin
in the salvaged blood might lead to renal
failure have not been realized. The renal
toxicity of free hemoglobin is questionable when incompatible red blood cell
stroma is not present. Collected blood is
reinfused through microaggregate filters
within 4 to 6 hours after collection. Suction pressure is usually limited to 100
mmHg negative pressure (or 15 to 20
cmH_2O for chest drainage systems) to
limit the extent of red blood cell hemolysis.

While most studies on postoperative
blood salvage have dealt with cardiovascular surgery, a few have studied this
technique in orthopedic patients. In total
joint arthroplasties, more blood is frequently lost through postoperative drains
than through intraoperative hemorrhage.[120,180] Bengston et al,[179] studying
18 patients undergoing total hip or total
knee arthroplasty, found that 12 patients
required transfusion of autologous blood
postoperatively. Blood was collected
with a Solcotrans system and the blood
was anticoagulated with citrate–dextrose
solution in the suction equipment. Faris
et al[96] studied postoperative salvage in
patients after total hip and total knee ar-

throplasty and found few hematologic changes but a higher febrile reaction rate in patients receiving unwashed autologous blood collected more than 6 hours after surgery (compared to those receiving blood collected 6 hours or less after surgery). Slagis et al[122] found postoperative salvage effective in bilateral total knee arthroplasty patients but not total hip or single total knee arthroplasty patients. An innovative study from Stanford by Semkiw et al[120] reported 74 patients receiving postoperative blood salvage and other autologous techniques for total joint arthroplasty. A cell washing device was connected to the patient's drains as soon as they were inserted in the operating room. The autotransfusion device was then transported with the patient to the recovery room so that blood shed from the wound could be washed and reinfused as it was collected in the early postoperative period. Slightly greater quantities of blood were collected in the postoperative period than during intraoperative salvage, even from total hip arthroplasties where it was not possible to use a tourniquet. Although the average time in the recovery room was approximately 3 hours, an average of 428 ml of blood was salvaged during this period (range 100 to 2,385 ml).[120] Although 83 percent of the patients received only autologous blood, the only significant difference between patients who received homologous blood and those who received autologous blood was that the latter group had a much higher mean predeposit autologous donation volume.

OTHER MEANS OF AVOIDING TRANSFUSION

Physiologic

Since its first description in 1946, many have used the technique of *induced hypotension* (also known as controlled or deliberate hypotension) in an attempt to reduce blood loss during surgery.[181] Techniques and drugs used to lower blood pressure include arteriotomy, spinal anesthesia, epidural anesthesia, halothane, enflurane, isoflurane, trimethaphan, nitroprusside, nitroglycerin, esmolol, labetalol, phentolamine, nicardipine, and adenosine.[182] In theory, a lower blood pressure should decrease the rate of blood flow through open arterial vessels and possibly capillaries intraoperatively. In the section on the physiology of hemodilution earlier in this chapter, the ability of the body to transport three to four times more oxygen than was used in the tissues was discussed. Increased extraction can compensate for lower blood flow in some circumstances. Many drugs, such as isoflurane and nitroprusside, are known to lower arterial blood pressure without decreasing blood flow to critical organs. The well-known phenomenon of autoregulation maintains a normal cerebral blood flow over a wide range of perfusion pressures. In theory, these drugs should be safer than those that decrease cardiac output and organ perfusion. While the risk of ischemia makes induced hypotension relatively contraindicated for patients with myocardial, cerebrovascular, and renal disease, few complications have actually been reported.[182,183] Although it is also used to decrease the transmural pressure and thus the risk of hemorrhage during neurosurgical procedures for clipping of intracerebral aneurysms, induced hypotension is probably used in orthopedic anesthesia more often than in other subspecialties.

Many reports purport the efficacy of induced hypotension in orthopedics, usually claiming 40 to 50 percent reductions in blood loss in patients undergoing total hip arthroplasty or scoliosis surgery.[182,184,185] Yet not all the literature supports the use of induced hypotension as a means of decreasing blood loss. Donald[184] has criticized the literature on this subject as containing "no lack of reports of clinical impressions, technical minutiae and unsubstantiated claims for particular techniques." Petroza[182] pointed out that "a reproducible and predictable relationship between degree of blood pressure reduction and operative blood loss remains to be elucidated." Every clinician knows the importance of the surgeon's dexterity and technique in limiting blood loss. Many studies claiming the efficacy of induced hypotension do not account for the importance of the operating surgeon in limiting hemorrhage. A 1986 study reported a 43 percent reduction in blood loss in Jehovah's Witnesses undergoing total hip arthroplasty with sodium nitroprusside-induced hypotension when compared to a control group; operative time was 160 minutes for the control group as compared to 115 minutes for the study group, however.[183] The authors even reported a 35 percent reduction in blood loss as compared to the control group when 11 Jehovah's Witnesses underwent normotensive total hip arthroplasty (because of contraindications to induced hypotension), offering further proof that meticulous surgical technique is just as effective as controlled hypotension.[183]

Even when attempts are made to do controlled, prospective studies on induced hypotension, results can be affected by the inaccuracy of blood loss estimation. Although anesthesia care providers must always attempt to estimate intraoperative blood loss, the inaccuracy of these estimations, even when performed by experienced personnel, is well documented in the literature.[186]

The effects of different anesthetic techniques on blood loss have been studied and might be at least as important as the actual blood pressure. Regional anesthesia is often believed to decrease intraoperative blood loss, and this effect has been documented in certain types of cases (see Ch. 4). Certain general anesthetics are known to affect platelet function differently from others, and this could affect blood loss during general anesthetic techniques.[187,188]

In a retrospective study, Lennon et al[189] found nearly identical intraoperative and total transfusion requirements in patients undergoing scoliosis surgery when the patients were grouped according to whether induced hypotension was used. Although it is generally accepted that induced hypotension can produce better operating conditions for the surgeon, another study from the Mayo Clinic showed that neither intraoperative blood loss nor the surgeon's evaluation of the operative field correlated with the use of induced hypotension in patients undergoing oral surgery procedures.[190]

Pharmacologic

1-Desamino-8-D-arginine vasopressin (desmopressin, DDAVP) is a synthetic vasopressin analog lacking vasoconstrictor activity that acts on the vascular endothelium through the vasopressin-2 or antidiuretic receptor to increase factor VIII coagulant (VIIIC), factor VIII-related antigen (VIIIr:Ag), and factor VIII von Willebrand factor activity (VIIIvWF). It causes these coagulation proteins to be released from endothelial storage sites soon after infusion so that platelet function is improved. It has been used effectively in uremia, mild hemophilia (VIII deficiency), and type I von Willebrand's disease to improve coagulation. Early studies in cardiac surgical patients claimed that DDAVP was effective in reducing blood loss; blood loss was excessive in the control group in an early study that made this claim,[191] however, and subsequent studies have found DDAVP to be ineffective in reducing blood loss in uncomplicated cardiac surgery.[192,193]

Two studies have evaluated the effectiveness of DDAVP in decreasing blood loss in orthopedic patients. Three days preoperatively Kobrinski et al[194] infused 10 μg/m² body surface area (maximum dose 20 μg) of DDAVP intravenously to 35 patients entering a randomized, double-blind trial of the drug during spinal fusion with Harrington rod instrumentation. Patients assigned to the DDAVP group received the same dose immediately after induction of anesthesia; a normotensive technique was used in all patients. The drug produced a 22.4 percent decrease in the bleeding time; normal bleeding times had been noted in all patients preoperatively. PTT was decreased and other studies of platelet function were improved. Intraoperatively, blood loss was decreased by 32.5 percent and red blood cell transfusions were reduced by 26.5 percent in the DDAVP group. Postoperatively, there was no difference in blood loss between the two groups.

In 1990, Johnson and Murphy[106] reported on a study in which 20 μg of DDAVP were given by slow infusion shortly after induction of anesthesia to 42 patients undergoing lumbar fusion procedures. Blood loss was identical (550 ml) in both the DDAVP group and the control group, but the authors speculated that DDAVP might be useful in patients in whom greater than 1,000 ml blood loss was expected or in patients in whom preoperative donation was not feasible. The authors also recommended the knee-to-chest position for reducing the amount of bleeding in lumbar fusions by preventing engorgement of the epidural venous plexus.

Aprotinin has been used to reduce blood loss in cardiovascular surgery. It works by inhibiting platelet aggregation and activation, the intrinsic clotting system, and thrombin and fibrinogen receptors. By inhibiting the coagulation system, aprotinin preserves soluble coagulation factors and platelets from consumption during cardiopulmonary bypass. During orthopedic surgery in which systemic heparinization is not used, aprotinin would be expected to increase bleeding.

Erythropoietin is a hormone that stimulates red blood cell production in the bone marrow. Human erythropoietin has been produced through genetic engineering and used to treat the anemia of chronic renal failure.[144] It has also been employed as a pharmacologic substance that can decrease homologous blood use by stimulating the patient to produce more red blood cells. It has been shown to be effective in increasing preoperative autologous donations (see earlier section in this chapter) and it might be effective in treating postoperative anemia, but thus far U.S. Food and Drug Administration approval for these indications has not been obtained.[145]

TRENDS

As the intricacies of immunohematology and antibody identification were slowly elucidated, transfusion became relatively safe and blood banking emerged in this country during the first half of the 20th century. During the last 40 years, multiple infectious risks of blood transfusion were identified. As many important technological advances were made, blood banking developed into the multidisciplinary speciality, transfusion medicine. Clinicians were slow to alter their practices because of the threat of hepatitis, but the AIDS epidemic got the attention of physicians and patients, motivating abrupt changes in practice trends during the last 5 years. While blood transfusions doubled between 1971 and 1980, the number of red blood cell transfusions started to decline by the late 1980s, in spite of increasing surgical complexity.[195] However, platelet transfusions continued to increase dramatically during this period. The increase in autologous blood transfusion of all types during the late 1980s has been most dramatic.[196]

There have been steady, step-wise improvements in the risks of transfusion and the shift from homologous to autologous blood. Not all improvements have come as the result of scientific breakthroughs; many have resulted from patient and physician education and administrative improvements. For example, maximum surgical blood ordering schedules (MSBOS) were introduced in the 1970s to minimize unnecessary crossmatching, increasing the efficiency of local blood banks.[20] These schedules list average transfusion needs for patients undergoing particular surgical procedures based on previous experience. More blood can still be ordered for complex procedures and patients with increased needs, but unnecessary crossmatches are reduced and blood bank resources are better utilized.

The promise of a safe oxygen-carrying blood substitute has been dangled before clinicians for many years. Stimulated by the dream of decreasing battlefield casualties, research has centered around perfluorochemicals and stroma-free hemoglobin. Fluosol-DA was an emulsion containing perfluorodecalin and perfluorotripropylamine, which was introduced into clinical trials in the early 1980s.[197] *Perfluorochemicals* have the ability to contain far more dissolved oxygen than can be dissolved in water. These are colorless, odorless, nonflammable, dense liquids that are poor solvents for most compounds and essentially insoluble in water.[198] A few toxic reactions were described, but the main reason they were withdrawn from the clinical trials was that they were found to be clinically ineffective. Because of their physical properties, it was impossible to introduce adequate quantities of these chemicals into humans to significantly affect oxygen transport.[199] In essence, the drugs were too "anemic" to help severely anemic patients.

Although it is hoped that a more effective perfluorochemical red blood cell substitute might still be found, *stroma-free hemoglobin* is being more actively pursued as an oxygen carrier at this time. It has long been established that hemoglobin is relatively nontoxic when free of incompatible red blood cell stroma. But outside the red blood cell, free hemoglobin dissociates from tetramer to dimer and is rapidly excreted. Also, free hemoglobin has a greater affinity for oxygen, impairing its ability to unload oxygen in the tissues. Biochemical manipulations have been used to solve many of the problems experienced with hemoglobin as it exists outside of the red blood cell.[200] An imaginative solution also circumvented the high oncotic pressure of free hemoglobin by encapsulating stroma-free hemoglobin in a lipid layer, creating microspherocytes.[201] Although clinical trials for a biochemically altered stroma-free hemoglobin are expected to take place in this decade, it would be wise not to anticipate the introduction of an oxygen-carrying wonder drug that is effective, safe, and inexpensive in the near future.

It is currently estimated that 14 million units of donated whole blood are collected in this country annually.[195] The number of units of homologous blood transfused should decline in the future to a fraction of the number currently transfused. By combining autotransfusion techniques, the potential to supply the majority has been repeatedly demonstrated (Table 2-4). Education and changing attitudes will be necessary to implement the successes in the autotransfusion literature into the standard of care in every operating room across the country. To avoid cost inefficiencies and waste of medical resources, accurate indications will have to be developed for each type of autotransfusion.[202,203] Since individual surgical practices vary so greatly, indications for autologous practices will have to be tailored for specific procedures and surgeons.

Technological advances will also aid in the trend away from homologous transfusion. A new concept in autotransfusion for cardiopulmonary bypass patients used a semicontinuous-flow centrifugation system to collect autologous platelet-rich plasma from patients during the early part of their cardiac surgical procedures.[204,205] These patients had 1,000 to 1,200 ml (15 to 20 percent of estimated blood volume) of whole blood withdrawn after anesthesia induction before going on cardiopulmonary bypass. The blood was processed intraoperatively to produce the equivalent to 2 to 4 U of platelet concentrate.

In addition to harvesting a patient's red blood cells and platelets pre- or postoperatively, coagulation proteins can also be collected before they might be needed. New autotransfusion devices that might be able to save elements of blood other than red blood cells through filtration are also being studied.[155] Although it is not practical at this time to predict a future medical practice without homologous blood, transfusion medicine is advancing with amazing rapidity in the last decade of this century. In the 21st century many current transfusion practices will surely seem archaic.

REFERENCES

1. Kalbfleisch JD, Lawless JF: Estimating the incubation time distribution and expected number of cases of transfusion-associated acquired immune deficiency syndrome. Transfusion 29:672, 1989
2. Peterman TA, Ward JW: What's happening to the epidemic of transfusion-associated AIDS? (editorial) Transfusion 29:659, 1989
3. Centers for Disease Control: HIV/AIDS surveillance report. April:1, 1992
4. Ward JW, Holmberg SD, Allen JR et al: Transmission of human immunodeficiency virus (HIV) by blood transfusions screened as negative for HIV antibody. N Engl J Med 318:473, 1988
5. Cumming PD, Wallace EL, Schorr JB, Dodd RY: Exposure of patients to human immunodeficiency virus through the transfusion of blood components that test antibody-negative. N Engl J Med 321:941, 1989
6. Busch MP, Eble BE, Khayam-Bashi H et al: Evaluation of screened blood donations for human immunodeficiency virus type 1 infection by culture and DNA amplification of pooled cells. N Engl J Med 325:1, 1991
7. Zuck TF: Greetings—a final look back with comments about a policy of a zero-risk blood supply. (editorial) Transfusion 27:447, 1987
8. Cordell RR, Yalon VA, Cigahn-Haskell C et al: Experience with 11,916 designated donors. Transfusion 26:484, 1986
9. Thaler M, Shamiss A, Orgad S et al: The role of blood from HLA-homozygous donors in fatal transfusion-associated graft-versus-host disease after open-heart surgery. N Engl J Med 321:25, 1989
10. Brecher ME, Taswell HF, Clare DE et al: Minimal-exposure transfusion and the committed donor. Transfusion 30:599, 1990
11. Faust RJ, Cucchiara RF, Messick JM Jr: Transfusion medicine and cardiovascular anesthesia. p. 527. In Tarhan S (ed): Cardiovascular Anesthesia and Postoperative Care. Year Book Medical Publishers, Chicago, 1989
12. Kuo G, Choo QL, Alter HJ et al: An assay for circulating antibodies to a major etiologic virus of human non-A, non-B hepatitis. Science 244:362, 1989
13. Consensus Conference: Perioperative

red blood cell transfusion. JAMA 260:2700, 1988

14. Alter HJ, Tegtmeier GE, Jett BW et al: The use of a recombinant immunoblot assay in the interpretation of anti-hepatitis C virus reactivity among prospectively followed patients, implicated donors, and random donors. Transfusion 31:771, 1991

15. Hoofnagle JH, Alter HJ: Chronic non-A, non-B heptatitis. Prog Clin Biol Res 182:63, 1985

16. Alter HJ: Posttransfusion hepatitis: clinical features, risk and donor testing. Prog Clin Biol Res 182:47, 1985

17. Nadelman RB, Sherer C, Mack L et al: Survival of *Borrelia burgdorferi* in human blood stored under blood banking conditions. Transfusion 30:298, 1990

18. Faust RJ, Warner MA: Transfusion risks. Int Anesthesiol Clin 28:184, 1990

19. Shulman IA: Parasitic infections, an uncommon risk of blood transfusion in the United States. Transfusion 31:479, 1991

20. American Society of Anesthesiologists, Committee on Transfusion Medicine: Questions and Answers on Transfusion Practices. 2nd Ed. American Society of Anesthesiologists, Chicago, 1992

21. Sazama K: Reports of 355 transfusion-associated deaths: 1976 through 1985. Transfusion 30:583, 1990

22. Morrow JF, Braine HG, Kickler TS et al: Septic reactions to platelet transfusions: A persistent problem. JAMA 266:555, 1991

23. Tipple MA, Bland LA, Murphy JJ et al: Sepsis associated with transfusion of red blood cells contaminated with *Yersinia enterocolitica*. Transfusion 30:207, 1990

24. Aber RC: Transfusion-associated *Yersinia entercolitica*. (editorial) Transfusion 30:193, 1990

25. Myhre BA: Fatalities from blood transfusion. JAMA 244:1333, 1980

26. Myhre BA, Bove JR, Schmidt PJ: Wrong blood—a needless cause of surgical deaths. (editorial) Anesth Analg 60:777, 1981

27. Pineda AA, Brzica SM Jr, Taswell HF: Hemolytic transfusion reaction: recent experience in a large blood bank. Mayo Clin Proc 53:378, 1978

28. Goldfinger D: Acute hemolytic transfusion reactions—a fresh look at pathogenesis and considerations regarding therapy. Transfusion 17:85, 1977

29. Popovsky MA, Abel MD, Moore SB: Transfusion-related acute lung injury associated with passive transfer of antileukocyte antibodies. Am Rev Respir Dis 128:185, 1983

30. Popovsky MA, Moore SB: Diagnostic and pathogenetic considerations in transfusion-related acute lung injury. Transfusion 25:573, 1985

31. Van Buren NL, Stroncek DF, Clay ME et al: Transfusion-related acute lung injury caused by an NB2 granulocyte-specific antibody in a patient with thrombotic thrombocytopenia purpura. Transfusion 30:42, 1990

32. Pineda AA, Taswell HF: Transfusion reactions associated with anti-IgA antibodies: report of four cases and review of the literature. Transfusion 15:10, 1975

33. Sloand EM, Fox SM, Banks SM, Klein HG: Preparations of IgA-deficient platelets. Transfusion 30:322, 1990

34. Opelz G, Terasaki PI: Improvement of kidney-graft survival with increased numbers of blood transfusions. N Engl J Med 299:799, 1978

35. Schriemer PA, Longnecker DE, Mintz PD: The possible immunosuppressive effects of perioperative blood transfusion in cancer patients. Anesthesiology 68:422, 1988

36. Blumberg N, Heal JM, Murphy P et al: Association between transfusion of whole blood and recurrence of cancer. Br Med J 293:530, 1986

37. Mezrow CK, Bergstein I, Tartter PI: Postoperative infections following autologous and homologous blood transfusions. Transfusion 32:27, 1992

38. Murphy P, Heal JM, Blumberg N: Infection or suspected infection after hip replacement surgery with autologous or homologous blood transfusions. Transfusion 31:212, 1991

39. Ness PM, Walsh PC, Zahurak ML et al: Prostate cancer recurrence in radical surgery patients receiving autologous or homologous blood. Transfusion 32:31, 1992

40. Collins JA: Problems associated with the massive transfusion of stored blood. Surgery 75:274, 1974

41. Faust RJ, Messick JM Jr: Blood component therapy: present and future. p. 553. In Tarhan S (ed): Cardiovascular Anesthesia and Postoperative Care. 2nd Ed. Year Book Medical Publishers, Chicago, 1989

42. American Association of Blood Banks, Committee on Technical Manual: Technical Manual. 10th Ed. American Association of Blood Banks, Arlington, VA, 1990

43. American Association of Blood Banks, American Red Cross, Council of Community Blood Centers: Circular of information: for the use of human blood and blood components. 1991

44. Pulsinelli WA, Levy DE, Sigsbee et al: Increased damage after ischemic stroke in patients with hyperglycemia with or without established diabetes mellitus. Am J Med 74:540, 1983

45. Lanier WL, Stangland KJ, Scheithauer BW et al: The effects of dextrose infusion and head position on neurologic outcome after complete cerebral ishcemia in primates: examination of a model. Anesthesiology 66:39, 1987

46. Longstreth WT Jr, Inui TS: High blood glucose level on hospital admission and poor neurological recovery after cardiac arrest. Ann Neurol 15:59, 1984

47. Tranbaugh RF, Lewis FR: Mechanisms and etiologic factors of pulmonary edema. Surg Gynecol Obstet 158:193, 1984

48. Poole GV, Meredith JW, Pennell T, Mills SA: Comparison of colloids and crystalloids in resuscitation from hemorrhagic shock. Surg Gynecol Obstet 154:577, 1982

49. Dawidson I: Fluid resuscitation of shock: current controversies. Crit Care Med 17:1078, 1989

50. Strauss RG: Review of the effects of hydroxyethyl starch on the blood coagulation system. Transfusion 21:299, 1981

51. Tuman KJ: Tissue oxygen delivery: the physiology of anemia. Anesthesiol Clin North Am 8:451, 1990

52. Robertie PG, Gravlee GP: Safe limits of isovolemic hemodilution and recommendations for erythrocyte transfusion. Int Anesthesiol Clin 28:197, 1990

53. Stehling L, Zauder HL: How long can we go? Is there a way to know? (editorial) Transfusion 30:1, 1990

54. Messmer K: Hemodilution—possibilities and safety aspects. Acta Anesthesiol Scand 32:49, 1988

55. Lundsgaard-Hansen P: Hemodilution—new clothes for an anemic emperor. Vox Sang 36:321, 1979

56. Crowell JW, Smith EE: Determinant of the optimal hematocrit. J Appl Physiol 22:501, 1967

57. Crystal GJ, Salem MR: Myocardial and systemic hemodynamics during isovolemic hemodilution alone and combined with nitroprusside-induced controlled hypotension. Anesth Analg 72:227, 1991

58. Crystal GJ, Rooney MW, Salem MR: Myocardial blood flow and oxygen consumption during isovolemic hemodilution alone and in combination with adenosine-induced controlled hypotension. Anesth Analg 67:539, 1988

59. Michenfelder JD, Theye RA: The effects of profound hypocapnia and dilutional anemia on canine cerebral metabolism and blood flow. Anesthesiology 31:499, 1969

60. Milde LN: Cerebral protection, p. 171. In Cucchiara RF, Michenfelder JD (eds): Clinical Neuroanesthesia. Churchill Livinstone, New York, 1990

61. Trouwborst A, Tenbrinck R, van Woerkens ECSM: Blood gas analysis of mixed venous blood during normoxic acute isovolemic hemodilution in pigs. Anesth Analg 70:523, 1990

62. Theye RA, Tuohy GF: The value of venous oxygen levels during general anesthesia. Anesthesiology 26:49, 1965

63. Suillivan SF: Oxygen transport. Anesthesiology 37:140, 1972

64. Crystal GJ, Levy PS, Eckel PK et al: Effect of coronary stenosis on cardiac compensation during hemodilution. Anesthesiology 75:A516, 1991

65. Crystal GJ, Salem MR: Myocardial oxygen consumption and segmental short-

ening during selective coronary hemodilution in dogs. Anesth Analg 67:500, 1988

66. Hagl S, Heimisch W, Meisner H et al: The effect of hemodilution on regional myocardial function in the presence of coronary stenosis. Basic Res Cardiol 72:344, 1977

67. Estafanous FG, Smith CE, Selim WM, Tarazi RC: Cardiovascular effects of acute normovolemic hemodilution in rats with disopyramide-induced myocardial depression. Basic Res Cardiol 85:227, 1990

68. Escobar E, Jones NL, Rapaport E, Murray JF: Ventricular performance in acute normovolemic anemia and effects of beta-blockade. Am J Physiol 211:877, 1966

69. Plewes JL, Farhi LE: Cardiovascular responses to hemodilution and controlled hypotension in the dog. Anesthesiology 62:149, 1985

70. Weisel RD, Charlesworth DC, Mickleborough LL et al: Limitations of blood conservation. J Thorac Cardiovasc Surg 88:26, 1984

71. Rao TLK, Montoya A: Cardiovascular, electrocardiographic and respiratory changes following acute anemia with volume replacement in patients with coronary artery disease. Anesth Rev 12:49, 1985

72. Rosberg B, Wulff K: Hemodynamics following normovolemic hemodilution in elderly patients. Acta Anaesthesiol Scand 25:402, 1981

73. Zauder HL: Preoperative hemoglobin requirements. Anesthesiol Clin North Am 8:471, 1990

74. Miller RD: Complications of massive blood transfusions. Anesthesiolgy 39:82, 1973

75. Reed RL II, Heimbach DM, Counts RB et al: Prophylactic platelet administration during massive transfusion: a prospective, randomized, double-blind clinical study. Ann Surg 203:40, 1986

76. Counts RB, Haisch C, Simon TL et al: Hemostasis in massively transfused trauma patients. Ann Surg 190:91, 1979

77. Murray DJ, Olson J, Strauss R, Tinker JH: Coagulation changes during packed red blood cell replacement of major blood loss. Anesthesiology 69:839, 1988

78. McNamara JJ, Buran EL, Stremple JF, Molot MD: Coagulopathy after major combat injury: occurrence, management, and pathophysiology. Ann Surg 176:243, 1972

79. Consensus Conference: Platelet transfusion therapy. JAMA 257:1777, 1987

80. Martin DJ, Lucas CE, Ledgerwood AM et al: Fresh frozen plasma supplement to massive red blood cell transfusion. Ann Surg 202:505, 1985

81. Turnage WS: Causes and evaluation of functional platelet disorders. p. 403. In Faust RJ (ed): Anesthesiology Review. Churchill Livingstone, New York, 1991

82. Lind SE: The bleeding time does not predict surgical bleeding. Blood 77:2547, 1991

83. Litwin MS, Smith LL, Moore FD: Metabolic alkalosis following massive transfusion. Surgery 45:805, 1959

84. Denlinger JK, Nahrwold ML, Gibbs PS, Lecky JH: Hypocalcaemia during rapid blood transfusion in anesthetized man. Br J Anaesth 48:995, 1976

85. Kahn RC, Jascott D, Carlon GC et al: Massive blood replacement: correlation of ionized calcium, citrate, and hydrogen ion concentration. Anesth Analg 58:274, 1979

86. Fernandez-del Castillo C, Harringer W, Warshaw AL et al: Risk factors for pancreatic cellular injury after cardiopulmonary bypass. N Engl J Med 325:382, 1991

87. Williamson KR, Taswell HF: Intraoperative blood salvage: a review. Transfusion 31:662, 1991

88. Ahlberg A, Nillius A, Rosberg B, Wulff K: Preoperative normovolemic hemodilution in total hip arthroplasty. A clinical study. Acta Chir Scand 143:407, 1977

89. Bailey TE Jr, Mahoney OM: The use of banked autologous blood in patients undergoing surgery for spinal deformity. J Bone Joint Surg [Am] 69:329, 1987

90. Barbier-Bohm G, Desmonts JM, Couderc E et al: Comparative effects of induced hypotension and normovolaemic

haemodilution on blood loss in total hip arthroplasty. Br J Anaesth 52:1039, 1980

91. Bernstein RL, Rosenberg AD: Predonation of autologous blood—its effect on decreasing the risk of homologous transfusion. Anesthesiology 67:A478, 1987

92. Bovill DF, Norris TR: The efficacy of intraoperative autologous transfusion in major shoulder surgery. Clin Orthop 240:137, 1989

93. Elawad AAR, Jonsson S, Laurell M, Fredin H: Predonation autologous blood in hip arthroplasty. Acta Orthop Scand 62:218, 1991

94. Elawad AA, Fredin HO, Laurell M, Jonsson S: Elderly patients' responses to preoperative autologous blood collection. Med J Aust 155:147, 1991

95. Endresen GKM, Spiechowicz J, Pahle JA, Espeland B: Intraoperative autotransfusion in reconstructive hip joint surgery of patients with rheumatoid arthritis and ankylosing spondylitis. Scand J Rheumatol 20:28, 1991

96. Faris PM, Ritter MA, Keating EM, Valeri CR: Unwashed filtered shed blood collected after knee and hip arthroplasties. A source of autologous red blood cells. J Bone Joint Surg [Am] 73:1169, 1991

97. Gannon DM, Lombardi AV Jr, Mallory TH et al: An evaluation of the efficacy of postoperative blood salvage after total joint arthroplasty. A prospective randomized trial. J Arthroplasty 6:109, 1991

98. Goodnough LT, Shafron D, Marcus RE: Utilization and effectiveness of autologous blood donation for arhtroplastic surgery. J Arthroplsty 5:S89, 1990

99. Goodnough LT: Directed blood procurement does not benefit patients who are enrolled in an autologous blood predeposit program. Am J Clin Pathol 92:484, 1989

100. Goodnough LT, Shafron D, Marcus RE: The impact of preoperative autologous blood donation on orthopaedic surgical practice. Vox Sang 59:65, 1990

101. Goodnough LT, Wasman J, Corlucci K, Chernosky A: Limitations to donating adequate autologous blood prior to elective orthopedic surgery. Arch Surg 124:494, 1989

102. Groh GI, Buchert PK, Allen WC: A comparison of transfusion requirements after total knee arthroplasty using the Solcotrans autotransfusion system. J Arthroplasty 3:281, 1990

103. Haberkern M, Dangel P: Normovolaemic haemodilution and intraoperative autotransfusion in children: experience with 30 cases of spinal fusion. Eur J Pediatr Surg 1:30, 1991

104. Hansen HL: A pre-operative autologous blood donation programme in a small hospital. Arctic Med Res 48:16, 1989

105. Haugen RK, Hill GE: A large-scale autologous blood program in a community hospital: a contribution to the community's blood supply. JAMA 257:1211, 1987

106. Johnson RD, Murphy JM: The role of desmorpressin in reducing blood loss during lumbar fusions. Surg Gynecol Obstet 171:223, 1990

107. Kafer ER, Isley MR, Hansen T et al: Automated acute normovolemic hemodilution reduces blood transfusion requirements for spinal fusion. Anesth Analg 65:S76, 1986

108. Kay LA, Noble RS: Systematic pre-deposit autologous blood provision for elective surgery: an important contribution to hospital blood supply. Vox Sang 59:23, 1990

109. Komatsu F: Autologous blood transfusion in orthopedic and oral surgical patients. Bull Tokyo Med Dent Univ 37:51, 1990

110. Kruger LM, Colbert JM: Intraoperative autologous transfusion in children undergoing spinal surgery. J Pediatr Orthop 5:330, 1985

111. Law JK, Wiedel JD: Autotransfusion in revision total hip arthroplasties using uncemented prostheses. Clin Orthop 245:145, 1989

112. Lchner JT, Van Peteghem PK, Leatherman KD, Brink MA: Experience with an intraoperative autogenous blood recovery system in scoliosis and spinal surgery. Spine 6:131, 1981

113. Lichtiger B, Huh YO, Armintor M, Fischer HE: Autologous transfusions for cancer patients undergoing elective ablative surgery. J Surg Oncol 43:19, 1990

114. MacEwen GD, Bennett E, Guille JT: Autologous blood transfusions in children and young adults with low body weight undergoing spinal surgery. J Pediatr Orthop 10:750, 1990

115. MacFarlane BJ, Marx L, Anquist K et al: Analysis of a protocol for an autologous blood transfusion program for total joint replacement surgery. Can J Surg 31:126, 1988

116. Mann DC, Wilham MR, Brower EM, Nash CL Jr: Decreasing homologous blood transfusion in spinal surgery by use of the cell saver and predeposited blood. Spine 14:1296, 1989

117. Martin E, Ott E: Extreme hemodilution in the Harrington procedure. Biblthca Haemat 47:322, 1981

118. McMurray MR, Birnbaum MA, Walter NE: Intraoperative autologous transfusion in primary and revision total hip arthroplasty. J Arthroplasty 5:61, 1990

119. Novak RW: Autologous blood transfusion in a pediatric population: safety and efficacy. Clin Pediatr 27:184, 1988

120. Semkiw LB, Schurman DJ, Goodman SB, Woolson ST: Postoperative blood salvage using the cell saver after total joint arthroplasty. J Bone Joint Surg [Am] 71:823, 1989

121. Silvergleid AJ: Safety and effectiveness of predeposit autologous transfusions in preteen and adolescent children. JAMA 257:3403, 1987

122. Slagis SV, Benjamin JB, Volz RG, Giordano GF: Postoperative blood salvage in total hip and knee arthroplasty. A randomised controlled trial. J Bone Joint Surg [Br] 73:591, 1991

123. Thomson JD, Callaghan JJ, Savory CG et al: Prior deposition of autologous blood in elective orthopaedic surgery. J Bone Joint Surg [Am] 69:320, 1987

124. Trammel TR, Fisher D, Brueckmann FR, Haines N: Closed-wound drainage systems. The Solcotrans Plus versus the Stryker-CBC ConstaVAC. Orthop Rev 20:536, 1991

125. Turner RH, Capozzi JD, Kim A et al: Blood conservation in major orthopedic surgery. Clin Orthop 256:299, 1990

126. Viviani GR, Sadler JT, Ingham GK: Autotransfusions in scoliosis surgery. Review of 20 Harrington fusions. Clin Orthop 135:74, 1978

127. Wasman J, Goodnough LT: Autologous blood donation for elective surgery: effect on physician transfusion behavior. JAMA 258:3135, 1987

128. Wilson WJ: Intraoperative autologous transfusion in revision total hip arthroplasty. J Bone Joint Surg [Am] 71:8, 1989

129. Woolson ST, Watt M: Use of autologous blood in total hip replacement. J Bone Joint Surg [Am] 73:76, 1991

130. Woolson ST, Marsh JS, Tanner JB: Transfusion of previously deposited autologous blood for patients undergoing hip-replacement surgery. J Bone Joint Surg [Am] 69:325, 1987

131. Toy PTCY, Strauss RG, Stehling LC et al: Predeposited autologous blood for elective surgery: a national multicenter study. N Engl J Med 316:517, 1987

132. Greenwalt TJ: Autologous and aged blood donors. (editorial) JAMA 257:1220, 1987

133. Owings DV, Kruskall MS, Thurer RL, Donovan LM: Autologous blood donations prior to elective cardiac surgery: safety and effect on subsequent blood use. JAMA 262:1963, 1989

134. Pindyck J, Avorn J, Kuriyan M et al: Blood donation by the elderly: clinical and policy considerations. JAMA 257:1186, 1987

135. McVay PA, Andrews A, Hoag MS et al: Moderate and severe reactions during autologous blood donations are no more frequent than during homologous blood donations. Vox Sang 59:70, 1990

136. Mann M, Sacks HJ, Goldfinger D: Safety of autologous blood donation prior to elective surgery for a variety of potentially "high-risk" patients. Transfusion 23:229, 1983

137. Spiess BD, Narbone RF, Sassetti R et al: Autologous blood donation service for high-risk patients. Anesth Analg 68:S272, 1989

138. Spiess BD, Sassetti R, McCarthy RJ et al: Autologous blood donation: hemodynamics in a high-risk patient population. Transfusion 32:17, 1992

139. Council on Scientific Affairs: Autologous blood transfusions. JAMA 256:2378, 1986

140. Druzin ML, Wolf CFW, Edersheim TG et al: Donation of blood by the pregnant patient for autologous transfusion. Am J Obstet Gynecol 159:1023, 1988

141. Zuck TF: Donor response to predeposit autologous transfusion phlebotomy, p. 51. In Dawson RB (ed): Autologous Transfusion. American Association of Blood Banks, Washington, DC, 1976

142. Kickler TS, Spivak JL: Effect of repeated whole blood donations on serum immunoreactive erythropoietin levels in autologous donors. JAMA 260:65, 1988

143. Birgegard G, Danersund A, Hogman C et al: Physiological response to phlebotomies for autologous transfusion at elective hi-joint surgery. Eur J Haematol 46:136, 1991

144. Eschbach JW, Kelly MR, Haley NR et al: Treatment of the anemia of progressive renal failure with recombinant human erythropoietin. N Engl J Med 321:158, 1989

145. Goodnough LT, Rudnick S, Price TH et al: Increased preoperative collection of autologous blood with recombinant human erythropoietin therapy. N Engl J Med 321:1163, 1989

146. Stehling L, Zauder HL: Acute normovolemic hemodilution. Transfusion 31:857, 1991

147. Leach PZ, Friedman LI, Stromberg RR: Blood cell salvage equipment. p. 164. In Taswell HF, Pineda AA (eds): Autologous Transfusion and Hemotherapy. Blackwell Scientific Publications, Boston, 1991

148. Yawn DH: Properties of salvaged blood. p. 194. In Taswell HF, Pineda AA (eds): Autologous Transfusion and Hemotherapy. Blackwell Scientific Publications, Boston, 1991

149. Davies MJ, Cronin KC, Moran P et al: Autologous blood transfusion for major vascular surgery using the Sorenson Receptal device. Anaesth Intens Care 15:282, 1987

150. McShane AJ, Power C, Jackson JF et al: Autotransfusion: quality of blood prepared with a red cell processing device. Br J Anaesth 59:1035, 1987

151. Sharp WV, Stark M, Donovan DL: Modern autotransfusion: experience with a washed red cell processing technique. Am J Surg 142:522, 1981

152. Kingsley JR, Valeri CR, Peters H et al: Citrate anticoagulation and cell washing for intraoperative autotransfusion in the baboon. Am J Surg 31:717, 1976

153. Stillman RM, Wrezlewicz WW, Stanczewski B et al: The haematological hazards of autotransfusion. Br J Surg 63:651, 1976

154. Lawrence-Brown MMD, Couch C, Halliday M et al: D-dimer levels in blood salvage for autotransfusion. Aust NZ Surg 59:67, 1989

155. Boldt J, Kling D, von Bormann B et al: Blood conservation in cardiac operations: cell separation versus hemofiltration. J Thorac Cardiovasc Surg 97:832, 1989

156. Gorsky BH: Alteration of blood components with hemodilution and administration of washed shed red cells. Anesth Analg 67:S79, 1988

157. Schwieger IM, Gallagher CH, Finlayson DC et al: Incidence of cell-saver contamination during cardiopulmonary bypass. Ann Thorac Surg 48:51, 1989

158. Boudreaux JP, Bornside GH, Cohn I Jr: Emergency autotransfusion: partial cleansing of bacteria-laden blood by cell washing. J Trauma 23:31, 1983

159. Griswold RA, Ortner AB: The use of autotransfusion in surgery of the serous cavities. Surg Gynecol Obstet 77:167, 1943

160. Andrews NJ, Bloor K: Autologous blood collection in abdominal vascular surgery. Assessment of a low pressure blood salvage system with particular reference to the preservation of cellular elements, triglyceride, complement and bacterial content in the collected blood. Clin Lab Haematol 5:361, 1983

161. Glover JL, Smith R, Yaw PB et al: Autotransfusion of blood contaminated by intestinal contents. JACEP 7:142, 1978

162. Yaw PB, Sentany M, Link WJ et al: Tumor cells caused through autotrans-

fusion: contraindication to intraoperative blood recovery? JAMA 231:490, 1975

163. Cole WH: The mechanisms of spread of cancer. Surg Gynecol Obstet 137:853, 1973

164. Salsbury AJ: The significance of the circulating cancer cell. Cancer Treat Rev 2:55, 1975

165. Griffiths JD, McKinna JA, Rowbotham HD et al: Carcinoma of the colon and rectum: circulating malignant cells and five-year survival. Cancer 31:226, 1973

166. Hart OJ III, Klimberg IW, Wajsman Z: Intraoperative autotransfusion in radical cystectomy for carcinoma of the bladder. Surg Gynecol Obstet 168:302, 1989

167. Klimberg I, Sirois R, Wajsman Z, Baker J: Intraoperative autotransfusion in urologic oncology. Arch Surg 121:1326, 1986

168. Miller GV, Ramsden CW, Primrose JN: Autologous transfusion: an alternative to transfusion with banked blood during surgery for cancer. Br J Surg 78:713, 1991

169. Smith DF, Mihm FG, Mefford I: Hypertension after intraoperative autotransfusion in bilateral adrenalectomy for pheochromocytoma. Anesthesiology 58:182, 1983

170. Robicsek F, Duncan GD, Born GVR et al: Inherent dangers of simultaneous application of microfibrillar collagen hemostat and blood-saving devices. J Thorac Cardiovasc Surg 92:766, 1986

171. Miller AC, Scherba-Krugliak L, Toy PT, Drasner K: Hypotension during transfusion of autologous blood. Anesthesiology 74:624, 1991

172. Cregan P, Donegan E, Gotelli G: Hemolytic transfusion reaction following transfusion of frozen and washed autologous red cells. Tranfusion 31:172, 1991

173. The National Blood Resource Education Program Expert Panel: The use of autologous blood. JAMA 263:414, 1990

174. Bull BS, Bull MH: The salvaged blood syndrome: a sequel of mechanochemical activation of platelets and leukocytes? Blood cells 16:5, 1990

175. Bull MH, Bull BS: The use of autologous blood. JAMA 263:3150, 1990

176. Chavez AM, Tarazi RY, Cosgrove DM III: Postoperative blood salvage. p. 155. In Taswell HF, Pineda AA (eds): Autologous Transfusion and Hemotherapy. Blackwell Scientific Publications, Boston, 1991

177. Kongsgaard UE, Tollofsrud S, Brosstad F, Ovrum E, Bjornskau L: Autotransfusion after open heart surgery: characteristics of shed mediastinal blood and its influence on the plasma proteases in circulating blood. Acta Anaesthesiol Scand 35:71, 1991

178. Fuller JA, Buxton BF, Picken J et al: Haematological effects of reinfused mediastinal blood after cardiac surgery. Med J Aust 154:737, 1991

179. Bengston J-P, Backman L, Stenqvist O et al: Complement activation and reinfusion of wound drainage blood. Anesthesiology 73:376, 1990

180. Berman AT, Geissele AE, Bosacco SJ: Blood loss with total knee arthroplasty. Clin Orthop 234:137, 1988

181. Gardner WJ: The control of bleeding during operation by induced hypotension. JAMA 132:572, 1946

182. Petrozza PH: Induced hypotension. Int Anesthesiol Clin 28:223, 1990

183. Nelson CL, Bowen S: Total hip arthroplasty in Jehovah's Witnesses without blood transfusion. J Bone Joint Surg 68A:350, 1986

184. Donald JR: Induced hypotension and blood loss during surgery. (editorial) J R Soc Med 75:149, 1982

185. Mandel RJ, Brown MD, McCollough NC III et al: Hypotensive anesthesia and autotransfusion in spinal surgery. Clin Orthop 154:27, 1981

186. Landmark SJ, Muldoon SM, Nolan NG, Coventry MB: Sequential blood volume changes in patients undergoing total hip arthroplasty. Anesth Analg 54:391, 1975

187. Ueda I: The effects of volatile general anesthetics on adenosine diphosphate-induced platelet aggregation. Anesthesiology 34:405, 1971

188. Bertha BG, Folts JD, Nugent M, Rusy BF: Halothane, but not isoflurane or enflurane, protects against spontaneous and epinephrine-exacerbated acute

thrombus formation in stenosed dog coronary arteries. Anesthesiology 71:96, 1989

189. Lennon RL, Hosking MP, Gray JR et al: The effects of intraoperative blood salvage and induced hypotension on transfusion requirements during spinal surgical procedures. Mayo Clin Proc 62:1090, 1987

190. Fromme GA, MacKenzie RA, Gould AB Jr et al: Controlled hypotension for orthognathic surgery. Anesth Analg 65:683, 1986

191. Salzman EW, Weinstein MJ, Weintraub RM et al: Treatment with desmopressin acetate to reduce blood loss after cardiac surgery. N Engl J Med 314:1402, 1986

192. Hackmann T, Gascoyne RD, Naiman SC et al: A trial of desmopressin (1-desamino-8-D-arginine vasopressin) to reduce blood loss in uncomplicated cardiac surgery. N Engl J Med 321:1437, 1989

193. Rocha E, Llorens R, Paramo JA et al: Does desmopressin acetate reduce blood loss after surgery in patients on cardiopulmonary bypass? Circulation 77:1319, 1988

194. Kobrinsky NL, Letts M, Patel LR et al: 1-Desamini-8-D-arginine vasopressin (desmopressin) decreases operative blood loss in patients having Harrington rod spinal fusion surgery. Ann Int Med 107:446, 1987

195. Stehling L: Trends in transfusion therapy. Anesthesiol Clin North Am 8:519, 1990

196. Taswell HF: The future of autologous blood transfusion and hemotherapy. p. 256. In Taswell HF, Pineda AA (eds): Autologous Transfusion and Hemotherapy. Blackwell Scientific Publications, Boston, 1991

197. Tremper KK, Friedman AE, Levine EM et al: The preoperative treatment of severely anemic patients with a perfluorochemical oxygen-transport fluid, Fluosol-DA. N Engl J Med 307:277, 1982

198. Hershey SG: Airless respiration—bloodless circulation. (editorial) Anesthesiology 34:305, 1971

199. Gould SA, Rosen AL, Sehgal LR, Sehgal HL et al: Fluosol-DA as a red-cell substitute in acute anemia. N Engl J Med 314:1653, 1986

200. Winslow RM: Blood substitutes: current status. (editorial) Transfusion 29:753, 1989

201. Hunt CA, Burnette RR, MacGregor RD et al: Synthesis and evaluation of a prototypal artificial red cell. Science 230:1165, 1985

202. Kruskall MS: On measuring the success of an autologous blood donation program. Transfusion 31:481, 1991

203. Silvergleid AJ: Preoperative autologous donation: what have we learned? Transfusion 31:99, 1991

204. Giordano GF, Rivers SL, Chung GKT et al: Autologous platelet rich plasma in cardiac surgery: effect on intraoperative and postoperative transfusion requirements. Ann Thorac Surg 46:416, 1988

205. Girodano GF, Giordano GF Jr, Rivers SL et al: Determinants of homologous blood usage utilizing autologous platelet-rich plasma in cardiac operations. Ann Thorac Surg 47:897, 1989

3

Coagulation Problems

Terese T. Horlocker

Regional anesthesia provides several advantages over general anesthesia for patients undergoing orthopedic procedures, including decreased incidence of cardiopulmonary complications and reduced blood loss and need for transfusion, as well as the benefits of postoperative analgesia.[1,2] In addition, patients experiencing chronic pain syndromes such as reflex sympathetic dystrophy or causalgia may improve with prolonged sympathetic blockade.[3] However, patients hospitalized for major orthopedic surgery frequently receive an anticoagulant or antiplatelet agent perioperatively to prevent venous thrombosis and embolism, and are therefore not considered candidates for regional anesthesia because of a theoretically greater risk of hemorrhagic complications. The decision to perform regional anesthesia on these patients must be made on an individual basis, weighing the potentially increased risk of iatrogenic hematoma from needle placement against the theoretical benefits gained. To reduce the risk of hemorrhagic complications associated with regional anesthesia, it is necessary to understand the mechanisms of blood coagulation, the pharmacologic properties of the anticoagulant and antiplatelet agents, and also the clinical studies involving patients undergoing regional anesthesia while receiving these medications.

Hemorrhagic complications can occur after virtually all regional techniques and may result in neurologic or vascular compromise. Bleeding into the spinal canal is perhaps the most serious hemorrhagic complication associated with regional anesthesia because the spinal canal is a concealed and nonexpandable space. Spinal cord compression from intraspinal hematoma may result in irreversible neurologic ischemia and paraplegia. Because of the catastrophic nature of intraspinal hematomas, this chapter deals mainly with central neuraxial blockade; however, the same principles apply to all regional techniques. Evaluation of the indications and contraindications for a specific patient will aid in the selection of an anesthetic.

TREATMENT OF THROMBOEMBOLIC DISEASE

Venous thromboembolic disease is the most common fatal complication following surgery or trauma to the lower extremities. Without prophylactic protection, 40 to 70 percent of orthopedic patients will develop venous thrombosis and 2 to 16 percent will show clinical or

55

laboratory evidence of pulmonary embolism. Fatal pulmonary embolism occurs in 1.8 to 3.4 percent of patients.[4] The incidence of fatal pulmonary embolism is highest in patients who have undergone surgery for hip fracture.[5]

Deep venous thrombosis (DVT) can occur in any vessel; however, 80 to 90 percent of DVTs develop in the operative limb of orthopedic patients, usually originating in the calf muscle and extending proximally. Pulmonary emboli generally arise from proximal vein thromboses; 75 percent of fatal pulmonary emboli originate from femoral DVTs. Thrombus formation begins intraoperatively in 50 percent of cases, and nearly all pulmonary emboli following total hip arthroplasty occur in the first week.[4]

Because of the high incidence of venous thrombosis and the severity of its complications, prophylactic measures are often initiated perioperatively on patients who are hospitalized for major orthopedic procedures. There are essentially two categories of prophylaxis for venous thromboembolism: mechanical and pharmacologic. Mechanical prophylaxis, such as continuous passive motion of the lower extremities and the use of thigh-high antiembolic stockings (TED hose) or thigh-high pneumatic compression stockings has been shown to significantly decrease the incidence of DVT following total hip or knee arthroplasty.[4,6] However, these methods are generally considered adjunctive to pharmacologic prophylaxis.

Of these agents used for thromboembolic prophylaxis—aspirin, low-dose heparin, and heparin/dihydroergotamine (DHE)—aspirin remains the most popular agent. Total daily aspirin dose ranges from 0.3 to 3.6 g. While some studies have demonstrated a modest decrease in the incidences of DVT and pulmonary embolism, most series do not show a significant reduction, and its use as a prophylactic agent in the prevention of venous thromboembolism remains controversial.[5] Likewise, subcutaneous low-dose heparin, while of benefit in other surgical settings, is ineffective in preventing DVT in patients undergoing total knee or hip arthroplasty.[4,6]

The use of adjusted-dose heparin maintains the partial thromboplastin time (PTT) at the upper limit of normal (31.5 to 36 seconds) and has been shown to significantly reduce the incidence of postoperative thrombosis to 13 percent in patients undergoing total hip arthroplasty.[4] It is not commonly used because of the difficulty in monitoring dosage and the logistic difficulties of the heparin pump during ambulation and rehabilitation.

Heparin/DHE is a combination drug. The addition of DHE reduces venous stasis and improves venous tone. Heparin/DHE is administered in a dose of 5,000 U heparin with 0.5 mg DHE subcutaneously every 8 to 12 hours. In a combined series of 718 patients receiving heparin/DHE thromboembolism prophylaxis who underwent total hip arthroplasty, the incidence of DVT decreased from 66 to 23 percent. The incidence of fatal pulmonary embolism also decreased to 0.3 percent (compared to 1.7 percent in untreated control subjects).[5]

Use of oral anticoagulants such as warfarin (Coumadin) is the most effective method of reducing venous thrombosis and pulmonary embolism. Several studies have reported zero percent incidence of pulmonary embolism when oral anticoagulants were begun preoperatively. Traditionally, the prothrombin time (PT) was maintained at 1.5 to 2 times normal levels. However, the therapeutic anticoagulation occasionally resulted in hemarthrosis and wound hematoma, and led to the practice of low-dose warfarin administration. Low-dose warfarin produces a PT of 1.2 to 1.5 times the control value and has been shown to be equally efficacious in reducing venous thromboembolism as traditional warfarin therapy. The main advantage of the low dosage is the fivefold reduction in hemorrhagic complications.[4]

Dextran, a branched polymer of glucose, has been found to be an effective prophylactic agent that consistently reduces the frequency of postoperative DVT and pulmonary embolism. Dextran is available in low- and high-molecular-weight forms: dextran 40 (molecular weight 40,000) and dextran 70 (molecular weight 70,000). Low-molecular-weight dextran is more commonly used because of the lower incidence of severe anaphylactoid reactions compared to high-molecular-weight dextran. Dextrans' anticoagulant effect is by inhibition of platelet aggregation, reduction of blood viscosity, and increase of thrombolysis. In a combined series, dextran 40 (low-molecular-weight dextran) infused intraoperatively at a dose of 10 ml/kg and followed by 7.5 ml/kg on the first and third day decreased the incidence of DVT to 14 percent (compared to 20 percent in control subjects).[5] Several studies have indicated that dextran effectively reduces the incidence of fatal pulmonary embolism to approximately 1 percent.[4] Complications of dextran include congestive heart failure from volume overload, anaphylactic reactions, renal damage, and hemorrhage.

In summary, low-dose heparin is ineffective in reducing the incidence of venous thromboembolic disease in patients undergoing orthopedic procedures, while the effectiveness of aspirin remains controversial.[4–6] Adjusted-dose heparin, heparin/DHE, dextran, and warfarin all appear to be effective in decreasing the incidence of venous thrombosis and pulmonary embolism.[4,5] Patients hospitalized for major orthopedic procedures may therefore receive heparin or warfarin perioperatively to prevent venous thromboembolic complications. The decision to perform spinal or epidural anesthesia on these patients must be made on an individual basis after a proper evaluation of medications and contraindications.

DIRECT ANTICOAGULANTS (HEPARIN)

Heparin is a complex polysaccharide that exerts its anticoagulant effect by accelerating the inhibition of activated coagulation factors by antithrombin III. There are at least six activated clotting factors that are inhibited by antithrombin III (thrombin, factors XII, XIa, Xa, IXa, and kallikrein).[7] Heparin also potentiates the action of activated factor X inhibitors (anti Xa).[8] The key position of factor X in the coagulation cascade enables it to generate thrombin through the intrinsic or extrinsic pathway (Fig. 3-1). Therefore inhibitors of this enzyme's activation will prevent thrombin formation.

Patients react with different sensitivities to heparin. Highly sensitive patients exhibit a greater increase in coagulation time and prolonged effect after intravenous or subcutaneous heparin administration. These patients may be at higher risk for hemorrhagic complications compared to patients with normal or low sensitivity. A number of factors affect an individual's sensitivity to heparin, including general medical condition, diet, cardiac status, renal function, and liver disease.[7]

Five minutes after intravenous injection of 10,000 U heparin, coagulation time is prolonged 2 to 4 times the control level. Heparin has a half-life in circulating blood of 1.5 to 2 hours.[7] Patients with acute thromboembolic disease may clear heparin even more rapidly. Within 4 to 6 hours of the administration of a therapeutic dose of heparin, its effect has ceased.

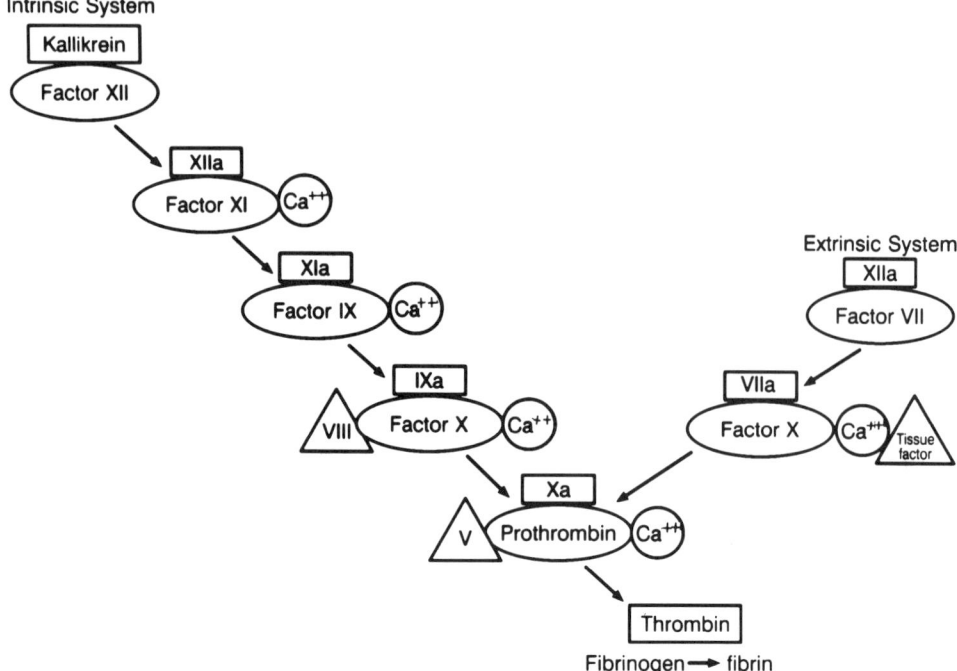

Fig. 3-1. Schematic diagram of the clotting mechanism. The blood coagulation system can be visualized as a cascade of distinct reaction stages in which a precursor protein is converted from its inactive circulating form into an active form. The clotting system consists of two pathways: the *intrinsic system*, which involves components formally formed in the circulation, and the *extrinsic system*, which uses a tissue factor in addition to blood components. Heparin enhancement of antithrombin III inactivation occurs with all components enclosed in rectangles except factor VII. Vitamin K-antagonist drugs will affect factors VII, IX, X, and prothrombin. (From Horlocker & Wedel,[34] with permission.)

Intravenously administered heparin can be promptly neutralized by protamine. A standard regimen would be 1 mg protamine for every 100 U heparin, although careful titration is advised.

The therapeutic basis of low-dose subcutaneous heparin (5,000 U every 8 to 12 hours) is based on heparin-mediated inhibition of activated factor X. Inhibition of small amounts of activated factor X prevents amplification of the coagulation cascade. Smaller doses of heparin are therefore required when administered as prophylaxis rather than as treatment for thromboembolic disease. Following intramuscular or subcutaneous injection of 5,000 U heparin, maximum anticoagula-

tion effect is observed in 40 to 50 minutes and usually returns to baseline within 4 to 6 hours.[9] The aPTT may remain in the normal range and often is not monitored.[10] The heparin effect is also detectable using a sensitive chromogenic heparin assay based on inhibition of activated factor X.

INDIRECT ANTICOAGULANTS

Oral anticoagulants are occasionally administered before major joint surgery in anticipation of continuing these agents during the postoperative period for venous thrombosis prophylaxis. Vitamin K-antagonist drugs such as warfarin or dicumarol exert their anticoagulant effect by interfering with the synthesis of the vitamin K-dependent clotting factors (VII, IX, X, and thrombin). As with heparin, patients show varying sensitivities to indirect anticoagulants. Sensitivity to warfarin-type drugs was normal in 60 percent and increased in 20 percent of patients, while the remaining 20 percent showed resistance.[9] In contrast to the immediate anticoagulant effects of heparin, the effects of indirect anticoagulants are not apparent until a significant amount of biologically inactive factors are synthesized. Since factor VII has a relatively short half-life (6 to 8 hours), the PT may be prolonged into the therapeutic range (1.5 to 2 times normal) in 24 to 36 hours. However, since factor VII participates only in the extrinsic pathway, adequate anticoagulation is not achieved until the levels of biologically active factors II and X are sufficiently depressed, which, because of their longer half-lives, requires 4 to 6 days.[7] With initial high loading doses of warfarin (15 to 30 mg) for the first 2 to 3 days of therapy the desired anticoagulant effect is achieved within 48 to 72 hours.[8] Similarly, the anticoagulant effects persist for 4 to 6 days after termination of therapy while new biologically active vitamin K factors are synthesized. In an emergent situation, the anticoagulant effects can be reversed by transfusing fresh frozen plasma and injecting vitamin K.

ANTICOAGULANTS IN CENTRAL NEURAXIAL BLOCKADE

Intraspinal hematoma is a rare and potentially catastrophic complication of spinal or epidural anesthesia. The actual incidence of neurologic dysfunction resulting from hemorrhagic complications associated with neuraxial blockade is unknown; however, the incidence cited in the literature is less than 1 in 10,000 procedures.[11] Hemorrhage into the spinal canal most commonly occurs in the epidural space because of the prominent epidural venous plexus. Spinal subdural hematomas are less common and, unlike epidural bleeding, the cause of subdural bleeding is unclear. Subarachnoid hematomas are the rarest form of intraspinal bleeding, presumably because the diluting and redistributing effect of CSF prevents subarachnoid blood from clotting.[12]

While intraspinal hematoma may occur as a result of vascular trauma from needle or catheter placement into the subarachnoid or epidural space, it may also occur in association with neoplastic disease or pre-existing vascular abnormalities. Of special interest to the anesthesia care provider are those intraspinal hematomas that have occurred spontaneously with or without the presence of antiplatelet or anticoagulation therapy. Over 100 spontaneous epidural hematomas have been reported, 25 percent of which are associated with anticoagulation therapy.[13]

In a review of the literature, Owens et al[14] reported 34 cases of intraspinal hematoma after lumbar puncture, 6 of which involved the administration of an anesthetic. Fourteen of the patients had received anticoagulants, though only 2 were given anticoagulants prior to needle placement. Another 2 patients were treated with antiplatelet therapy immediately before or after lumbar puncture. In addition, 11 patients had evidence of coagulopathy or significant thrombocytopenia. Thus, in 27 of the 34 patients (79 percent), the intraspinal hematomas associated with lumbar puncture occurred in patients with evidence of hemostatic abnormality.

ANTICOAGULATION THERAPY

Rao and El-Etr[15] reported on 3,164 patients who had continuous epidural anesthesia and 847 patients who had continuous spinal anesthesia for lower extremity vascular procedures. Patients with known coagulation abnormalities or those receiving preoperative anticoagulants were excluded. All catheters were placed through a 17-gauge Tuohy needle. In 4 patients, following insertion of the needle into the epidural space, blood was freely aspirated. The needle was withdrawn and the patients were given general anesthesia the following day. Heparin was administered 50 to 60 minutes after catheter placement to maintain the activated clotting time at twice the baseline value. The catheters were removed the following day 1 hour prior to administration of the maintenance dose of heparin. No patient developed signs or symptoms of epidural or subarachnoid hematoma, including the 4 patients who had traumatic needle placement and subsequently received general anesthesia. Similar findings have been reported by Matthews and Abrams,[16] who administered intrathecal morphine through a 20- to 25-gauge needle to 40 cardiac surgical patients 50 minutes prior to complete heparinization and cardiopulmonary bypass. Again, no neurologic sequelae were noted postoperatively.

Ruff and Dougherty[17] studied 342 patients who underwent a diagnostic lumbar puncture with a 20-gauge needle for evaluation of cerebral ischemia and were subsequently anticoagulated with intravenous heparin. The amount of heparin used and the coagulation studies performed were not reported. Patients were followed neurologically. Five patients developed paraparesis. (Two patients had subarachnoid hematomas and one patient had an epidural hematoma; all were surgically removed with good neurologic recovery. One additional patient had a documented epidural hematoma that was decompressed with a spinal needle. One patient refused myelography and remained paraparetic and died 3 months later. Autopsy revealed a chronic subdural hematoma.) There were also 18 patients with severe or radicular back pain lasting more than 48 hours. Seven of these patients subsequently died of unrelated causes, and at autopsy, one patient had findings of chronic epidural hematoma while another showed an organized subdural hematoma. Thus 7 of 342 (2.0 percent) of patients who received a lumbar puncture and were subsequently heparinized had documented intraspinal hematomas. The authors identified traumatic needle placement, initiation of anticoagulation within 1 hour of lumbar puncture, and concomitant aspirin therapy as being risk factors in the development of intraspinal hematoma in anticoagulated patients.

The risk of intraspinal hematoma in patients on low-dose heparin (5,000 U subcutaneously every 8 to 12 hours) remains controversial and largely unstudied. In a study of 30 patients hospitalized for operative treatment of femur fracture who received 5,000 U heparin subcutaneously every 8 hours, the aPTT was measured daily 4 hours after a heparin dose for 9 days. The authors reported a wide variation in the percentage of patients with aPTT prolongation to greater than 50 seconds (normal 38 to 45 seconds), ranging from 5 to 37 percent of patients with a mean of 21 percent.[18] Anti-Xa activity was also measured and found to be greater than 0.05 U/ml in 63 percent of patients, a level consistent with therapeutic anticoagulation.

This wide variation in response to subcutaneous low-dose heparin makes it difficult to formulate a generalized recommendation regarding regional anesthesia in these patients. Lowson and Goodchild[19] reviewed their 5-year retrospective experience of 99 epidural and 37 spinal anesthetics performed on patients who received 5,000 U heparin 2 hours prior to elective abdominal procedures. Heparin prophylaxis was continued into the postoperative period. The spinal anesthetics were performed with a 22-gauge needle, while the epidural anesthetics used a 16-gauge Tuohy needle. Epidural catheters were placed in some patients and were left in place up to 72 hours postoperatively. Epidural blood vessel puncture occurred in 5 percent. If vessel puncture occurred, the needle or catheter was replaced at a different interspace. There were no neurologic complications.

Allemann et al[20] studied 82 spinal and 105 epidural anesthetics (66 of which involved an epidural catheter) performed on patients undergoing orthopedic procedures who had received 5,000 U heparin subcutaneously 2 hours postoperatively. Heparin prophylaxis was continued postoperatively. There were no reported cases of intraspinal hematoma.

However, there are at least two reported cases of epidural hematoma occurring in patients on low-dose heparin who underwent lumbar puncture or epidural blockade. In the first case, a patient receiving 5,000 U heparin every 12 hours for prophylaxis had an epidural catheter placed through a 16-gauge Tuohy needle for chronic pain relief. Pain and blood were encountered during catheter placement and an epidural hematoma with complete paraplegia developed within hours. Surgery to improve neurologic function was unsuccessful.[21] In another patient, a diagnostic lumbar puncture was performed on a renal allograft recipient receiving 5,000 U heparin subcutaneously every 8 hours as prophylaxis for ve-

nous thromboembolism. Lumbar puncture was performed 6 hours after a heparin injection. Platelet count and aPTT were normal at the time of lumbar puncture, which was described as difficult. Initial cerebrospinal fluid return yielded bloody fluid that subsequently cleared. Twenty-four hours later, the patient complained of inability to void and bilateral leg weakness. A myelogram performed 2 weeks later showed a defect of the posterior lumbosacral spinal cord consistent with spinal hematoma. No surgical procedure was performed and the patient died several weeks later of a myocardial infarction.[22]

Most of the previously mentioned studies involved patients who received spinal or epidural blockade prior to anticoagulation. However, Odoom and Sih[23] performed 1,000 continuous lumbar epidural anesthetics (using an 18-gauge Tuohy needle to place the catheter) in 950 patients undergoing vascular procedures who were receiving oral anticoagulants preoperatively. The thrombotest (a test measuring factor IX activity) was decreased and the aPTT was prolonged in all patients prior to epidural puncture. Excluded from their study were patients with known coagulopathies, preoperative heparin or aspirin therapy, or a thrombotest below 10 percent. Patients received a continuous heparin infusion at a rate of 250 to 300 μg/min for 30 to 180 minutes intraoperatively. Coagulation status was monitored with serial aPTT and thrombotest determinations. Epidural catheters remained in place for 48 hours postoperatively for analgesia. The coagulation status at time of catheter removal was not described. There were no neurologic complications. The authors concluded that, provided adequate precautions are taken, epidural anesthesia can be safely performed in patients receiving anticoagulant therapy.

The conflicting results of these studies

and the rarity of this complication make it difficult to assess the relative risk and contributing variables of intraspinal hematoma associated with regional anesthesia in anticoagulated patients. However, possible factors contributing to increased risk in these patients appear to be pre-existing coagulopathy or thrombocytopenia, concomitant aspirin therapy, traumatic or difficult needle placement, heparinization within 1 hour of spinal or epidural puncture, and absence of monitoring of the anticoagulant activity.[14,15,17,23]

ANTIPLATELET THERAPY

Orthopedic patients undergoing major joint surgery often have chronic musculoskeletal pain or underlying inflammatory disease such as rheumatoid arthritis and are frequently medicated with antiplatelet drugs preoperatively. Antiplatelet therapy, including such medications as aspirin, naproxen, piroxicam, and dipyridamole, has been considered a relative contraindication to regional anesthesia by some authors because of the associated prolongation of the bleeding time and theoretically greater risk of hematoma formation.[4]

Antiplatelet agents inhibit platelet cyclo-oxygenase and prevent the synthesis of thromboxane A_2. Thromboxane A_2 not only is a potent vasoconstrictor, but also facilitates secondary platelet aggregation and release reactions (Fig. 3-2). Platelets from patients who have been taking these medications have normal platelet adherence to subendothelium and normal primary hemostatic plug formation. Thus an adequate, although potentially fragile, clot may form. While such plugs may be satisfactory hemostatic barriers for smaller vascular lesions, they

may not ensure adequate perioperative hemostatic clot formation.

It has been suggested that the Ivy bleeding time is the most reliable predictor of abnormal bleeding in patients receiving antiplatelet therapy.[24] However, the "postaspirin" bleeding time is not always a reliable indicator of platelet function.[25] Although the bleeding time may normalize within 3 days after aspirin ingestion, platelet function as measured by platelet response to adenosine diphosphate (ADP), epinephrine, and collagen may take up to 1 week to return to normal. Conversely, several studies have failed to show a correlation between aspirin-induced prolongation of the bleeding time and surgical blood loss.[26] Therefore, measurement of an Ivy bleeding time before induction of spinal or epidural anesthesia may not necessarily identify those patients at increased risk for epidural or spinal hematoma. Other nonsteroidal analgesics (naproxen, piroxicam, ibuprofen) produce a short-term defect that normalizes within 3 days.[27]

The risk associated with administration of spinal or epidural anesthesia to a patient receiving antiplatelet therapy also remains controversial and largely unstudied. Owens et al[14] implicated antiplatelet therapy in 2 of 34 cases of spinal hematoma occurring after attempted lumbar puncture. Horlocker et al[28] reported 1,013 spinal and epidural anesthetics in which antiplatelet medications were taken by 39 percent of the patients, of whom 11 percent were on multiple antiplatelet drugs. No patient developed signs of spinal hematoma. However, patients on antiplatelet medication showed a higher incidence of minor hemorrhagic complications (blood aspirated through the spinal or epidural needle or catheter). In addition, increased age and an epidural (but not a spinal) anesthetic technique, when occurring simultaneously, were also associated with an increase in

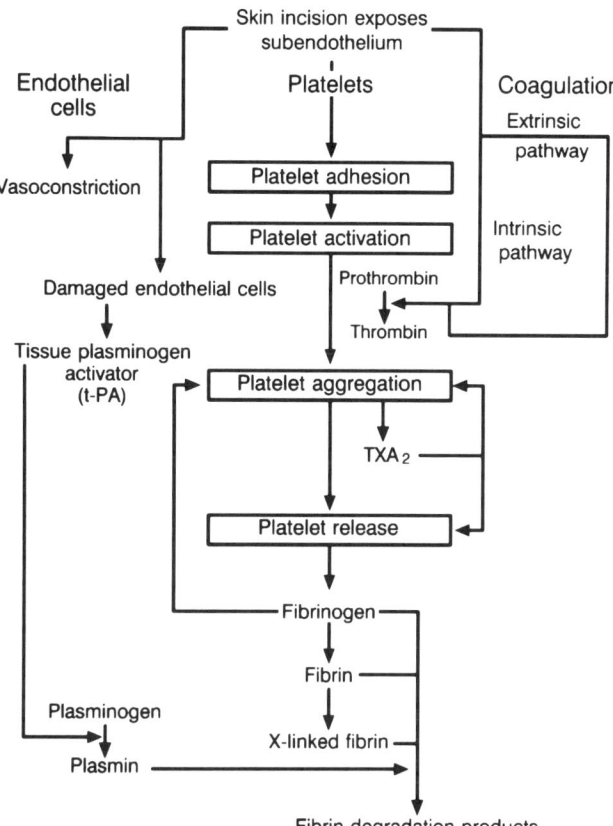

Fig. 3-2. Platelet, coagulation factor, and vessel wall interactions in hemostasis. Platelets exposed to subendothelial collagen adhere to it and each other and become activated. Thrombin and collagen, as well as ADP in high concentration, cause platelets in the primary plug to degranulate and release vasoactive amines and additional ADP, and generate thromboxane A_2. The platelet plug is now fused into a tightly packed mass or secondary hemostatic plug. (From Hirsch & Goldhaber,[35] with permission.)

the incidence of minor hemorrhagic events. Although aspiration of blood through the spinal or epidural needle may not imply an increased risk for spinal hematoma, 80 percent of spinal hematomas occurring after lumbar puncture occurred in patients with evidence of hemostatic abnormality, and in 62 percent the needle placement was described as difficult and/or traumatic.[14]

There has also been a single reported case of spontaneous epidural hematoma formation (in the absence of regional anesthesia) in a patient with a history of excessive aspirin ingestion.[29] The patient self-administered 1,500 mg of aspirin in the form of an aspirin-containing antacid and a short time later complained of severe lower extremity weakness. A myelogram revealed complete epidural block at the T5-T6 level. The cerebrospinal fluid was clear, although prolonged bleeding from the lumbar puncture site was noted after myelography. A laminectomy was performed and the hematoma removed. Neurologic function improved and 9 weeks later the patient could ambulate with a walker. Perioperative bleeding time was prolonged to 12.5 minutes (normal, 4 to 7 minutes) and did not normalize until the fourth postoperative day. PT, aPTT, and platelet count and morphology were all normal. Also of interest in this case is that the patient initially denied taking aspirin and was unaware of the high aspirin content of the antacid. Aspirin is the most frequently taken nonprescription medication and is found in more than 200 over-the-counter remedies. Patients must be specifically questioned as to which medications, both prescription and nonprescription, they have been using if preoperative aspirin or other antiplatelet ingestion is to be determined.

THROMBOLYTIC THERAPY

Thrombolytic therapy is frequently used in the treatment of myocardial infarction, pulmonary embolism, DVT, and peripheral artery occlusion. In addition to the fibrinolytic agent, these patients frequently receive intravenous heparin to maintain an aPTT of 1.5 to 2 times normal.[30] While epidural or spinal needle and catheter placement with subsequent heparinization appears relatively safe, the risk of intraspinal hematoma in patients who receive thrombolytic therapy is less well defined.[15,23,31]

The site of action of thrombolytic agents such as plasminogen activators differs from that of heparin. In contrast to anticoagulants, these agents actively dissolve fibrin clots that have already been formed. Exogenous plasminogen activators such as streptokinase and urokinase not only dissolve thrombus but also affect circulating plasminogen as well, leading to decreased levels of both plasminogen

and fibrin. Recombinant tissue-type plasminogen activator (rt-PA), an endogenous agent, is more fibrin-selective and has less effect on circulating plasminogen levels.[32] Clot lysis leads to elevation of fibrin degradation products, which themselves have an anticoagulant effect by inhibiting platelet aggregation (Fig. 3-3). In a study involving 290 patients with acute myocardial infarction who were treated with thrombolytic therapy (streptokinase or rt-PA) and subsequently heparinized, fibrinogen and plasminogen were maximally depressed at 5 hours after thrombolytic therapy and remained significantly depressed at 27 hours.[30] Hemorrhagic events occurred in 33 percent of the rt-PA patients and 31 percent of the streptokinase patients. Major hemorrhagic events, defined as a decrease in the hemoglobin level of 5 g/dl, occurred in approximately half of these cases. For more than 70 percent of the patients with hemorrhagic events in each group, the primary bleeding site was the catheterization or other puncture site. The authors recommended avoiding invasive procedures in patients receiving thrombolytic therapy.

Dickman et al[31] reported a case of a patient with femoral artery occlusion who received an epidural anesthetic for surgical placement of an intra-arterial catheter. A urokinase infusion was initiated through the femoral artery catheter postoperatively. The patient complained of back pain 3 hours postoperatively. A large groin hematoma was also noted at the arterial catheter placement site. Both the epidural and intra-arterial catheters were removed; however, the back pain persisted and paraplegia developed. Myelography revealed an epidural hematoma extending from T12 to L4. An emergency decompressive laminectomy was performed, and a large solidified hematoma compressing the thecal sac was evacuated. The patient recovered full neurologic function within 3 days.

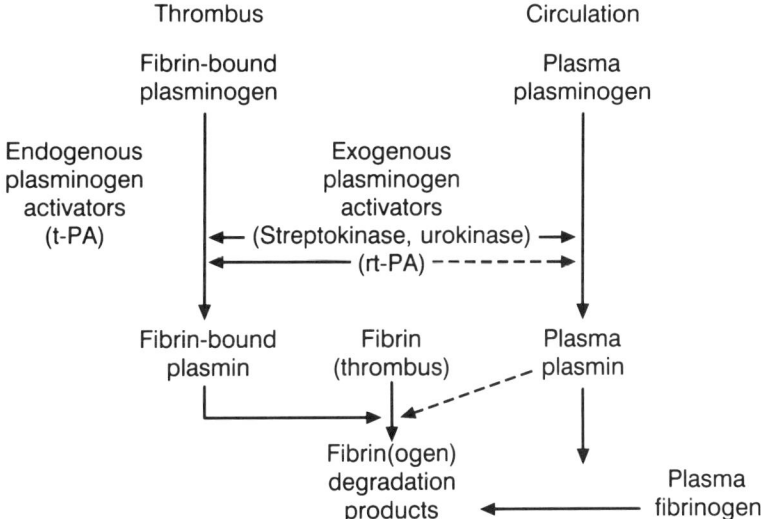

Fig. 3-3. The mechanism of action of thrombolytic agents. Solid arrows represent the usual pathways of the activation of plasminogen. Dashed arrows represent less important activity. Endogenous plasminogen activators convert fibrin-bound plasminogen to fibrin and thereby dissolve thrombus. Exogenous plasminogen activators not only affect fibrin-bound plasminogen, but have systemic effects as well and deplete circulating plasminogen and fibrinogen. rt-PA is more fibrin-selective but has systemic effects at high doses. (From Hirsch & Goldhaber,[32] with permission.)

In summary, spinal and epidural anesthesia can be safely performed on patients receiving anticoagulant or antiplatelet therapy as attested by studies reported by Rao and El-Etr,[15] Horlocker et al,[28] and Odoom and Sih.[23] However, it is important to note that even in a large series, the finding of zero events does not mean the risk is zero, but rather indicates the expected variable incidence of a relatively infrequent event.

The decision to perform spinal or epidural anesthesia on a patient receiving these medications should be made on an individual basis, weighing the risk of intraspinal hematoma and benefits of regional anesthesia for a specific patient. The patient's history should be reviewed for medical conditions associated with bleeding tendencies. Since it is difficult to predict an individual's response to antiplatelet or anticoagulant therapy, laboratory verification may be helpful prior to initiation of regional anesthesia. It is clinically most useful to evaluate the coagulation parameter(s) specific to the clotting defect expected, such as the PT in warfarinized patients or bleeding time in patients on antiplatelet therapy (Table 3-1). While tests such as the thromboelastogram or sonoclot, which measure overall coagulation function, may prove useful in the future, their role has not been defined at this time. However, the following statements will guide the anesthesia care provider faced with this difficult decision.

1. It is generally agreed, although difficult to prove, that in the absence of extraordinary indications, spinal and epidural anesthesia are contraindicated in patients within 24 hours of receiving thrombolytic therapy, with known coagulopathies, or with significant thrombocytopenia.

Table 3-1. Pharmacologic Activities of Anticoagulants and Antiplatelet Agents

Agent	Effect on Coagulation Variables			Time to Peak Effect	Time to Normal Hemostasis Post-therapy	Comments
	BT	PT	aPTT			
Intravenous heparin	↑	↑	↑ ↑ ↑	Minutes	4–6 hours	Monitor ACT, aPTT; delay heparinization for 1 hour after needle placement
Subcutaneous heparin	↑	↑	↑ ↑	40–50 minutes	4–6 hours	Monitor aPTT, anti-Xa activity
Warfarin	—	↑ ↑ ↑	↑	4–6 days (3 days with loading dose)	4–6 days	Monitor PT
Aspirin	↑ ↑ ↑	—	—	Hours	7 days	Increased age with epidural technique may increase incidence of minor hemorrhage following needle placement
Other NSAID	↑ ↑ ↑	—	—	Hours	3–5 days	
Thrombolytic agent	↑ ↑ ↑	↑	↑	Minutes	1–2 days	Usually heparinized in addition; monitor closely

BT, bleeding time; PT, prothombin time; aPTT, acitvated partial thromboplastin time; ACT, activated clotting time; NSAID, nonsteroidal anti-inflammatory drug; ↑, clinically insignificant increase; ↑ ↑, possibly clinically significant increase; ↑ ↑ ↑, clinically significant increase. (From Horlocker & Wedel,[34] with permission.)

2. Although the data by Odoom and Sih[23] are reassuring, central neuraxial blockade should probably be avoided in fully anticoagulated patients. However, patients who have received only one or two doses of an oral anticoagulant (i.e., 5 to 10 mg) will generally not have an increased PT and may safely undergo regional anesthesia. A PT may be measured prior to needle placement.

3. Patients fully anticoagulated with a continuous heparin infusion should have the infusion discontinued 4 to 6 hours before needle or catheter placement. Subcutaneous low-dose heparin should also not be administered within 4 to 6 hours of a spinal or epidural anesthetic to allow for normalization of the aPTT. Laboratory verification may be performed before initiation of regional blockade.

4. Epidural or spinal anesthesia followed by systemic heparinization is probably safe, provided adequate precautions are taken.[15,16] Heparinization should not be initiated for at least 1 hour after needle placement.[15–17] In addition, patients receiving antiplatelet medications who will undergo subsequent heparinization appear to be at increased risk for spinal hematoma and need to be followed closely.[17] Rao and El-Etr[15] and Odoom and Sih[23] recommended careful monitoring of the aPTT during heparinization. If needle placement is traumatic or difficult, the decision to proceed with surgery should be re-evaluated. Removal of an indwelling epidural catheter in a patient receiving intravenous or subcutaneous heparin should occur 4 to 6 hours after the last heparin dose and anticoagulation should not be reinsti-

tuted for at least 1 hour after catheter removal. An indwelling epidural or spinal catheter in a patient with a perioperative coagulopathy, such as disseminated intravascular coagulation or dilutional thrombocytopenia, should be removed only after normalization of coagulation status.

5. Epidural and spinal anesthesia can be safely performed in a patient receiving antiplatelet therapy.[28] Patients with a history of bleeding or bruising may be further evaluated with a preoperative bleeding time.

6. Use of small-gauge needles and the midline approach may allow more atraumatic needle placement (a paramedian or lateral approach may increase the risk of puncturing the epidural veins). Epidural catheters should not be inserted more than 3 to 4 cm into the epidural space to minimize trauma to the epidural venous structures.

7. Short-acting local anesthetics should be used in patients at increased risk so that their neurologic status may be evaluated immediately postoperatively. Likewise, an epidural block should be allowed to regress sufficiently to allow neurologic evaluation before initiating a continuous local anesthetic infusion for postoperative anaglesia. A narcotic rather than local anesthetic infusion would allow continuous monitoring of neurologic function and may be a more prudent choice in these patients.

8. The patient should be monitored closely in the perioperative period for early signs of cord compression such as severe back pain, local tenderness, meningismus, or neurologic dysfunction. If intraspinal hematoma is suspected, myelography, computed tomography scan, or magnetic resonance imaging should be performed immediately since delay may lead to irreversible cord ischemia. The treatment of choice is immediate decompressive laminectomy. Recovery is unlikely if surgery is postponed for more than 12 hours; only 45 percent of the patients in Owens' series had partial or good recovery of neurologic function.[14,33]

REFERENCES

1. Keith I: Anaesthesia and blood loss in total hip replacement. Anaesthesia 32:444, 1977
2. Modig J, Borg T, Karlström G et al: Thromboembolism after total hip replacement: role of epidural and general anesthesia. Anesth Analg 62:147, 1983
3. Raj PP, Denson DD, Joyce TH: Evaluation of continuous extravascular infusion of bupivacaine for prolonged pain relief. Pain 11:S251, 1981
4. O'Meara PM, Kaufman EE: Prophylaxis of venous thromboembolism in total hip arthroplasty: a review. Orthopedics 13:173, 1990
5. Haake DA, Berkman SA: Venous thromboembolic disease after hip surgery: risk factors, prophylaxis, diagnosis. Clin Orthop 242:212, 1989
6. Lynch JA, Baker PL, Polly RE et al: Mechanical measures in the prophylaxis of postoperative thromboembolism in total knee arthroplasty. Clin Orthop 260:24, 1990
7. Joist JH, Sherman LA (eds): Venous and Arterial Thrombosis: Pathogenesis, Diagnosis, Prevention, and Therapy. Grune & Stratton, Orlando, 1979
8. Linn BJ, Mazza JJ, Friedenberg WR: The treatment of venous thromboembolic disease. Postgrad Med 79:171, 1986
9. Malinovsky NN, Kozlov VA (eds): Anticoagulant and Thrombolytic Therapy in Surgery. CV Mosby, St. Louis, 1979
10. Ockelford P: Heparin: 1986 indications and effective use. Drugs 31:81, 1986
11. Gustafson H, Rutberg H, Bengtsson M: Spinal haemotoma following epidural analgesia. Anaesthesia 43:220, 1988

12. Kirkpatrick D, Goodman SJ: Combined subarachnoid and subdural spinal hematoma following spinal puncture. Surg Neurol 3:109, 1975
13. Spurny OM, Rubin S, Wolff JW et al: Spinal epidural hematoma during anticoagulant therapy. Arch Intern Med 114:103, 1964
14. Owens EL, Kasten GW, Hessel EA: Spinal hematoma after lumbar puncture and heparinization. Anesth Analg 65:1201, 1986
15. Rao TLK, El-Etr AA: Anticoagulation following placement of epidural and subarachnoid catheters: an evaluation of neurologic sequelae. Anesthesiology 55:618, 1981
16. Matthews ET, Abrams LO: Intrathecal morphine in open heart surgery. Lancet 2:543, 1980
17. Ruff RL, Dougherty JH: Complications of lumbar puncture followed by anticoagulation. Stroke 12:879, 1981
18. Poller L, Taberner DA, Sandilands DG, Galasko CSB: An evaluation of aPTT monitoring of low-dose heparin dosage in hip surgery. Thromb Haemost 47:50, 1982
19. Lowson SM, Goodchild CS: Low-dose heparin therapy and spinal anesthesia. Anaesthesia 44:67, 1989
20. Allemann BH, Gerber H, Gruber UF: Rückenmarksnahe Anaesthesie und subkutan verabreichtes low-dose heparin-dihydergot zur thromboembolieprophylaxe. (Perispinal anesthesia and subcutaneous administration of low-dose heparin-dihydergot for prevention of thromboembolism.) Anaesthetist 32:80, 1983
21. Darnat S, Guggiari M, Grob R et al: Lumbar epidural haematoma following the setting-up of an epidural catheter. Ann Fr Anesth Reanim 5:550, 1986
22. Dean WM, Woodside JR: Spinal hematoma compressing cauda equina. Urology 13:575, 1979
23. Odoom JA,. Sih IL: Epidural anaglesia and anticoagulant therapy. Anaesthesia 38:254, 1983
24. Rapaport SI: Preoperative hemostatic evaluation: which tests if any? Blood 61:229, 1983
25. Hindman BJ: Usefulness of the post-aspirin bleeding time. Anesthesiology 64:368, 1986
26. Ferraris VA, Swanson E: Aspirin usage and perioperative blood loss in patients undergoing unexpected operations. Surg Gynecol Obstet 156:439, 1983
27. Cronberg S, Wallmark E, Soderberg I: Effect on platelet aggregation of oral administration of 10 non-steroidal analgesics to humans. Scand J Haematol 33:155, 1984
28. Horlocker TT, Wedel DJ, Offord KP: Does preoperative antiplatelet therapy increase the risk of hemorrhagic complications associated with regional anesthesia? Anesth Analg 70:631, 1990
29. Locke GE, Giorgio AJ, Biggers SL et al: Acute spinal epidural hematoma secondary to aspirin-induced prolonged bleeding. Surg Neurol 4:293, 1976
30. Rao AK, Pratt C, Berke A et al: Thrombolysis in myocardial infarction trial—phase I. J Am Coll Cardiol 11:1, 1988
31. Dickman CA, Shedd SA, Spetzler RF et al: Spinal epidural hematoma associated with epidural anesthesia: complications of systemic heparinization in patients receiving peripheral vascular thrombolytic therapy. Anesthesiology 72:947, 1990
32. Hirsch DR, Goldhaber SZ: Bleeding time and other laboratory tests to monitor the safety and efficacy of thrombolytic therapy. Chest 97:1245, 1990.
33. Harik SI, Raichle ME, Reiss DJ: Spontaneously remitting spinal epidural hematoma in a patient on anticoagulants. N Engl J Med 284:1355, 1971
34. Horlocker TT, Wedel DJ: Anticoagulants and antiplatelet therapy and neuraxis blockade. Anesth Clin North Am 10(1):1, 1992
35. Hirsch DR, Goldhaber SZ: The bleeding time: its potential utility among patients receiving thrombolytic therapy. Am Heart J 119:158, 1990

4

A Comparison of Regional and General Anesthesia

Steven H. Rose

When discussing the option of regional or general anesthesia during the preoperative interview, patients often ask which type is "best." Unfortunately, in many instances there is no clear answer to this important question. It is difficult to compare the techniques because of the large number of variables that may have an influence (type of regional or general anesthesia used, which intravenous and/or volatile agents are selected, type of surgery, patient's medical history, etc.). Since the incidence of major morbidity and mortality is very low with either technique, extremely large numbers of patients must be studied for subtle influences to become apparent. A comparison of regional and general anesthesia is further confounded by the lack of a rigid separation between the techniques. In fact, there are situations in which a combination of both has been shown to be beneficial.[1,2] An awareness of the relative risks and benefits of regional and general anesthesia allows the practitioner to "tailor" the anesthetic to meet the specific needs of the patient and surgeon. This chapter compares the advantages and disadvantages of regional and general anesthesia and focuses on those aspects most applicable to the anesthetic care of orthopedic surgical patients.

Regional anesthesia is well suited to the needs of many orthopedic surgical patients. Extremity surgery can often be performed with peripheral nerve blocks, avoiding the major physiologic trespass associated with the induction of general anesthesia or central neuraxial blockade. Advantages of regional anesthesia often include avoidance of airway instrumentation, rapid recovery, and excellent postoperative analgesia. A range of techniques and local anesthetics allows the practitioner to choose a regional procedure appropriate for the clinical circumstance. For example, a long-acting local anesthetic (or a continuous technique) may be used for a patient undergoing an inpatient procedure associated with considerable postoperative pain. Similarly, a short-acting local anesthetic may be selected for a patient undergoing an outpatient procedure, allowing rapid resolution of the block and an early return to normal function.

Patients generally experience less nausea and are able to tolerate oral intake more quickly after regional anesthesia. Regional techniques allow communication with the patient, which is important under some circumstances. A diabetic patient, for example, could convey symptoms of hypoglycemia or a patient with atherosclerotic heart disease could inform the anesthesia provider of chest pain. Neurologic deterioration, such as an altered level of consciousness, is more easily detected using regional techniques as well. Some patients prefer being "awake" to avoid the loss of autonomy that accompanies heavy sedation or general anesthesia. Continuous regional techniques may be extended into the postoperative period to provide analgesia and sympathetic blockade, and to allow tolerance of passive joint motion devices. Low concentrations of local anesthetics and/or narcotics can provide postoperative analgesia without the profound anesthesia and motor block necessary for the procedure itself. Sympathetic blockade is particularly useful when vasodilation is desired, such as after limb replantation procedures.

Still, regional anesthesia is not without problems. There are situations in which

Table 4-1.   Preoperative Assessment for Regional Anesthesia

Relative Contraindications	Medical Conditions That May Affect Anesthetic Choice
Progressive neurologic disease, (e.g., multiple sclerosis)	Stable pre-existing neurologic disease (e.g., documented peripheral neuropathy, cerebral vascular accident)
Aortic or mitral valve stenosis (central neural blockade)	
Severe or unstable psychiatric disease	Diabetes mellitus
Severe emotional instability	Medications (e.g., antihypertensives and antiplatelet drugs)
Clotting disorders (uncompensated)	Cardiovascular disease
	Stable psychiatric and/or emotional disorders

(From Wedel,[123] with permission.)

it is absolutely or relatively contraindicated (Table 4-1). A significant number of orthopedic surgical procedures are ill-suited for regional anesthesia alone because of positioning and airway considerations. Regional anesthesia can be time-consuming and it does not always work. Clearly, the administration of a particular anesthetic to any given patient depends on a number of patient, surgical, and practitioner factors. In this chapter the effects of regional and general anesthesia on several important clinical variables are reviewed.

INFLUENCE OF ANESTHETIC CHOICE ON BLOOD LOSS

There has been a widespread increase in concern about homologous blood transfusion among health care professionals and the general public. Accordingly, transfusion therapy has been an increasingly important issue for anesthesia providers to consider, especially when elective rather than emergent surgery is planned. Strategies to decrease the need for homologous transfusion include autologous predonation, intraoperative salvage techniques, and administration of nonblood colloids. There is also substantial evidence that the choice of regional or general anesthesia may influence perioperative blood loss. This issue has been addressed by several authors studying orthopedic surgical patients (Table 4-2). Three studies examining the influence of regional anesthesia on perioperative blood loss have been reported by Modig et al.[3–5] Each study compared intraoperative blood loss in patients undergoing elective total hip arthroplasty. One studied postoperative blood loss as well.[3] A total of 120 patients (60 in one study, 30 in each of the others) were randomly al-

Table 4-2. Influence of Anesthetic Technique on Perioperative Blood Loss During Elective Total Hip Arthroplasty

Study/Year	Anesthetic Technique/ Postoperative Pain Therapy	No. of Patients	Intraoperative Blood Loss	Postoperative Blood Loss
Modig (1981)	General/ketobemidone	15	$757^b \pm 426$	
	Epidural/epidural	15	100 ± 316	
Modig (1983)	General/ketobemidone	16	$1616^a \pm 313$	
	Epidural/epidural	14	1100 ± 316	
Modig (1983)	General/ketobemidone	30	$1548^b \pm 410$	$427^b \pm 175$
	Epidural/epidural	30	1148 ± 446	294 ± 64
Keith (1977)	Epidural/parenteral	10	$341^a \pm 59$	393 ± 96
	Halothane/parenteral	9	648 ± 58	338 ± 61
	Neurolept anesthesia/ parenteral	8	744 ± 99	424 ± 98
Wille-Jorgensen (1989)	Epidural or spinal/ parenteral	33	450^a	510
	General/parenteral	65	899	450

^{a} $P < 0.01$.
^{b} $P < 0.001$.

located to receive regional or general anesthesia. The regional anesthesia groups received intraoperative epidural anesthesia and postoperative epidural analgesia. The general anesthesia groups received narcotics and nitrous oxide intraoperatively and parenteral narcotics for postoperative pain. All three studies demonstrated a statistically significant decrease in intraoperative blood loss in the epidural groups. A statistically significant decrease in postoperative blood loss was also demonstrated in the single study in which it was measured.

In a similar study of 98 patients undergoing elective total hip arthroplasty using regional (epidural or spinal) or general anesthesia, Wille-Jorgensen et al[6] reported a statistically significant decrease in intraoperative blood loss when the regional anesthesia group was compared to the group receiving general anesthesia. No difference in postoperative blood loss was apparent. This is of interest because, in contrast with the studies by Modig et al (in which the patients in the regional

anesthesia group received postoperative epidural analgesia), the postoperative pain management in both of Wille-Jorgensen's groups was the same (parenteral narcotics). Whether postoperative blood loss in the regional anesthesia group would have been less if postoperative pain had been managed by a continuous epidural technique is not known.

In a third study of patients undergoing elective total hip arthroplasty Keith[7] studied the effect of anesthetic choice on blood loss prospectively in 27 patients. He divided the patients into three groups: one received epidural anesthesia, one received a halothane-based general anesthetic, and the third received modified neuroleptanesthesia (droperidol, fentanyl, and nitrous oxide). Again, a statistically significant decrease in intraoperative blood loss between the epidural and either of the general anesthesia groups was demonstrated. There was no comment on postoperative pain management but no significant difference in postoperative blood loss was reported.

A number of possible explanations for these results have been forwarded. Regional anesthesia is associated with a reduction in mean arterial pressure, a redistribution of blood flow favoring increased volume in the larger vessels, and decreased local venous pressures (perhaps influenced by the elimination of the need for positive pressure ventilation).[3,7,8] It is likely that each of these factors may play a role.

On balance, central neuraxial blockade for hip procedures seems to decrease intraoperative blood loss, and pain management using regional techniques may decrease postoperative bleeding as well.

INFLUENCE OF ANESTHETIC CHOICE ON THE INCIDENCE OF DEEP VENOUS THROMBOSIS AND PULMONARY THROMBOEMBOLIC DISEASE

Pulmonary thromboembolic disease (PTE) is an important cause of major morbidity and mortality in orthopedic surgical patients. Fatal pulmonary thromboemboli have been reported to develop in 0.3 to 2.4 percent of patients undergoing hip arthroplasty and in 4 to 7 percent of patients after surgery for hip fractures.[9] Autopsy studies performed on patients who died shortly after total hip replacement have revealed PTE to be the most common cause of death.[10] Total knee arthroplasty is another commonly performed orthopedic procedure having a relatively high incidence of postoperative deep venous thrombosis (DVT) and PTE. DVT has been reported to occur in 40 to 88 percent of patients undergoing total knee arthroplasty.[11-16] Perioperative thrombotic risk is increased by advanced age, obesity, malignancy, congestive

heart failure, acute myocardial infarction, prior DVT or PTE, estrogen use, and immobilization.[17-19] Unfortunately these predispositions are relatively common in orthopedic surgical patients. A variety of physical and pharmacologic approaches to DVT/PTE prophylaxis have been attempted and are reviewed elsewhere in this text (Ch. 3). Consequently, this section mainly deals with one central clinical issue, the influence of the choice of regional or general anesthesia on the incidence of DVT/PTE.

Several studies have shown that the incidence of DVT/PTE can be significantly reduced by using epidural anesthesia (with or without postoperative epidural analgesia) or spinal anesthesia instead of general anesthesia.[3,4,20,21] The influence of anesthetic choice on the incidence of DVT and PTE in elective total hip arthroplasty has been determined by several investigators (Table 4-3). Modig et al prospectively studied the influence of epidural anesthesia (and postoperative epidural analgesia) or general anesthesia (with parenteral narcotics for postoperative pain relief) on the incidence of DVT/PTE in two randomized studies. The first included 30 patients and showed a statistically significant decrease in the incidence of DVT when the epidural group (3 of 15, 20 percent) was compared to the group receiving general anesthesia (11 of 15, 73 percent). Pulmonary embolism was also less common in the epidural group (2 of 15, 13 percent) than in the general anesthesia group (7 of 15, 47 percent) but did not reach statistical significance.[4] In their second study (which was of similar design),[3] 60 patients undergoing elective total hip arthroplasty were randomized to receive epidural or general anesthesia. Statistically significant decreases were reported in the incidence of thrombosis involving the popliteal and femoral veins (13 vs. 67 percent), thrombosis of calf and thigh veins (40 vs. 77 percent), and pul-

Table 4-3. Incidence of DVT/PTE Associated With Certain Orthopedic Procedures

Procedure	Study/Year	Anesthetic	No. of Patients	DVT		PTE
Total hip arthroplasty	Modig (1981)	General	15	73%[a]		47%
		Continuous epidural	15	20%		13%
				Pop & fem	*Calf & thigh*	
	Modig (1983)	General	30	67%[a]	77%[a]	33%[a]
		Continous epidural	30	13%	40%	10%
	Wille-Jorgensen (1989)	General	65	31%[a]		9%
		Regional (epidural or spinal)	33	9%		1%
	Davis (1989)	General	71	27%[a]		
		Spinal	69	13%		
Hip fracture	McKenzie (1985)	General	20	75%[a]		
		Regional	20	40%		
Total knee arthroplasty	Nielsen (1990)	General	18	62.5%[a]		
		Continuous epidural	18	12.5%		
	Sharrock (1991)	General	264	64%[a]		
		Epidural	227	48%		

[a] $P < 0.01$.

monary embolization (10 vs. 33 percent) when the patients receiving epidural anesthesia were compared to those receiving general anesthesia.

The influence of central neuraxial blockade or general anesthesia on the incidence of DVT/PTE in patients undergoing total hip arthroplasty was also studied prospectively in 98 patients by Wille-Jorgensen et al.[6] Sixty-five patients were included in the general anesthesia group. Twenty of them (31 percent) developed DVT and 6 (9 percent) developed PTE. In the 33 patients receiving spinal or epidural anesthesia, 3 (9 percent) developed DVT and 1 (3 percent) developed PTE. The difference in the incidence of DVT (but not PTE) between the groups reached statistical significance.

Another prospective comparison of regional (spinal) and general anesthesia on the incidence of DVT in 140 elective total hip arthroplasty patients was performed by Davis et al.[22] DVT developed in 9 of the 69 patients receiving spinal anesthesia (13 percent) and in 19 of the 71 patients receiving general anesthesia (27 percent). This difference was statistically significant. The presence of varicose veins was shown to increase the likelihood of DVT in this study and, oddly, being a nonsmoker and having a low body mass index did as well.

In a comparison of the incidence of DVT in 40 hip fracture (rather than hip arthroplasty) patients, McKenzie et al[23] reported a 75 percent incidence (15 of 20) of DVT in a group randomized to receive general anesthesia. In a second group randomized to receive regional anesthesia, 40 percent (8 of 20) developed DVT (a statistically significant decrease). It is noteworthy that regional anesthesia was shown to be efficacious in lowering the risk of DVT in hip fracture patients who suffered the traumatic insult predisposing them to DVT before the administration of either regional or general anesthesia.

At least two studies have addressed this question in patients undergoing knee rather than hip procedures. In a large retrospective study, Sharrock et al[24] reviewed the records of over 700 patients undergoing unilateral or bilateral total knee arthroplasty. They compared the incidence of DVT in patients anesthetized with either epidural or general anesthesia. The diagnosis of DVT was established by performance of pre- and postoperative lung perfusion scans and postoperative venography of the leg (or legs if bilateral) that were operated on. All of the procedures were performed by the same surgeon using a single operative technique and similar thromboembolic prophylaxis (650 mg aspirin twice a day). The patients were not randomly selected to receive a given anesthetic. Patients included in the first 2 years of the study period usually had general anesthesia and those in the last 2 years were usually managed with epidural anesthesia. A statistically significant difference in the incidence of DVT was reported between the groups. The incidence of DVT was 64 percent (170 of 264) in the general anesthesia group and 48 percent (133 of 277) in the epidural anesthesia group. A positive lung scan was present in 9 percent (23 of 264) of the patients in the general anesthesia group and 6 percent (17 of 277) of the patients receiving epidural anesthesia. This difference was not statistically significant. Two patients in each group had clinically symptomatic pulmonary emboli.

Nielsen et al[25] also addressed this issue with a prospective but much smaller study. Thirty-six patients scheduled for elective total knee arthroplasty were randomly assigned to receive general or epidural anesthesia. The patients randomized to receive epidural anesthesia also received epidural analgesia for postoperative pain management. The patients randomized to receive general anesthesia were administered parenteral narcotics for postoperative pain. The diagnosis of DVT was established using bilateral ascending venography 9 to 11 days after surgery. A statistically significant decrease in DVT was shown when the epidural group (2 of 13, 15 percent) was compared to the general anesthesia group (10 of 16, 63 percent). Seven patients were excluded from the study after allocation for a variety of reasons. Despite the weaknesses of each study, it appears that thromboembolic complications may be reduced in patients undergoing total knee arthroplasty receiving epidural anesthesia.

The mechanisms responsible for the decreased incidence of thromboembolic phenomena associated with regional anesthesia are uncertain, although a variety have been suggested. Clearly, rheologic considerations may be important. Modig et al[26] performed studies indicating arterial inflow, venous emptying rate, and venous capacitance were all significantly greater in patients receiving intraoperative epidural anesthesia and postoperative epidural analgesia than in patients managed with intraoperative general anesthesia and parenteral narcotics postoperatively for pain. Davis[27] demonstrated increases in leg blood flow in a group of total hip arthroplasty patients anesthetized with spinal rather than general anesthesia, but no clear association between the increases in lower limb blood flow and the occurrence of DVT in individual patients was apparent. Other investigators[24,28] have shown substantial increases in leg blood flow during the early postoperative period in patients receiving regional anesthesia as well. Systemic hemodynamic differences may also be of importance. The onset of vasodilation associated with central neuraxial blockade results in well-recognized decreases in arterial and venous pressures, which may affect the incidence of DVT.

Other mechanisms that may play a contributing role in the decreased incidence of thromboembolic disease include altered coagulation in response to surgery.[2,29–31] improved fibrinolysis, and perhaps an antithrombotic effect of lidocaine and presumably other local anesthetics as well.[32–35] These complex issues have been studied by several investigators. Donadoni et al[36] studied coagulation and fibrinolysis in 80 patients undergoing total hip arthroplasty. The patients were randomly allocated to one of three groups: one group received general anesthesia, one epidural anesthesia, and the third, combined epidural and general anesthesia. Coagulation and fibrinolysis were assessed by measuring the prothrombin time, the activated partial thromboplastin time, fibrinogen, plasminogen, antithrombin III, protein C, α_2-antiplasmin, factor VIII coagulating activity, von Willebrand factor antigen, von Willebrand ristocetin cofactor, and tissue plasminogen activator before anesthetic induction, at the end of surgery, on the first postoperative morning, and 7 days postoperatively. Though several parameters of coagulation differed significantly between the groups, the indicator thought to be most important by the authors was the demonstration that antithrombin III, which was depressed immediately after surgery in each group, returned to normal more quickly in the group receiving epidural anesthesia (Fig. 4-1).

Differing results were reported by Davis et al,[37] who in a prospective randomized study of 101 total hip arthroplasty patients receiving spinal or general anesthesia were unable to demonstrate a difference in antithrombin III between the groups. They did, however, report

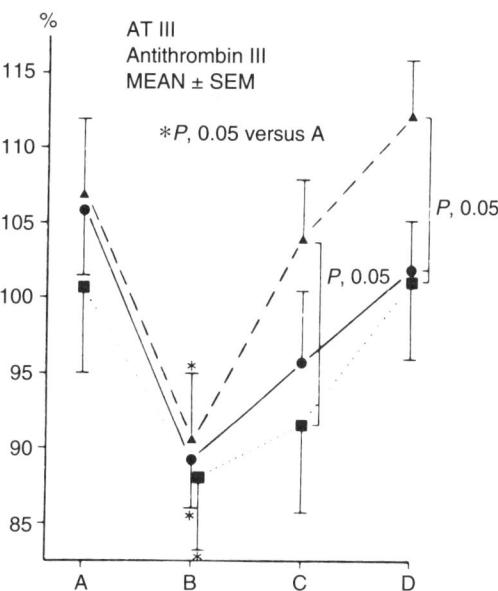

Fig. 4-1. Changes of antithrombin III at different examination times (A, preinduction; B, end of surgery; C, first postoperative morning; D, seventh postoperative day). General anesthesia (solid circles): n = 29; epidural anesthesia (triangles): n = 29; combined anesthesia (solid squares): n = 22. (From Donadoni et al,[36] with permission.)

significant differences between the groups in platelet count, thrombin production, and factor VIII-related antigen perioperatively and in the immediate postoperative period. In Davis et al's study, intraoperative fibrinolysis was shown to be decreased in the group receiving spinal anesthesia. By contrast, Modig et al[5] and Simpson et al[38] reported enhanced fibrinolysis in association with lumbar epidural anesthesia. In the study by Modig et al, 30 patients scheduled for total hip arthroplasty were given the option of epidural or general anesthesia for the procedure. Fourteen patients chose epidural anesthesia and 16 chose general anesthesia. Venous samples were drawn before the anesthetic was administered, immediately before the surgical incision, and daily for 1 week postoperatively. The samples were analyzed for fibrinolysis inhibition activity, plasminogen activators, and capacity for activation of factor VIII. Fibrinolysis inhibition activity increased in both groups after surgery but was significantly lower in the epidural group (Fig. 4-2). Plasminogen activators and the capacity of the venous epithelium to release them significantly differed between the groups (Fig. 4-3), and factor VIII activity was significantly increased in both groups but lower in the group receiving epidural anesthesia (Fig. 4-4).

In a recent study addressing this issue by Tuman et al[2] coagulation was assessed in two groups of patients undergoing major vascular surgery. One group received general anesthesia combined with postoperative epidural analgesia and the other received general anesthesia with patient controlled narcotic analgesia for postoperative pain. Coagulability was assessed via thromboelastography after the induction of anesthesia and on the first postoperative day. Patients in the epidural group collectively had significantly decreased α and maximum amplitude (MA) values as measured by thromboelastography postoperatively. In addition, they had a significantly decreased rate of postoperative thrombotic complications (thrombosis of a coronary artery, deep vein, or vascular graft).

Other factors that may account for the differences in the incidence of thromboembolic disease based on anesthetic choice include an altered neuroendocrine–metabolic response, an effect of the local anesthetic per se, decreased blood loss and transfusion requirements in the regional groups, and a host of other fac-

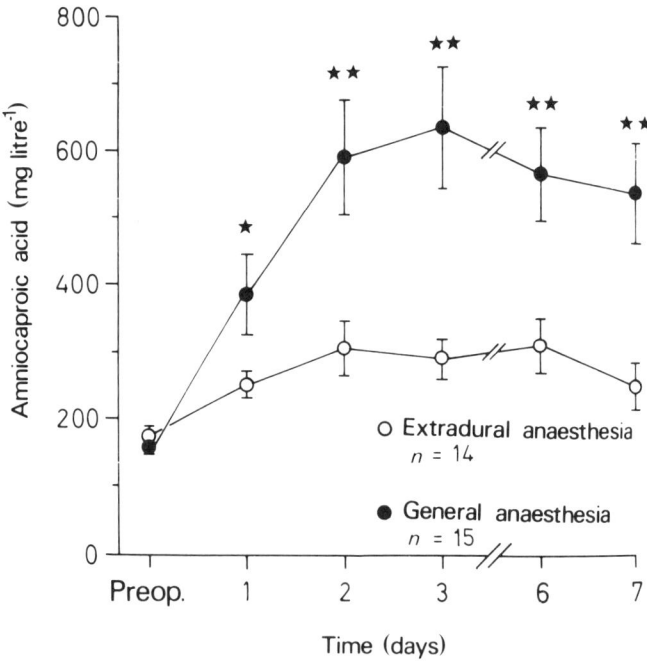

Fig. 4-2. Fibrinolysis inhibition activity in serum associated with the two different anesthetic techniques. Mean ± SEM. Asterisks indicate level of significance between the anaesthetic groups: *P <0.05; **P <0.01. (From Modig et al,[5] with permission).

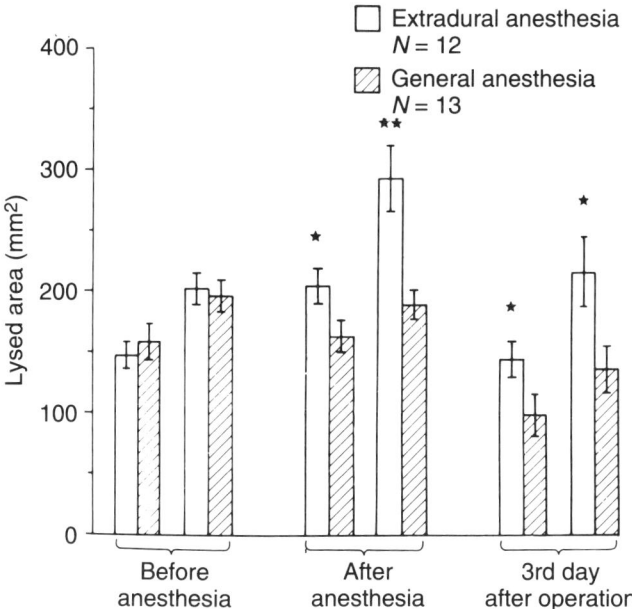

Fig. 4-3. Resting concentration of plasminogen activators (left bars) and capacity for release of plasminogen activators after venous occlusion (right bars) associated with the two anesthetic techniques. Mean ± SEM. Asterisks indicate level of significance between the anesthetic groups: *P <0.05; **P <0.01. (From Modig et al,[5] with permission.)

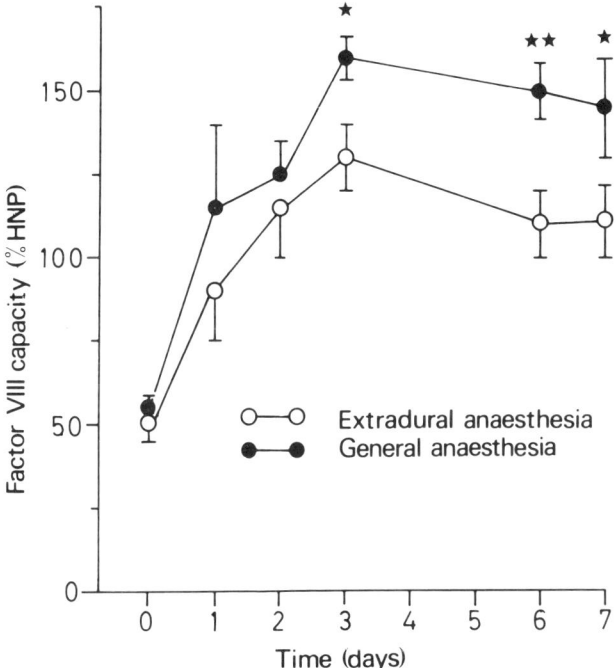

Fig. 4-4. Factor VIII capacity associated with the two anesthetic techniques. Mean ± SEM. Asterisks indicate level of significance between the anesthetic groups: *P <0.05; **P <0.01. HNP, human normal plasma. (From Modig et al,[5] with permission.)

tors. Further studies are necessary to fully elucidate the reasons for the decreased incidence of thromboembolic phenomena associated with regional anesthesia.

A serious problem in applying the results of these studies to contemporary orthopedic surgical practice stems from the fact that most of the patients in the studies received no pharmacologic prophylaxis to avoid DVT/PTE. Currently, it is common for patients to receive some type of anticoagulant prior to the performance of total hip or (to a lesser extent) total knee arthroplasty. Insufficient data are presently available to ascertain whether regional anesthesia would lower the incidence of thromboembolic complications in patients receiving prophylactic anticoagulants. Study of this issue is complicated because some authorities consider preoperative anticoagulant thrombosis prophylaxis to be a contraindication to the performance of central neuraxial blockade[9,39,40] (especially in the presence of minidose heparin because of the wide variability in patient response[41,42]), but at least one study in addition to that by Sharrock has been reported. Planes et al[43] investigated the incidence of DVT after regional or general anesthesia for orthopedic procedures in patients receiving DVT prophylaxis with low-molecular-weight heparin and failed to show significant differences. However, problems have been identified with the design of the study, including inconsistent heparin dose schedules.[44]

The issue of the appropriateness of regional anesthesia in patients receiving perioperative anticoagulants is addressed in more detail elsewhere in this text (Ch. 3). Unfortunately, since hemorrhagic complications of spinal or epidural anesthesia may be catastrophic,[45] very large numbers of patients must be studied before confident recommendation of central neuraxial blockade in patients receiving a variety of anticoagulant regimens would

be warranted. At present, the risks and benefits of regional anesthesia must be weighed in choosing the appropriate anesthetic for any given patient based on concerns of thrombotic or hemorrhagic complications.

In summary, in patients not receiving pharmacologic DVT/PTE prophylaxis, central neuraxial blockade is efficacious in reducing thromboembolic complications after operative fixation of hip fractures and after total hip or knee arthroplasty. Whether there is a clinically significant difference in the incidence of thromboembolic complications after these orthopedic surgical procedures in patients receiving a variety of anticoagulants is not known.

INFLUENCE OF ANESTHETIC CHOICE ON PSYCHOLOGICAL AND COGNITIVE FACTORS

There is considerable concern about possible deleterious effects of anesthesia and surgery on postoperative mental function, especially among elderly patients.[46] Patients often describe psychological and cognitive difficulty after major surgery, and postoperative mental problems have been documented in some studies.[47,48] An issue of interest to anesthesia providers is whether the choice between regional and general anesthesia can influence mental or psychological outcome postoperatively. This issue has been addressed by many authors, often with conflicting results. Some studies suggest there may be a variety of subtle to gross deleterious effects on mental and/or psychological function when general anesthesia is compared to regional anesthesia for a variety of procedures,[49] while others fail to show a difference.[47,50,51]

Five recent well-controlled prospective studies that include orthopedic surgical patients have examined the influence of the choice between regional and general anesthesia on postoperative psychological, cognitive, and social function (Table 4-4). Ghonheim and associates[52] studied 105 patients; 20 underwent vaginal hysterectomy, 34 underwent transurethral resection of the prostate, and 50 underwent total knee or total hip arthroplasty. Patients were randomly assigned to a regional anesthesia group (38 subarachnoid blocks, 14 epidural blocks) or a balanced general anesthesia group. A variety of sensitive indicators of mental function were assessed before, 1 to 7 days after, and 3 months after surgery. No important differences in mental or psychological outcome were found between the groups. In a similar study Nielson et al[51] prospectively examined the effects of spinal or balanced general anesthesia on postoperative mental function in 64 patients aged 60 to 86 years who underwent total knee arthroplasty. Again a variety of sensitive mental and psychological indicators were assessed preoperatively and about 3 months postoperatively. No important differences between the regional and general anesthetic groups were apparent.

Hughes et al[53] studied patients who underwent total hip arthroplasty using spinal or general anesthesia. They were specifically investigating relatively sophisticated and subtle effects on memory. Although there was little overall change in memory, a significant decrease in the ability to recognize words was noted in the spinal anesthesia group. The importance of this finding is questionable.

A study comparing cognitive performance in older (more than 60 years) orthopedic surgical patients (elective total knee or total hip arthroplasty) by Jones et al[54] failed to show a detectable impairment of cognitive or functional competence 3 months postoperatively in groups of patients receiving spinal or general

Table 4-4.   Influence of Anesthetic Choice on Mental Function

Study/Year	Anesthetic		Procedures		No. of Patients	Outcome
Ghonheim (1988)	Spinal	38	Vaginal hysterectomies	20	105	No important differences
	Epidural	14	TURP	34		
	General	53	TKA/THA	50		
Nielsen (1990)	Spinal	25	TKA		64	No important differences
	General	39				
Hughes (1988)	Spinal		THA		30	Little overall change in memory but significant decrease in word recognition in spinal group
	General					
Jones (1990)	Spinal	74	TKA		146	Improved recognition and response components of choice reaction time in general group
	General	72	THA			
Bigler (1985)	Spinal	20	Hip fractures		40	No important differences
	General	20				

TURP, Transurethral resection of the prostate; TKA, Total knee arthroplasty; THA, Total hip arthroplasty.

anesthesia. The only significant difference was an improvement in the response component of the choice reaction time in the group receiving general anesthesia, a finding that is again of questionable importance. Interestingly, a nearly equal number of patients in each group reported a subjective loss in memory and concentration that was not confirmed by testing.

Finally, Bigler et al[55] studied 40 elderly patients (mean age 78.9 years) who underwent surgery for hip fractures under spinal or general anesthesia. They were unable to determine any persistent mental impairment in either group.

On balance, the available literature does not clearly support a difference in mental or psychological outcome in orthopedic surgical patients receiving regional or general anesthesia. A variety of other factors such as perioperative medications and disorientation due to hospitalization may be more important than the choice of regional or general anesthesia in this regard.

INFLUENCE OF ANESTHETIC CHOICE ON CONVALESCENCE AND COST

With the ever-increasing pressure to control the cost of medical care there is considerable interest in shortening hospital stays. There are numerous reports comparing length of hospitalization for a variety of procedures performed under regional or general anesthesia. Most show a decrease in hospital stay in the regional anesthesia group that falls short of statistical significance.[56–61] But at least three studies have shown a significant decrease in hospital stay or costs. Pflug et al[62] reported a significantly decreased hospital stay in patients who underwent upper ab-

dominal or hip fracture surgery when a group of patients receiving epidural anesthesia was compared to a group receiving general anesthesia. In fact, the difference was more pronounced if only the hip fracture patients were considered. They defined convalescence as the day of operation subtracted from the day the patient was afebrile, capable of independent ambulation, and not in need of parenteral fluids or analgesics. Whether the actual day of discharge was less in the group that received epidural anesthesia was not stated. A more recent study addressed this issue in high-risk patients undergoing intrathoracic, intra-abdominal, or major vascular surgery. Yeager et al[1] reported a significant decrease in hours of intubation, intensive care unit stay, and physician costs when a group receiving intraoperative combined epidural and general anesthesia and postoperative epidural analgesia was compared to a group receiving intraoperative general anesthesia and parenteral narcotics postoperatively for pain. Hospital stay did not differ significantly between the groups.

In a similar study of patients undergoing major vascular surgery, Tuman et al[2] reported a significant decrease in intensive care unit stay when patients receiving combined general and epidural anesthesia were compared to a group receiving general anesthesia alone. It is of interest to note that the studies by Pflug et al,[62] Yeager et al,[1] and Tuman et al[2] included the use of epidural analgesia rather than parenteral narcotics for postoperative pain management in the combined epidural plus general anesthesia groups.

A study by Baron et al[63] suggests that postoperative pain management may be more important in terms of outcome than the choice of anesthetic for the procedure itself. They studied 173 patients undergoing abdominal aortic reconstruction. One group (86 patients) received a "balanced" general anesthetic for the procedure. The second (87 patients) received thoracic epidural and "light general" anesthesia. Postoperative pain was managed similarly in each group (subcutaneous morphine, epidural bupivacaine, or epidural fentanyl). Their results did not support a major advantage or disadvantage between the groups. This is clearly an important issue deserving more study, including trials in lower risk patients.

The costs related to the provision of regional anesthesia are highly competitive when compared to general anesthetic techniques. Spinal anesthesia in particular is cheap and time efficient. Regional anesthesia may be conducted safely with basic resuscitation equipment and is well suited to the provision of care to large numbers of patients in circumstances of limited resources. Further study of this issue is likely as the cost of medical care is increasingly scrutinized.

INFLUENCE OF ANESTHETIC CHOICE ON IMMUNOLOGIC RESPONSE

It is well established that immunologic function may be impaired after surgery (or after other forms of trauma).[64] Perioperative immunocompetence is important since the occurrence of a significantly impaired immune response could have implications regarding the incidence of perioperative infections (a particularly troublesome complication in orthopedic surgical patients) or on possible metastatic spread in patients with malignancies.

Lymphocytopenia and leukocytosis occur commonly after total hip arthroplasty performed under general anesthesia. Epidural anesthesia has been shown to modify this response and the improved immunologic function attributed to blockade of the "stress" response to surgery.[65] The clinical importance of this issue is emphasized by Meakins et al,[66] who have demonstrated a correlation between the severity of lymphocytopenia and postoperative septicemia. However, other investigators have not reported consistent results. For example, Jakobsen et al[67] compared two groups of hip arthroplasty patients anesthetized with epidural or general anesthesia. They reported significant leukocytosis and lymphocytopenia in both groups and no significant difference between them. Similarly, Salo and Nissila[68] recently studied immunologic function in hip arthroplasty patients anesthetized with spinal or general anesthesia. Their study involved extensive testing of cell-mediated and humoral immunity. They also reported leukocytosis with a significant increase in the percentage of neutrophils and a significant decrease in the percentage of basophils and lymphocytes (Table 4-5). Lymphocyte subpopulations were measured and no significant changes in the percentage of T-, T-helper, T-suppressor, B-lymphocytes, or NK-cells were observed postoperatively. The absolute numbers of T-lymphocytes and T-suppressor lymphocytes significantly decreased postoperatively without differences between the spinal and general anesthesia groups (Table 4-6). In fact, the only difference between the spinal and general anesthesia groups in this study was an increase in the phytohemagglutinin-induced lymphocyte proliferative response in the spinal anesthesia group that was not seen in the general anesthesia group. The clinical importance of this single difference is questionable.

In summary, the data that are available currently do not firmly support a clinically important difference between general and regional anesthesia in terms of immunocompetence.

Table 4-5. Leukocyte and Differential Counts (Means ± SD)

	Anesthetic	Postoperative Day	Postoperative Day		
			1	*3–4*	*6–7*
Leukocytes (× 10^9/L)	Spinal	5.1 ± 1.3	8.1 ± 2.4[b]	6.2 ± 2.6	6.6 ± 1.6
	General	6.2 ± 1.2	7.8 ± 2.2[b]	6.6 ± 2.0	5.3 ± 1.7
Neutrophils (%)	Spinal	55.5 ± 11.7	73.0 ± 9.8[b]	68.2 ± 6.8[b]	60.9 ± 6.8
	General	59.9 ± 8.3	74.6 ± 9.2[b]	71.2 ± 11.0[b]	62.5 ± 9.0
Eosinophils (%)	Spinal	3.5 ± 2.6	0.7 ± 0.8[b]	3.9 ± 2.3	4.4 ± 3.0
	General	3.4 ± 2.8	0.5 ± 0.7[b]	4.5 ± 1.9	5.0 ± 3.4
Basophils (%)	Spinal	0.2 ± 0.5	0.1 ± 0.2	0.2 ± 0.3	0.0 ± 0.2
	General	0.0 ± 0.0	0.0 ± 0.0	0.1 ± 0.2	0.1 ± 0.2
Lymphocytes (%)	Spinal	39.5 ± 11.3	25.5 ± 8.8[b]	26.2 ± 5.7[b]	32.8 ± 6.0[a]
	General	35.7 ± 9.7	23.5 ± 9.4[b]	23.2 ± 9.8[b]	31.1 ± 7.3[a]
Monocytes (%)	Spinal	1.2 ± 0.8	0.6 ± 0.8	1.3 ± 0.8	1.8 ± 1.1
	General	1.1 ± 0.8	1.5 ± 1.4	1.0 ± 0.9	1.3 ± 0.6

[a] $P < 0.05$, [b] $P < 0.01$ compared with preoperative values. No differences between groups. (From Salo & Nissila,[68] with permission.)

Table 4-6. Lymphocyte Subpopulation (Means ± SD)

	Anesthetic	Postoperative Day	Postoperative Day		
			1	*3–4*	*6–7*
Lymphocytes (× 10^9/L)	Spinal	1.9 ± 0.6	1.9 ± 0.5	1.5 ± 0.4[a]	2.1 ± 0.5
	General	2.3 ± 0.7	1.7 ± 0.5	1.5 ± 0.6[a]	1.7 ± 0.6
T-lymphocytes (OKT$_3$+) (%)	Spinal	59.3 ± 9.5	52.6 ± 10.7	57.5 ± 14.2	53.5 ± 8.4
	General	63.2 ± 10.9	61.2 ± 15.3	66.5 ± 12.2	65.5 ± 11.7
T-helper (OKT$_4$+) (%)	Spinal	38.3 ± 9.0	34.5 ± 9.2	36.7 ± 8.2	32.8 ± 10.7
	General	45.5 ± 13.0	47.1 ± 13.6	53.9 ± 13.2	49.7 ± 10.1
T-suppressor (OKT$_8$+) (%)	Spinal	24.6 ± 6.1	20.8 ± 5.3	21.2 ± 5.1	18.6 ± 6.8
	General	23.3 ± 6.9	22.5 ± 10.1	20.4 ± 7.0	22.7 ± 11.6
B-lymphocytes (anti-Ig+) (%)	Spinal	9.3 ± 3.6	8.0 ± 3.5	9.9 ± 4.1	8.4 ± 3.9[a]
	General	8.4 ± 4.2	8.0 ± 4.7	9.4 ± 8.2	8.0 ± 6.6
NK-cells (Leu$_7$+) (%)	Spinal	10.9 ± 5.9	9.1 ± 5.0	11.1 ± 3.7	10.7 ± 5.0
	General	13.2 ± 7.2	10.5 ± 5.2	11.1 ± 6.1	11.5 ± 6.8

[a] $P < 0.05$, [b] $P < 0.01$ compared with preoperative values. No differences between groups. (From Salo & Nissila,[68] with permission.)

INFLUENCE OF ANESTHETIC CHOICE ON THE ENDOCRINE–METABOLIC RESPONSE TO SURGERY

The physiologic response to surgery or other traumatic injury is an enormously complex interaction of neural and humoral events referred to collectively as the *stress response*. The response is generally initiated by afferent neural activity triggered by a noxious stimulus. The noxious stimulus may also locally affect the levels of a variety of vasoactive tissue factors such as prostaglandins, substance P, histamine, and serotonin.[69] An additional systemic endocrine–metabolic response occurs with hemorrhage, sepsis, hypoxia, and acidosis (among others).[70] Though perhaps teleologically a protective reaction to injury, the stress response may at times be detrimental to the care of surgical patients.[71]

The stress response to surgery is characterized by a general increase in catabolism (associated with an increase in catabolic hormones such as adrenocorticotropic hormone, cortisol, antidiuretic hormone, growth hormone, etc.) and a decrease in anabolism (associated with a decrease in anabolic hormones). Carbohydrate metabolism is altered and hyperglycemia associated with impaired insulin release is common.[72] Hepatic glycogenolysis and gluconeogenesis increase in response to a number of hormonal influences including cortisol, epinephrine, growth hormone, and others. Catabolic effects on protein include breakdown of muscle and increased lipolysis causes breakdown of fat. The focus of this section is the influence of regional and general anesthesia on the stress response to surgery rather than a detailed analysis of the stress response itself.

Anesthesia clearly is an important modulator of the stress response to surgery. In usual clinical concentrations, most intravenous and volatile anesthetic agents have a comparatively small influence on the endocrine–metabolic response to surgery.[73,74] Notable exceptions to this rule include the rarely used explosive volatile anesthetics, ether and cyclopropane, which have stimulatory effects on the sympathetic nervous system and the adrenal cortex, and the more commonly used intravenous anesthetics, etomidate and narcotics (in high doses), which have an inhibitory effect. Etomidate selectively interferes with cortisol synthesis via inhibition of the enzyme 11-β-hydroxylase,[75] an effect that has limited its general clinical use. "High-dose" narcotic anesthesia, presently used primarily for cardiovascular surgery, has a well-documented ability to suppress most of the endocrine–metabolic stress response to surgery,[73,74,76] but requires prolonged mechanical ventilation postoperatively, precluding its use in the vast majority of orthopedic surgical patients.[77]

Several studies have addressed the effect of central neuraxial blockade on the stress response to surgery.[78–84] There is ample evidence that spinal or epidural anesthesia can attenuate or abolish this response. At least two studies have included orthopedic surgical patients.

A study by Davis et al[85] examined the metabolic response to total hip arthroplasty in 101 patients randomized to receive either spinal or general anesthesia. In 93 of these patients, whole blood glucose concentrations were measured before and after surgery and in 77 plasma cortisol levels were measured pre- and postoperatively as well. No preoperative differences were identified between the groups. Whole blood glucose concentrations were slightly increased following anesthetic induction in both groups (the transient increase in blood glucose concentration in the group receiving spinal anesthesia was attributed to the stress of the spinal anesthetic procedure itself). However, subsequent blood glucose levels decreased in the spinal anesthesia group, while in the general anesthesia group they continued to significantly rise (Fig. 4-5). Plasma cortisol concentrations did not differ preoperatively between the two groups, but when measured 30 minutes postoperatively, the level was unchanged in the spinal anesthesia group and markedly increased in the group receiving general anesthesia (Fig. 4-6). These results are of particular interest to the practitioner of orthopedic anesthesia since they were assessed in patients undergoing total hip arthroplasty with relatively low sensory dermatomal levels and differ from results of other investi-

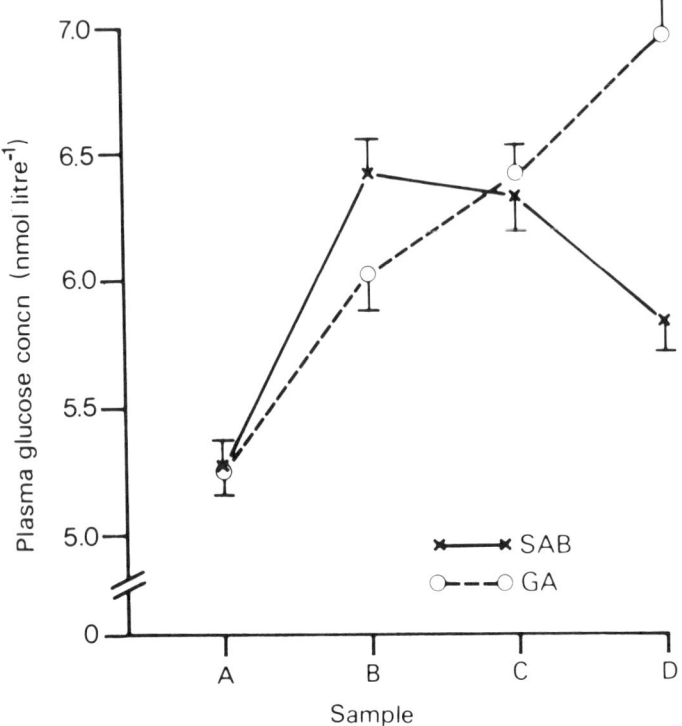

Fig. 4-5. Whole blood glucose concentrations (mean, SEM) in 93 patients during total hip arthroplasty under either spinal (SAB) or general (GA) anesthesia. See text for timing of samples and statistical analysis. (From Davis et al,[85] with permission.)

gators studying patients undergoing intra-abdominal procedures where suppression of the neuroendocrine response required extensive afferent blockade.[86,87]

A second study that included orthopedic surgical procedures (as well as urologic, inguinal herniorrhaphy, and perineal procedures) performed by Halter and Pflug[72] examined the influence of spinal or general anesthesia on perioperative metabolic function. Hyperglycemia and impaired insulin responses to intravenous glucose occurred in the general anesthesia group but not in the group that received spinal anesthesia. These results

were at least in part attributable to an increased level of circulating catecholamines in the general anesthesia group. The catecholamine response was abolished in the patients undergoing spinal anesthesia.

In summary, it is clear that anesthetic choice may have a profound influence on perioperative endocrine–metabolic function, the clinical significance of which remains to be fully elucidated. The endocrinologic–metabolic implications of continuous neuraxial blockade for postoperative pain management are largely unexplored in orthopedic surgical patients and may be significant.

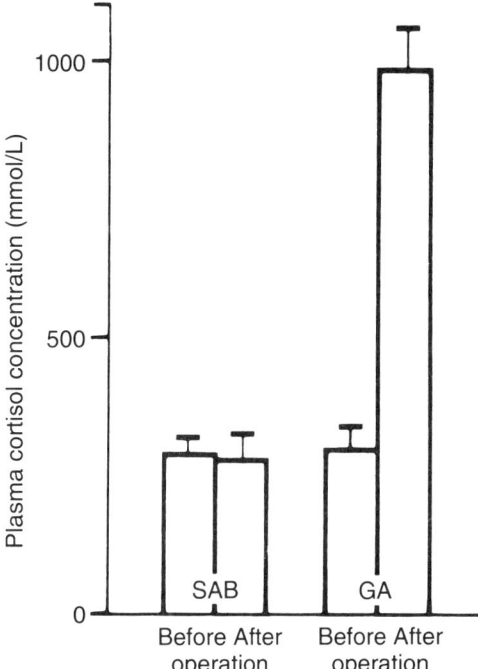

Fig. 4-6. Plasma cortisol concentrations (mean, SEM) preinduction and 30 minutes after surgery in 77 patients undergoing total hip arthroplasty under either spinal (SAB, n = 38) or general (GA, n = 39) anesthesia. See text for statistical analysis. (From Davis et al,[85] with permission.)

INFLUENCE OF ANESTHETIC CHOICE ON PULMONARY FUNCTION

Many anesthesia providers believe that central neuraxial blockade is associated with improved perioperative pulmonary function and prefer regional techniques in patients with pulmonary compromise. Avoidance of endotracheal intubation, a potent stimulus of bronchospasm, is often cited as an advantage and the decrease in functional residual capacity associated with general anesthesia may be reduced or avoided. Despite these commonly held beliefs, the available literature suggests, but does not unequivocally support, a significant advantage of regional over general anesthesia as the choice for intraoperative anesthesia based on pulmonary function.[88,89]

By contrast, there is considerable evidence that postoperative regional analgesia is efficacious in preventing pulmonary complications. Postoperative regional analgesia is associated with improved diaphragmatic function and improved pulmonary volumes and flows when compared with pain management using parenteral narcotics.[90,91] Pulmonary infections have also been shown to be reduced in some[1,92] but not all series.[93,94]

It must be recognized, however, that the studies that demonstrated an improved pulmonary outcome primarily involved relatively high-risk patients undergoing upper abdominal, vascular, and thoracic operations.[1,95,96] Since some studies examined combined intraoperative regional and general anesthesia, with regional analgesia continued postoperatively, interpretation of cause and effect is difficult. An important question to answer is whether an improvement in pulmonary outcome is caused by the choice of intraoperative anesthesia, postoperative pain management, or both. At present, the answer to this question is not established. Direct application of these results to orthopedic surgical patients is confounded by differences in the physical status of the studied patients; complexity, site, and extent of the operations; exact anesthetic and analgesic regimens; use of central local anesthetics and/or narcotics for pain; and the measures of pulmonary function examined. Whether the improved pulmonary function associated with central neuraxial anesthesia/analgesia in some studies is specifically transferable to orthopedic surgical patients and procedures is of considerable interest.

Peripheral nerve blocks may also influence respiratory function. Interscalene blocks usually block the phrenic nerve, and concerns have been raised about respiratory failure if bilateral phrenic blockade occurs. Certainly patients should be informed about the possible sensation of dyspnea that may occur even with unilateral blockade.[97] Simple reassurance about the adequacy of respiration is often all that is required, although judicious sedation may be advisable and, in rare instances, positive pressure ventilation may be necessary. Horner syndrome may also occur, especially if large volumes of local anesthetic are used.

Respiratory compromise may also be caused by pneumothorax, the most common serious complication of supraclavicular blockade. Pneumothorax occurs with an incidence of 0.5 to 6 percent depending primarily on the experience of the practitioner.[97] Most pneumothoraces develop slowly (over several hours) and may be undetected during the early postoperative period. If the pneumothorax is clinically significant, chest tube placement may be necessary. This is a particularly troublesome complication if the patient would otherwise not have required hospitalization. As with interscalene blocks, the phrenic nerve may be blocked during a supraclavicular block (in 40 to 60 percent of cases) with potential for respiratory compromise.[98]

Intercostal nerve blocks and interpleural techniques may improve pulmonary function after intrathoracic surgery such as spinal surgery using an anterior approach. However, these techniques have often been replaced by postoperative epidural analgesia using narcotics and/or local anesthetics.[99]

A clinical controversy exists about the appropriateness of regional anesthesia in patients who have difficult airways. Many practitioners recommend regional anesthesia for these patients so that laryngoscopy and intubation can be avoided. Others argue that since the avoidance of intubation cannot be guaranteed, a secure airway and general anesthesia is indicated. If the decision is made to proceed with regional anesthesia, caution is warranted. Continuous spinal anesthesia has the advantage of avoiding the possibility of local anesthetic toxicity and allowing careful titration of the block to the lowest dermatomal level consistent with the operative requirements. In situations where a larger volume of local anesthetic is required (such as epidural or axillary anesthesia), repeated aspiration and incremental dosing is suggested. If regional anesthesia is chosen, it is very important to establish that the block is sufficient for the procedure, especially if the positioning of the patient will impede airway access. An alternative to consider is to combine regional with "light general" anesthesia, thus allowing the airway to be secured.

INFLUENCE OF ANESTHETIC CHOICE ON CARDIOVASCULAR FUNCTION

Central neuraxial blockade has predictable cardiovascular consequences that are greatly influenced by the anesthetic dermatomal level. Preload and afterload are generally unchanged or decreased, due primarily to the vasodilation associated with sympathetic blockade. Though these decreases in preload and afterload decrease myocardial oxygen demand, there is conflicting evidence regarding their influence in patients at risk for myocardial ischemia. For example, Baron et al[63] reported an improvement in cardiac function using radionuclide imaging of myocardial wall motion abnormalities associated with lumbar epidural anesthesia, while Saada et al[100] reported the opposite (an increased number of echocardiographically visualized wall motion abnormalities associated with a decrease in diastolic pressure in patients undergoing lumbar epidural blockade). It is also important to note that in patients who have relatively fixed cardiac outputs (e.g., aortic stenosis or hypertrophic obstructive cardiomyopathy) the decrease in preload and afterload associated with central neuraxial blockade may critically impair overall cardiac performance.

Heart rate, another major determinant of myocardial oxygen supply and demand, may be decreased by central neuraxial blockade because of blockade of the cardioaccelerator fibers (sympathetic blockade), a decrease in the neurohumoral response to pain, or increased vagal tone. The dermatomal level is a critical factor influencing the heart rate response since the cardioaccelerator fibers originate from the upper thoracic spinal cord (T1–T4). The physiologic effects of central neuraxial blockade on the cardiovascular system must be understood and carefully assessed before proceeding with the choice of a given anesthetic.

Cardiovascular disease is the single most important cause of surgical mortality in high-risk patients,[101] and many questions about the cardiovascular effects of anesthetic choice remain unanswered. Examination of the incidence of perioperative myocardial reinfarction comparing regional and general anesthetic techniques by Rao et al,[102] Steen et al,[103] and Backer et al[104] have shown no difference in myocardial reinfarction rate between groups anesthetized with regional or general anesthesia.

Rao et al[102] studied the incidence of and factors related to recurrent perioperative myocardial infarction in noncardiac surgical patients. Their study was designed to evaluate the effect of advanced hemodynamic monitoring and aggressive pharmacologic intervention in a group of patients who had a history of myocardial infarction and were scheduled for noncardiac surgery. They compared this group to a historical control group of similar patients whose anesthetic management did not involve sophisticated monitoring and vasoactive pharmacologic therapy. The cardiovascular effects of regional anesthesia and five different types of general anesthesia were also evaluated. No significant differences between the regional anesthesia group and all but one of the general anesthesia groups were apparent (Table 4-7). The general anesthesia group, consisting of patients receiving nitrous oxide, oxygen, a muscle relaxant, and narcotics, had a statistically significant increase in the incidence of reinfarction when compared to the regional group and each of the other three general anesthesia groups.

Backer et al[103] retrospectively studied 195 patients with history of a previous documented myocardial infarction who underwent 288 ophthalmic procedures under local or retrobulbar block anesthesia and compared this group to a much smaller group (26 procedures performed on 21 patients) receiving general anesthesia for similar procedures. They reported no myocardial reinfarctions in either group. Although their data did not support a significant difference between the groups they speculated that local anesthesia may be associated with a lesser risk of perioperative reinfarction than general or central neuraxial anesthesia based on their incidence in other studies. It is possible the low incidence of reinfarction was due to the relatively minor nature of the surgery rather than the type of anesthetic.

Steen et al[104] reviewed the records of 587 patients with a documented history of prior myocardial infarction who required anesthesia for a subsequent procedure. Thirty-six patients had another myocardial infarction (6.1 percent) and 25

Table 4-7. Relation Between Anesthetic Drugs Used and Incidence of Reinfarction

	Group 1		Group 2	
Anesthetic Used	No. of Patients	No. of Patients	No. of Patients	No. of Patients
Nitrous oxide, oxygen, relaxant, and halothane	99	8	146	1[a]
Nitrous oxide, oxygen, relaxant, and enflurane	75	7	196	3[a]
Nitrous oxide, oxygen, relaxant, and narcotics	112	8	101	7[c]
Oxygen, relaxant, and narcotics	31	3	216	1[b]
Regional anesthesia	47	2	74	2

Reinfarction incidence for the same anesthetic compared with group 1; [a] $P < 0.05$; [b] $P < 0.005$.

Reinfarction incidence in nitrous oxide + oxygen + relaxant + narcotic subgroup compared with other anesthetics in group 2; [c] $P < 0.005$.

(From Rao et al,[102] with permission.)

of the 36 (69 percent) died. Sixty-six of the 587 patients received regional anesthesia (50 spinals, 3 epidurals, 8 caudals, and 5 brachial plexus blocks) and the balance received general anesthesia. No differences in reinfarction rate occurred between the groups (Table 4-8). Both cases of reinfarction that occurred in the group receiving regional anesthesia were in patients undergoing spinal anesthesia for transurethral resection of the prostate (TURP). When only TURP cases were considered, 44 received spinal anesthesia and 52 received general anesthesia. Two reinfarctions occurred in the group receiving spinal anesthesia and one in the group receiving general anesthesia. The difference was not statistically significant.

Prough et al reported a series of patients who underwent carotid endarterectomy under regional anesthesia (superficial cervical plexus block). As might be expected, there was a high incidence of

Table 4-8. Relation of Myocardial Reinfarction to Anesthetic Technique

Thiopental Sodium, Oxygen, and Nitrous Oxide	No. of Patients	No. of Patients
With enflurane	234	14 (6.4)
With halothane	68	5 (7.4)
With fentanyl citrate or droperidol	146	10 (6.8)
With diethyl ether	11	1 (9.1)
Subarachnoid block (spinal)	50	2 (4.0)
Other	78	3 (3.8)

(From Steen et al,[103] with permission.)

previous myocardial infarction in this series (38 of 153 patients, 25 percent). There were no apparent myocardial infarctions in any of the 105 patients, who collectively underwent 185 carotid endarterectomies. The lack of a control group that received general anesthesia makes interpretation of this study difficult.

Dysrhythmias, usually benign, often occur during the perioperative period. The incidence of dysrhythmias in patients undergoing regional or general anesthesia has been compared by Goldman et al[105] and McGowan et al.[59] Neither investigator showed a significant difference between the groups.

There is some evidence that anesthetic choice may influence patients with congestive heart failure (CHF). Yeager et al[1] in a study of high-risk patients undergoing thoracic, upper abdominal, and vascular surgery showed a significant difference in the development of heart failure (1 of 28 patients receiving epidural plus "light general" anesthesia developed perioperative CHF compared to 10 of 25 patients receiving general anesthesia). It is important to note, however, that postoperative pain was also managed differently in these patients (epidural narcotics compared to conventional parenteral narcotic therapy), making precise interpretation of the results more difficult. Goldman et al[105] similarly compared patients undergoing spinal or general anesthesia for a variety of procedures and also showed a significant increase in the rate of development of new CHF or worsening of existent CHF in the group receiving general anesthesia.

On balance, although it is likely anesthetic choice may influence cardiovascular morbidity in some patients, there remain few certain indications of the superiority of any regional or general anesthetic technique regarding cardiovascular outcome. This is clearly an extremely important issue to practitioners

of orthopedic anesthesia because of the high prevalence of older patients, many of whom have occult or overt heart disease, undergoing procedures that can often be readily managed by either regional or general anesthesia.

INFLUENCE OF ANESTHETIC CHOICE ON TOURNIQUET PAIN

Tourniquet pain is a troublesome problem in some orthopedic surgical patients, associated with inflation of an extremity tourniquet to technically facilitate surgery and decrease blood loss. Patients complain of an ill-defined aching or burning sensation generally beginning 45 to 60 minutes after tourniquet inflation. It is believed to be mediated by small, unmyelinated C fibers and is relieved by deflation of the tourniquet for 10 to 15 minutes, after which the tourniquet may be reinflated. It also may be relieved by increased sedation but at times is so severe that administration of general anesthesia is required. A physiologic response to tourniquet use has been described in patients under general anesthesia as well, presumably caused by the same mechanisms as tourniquet pain. Valli and Rosenberg studied 51 patients undergoing lower extremity surgery that included use of a thigh tourniquet for 60 minutes or longer. They reported an increase in systolic or diastolic arterial pressures of more than 30 percent[106] in 8 of the 15 patients undergoing enflurance general anesthesia, 1 of the 15 patients receiving bupivacaine epidural anesthesia, and none of the 15 patients receiving bupivacaine subarachnoid anesthesia. Rocco et al[107] also demonstrated a significant hypertensive response in patients anesthetized with enflurance or halothane but not with spinal or epidural anesthesia. Central neuraxial blockade may be an effective technique to avoid tourniquet pain and its physiologic consequences.

INFLUENCE OF ANESTHETIC CHOICE ON MORTALITY AFTER HIP SURGERY

The most important issue to consider when comparing regional and general anesthesia for orthopedic surgery is outcome. This issue has been addressed in prospective randomized studies of patients undergoing hip surgery performed by several investigators. The results of some of these studies for femoral fracture and total hip arthroplasty patients are reviewed.

Mortality After Operative Fixation of Femur Fracture

Fracture of the upper femur is a common orthopedic injury, the incidence of which increases with age. The mean age of patients suffering upper femoral fractures is 75 to 80 years.[108,109] Women represent 70 to 80 percent of these patients, due in part to the predominance of women in the elderly age groups and in part to the prevalence of osteoporosis in older women.[110] Increased longevity will probably make this condition increasingly common. Many of these patients present with numerous medical problems and performance designations of ASA III or IV occur in about 60 percent of the patients in some series.[111] Serious cardiopulmonary disease is common. Berggren et al[50] report a history of ischemic heart disease in about half of these patients and preoperative hypoxemia (arterial oxygen tension less than 60 mmHg) while breathing room air in nearly one-quarter. Internal fixation of upper femoral fractures is frequently performed under regional (spinal or epidural) or general anesthesia. Mortality may be significant, with published hospital mortality rates of 2.7 to 28 percent.[112,113] Since mortality is the best-defined morbid outcome, we review the results of several investigators who have studied its incidence in patients undergoing internal fixation of hip fractures.

Valentin et al[114] performed a randomized prospective study including 578 patients over 50 years of age undergoing internal fixation or hip replacement for management of upper femoral fractures. The patients were randomized to receive spinal or general anesthesia and patient survival was studied until 10 months after inclusion of the last patient in the study. Although patients in the spinal anesthesia group had significantly less blood loss, no difference in early (up to 30 days) or long-term (2 years) survival was apparent. Mortality was significantly less in women and among patients with femoral neck fractures rather than trochanteric fractures. Mortality significantly increased with increased age. No difference in mortality was apparent between the two general anesthesia groups (enflurane/nitrous oxide or neuroleptanesthesia).

In another prospective randomized study, Davis et al[115] compared spinal and general anesthesia in a multicenter study of 538 patients age 55 and older undergoing internal fixation of upper femoral fractures. After follow-up of 3 to 30 months, no difference in short- or long-term mortality was shown. Increased age, ischemic heart disease, congestive heart failure, preoperative dysrhythmias, and poorer ASA status were associated with increased mortality.

Similarly, McKenzie et al[116] in a randomized prospective investigation studied 148 patients receiving spinal or general anesthesia for internal fixation of upper femoral fractures. Interestingly, they reported a statistically significant decreased mortality 14 days postoperatively in the spinal anesthesia group but no such difference at the end of 2 months (patients were followed for at least 12 months postoperatively) (Fig. 4-7). Although a number of other outcome studies have been performed (Table 4-9), the only other prospective randomized trial showing a difference in mortality comparing spinal and general anesthesia for internal fixation of hip fracture was reported by McLaren et al.[117] Their study was conducted on 55 patients comparing spinal and general anesthesia and re-

ported a 1-month mortality of 31 percent in the general anesthesia group and 3.6 percent in the spinal anesthesia group. This study has been criticized for both the small sample size and the surprisingly high mortality in the general anesthesia group.

Epidural anesthesia has also been compared to general anesthesia in hip fracture patients. Wickstrom et al[118] compared mortality after internal fixation of hip fractures using epidural anesthesia or one of four general anesthetic techniques. No differences in mortality were apparent based on the type of anesthesia.

On balance, the literature does not support a difference in long-term mortality in

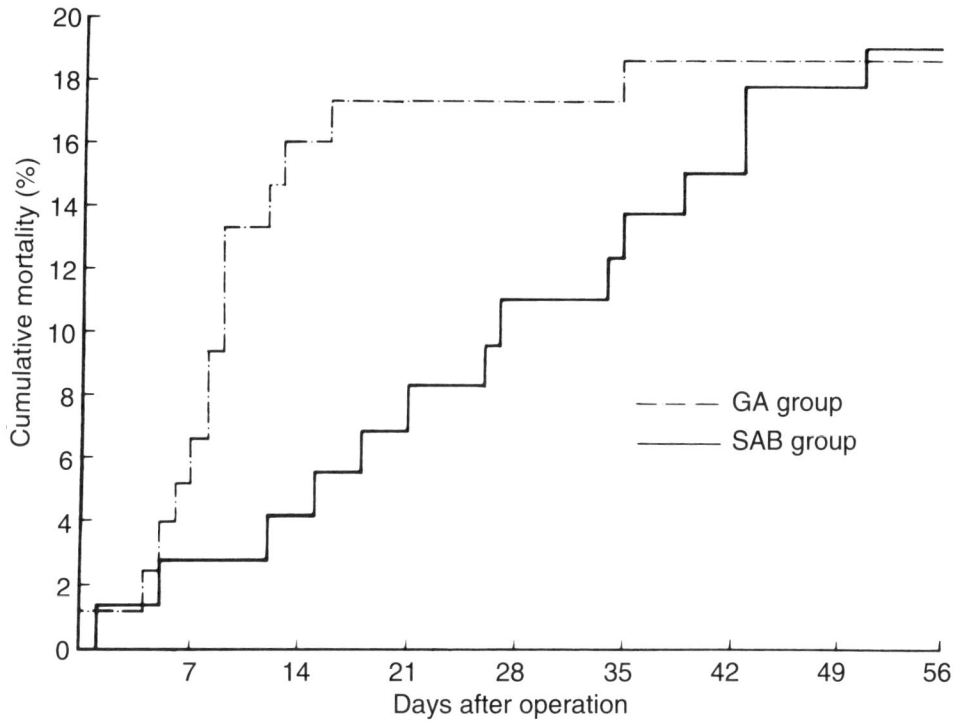

Fig. 4-7. Cumulative total mortality in each group in first 56 days after operation. Individual deaths occurred on the following days after operation: General anesthesia (GA) group (n = 75; 14 deaths): 0, 4, 5, 6, 7, 8, 8, 9, 9, 9, 12, 13, 16, 35; subarachnoid blockade (SAB) group (n = 73; 14 deaths): 1, 5, 12, 15, 18, 21, 26, 27, 34, 35, 36, 43, 43, 43, 51. (From McKenzie et al,[116] with permission.)

Table 4-9. Randomized, Prospective Studies of the Effect of Anesthetic Technique on Mortality After Hip Fracture Surgery

Study	Techniques Compared	Observation Time	Significant Mortality Difference
McLaren et al	SA, GA	1 mo	Yes (GA > SA)
McKenzie et al	SA, GA	1 mo	No
White et al	SA, GA, psoas block	1 mo	No
Davis et al	SA, GA	1 mo	No
Wickstrom et al	EA, GA	1 mo	No
McKenzie et al	SA, GA	2 wk	Yes (GA > SA)
		2 mo	No
Valentin et al	SA, GA	1 mo	No
Davis et al	SA, GA	1 mo	No

SA, spinal anesthesia; GA, general anesthesia; EA, epidural anesthesia.
(From Covert & Fox,[124] with permission.)

patients undergoing surgery for upper femoral fracture when regional and general anesthesia are compared.

Mortality After Total Hip Arthroplasty

Elective total hip arthroplasty is a commonly performed procedure usually indicated by chronic arthritis of the hip. Nearly half of the patients who undergo total hip arthroplasty have degenerative arthritis and about 7 percent have rheumatoid arthritis.[119] It is a procedure commonly performed on older patients (about 60 percent are over 65 years),[120] who are generally more healthy (about 80 percent are ASA I or II)[121] than those undergoing surgery for hip fractures. Spinal or epidural anesthesia (often via continuous techniques) are well suited for the anesthetic care of these patients. The major operative concerns include blood loss, bone cement implantation syndrome (and other embolic phenomena), and cardiovascular stability during the procedure. Airway difficulties are often encountered

as well, particularly in patients with rheumatoid arthritis or ankylosing spondylitis, who may have considerable limitation of neck and jaw movement. The appropriateness of regional anesthesia for these procedures has been debated. Some have expressed concern over the poor access to the airway in patients who are in the lateral decubitus position should heavy sedation or general anesthesia be required. Our experience has been that intubation of patients with normal airway anatomy in the lateral decubitus position is highly successful. Consideration of combined regional/general techniques with preoperative awake fiberoptic intubation may be appropriate in some patients with significant airway compromise. Advantages of regional anesthesia in these patients include the decreases in morbidity (decreased blood loss, decreased incidence of DVT/PTE, etc.) discussed earlier. Despite these decreases in morbidity, regional anesthesia has not been shown to significantly decrease perioperative mortality which is low[122] in patients undergoing this procedure.

In summary regional anesthesia is an

effective anesthetic for large numbers of orthopedic surgical patients. It offers advantages, both proven and assumed, over general anesthesia and is popular with our patients, surgeons, and nursing personnel. We consider mastery of the provision of regional anesthesia to be an important part of our training program. The potential benefit of regional techniques for postoperative pain relief is considerable and is increasingly recognized. We fully expect regional anesthesia to continue to play a fundamental role in the practice of anesthesiology for surgical anesthesia (both alone and in combination with general anesthesia) and postoperative care. It is important to continually assess the effect of anesthetic choice on medical and surgical outcome. A thoughtfully prepared anesthetic plan, derived after consideration of many factors, provides the patient with the best available care. The choice between regional and general anesthesia should be made on rational grounds. The techniques are not in opposition to one another and should be selected alone or together as the clinical situation dictates. Advances in the understanding of specific central receptors, agonists, and antagonists hold promise for the future.

REFERENCES

1. Yeager MP, Glass DD, Neff RK, Brinck-Johnsen T: Epidural anesthesia and analgesia in high-risk surgical patients. Anesthesiology 66:729, 1987
2. Tuman KJ, McCarthy RJ, March RJ et al: Effects of epidural anesthesia and analgesia on coagulation and outcome after major vascular surgery. Anesth Analg 73:696, 1991
3. Modig J, Borg T, Karlstrom G et al: Thromboembolism after total hip replacement: role of epidural and general anesthesia. Anesth Analg 62:174, 1983
4. Modig J, Hjelmsted A, Sahlstedt B, Maripuu E: Comparative influences of epidural and general anaesthesia on deep venous thrombosis and pulmonary embolism after total hip replacement. Acta Chir Scand 147:125, 1981
5. Modig J, Borg T, Bagge L, Saldeen T: Role of extradural and of general anaesthesia in fibrinolysis and coagulation after total hip replacement. Br J Anaesth 55:625, 1983
6. Wille-Jorgensen P, Christensen SW, Bjerg-Nielsen A et al: Prevention of thromboembolism following elective hip surgery. Clin Orthop 247:163, 1989
7. Keith I: Anaesthesia and blood loss in total hip replacement. Anaesthesia 32:444, 1977
8. Modig J, Malmberg P: Pulmonary and circulatory reactions during total hip replacement surgery. Acta Anaesthesiol Scand 19:219, 1975
9. Hull RD, Raskob GE, Hirsh J: Prophylaxis of venous thromboembolism: an overview. Chest 89(suppl):374, 1986
10. Johnson R, Green JR, Charnley J: Pulmonary embolism and its prophylaxis following the Charnley total hip replacement. Clin Orthop 127:123, 1977
11. Cohen SH, Ehrlich GE, Kauffman MS, Cope C: Thrombophlebitis following knee surgery. J Bone Joint Surg [Am] 55:106, 1973
12. Hull R, Delmore TJ, Hirsh J et al: Effectiveness of intermittent pulsatile elastic stockings for the prevention of calf and thigh vein thrombosis in patients undergoing elective knee surgery. Thromb Res 16:37, 1979
13. McKenna R, Bachmann F, Kaushal SP, Galante JO: Thromboembolic disease in patients undergoing total knee replacement. J Bone Joint Surg [Am] 58:928, 1976
14. McKenna R, Galante J, Bachmann F et al: Prevention of venous thromboembolism after total knee replacement by high-dose aspirin or intermittent calf and thigh compression. Br Med J 280:514, 1980
15. Stringer MD, Steadman CA, Hedges AR et al: Deep vein thrombosis after elec-

tive knee surgery. An incidence study in 312 patients. J Bone Joint Surg [Br] 71:492, 1989

16. Stulberg BN, Insall JN, Williams GW, Ghelman B: Deep-vein thrombosis following total knee replacement. An analysis of six hundred and thirty-eight arthroplasties. J Bone Joint Surg [Am] 66:194, 1984

17. Coon WW: Risk factors in pulmonary embolism. Surg Gynecol Obstet 143:385, 1976

18. Schafer AI: The hypercoagulable states. Ann Intern Med 102:814, 1985

19. Sevitt S, Gallagher N: Venous thrombosis and pulmonary embolism: a clinicopathological study in injured and burned patients. Br J Surg 48:475, 1961

20. Davis FM, Quince M, Laurenson VG: Deep vein thrombosis and anaesthetic technique in emergency surgery. Br Med J 182:1528, 1980

21. Thornburn J, Louden JR, Wallance R: Spinal and general anaesthesia in total hip replacement: frequency of deep vein thrombosis. Br J Anaesth 52:1117, 1980

22. Davis FM, Laurenson VG, Gillespie WJ et al: Deep vein thrombosis after total hip replacement. J Bone Joint Surg [Br] 71B:181, 1989

23. McKenzie PJ, Wishart HY, Gray J, Smith G: Effects of anesthetic technique on deep vein thrombosis. Br J Anaesth 57:853, 1985

24. Sharrock NE, Haas SB, Hargett MJ et al: Effects of epidural anesthesia on the incidence of deep-vein thrombosis after total knee arthroplasty. J Bone Joint Surg [Am] 73:502, 1991

25. Nielsen PT, Jorgensen LN, Albrecht-Beste E et al: Lower thrombosis risk with epidural blockade in knee arthroplasty. Acta Orthop Scand 61:29, 1990

26. Modig J, Malmberg P, Karlstrom G: Effect of epidural versus general anaesthesia on calf blood flow. Acta Anaesthesiol Scand 24:305, 1980

27. Davis FM, Laurenson VG, Gillespie WJ et al: Leg blood flow during total hip replacement under spinal or general anaesthesia. Anaesth Intensive Care 17:136, 1989

28. Foate JA, Horton H, Davis FM: Lower limb blood flow during transurethral resection of the prostate under spinal or general anaesthesia. Anaesth Intensive Care 13:383, 1985

29. Modig J, Malmberg P, Saldeen T: Comparative effects of epidural and general anesthesia on fibrinolysis function, lower limb rheology and thromboembolism after total hip replacement. Anesthesiology 53(suppl):S34, 1980

30. Modig J, Hjelmstedt A, Sahlstedt B et al: The influence of epidural versus general anaesthesia on the incidence of thromboembolism after total hip replacement. p. 121. In Wust HJ, Zindler M (eds): Anaesthesiologie und Intensivmedizin. Vol. 138. Springer-Verlag, Berlin, 1981

31. Modig J, Borg T, Karlstrom G et al: Epidural versus general anaesthesia. Influence on fibrinolysis and coagulation after total hip replacement. Br J Anaesth 55:625, 1983

32. Giddon DB, Lindhe J: In vivo quantitation of local anesthetic suppression of leukocyte adherence. Am J Pathol 68:327, 1972

33. Stewart GJ, Ritchie WGM, Lynch PR: Venous endothelial damage produced by massive sticking and emigration of leukocytes. Am J Pathol 74:507, 1974

34. Luostarinen V, Evers H, Lyytikainen M-T et al: Antithrombotic effects of lidocaine and related compounds on laser-induced microvascular injury. Acta Anaesthesiol Scand 25:9, 1981

35. Cooke ED, Bowcock SA, Lloyd MJ, Pilcher MF: Intravenous lignocaine in prevention of deep venous thrombosis after elective hip surgery. Lancet 2:797, 1977

36. Donadoni R, Baele G, Devulder J, Rolly G: Coagulation and fibrinolytic parameters in patients undergoing total hip replacement: influence of the anaesthesia technique. Acta Anaesthesiol Scand 33:588, 1989

37. Davis FM, McDermott E, Hickton C et al: Influence of spinal and general anaesthesia on haemostasis during total hip arthroplasty. Br J Anaesth 59:561, 1987

38. Simpson PJ, Radford SG, Forster SJ et al: The fibrinolytic effects of anaesthesia. Anaesthesia 37:3, 1982

39. Stoelting RK, Dierdorf SF, McCammon RL: Pulmonary embolism. p. 187. In Anesthesia and Co-existing Disease. Churchill Livingstone, New York, 1988

40. Murphy TM: Spinal, epidural, and caudal anesthesia. p. 1061. In Miller RD (ed): Anesthesia. 2nd Ed. Churchill Livingstone, New York, 1986

41. Gurewich V, Nunn T, Kuriakose X, Hume M: Hemostatic effects of uniform, low-dose subcutaneous heparin in surgical patients. Arch Intern Med 138:41, 1978

42. Gallus AS, Hirsh J, Tuttle RJ et al: Small subcutaneous doses of heparin in prevention of venous thrombosis. N Engl J Med 288:545, 1973

43. Planes A, Vochelle N, Ferre J et al: Efficacy and safety of enoxaparin in prevention of deep venous thrombosis after total hip replacement under spinal anesthesia. Comparison with general anesthesia. Thromb Haemost 62:489A, 1989

44. Prins MH, Hirsh J: A comparison of general anesthesia and regional anesthesia as a risk factor for deep vein thrombosis following hip surgery: a critical review. Thromb Haemost 64:497, 1990

45. Owens EL, Kasten GW, Hessell EA: Spinal subarachnoid hematoma after lumbar puncture and heparinization: a case report, review of the literature, and discussion of anesthetic implications. Anesth Analg 65:1201, 1986

46. Millar HR: Psychiatric morbidity in elderly surgical patients. Br J Psychiatry 138:17, 1981

47. Riis J, Lombholt B, Haxholdt O et al: Immediate and long-term mental recovery from general versus epidural anesthesia in elderly patients. Acta Anaesthesiol Scand 27:44, 1983

48. Blundell E: A psychological study of the effects of surgery on eighty six elderly surgical patients. Br J Soc Clin Psychol 6:297, 1967

49. Hole A, Tergesen T, Breivik H: Epidural vs general anaesthesia for total hip arthroplasty in elderly patients. Acta Anaesthesiol Scand 24:279, 1980

50. Berggren D, Gustafson Y, Eriksson B et al: Postoperative confusion after anaesthesia in elderly patients with femoral neck fractures. Anesth Analg 66:497, 1987

51. Nielson WR, Gelb AW, Casey JE et al: Long-term cognitive and social sequelae of general versus regional anesthesia during arthroplasty in the elderly. Anesthesiology 73:1103, 1990

52. Ghoneim MM, Hinrichs JV, O'Hara MW et al: Comparison of psychologic and cognitive functions after general or regional anesthesia. Anesthesiology 69:507, 1988

53. Hughes D, Bowes JB, Brown MW: Changes in memory following general or spinal anaesthesia for hip arthroplasty. Anaesthesia 43:114, 1988

54. Jones MJT, Piggott SE, Vaughan RS et al: Cognitive and functional competence after anesthesia in patients aged over 60: controlled trial of general and regional anaesthesia for elective hip or knee replacement. Br Med J 300:1683, 1990

55. Bigler D, Adelhoj B, Petring OU et al: Mental function and morbidity after acute hip surgery during spinal and general anaesthesia. Anaesthesia 40:672, 1985

56. Miller L, Gertel M, Fox GS, MacLean LD: Comparison of effect of narcotic and epidural analgesia on postoperative respiratory function. Am J Surg 131:291, 1976

57. Patel JM, Lanzafame RJ, Williams JS et al: The effect of incisional infiltration of bupivacaine hydrochloride upon pulmonary functions, atelectasis and narcotic need following elective cholecystectomy. Surg Gynecol Obstet 157:338, 1983

58. Hendolin H: The influence of continuous epidural analgesia and general anaesthesia on the peri- and postoperative course of patients subjected to retropubic prostatectomy. Thesis, University of Kuopio, Finland, 1980

59. McGowan SW, Smith GFN: Anaesthesia for transurethral prostatectomy: a comparison of spinal intradural analgesia with two methods of general anaesthesia. Anaesthesia 35:847, 1980

60. Tolksdorf W, Raiss G, Streibel J-P, Lutz H: Intra und postoperative Kardiopulmonale Komplikationen bei transurethralen Prostataresektionen in Intubationsnarkose und ruckenmarksnaher leitungsanasthesie. p. 146. In Wust HJ, Zindler M (eds): Neue Aspekte in der Regional-Anasthesie I. Springer-Verlag, Berlin, 1980

61. Crawford ED, Skinner DG: Intercostal nerve block with thoracoabdominal and flank incisions. Urology 14:25, 1982

62. Pflug AE, Murphy TM, Butler SH, Tucker GT: The effects of postoperative peridural analgesia on pulmonary therapy and pulmonary complications. Anesthesiology 41:8, 1974

63. Baron JF, Coriat P, Mundler O et al: Left ventricular global and regional function during lumbar epidural anesthesia in patients with and without angina pectoris. Influence of volume loading. Anesthesiology 66:621, 1987

64. Walton B: Anaesthesia, surgery and immunology. Anaesthesia 33:322, 1978

65. Rem J, Brandt MR, Kehlet H: Prevention of postoperative lymphopenia and granulocytosis by epidural analgesia. Lancet 1:283, 1980

66. Meakins JL, Pietsch JB, Bubenick O et al: Delayed hypersensitivity: indicator of acquired failure of host defenses in sepsis and trauma. Ann Surg 186:241, 1977

67. Jakobsen BW, Pedersen J, Egeberg BB: Postoperative lymphocytopenia and leucocytosis after epidural and general anaesthesia. Acta Anaesthesiol Scand 30:668, 1986

68. Salo M, Nissila M: Cell-mediated and humoral immune responses to total hip replacement under spinal or general ananaesthesia. Acta Anaesthesiol Scand 34:241, 1990

69. Yaksh TL, Hammond DL: Peripheral and central substrates involved in the rostrad transmission of nociceptive information. Pain 13:1, 1982

70. Kehlet H: Modification of responses to surgery by neural blockade: clinical implications. p. 145. In Cousins MJ, Bridenbaugh PO (eds): Neural Blockade. 2nd Ed. JB Lippincott, Philadelphia, 1988

71. Kehlet H, Schulze S: Modification of the general response to injury—Pharmacological and clinical aspects. p. 153. In Little RA, Frayn KN (eds): The Scientific Basis of Care of the Critically Ill. Manchester University Press, Manchester, UK, 1986

72. Halter JB, Pflug AE: Relationship of impaired insulin secretion during surgical stress to anesthesia and catecholamine release. J Clin Endocrinol 51:1093, 1980

73. Kehlet H: The stress response to anaesthesia and surgery: release mechanisms and modifying factors. Clin Anaesth 2:315, 1984

74. Kehlet H: The modifying effect of general and regional anesthesia on the endocrine-metabolic response to surgery. Reg Anaesth 7:S38, 1982

75. Longnecker DE: Stress free: to be or not to be? Anesthesiology 51:643, 1984

76. Bovill JG, Sebel PS, Stanley TH: Opioid analgesics in anesthesia: with special reference to their use in cardiovascular anesthesia. Anesthesiology 61:731, 1984

77. Blunnie WP, McIlroy PDA, Merrett JD, Dundee JW: Cardiovascular and biochemical evidence of stress during major surgery associated with different techniques of anaesthesia. Br J Anaesth 55:611, 1983

78. Halter JB, Pflug AE: Effect of sympathetic blockade by spinal anesthesia on pancreatic islet function in man. Am J Physiol 239:E151, 1980

79. Jensen CH, Berthelsen P, Kühl C, Kehlet H: Effect of epidural analgesia on glucose tolerance during surgery. Acta Anaesthesiol Scand 24:472, 1980

80. Newsome HH, Rose JC: The response of human adrenocorticotrophic hormone and growth hormone to surgical stress. J Clin Endocrinol Metab 33:481, 1971

81. Pflug AE, Halter JB: Effect of spinal anesthesia on adrenergic tone and the neuroendocrine response to surgical stress in humans. Anesthesiology 55:120, 1981

82. Stevens RA, Artuso JD, Kao T-C et al: Changes in human plasma catechol-

amine concentrations during epidural anesthesia depend on the level of block. Anesthesiology 74:1029, 1991

83. Kehlet H, Brandt MR, Hansen AP, Alberti KGMM: Effect of epidural analgesia on the metabolic profiles during and after surgery. Br J Surg 66:543, 1979

84. Brandt M, Kehlet H, Binder C et al: Effect of epidural analgesia on the glycoregulatory endocrine response to surgery. Clin Endocrinol 5:107, 1976

85. Davis FM, Laurenson VG, Lewis J et al: Metabolic response to total hip arthroplasty under hypobaric subarachnoid or general anaesthesia. Br J Anaesth 59:725, 1987

86. Brandt MR, Fernandes A, Mordhorst R, Kehlet H: Epidural analgesia improves postoperative nitrogen balance. Br Med J 1:1106, 1978

87. Engquist A, Brandt MR, Fernandes A, Kehlet H: The blocking effect of epidural analgesia on the adrenocortical and hyperglycemic responses to surgery. Acta Anaesthesiol Scand 21:330, 1977

88. Ringsted C, Pedersen T, Eliasen K, Henriksen E: Estimated risk of postoperative pulmonary complications in relation to general and regional anesthesia. Anesthesiology 69:A715, 1988

89. McKenzie PJ, Wishart HY, Dewar KMS et al: Comparison of the effects of spinal anesthesia and general anaesthesia on postoperative oxygenation and perioperative mortality. Br J Anaesth 52:49, 1980

90. Mankikian B, Cantineau JP, Bertrand M et al: Improvement of diaphragmatic function by a thoracic extradural block after upper abdominal surgery. Anesthesiology 68:379, 1988

91. Dureuil B, Viires N, Cantineau J-P et al: Diaphragmatic contractility after abdominal surgery. J Appl Physiol 61:1775, 1986

92. Cuschieri RJ, Morran CG, Howie DC, McArdle CS: Postoperative pain and pulmonary complications: comparison of three analgesic regimens. Br J Surg 72:495, 1985

93. Hjortso NC, Neumann P, Frosig F et al: A controlled study on the effect of epidural analgesia with local anaesthetics and morphine on morbidity after abdominal surgery. Acta Anaesthesiol Scand 29:790, 1985

94. Jayr C, Mollie A, Bourgain JL et al: Postoperative complications: general anesthesia with postoperative parenteral morphine compared with epidural analgesia. Surgery 104:57, 1988

95. Cook PT, Davis MJ, Cronin KD, Moran P: A prospective randomized trial comparing spinal anaesthesia using hyperbaric cinchocaine with general anaesthesia for lower limb vascular surgery. Anaesth Intensive Care 14:373, 1986

96. Pflug AE, Murphy TM, Butler SH, Tucker GT: The effects of postoperative peridural analgesia on pulmonary therapy and pulmonary complications. Anesthesiology 41:495, 1974

97. Kuman A, Battis GE, Froese AD et al: Bilateral cervical and thoracic epidural blockade complicating interscalene block: reports of two cases. Anesthesiology 35:650, 1971

98. Bridenbaugh LD: The upper extremity: somatic blockade. p. 387. In Cousins MJ, Bridenbaugh PO (eds): Neural Blockade. 2nd Ed. JB Lippincott, Philadelphia, 1988

99. Seltzer JL, Larijani GE, Goldberg ME, Marr AT: Intrapleural bupivacaine—a kinetic and dynamic evaluation. Anesthesiology 67:798, 1987

100. Saada M, Duval A-M, Bonnet F et al: Abnormalities in myocardial segmental wall motion during lumbar epidural anesthesia. Anesthesiology 71:26, 1989

101. Shoemaker WC, Appel PL, Kram HB et al: Prospective trial of supranormal values of survivors as therapeutic goals in high-risk surgical patients. Chest 94:1176, 1988

102. Rao TLK, Jacobs KH, El-Etr AA: Reinfarction following anesthesia in patients with myocardial infarction. Anesthesiology 59:499, 1983

103. Steen PA, Tinker JH, Tarhan S: Myocardial reinfarction after anesthesia and surgery. JAMA 239:2566, 1978

104. Backer CL, Tinker JH, Robertson DM, Vlietstra RE: Myocardial reinfarction

following local anesthesia for ophthalmic surgery. Anesth Analg 59:257, 1980

105. Goldman L, Caldera DL, Southwick FS et al: Cardiac risk factors and complications in non-cardiac surgery. Medicine 57:357, 1978

106. Valli H, Rosenberg PH: Effects of three anaesthesia methods on haemodynamic responses connected with the use of thigh tourniquet in orthopedic patients. Acta Anaesthesiol Scand 29:142, 1985

107. Rocco AG, Concepcion MA, Desai S et al: The effect of general and regional anesthesia on tourniquet induced blood pressure elevation. Reg Anesth 12:174, 1987

108. Jensen JS, Tondevold E: Mortality after hip fractures. Acta Orthop Scand 50:161, 1979

109. Cummings SR, Kelsey JL, Nevitt MC, O'Dowd KJ: Epidemiology of osteoporosis and osteoporotic fractures. Epidemiol Rev 7:178, 1985

110. Melton LJ III, Wahner HW, Richelson LS et al: Osteoporosis and the risk of hip fracture. Am J Epidemiol 124:254, 1986

111. Davis FM, Woolner DF, Frampton C et al: Prospective multi-centre trial of mortality following general or spinal anaesthesia for hip fracture surgery in the elderly. Br J Anaesth 59:1080, 1987

112. McLaren AD, Stockwell MC, Reid VT: Anaesthetic techniques for surgical correction of fractured neck of femur. A comparative study of spinal and general anaesthesia in the elderly. Anaesthesia 33:10, 1978

113. Goucke CR: Mortality following surgery for fractures of the neck of femur. Anaesthesia 40:578, 1985

114. Valentin N, Lomholt B, Jensen JS et al: Spinal or general anesthesia for surgery of the fractured hip? Br J Anaesth 58:284, 1986

115. Davis FM, Laurenson VG: Spinal anaesthesia or general anaesthesia for emergency hip surgery in elderly patients. Anaesth Intensive Care 9:352, 1981

116. McKenzie PJ, Wishart HY, Smith G: Long-term outcome after repair of fractured neck of femur. Br J Anaesth 56:581, 1984

117. McLaren AD, Stockwell MC, Reid VT: Anaesthetic techniques for surgical correction of fractured neck of femur. Anaesthesia 33:10, 1978

118. Wickstrom I, Holmberg I, Stefansson T: Survival of female geriatric patients after hip fracture surgery. A comparison of 5 anesthetic methods. Acta Anaesthesiol Scand 26:607, 1982

119. Melton JL III, Stauffer RN, Chao EY, Ilstrup DM: Rates of total hip arthroplasty. N Engl J Med 307:1242, 1982

120. Total hip-joint replacement in the United States. Consensus development conference of the National Institute of Health. JAMA 248:1817, 1982

121. Koide M, Pilone RN, Vandam LD, Lowell JD: Anaesthetic experience with total hip replacement. Clin Orthop 99:78, 1974

122. Soreide O, Molster A, Raugstad TS: Internal fixation versus primary prosthetic replacement in acute femoral neck fractures: a prospective, randomized clinical study. Br J Surg 66:56, 1979

123. Wedel D: Complications, p. 511. In Raj PP (ed): Clinical Practice of Regional Anesthesia. 2nd Ed. Churchill Livingstone, New York, 1991

124. Covert CR, Fox GS: Anesthesia for hip surgery in the elderly. Can J Anaesth 36:311, 1989

5

Positioning and Monitoring

Beth A. Elliott

POSITIONING

Proper positioning of patients for orthopedic surgery can be a challenging and time-consuming process. Communication between the surgical and anesthesia personnel involved is essential for a successful outcome. Frequently, a compromise must be reached to balance surgical requirements with patient tolerance.

Anesthesia not only obtunds patients' response to surgical stimulation, it also makes it difficult for them to object to nonanatomic or otherwise uncomfortable positions. This, coupled with the skeletal muscle relaxation provided by either regional or general anesthesia, creates the potential for a wide range of unfortunate sequelae.

Many orthopedic procedures are performed in a standard fashion as regards positioning, location of incision, and other factors, and therefore many of the potential adverse consequences for the patient can be anticipated and, it is hoped, prevented. However, one must still take into account variability among patients as to underlying pathology and physical limitations, which may require modification of the usual standard approach (e.g., the multiple-trauma patient having simultaneous surgical procedures,

for whom other injuries may preclude the usual surgical posture, or the patient with rheumatoid arthritis who has limited motion of multiple joints).

A thorough understanding of anatomy, the physiologic implications of various positions, and the underlying pathology and associated illness is needed, as well as an awareness of surgical intent, duration, and other idiosyncracies.

Over the years, a number of investigators have attempted to document the incidence of negative outcomes due to positioning during surgical procedures. Dhunér[1] in 1948 reviewed approximately 30,000 cases from a 5-year period to examine the incidence of peripheral nerve injuries in the postanesthetic postsurgical period. In these 30,000 cases, 31 patients were identified as having suffered paresis of one or more peripheral nerves. Twenty-six cases involved the upper extremity: brachial plexus, 11; radial nerve, 7; and ulnar nerve, 8. Of these 26 cases, 13 had a spinal anesthetic. All 5 patients with lower extremity problems experienced paresis of the peroneal nerve. Of these 5 patients, 4 had a spinal anesthetic. Regardless of the anesthetic technique used, the mechanism of these injuries appeared to be similar: direct trauma to the nerve most likely as a result of positioning during surgery.

99

Parks[2] in 1973 reported from a 13-year summary of 50,000 patients, 72 patients with postoperative peripheral nerve injuries that were attributed to malposition during anesthesia and surgery. Upper extremity problems (50) again outnumbered those involving the lower extremity (22). No comment was made as to the type of anesthetic administered. Duration of surgery (and hence position) was a factor. Most peripheral nerve complications occurred in patients whose surgery was of at least 6 hours duration or more. In these series and others, ischemia as a result of compression and stretching of peripheral nerves was implicated as the leading cause of the neurologic deficits uncovered.[3]

Although usually associated with sitting neurosurgical patients, venous air embolism has also been reported in patients undergoing total hip arthroplasty[4] and spinal instrumentation,[5,6] and is a theoretical consideration in sitting position shoulder surgery.

Vascular compromise leading to compartment syndrome and eventual amputation has been seen following total hip arthroplasty.[7] Compartment syndromes requiring fasciotomies and/or leading to renal failure have complicated the postoperative course of spinal fusion patients[8,9] (R. A. Klassen, M.D., personal communication, 1991).

Morbidity related to surgical posture is not limited to peripheral nerve injuries and can, on occasion, lead to mortality.

No surgical posture is immune from the potential for patient morbidity. It is up to the anesthesia and surgical teams involved to be aware of that potential and to take every precaution to prevent complications from occurring. In those situations in which a required surgical posture exposes a patient to a high risk of a positioning-related complication, this should be discussed with the patient preoperatively along with reassurance that

measures will be taken to avoid such a problem.

More frequently, the surgical posture is modified to accommodate the needs of the patient. Many patients who present for orthopedic surgery are elderly and have decreased flexibility or limited range of motion of various joints as a result of arthritic degeneration, trauma, congenital abnormalities, previous surgical procedures, or external fixation devices.

These factors may also have an impact on the choice of anesthetic technique to be administered. When planning a given anesthetic, one should always take into consideration the position in which the patient is to be placed (along with myriad other considerations). For example, a spinal anesthetic may work perfectly well for most patients presenting for total hip arthroplasty, but for the patient with severe multijoint arthritis, the pain produced in the dependent shoulder while in the lateral decubitus position may necessitate sedation to the point of airway compromise. In this situation, a better alternative may be general anesthesia, either alone or in combination with regional blockade.

Part of the preoperative interview and examination with each patient should include assessment of historical tolerance (if available) for the anticipated surgical posture, and evaluation of range of motion in whichever joints/extremities are to be manipulated in achieving that posture.

Awareness of the surgical posture may also influence decisions about intraoperative monitoring (i.e., need for precordial Doppler and right atrial catheter in sitting cases or others at risk for venous air embolism, or preoperative placement of an additional intravenous line or intra-arterial catheter when intraoperative access to the patient is limited by the position itself).

Proper positioning of a patient for a sur-

Table 5-1. Prepositioning Considerations

A history of patient intolerance for certain positions

Physical examination including joint range of motion

Documentation of pre-existing neurologic deficits

Assessment of surgical positioning needs

Estimated duration of surgical procedure

Thorough equipment check

---

gical procedure should also include preparation of the surgical bed or table. Unfamiliarity with, or malfunction of, equipment can lead to costly time delays and may compromise patient care. A thorough check of the equipment should be done prior to its use and experienced personnel should be available to assist with any difficulties encountered. Care should be taken to see that potential contact areas with the mattress, metal supports, and other equipment are covered. If the procedure is to be lengthy, additional padding such as "jelly pads" or "egg-crate" mattresses should be employed to prevent skin breakdown or nerve compression. In addition to experienced personnel, provisions for a sufficient number of personnel to help with lifting, moving, and turning patients should be made to avoid placing the patient at risk for injury or placing undue strain on the backs of those involved in positioning the patient (Table 5-1).

When moving or turning patients, care should be taken to avoid hyperextension of the joints, with special attention to the neck, and to see that extremities are not pinched, allowed to hang unsupported, or placed in any other nonanatomic or compromised position.

One person should assume responsibility for the head, neck, and airway during moving or turning and should be the one to provide the coordinating signals

for the effort. A member of the surgical team should assume responsibility for maintaining traction or a neutral position for fractured and unstable limbs during patient transfers and positioning.

Physiology

When a conscious subject changes body position (e.g., erect to supine), a variety of reflex physiologic responses occur to maintain homeostasis. Alterations of myocardial contractility, stroke volume, cardiac output, and autonomic tone occur in response to postural changes affecting gravitational distribution of the intravascular blood volume[10] (Fig. 5-1).

Just as assuming a supine posture results in an increased venous return to the heart, assuming an erect or head-up posture diminishes venous return to the heart by promoting venous pooling (Table 5-2). The presence of an anesthetic, with myocardial depressant or vasodilatory properties, can exacerbate the magnitude of effect that gravitational pooling has on cardiovascular response

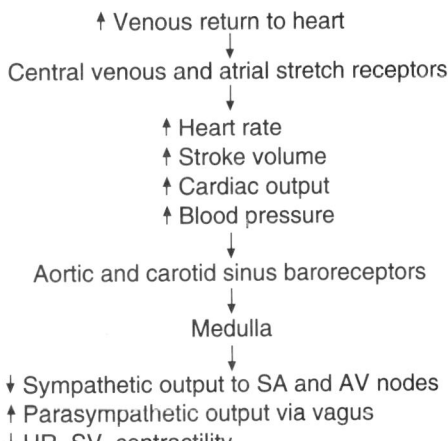

Fig. 5-1. Reflex cardiovascular response to change from upright to supine posture.

Table 5-2. Cardiovascular Changes
With Assumption of a Head-Elevated
Position

Decreased
    Left atrial pressure
    Cardiac output
    Stroke volume
    ± Systemic blood pressure
Increased
    Systemic vascular resistance
    Pulmonary vascular resistance
    Heart rate

---

and function. Elderly patients, patients with a history of cardiovascular disease, or hypovolemic patients may not tolerate rapid changes in position and should be carefully monitored during gradual positioning to avoid hypotension.

Pulmonary mechanics, ventilation/perfusion relationships, and gas exchange can be significantly affected by postural changes as well. The cephalad displacement of the diaphragm in the supine position can decrease functional residual capacity (FRC) by 0.5 to 1.0 L. In patients with abnormal airways, this reduction of lung volume may place FRC below closing capacity (CC), leading to airway closure, which results in an increase in the alveolar to arterial oxygen difference and shunt.[10] In normal patients, in whom FRC exceeds CC both erect and supine, one may actually see an improvement in gas exchange because of the greater overall uniformity of ventilation and perfusion in the supine position and increased cardiac output.[10]

Specific Positions

Supine Position

The most frequently requested surgical posture is the supine or recumbent position. This position generally confronts the patient with the least physiologic stress or challenge, provides easy access for both surgeon and anesthesia care provider, and requires minimal effort to achieve. It is not, however, without some potential problems.

Both general and regional anesthesia of the central neuraxis provide relaxation of the lumbar musculature and loss of the normal lordotic curve. This may result in stretch of the ligamentous structures of the lower back and present as low back pain in the postoperative period.[11] When possible, a slight degree of flexion at the hips and knees can minimize the stress on these structures and provide a more comfortable posture. This is also more comfortable for awake patients with upper or lower extremity peripheral block anesthesia. Particularly with procedures of long duration, additional efforts to ensure adequate padding on the operating room table to prevent pressure sores are crucial. An egg-crate mattress or jelly-pads can be used on top of the usual firm mattress to help disperse the patient's weight over a greater surface area. Special attention should be paid to avoid pressure on the heels, particularly in patients with compromised circulation to the feet (i.e., vascular disease, diabetes), and the occiput. Frequent turning of the head and, if possible, massage of the skin overlying the heels and occiput may help prevent skin injury or hair loss.[12]

Arm position in the supine patient is also of concern because of the potential for injury to neural elements.[13] The brachial plexus and its peripheral branches are by far the most vulnerable to position-related injuries. The brachial plexus is relatively fixed at both its origin along the vertebral and prevertebral fascia and at its insertion at the axillary fascia of the upper arm. It may be subjected to stretch at any of three points along its course: as it passes under the clavicle, under the head of the pectoralis muscle, and by the head of the humerus[14] (Fig. 5-2). Stretching oc-

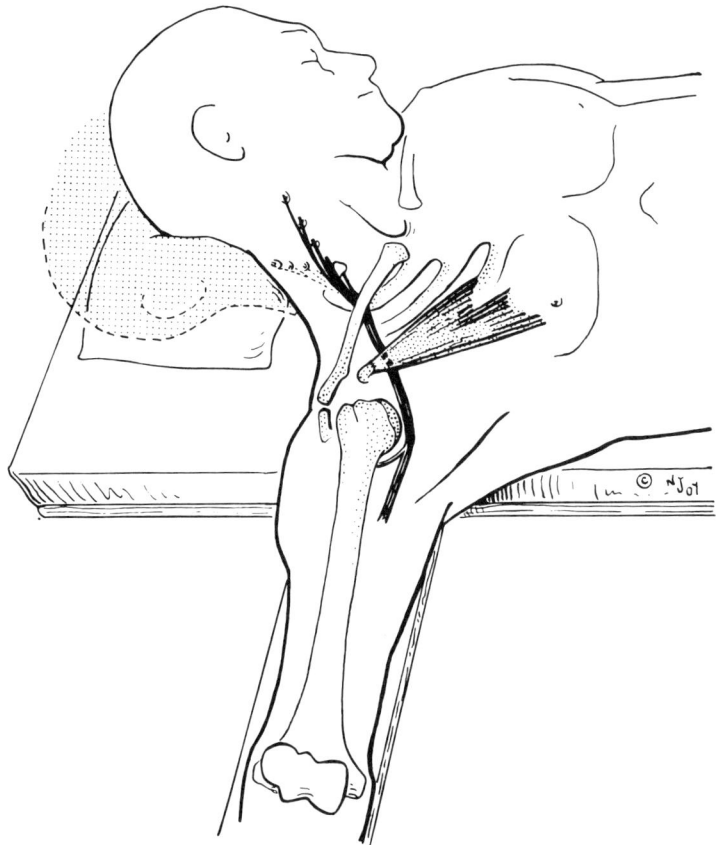

Fig. 5-2. The brachial plexus may be subjected to stretch injury at three points along its course: as it passes under the clavicle, under the head of the pectoralis muscle, and around the head of the humerus. (From Britt & Gordon,[18] with permission.)

curs with abduction, extension, and external rotation of the arm, such as might be seen with use of an arm board. The head should be kept in a neutral position, as additional strain on the plexus may be exerted if the head is turned to the contralateral side, or away from the abducted upper extremity. When an arm board is used, the arm should not be abducted beyond 90 degrees[15] (Fig. 5-3). Vascular compression with loss of the radial pulse occurred in 83 percent of healthy volunteers with arm abduction of greater than 90 degrees.[16] The padding on the arm board should be level with that of the operation room table to avoid dorsal exten-

sion of the arm with subsequent impingement by the humeral head on the neurovascular elements.[17]

If the arms are to be "tucked" or placed alongside the body of the patient, care should be taken to adequately protect the arm from compression by leaning surgeons and their assistants. The ulnar nerve is vulnerable to injury if the elbow is allowed to hang over the edge of the operating room table, where compression against the medial epicondyle can occur[18] (Fig. 5-4). Radial nerve injury may occur with compression against the posterolateral humerus by an unpadded ether screen support (Fig. 5-5).

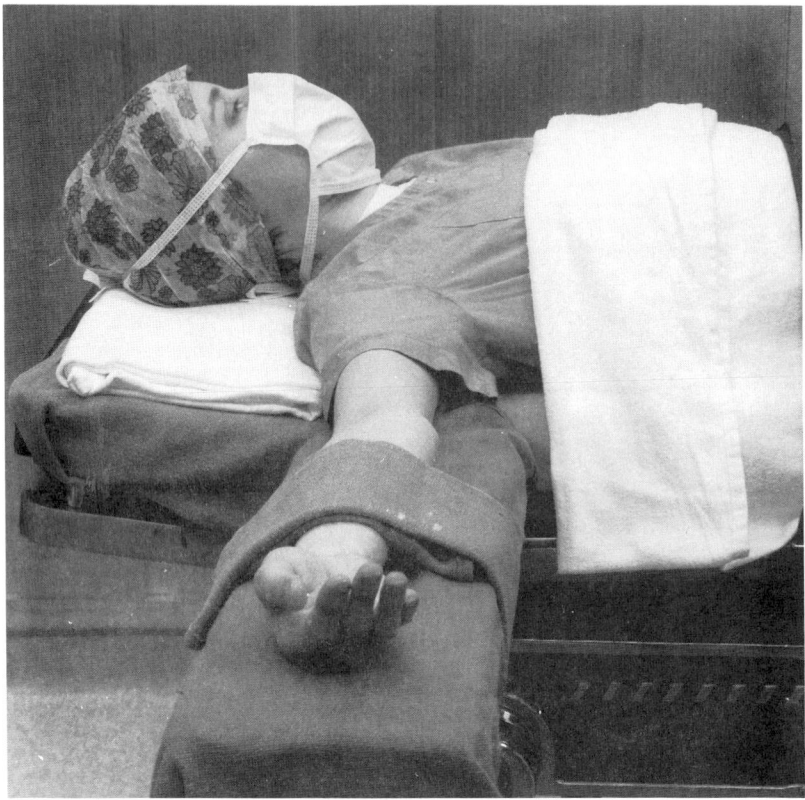

Fig. 5-3. Supine position. When using an armboard, the arm should be supinated, and not abducted more than 90 degrees. The level of the armboard should be even with the mattress on the operating room table. The head should be kept in a neutral position.

Lateral Decubitus Position

The lateral decubitus position is most frequently used in orthopedic surgery for total hip arthroplasty, anterior spinal fusion, and occasionally miscellaneous procedures on the lower extremities such as skin grafting, debridement, and tumor excision.

When turning the patient from a supine to a lateral decubitus position, care must be taken to maintain the neck, shoulders, and pelvis in the same plane to avoid injury to the spine. Ideally, one person should be responsible for turning the head, one the shoulders, one the hips, and one the legs and feet. Once turned, the patient should be physically held in place until stabilization can be achieved. A variety of mechanical aids for stabilization are available, including padded hip rests, bean bags, and chest rolls (Fig. 5-6).

The dependent arm should be abducted and rest on a padded arm board. The upper arm may rest on a padded over-arm board or pillows, or less satisfactorily, may be suspended from an ether screen. The arms should appear to lie in a natural position free of stretch and excessive abduction or rotation. Not infrequently, the presence of arthritic disease or trauma will require modification of arm placement. Patients having procedures under regional anesthesia can be of assistance in making adjustments to achieve

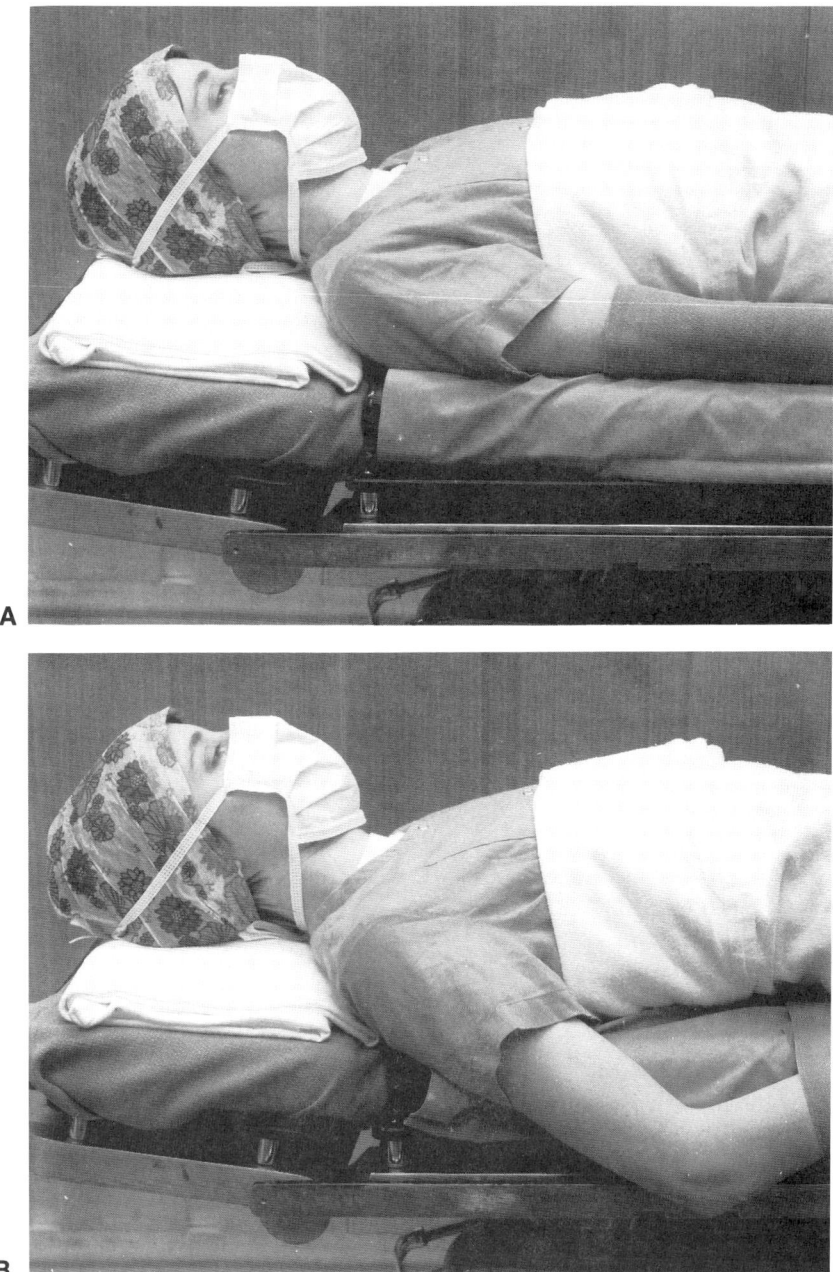

Fig. 5-4. When the arms are to be tucked along side the patient's body, the elbow should not be allowed to hang over the edge of the table, which exposes the ulnar nerve to injury. (**A**) Correct. (**B**) Incorrect.

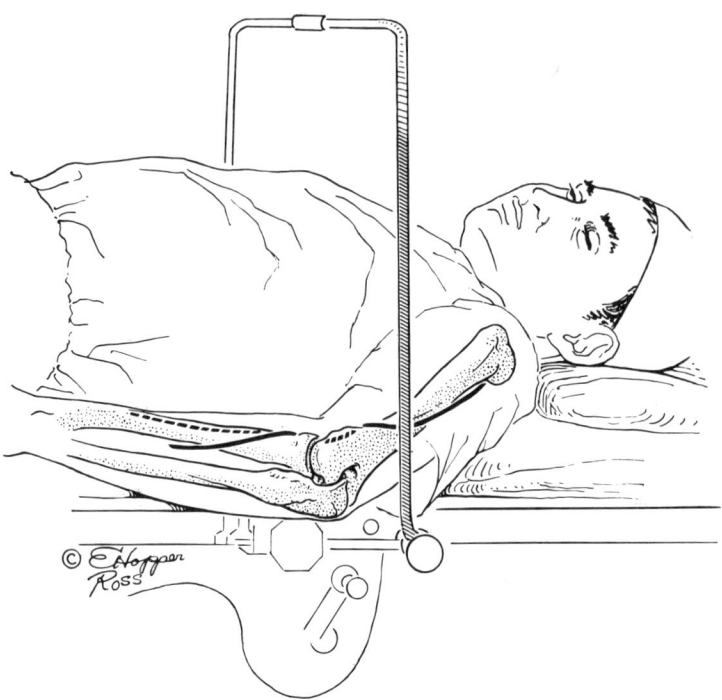

Fig. 5-5. As the radial nerve courses around the posterolateral aspect of the humerus it may be subject to compression against upright supports such as the ether screen. (From Britt & Gordon,[18] with permission.)

a position acceptable to both them and the surgeon. All bony prominences and potential contacts with metal supports should be well padded. An axillary or chest roll under the dependent chest wall just below the axilla can diminish the degree of weight bearing by the dependent shoulder and potential impingement of the humeral head upon the neurovascular bundle.[19] The dependent arm should be examined to ensure that adequate venous drainage and arterial pulsation are present.

The head and cervical spine should be supported with padding to maintain proper alignment with the thoracic spine. If the head is allowed to hang in exaggerated lateral flexion, undue stretch on the cervical sympathetic chain can result in a postoperative Horner syndrome.[20]

The dependent ear and eye should be free from pressure. There are a number of reports of postoperative blindness as a result of excess pressure on the eye leading to retinal ischemia. While patients in the prone position are perhaps at greater risk for this complication, the potential exists in the lateral decubitus position as well.[17,18,21]

Flexion of the dependent leg at the hip and knee (and extension of the uppermost leg) will provide greater stability for the patient in the lateral position. If the operative site does not include the lower extremities, pillows should be placed between the patient's legs to avoid pressure injury from the bony protuberances of the uppermost extremity. It is usually neither possible nor necessary to place pillows between the legs of patients having total hip arthroplasty as the operative leg is suspended and then dislocated and

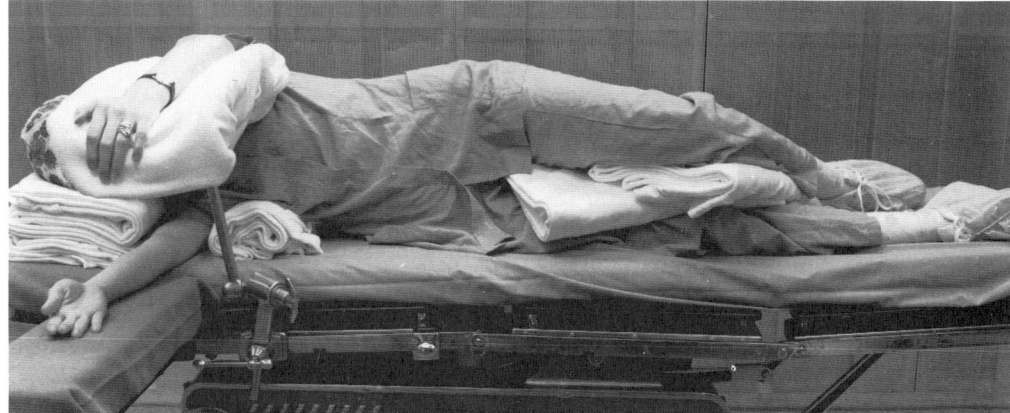

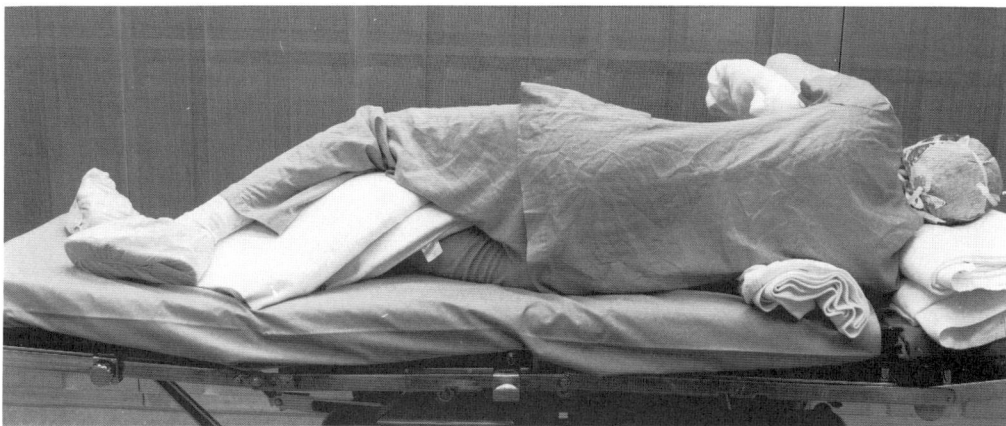

Fig. 5-6. The lateral decubitus position. The head is supported to align the central neuraxis, the eyes and ears are free of pressure, the arms are supported in a neutral position, the body is stabilized with padded hip rests, the dependent leg is flexed, and padding is placed between the legs. (**A**) Front view. (**B**) Back view.

placed anteriorly, and thus does not put pressure on the dependent leg for any length of time.

Once the patient is turned, adequately positioned, and padded, re-evaluation of the patient should take place to ascertain that equal breath sounds are heard over both lung fields, and that the endotracheal tube has not been displaced during the transition. Arterial pulses should be assessed in the upper extremities and the dependent eye should be re-checked each time the patient's position is shifted.

During the transition to the lateral position, some monitoring modalities may occasionally be temporarily suspended to avoid tangling of lines, wires, and catheters. If so, efforts to resume patient monitoring should be made as soon as possible. However, it is usually reasonable and prudent to maintain monitoring of oxygen saturation during transfers and positioning. Electrocardiogram electrodes should not be allowed to remain beneath the patient on a weight-bearing area to avoid pressure injury to the skin. Disagreement as to the correct arm on which to place a noninvasive blood pressure cuff in the lateral position is common. Discrepancies in blood pressures measured from the two arms may be as high as 36 mmHg because of gravitational forces and hydrostatic differences relative to the level of the heart.[22] Either arm may be used provided that these differences are remembered and vascular compromise does not occur.

To provide adequate surgical exposure for anterior spinal fusion in the lumbar area, the patient is placed in the nephrectomy position using the kidney rest. The patient should be placed on the table so that the kidney rest is supporting the crest of the ilium. Frequently the rest is inappropriately placed under the flank and lower ribs, which jeopardizes respiratory function and risks vena caval obstruction.[23,24] When properly placed beneath the ilium, the dependent crest functions as a fulcrum, allowing the pelvic brim to rotate away from the rib cage and open up the surgical exposure (Fig. 5-7).

Prone Position

The prone position is used primarily for spinal surgery, but may also be requested for tumor resection, pelvic stabilization, debridement, and miscellaneous other procedures.

Anesthetic management of a patient in the prone position requires strict attention to detail, careful planning, and anticipation of potential intraoperative events. Access to the airway and intravascular lines can be quite limited once the patient is turned prone, so these need to be reliable and adequately secured to avoid disruption or mishap.

Were the patient allowed to lie prone, without chest supports on the usual operating table, the abdominal contents would be subjected to compression, forcing the diaphragm cephalad and making ventilation more difficult. Increased pressure within the abdomen is also transmitted to the venous circulation, thereby increasing the volume and pressure within the confluent epidural venous plexus. To avoid these potential complicating factors, a number of devices have been designed to redistribute the weight-bearing burden to allow the abdomen to hang unencumbered.

These devices or variations of the prone posture can be divided into three categories:

1. Longitudinal rolls or arches that extend from just below the clavicle to the iliac crest (e.g., chest rolls, Walker frame) (Fig. 5-8)
2. System of pedestals at the iliac crests and infraclavicular chest wall (e.g., Relton frame, Tower table) (Fig. 5-9)
3. Variety of kneeling/tucking/sitting positions, which redistribute the weight to the chest wall, buttocks, and knees (e.g., tuck or knee–chest position, Tarlov seat, Hasting's frame) (Fig. 5-10 and 5-11)

Longitudinal chest rolls can be inexpensively constructed from sheets and blankets, or purchased. They should be firmly affixed to the operating table to prevent slipping. The cephalad end of the role should not place pressure on the clavicle to prevent compression of the brachial plexus between the clavicle and underlying first rib. A pillow or other soft padding should be placed over the caudal end of the rolls to minimize pressure on the groin. The abdomen should hang freely between the chest rolls, but if insufficient space is available, should be evenly distributed so that the patient does not list to one side. Male genitalia should be checked once the patient is positioned on the rolls to avoid distortion or compression injury. Breasts should be placed in a neutral or medial position to minimize the potential for tearing and pressure injury. Lateral breast placement

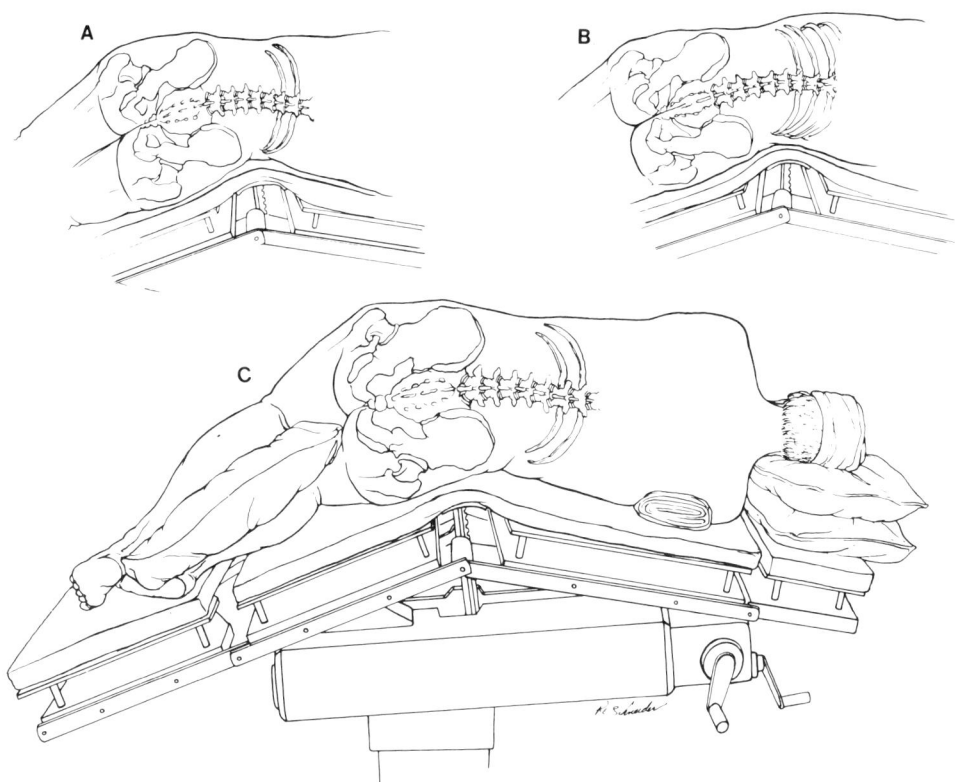

Fig. 5-7. (**A**) Incorrect placement. (**B**) Incorrect placement. (**C**) Correct placement of the kidney rest beneath the iliac crest, resulting in the least interference with functions of the dependent lung and diaphragm. (From Kropp,[54] with permission.)

may interfere with arm positioning and is more painful in the awake state than medial placement.[25]

Arms may be tucked against the body or supported on arm boards alongside the head with the arms abducted 90 degrees at the shoulder and flexed at the elbow. Padding should be placed beneath the arm just above and below the elbow to avoid pressure on the ulnar nerve. Our practice is to have one arm tucked and the other alongside the head. This allows for improved access to intravascular lines and assessment of arterial pulse, capillary refill, and other monitors. The head (if turned lateral) should always be facing the side with the "up" arm to avoid brachial plexus injury. As the plexus emerges from the intervertebral foramina it is relatively fixed in the vertebral and prevertebral fascia. It is subject to compression between the clavicle and first rib and must course around the humeral head, which is more prominent when the arm is abducted.[18] Turning the head away from the abducted arm tends to pull the plexus taut, increasing the risk of injury (Fig. 5-12). Compression of the axillary artery by the humeral head may also occur with hyperabduction of the shoulder.[19,26]

If patient mobility will allow, the head may be turned laterally and supported beneath the forehead and chin (as in the lateral decubitus position), being careful to avoid pressure on the dependent eye and

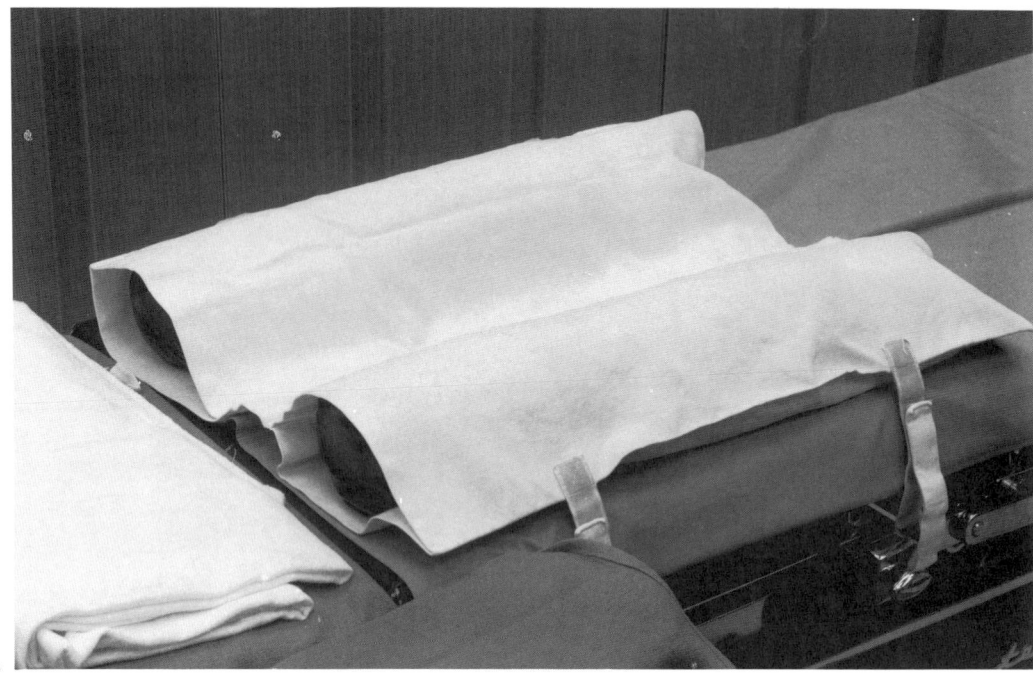

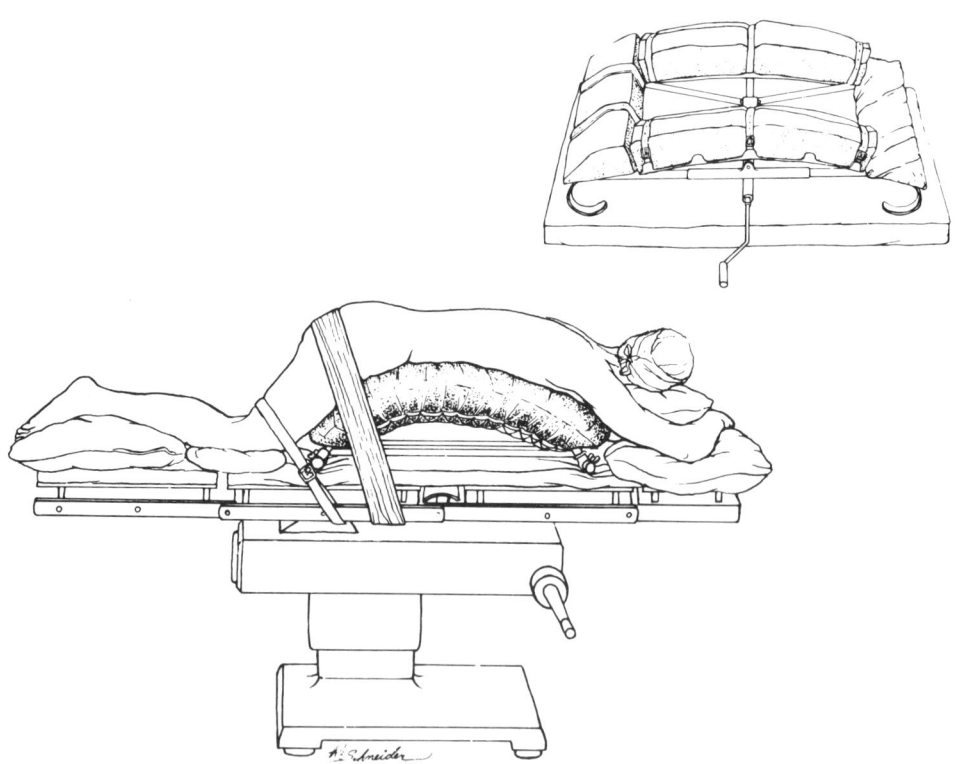

Fig. 5-8. Longitudinal support devices used in conjunction with a typical operating room table. (**A**) Chest rolls. (**B**) Walker frame. (Fig. B from Martin,[25] with permission.)

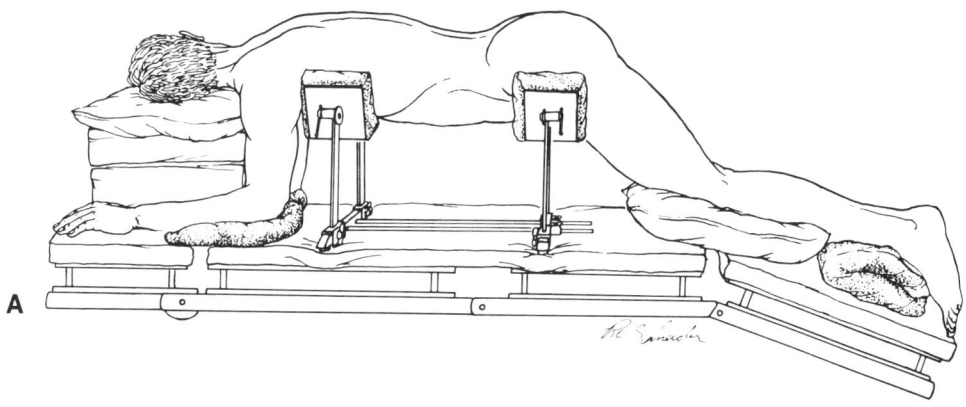

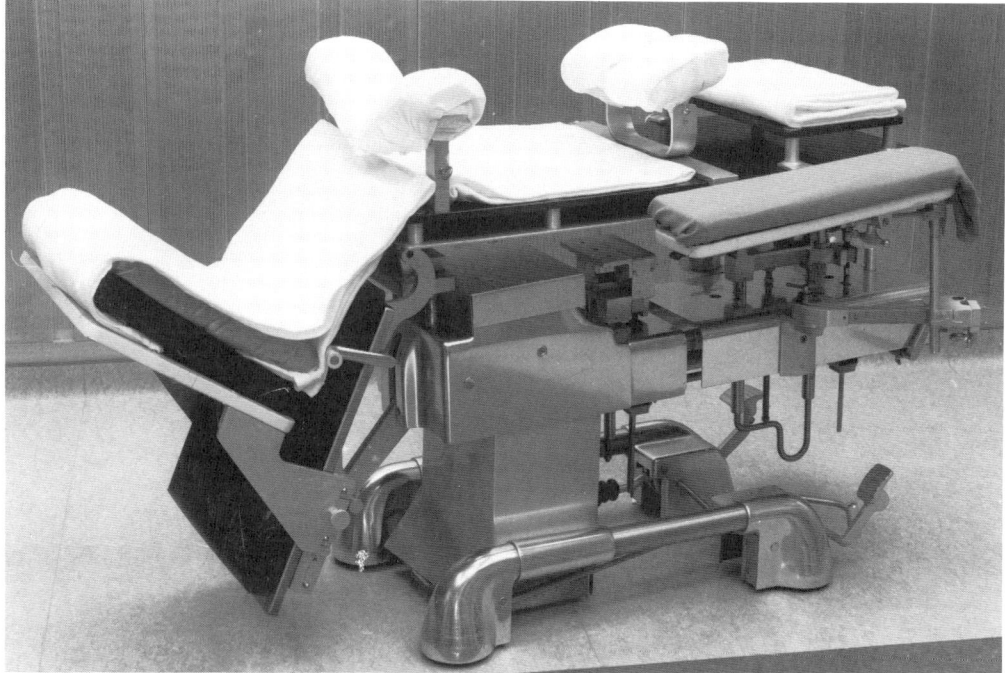

Fig. 5-9. Pedestal-type support devices. (**A**) Relton frame. (**B**) Tower table. (Fig. A from Singh,[55] with permission.)

ear. The endotracheal tube should be positioned so that it is not exerting pressure on the down side of the face, as the lingual and buccal nerves may be injured.[27] Legs should be wrapped or elastic stockings worn to minimize venous pooling. Knees should be flexed and supported by pillows or blankets. Frequently the operating table will be flexed to minimize the lumbar lordotic curve during spinal surgery. If this is done, a restraint or strap should be placed across the gluteal region to prevent slippage in a caudal direction.

A horseshoe headrest can be used to allow the head to remain in a neutral face-down position. The biggest problem with this device is the very real possibility of orbital compression. Even with careful

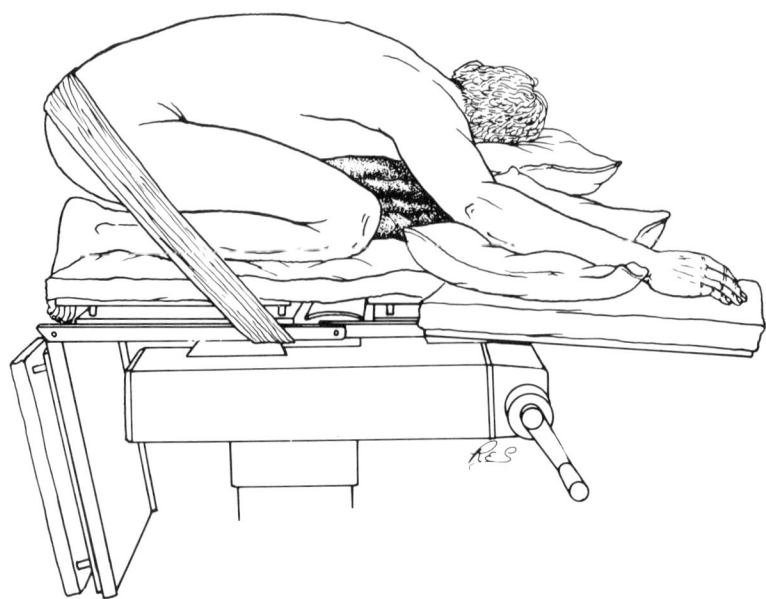

Fig. 5-10. Tuck position. (From Singh,[55] with permission.)

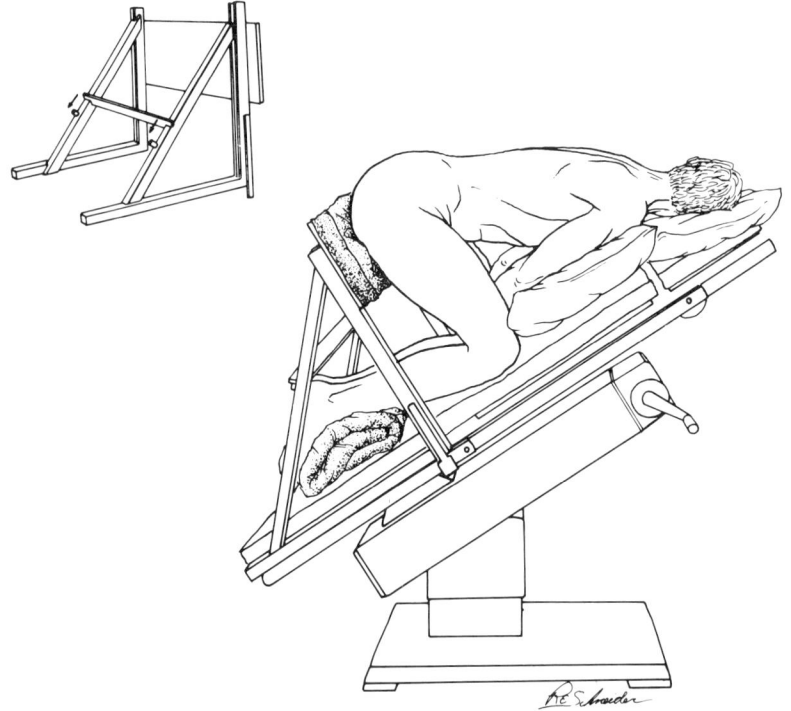

Fig. 5-11. Hasting's frame. (From Singh,[55] with permission.)

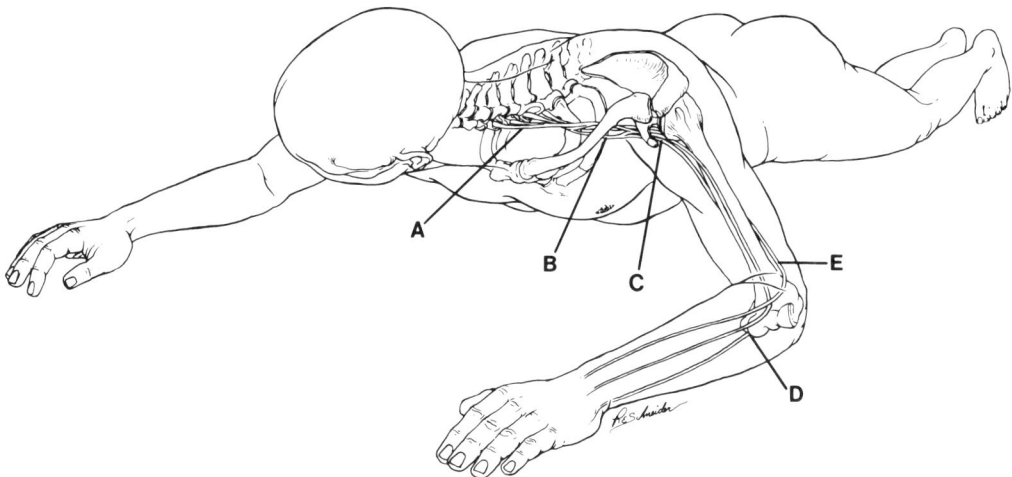

Fig. 5-12. The prone position exposes the brachial plexus and its peripheral branches to potential injury. A, lateral head position stretches the plexus; B, chest rolls may compress the neurovascular bundle between the clavicle and the first rib; C, pressure or tension on the arm may thrust the head of the humerus into the neurovascular bundle; D, compression of the ulnar nerve at the elbow, and E, compression of the radial nerve laterally above the elbow. (From Martin,[25] with permission.)

positioning, intraoperative movement by the patient or surgeon can cause the head to shift and compress the eye, leading to retinal ischemia and blindness (Fig. 5-13). If used, the position of the eyes relative to the headrest should be checked at frequent intervals intraoperatively.

The use of pinions and a head clamp avoids the problem of ocular compression, allows for a better stabilized cervical spine, and ensures relatively free access to the patient's face and airway.

If cervical range of motion is limited for any reason, it is important not to force the patient into what would be an intolerable position if awake. Management of the head position in a patient with an immobile or unstable cervical spine requires communication and coordination with the responsible surgical team. The longitudinal chest rolls are typically used in conjunction with the routine operating table and it is relatively easy to attach and use the pinion head rest.

The pedestal-type ventral supports may have an advantage for the obese patient in that they are less subject to compression than the longitudinal rolls and the abdomen may have more room to hang free. When thinner patients are positioned, there is frequently room between the abdomen and table surface for placement of one or both arms, thereby avoiding the need for cumbersome arm boards. This practice should, however, be avoided in the obese patient as the weight of the pendulous abdomen on the forearm can cause sufficient compression to result in compartment syndrome (R. A. Klassen, M.D., personal communication, 1991).

The Tower table, which is most commonly used for spinal instrumentation in our institution, is a pedestal support device. Weight bearing is on two movable padded chest supports, immobile iliac crest supports, and an adjustable-height knee support. The chest supports are placed below the level of the clavicle, and

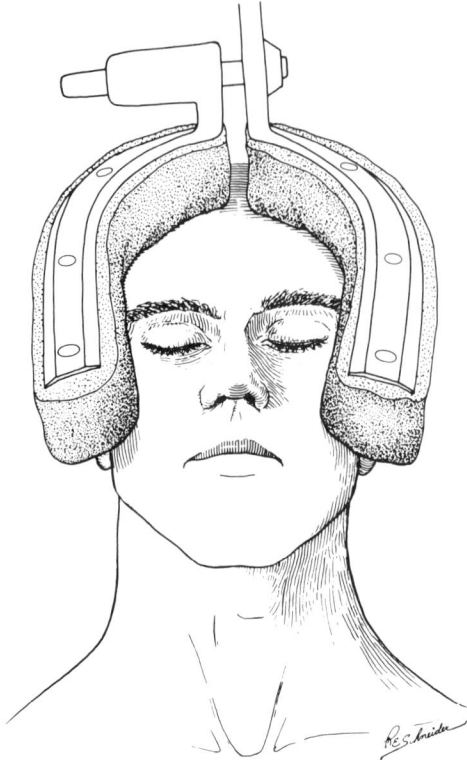

Fig. 5-13. Horseshoe head rest for prone position. (From Reid & Grundy,[56] with permission.)

breasts are directed medially. The weight-bearing of the lower half of the body should be roughly equally shared by the iliac crests and knees. It is not possible to attach the pinion head rest to the Tower table, however, and thus it is more challenging to position the patient with limited cervical range of motion. It may be necessary to build up the chest supports with additional padding to provide adequate clearance for the patient with a fixed flexion deformity of the cervical spine (i.e., ankylosing spondylitis) requiring a face down position.

Kneeling or tuck positions for spinal surgery are not used in our institution. Many potential problems exist with these positions. The extreme degree of hip and

knee flexion required to achieve the tuck position is not possible for a large number of patients and this position places the sciatic and obturator nerves at risk for stretch injury. Vascular compromise to the lower extremities has led to the development of compartment syndromes with subsequent rhabdomyolysis, renal failure, and even death.[8,9] It is our belief that there are superior alternative measures and positions that provide the same if not greater advantages for our patients.

For most elective surgical procedures performed in the prone position, induction of anesthesia occurs before positioning on the operating table. This allows for proper positioning for placement of monitoring devices and intravascular access lines, and maximizes patient comfort.

If appropriate for a specific patient or procedure, regional anesthesia is not contraindicated simply because of the prone position. One should, however, ascertain that an adequate level of blockade has developed prior to positioning to avoid the difficulties encountered with managing an unprotected airway in a patient with inadequate or excessive regional anesthesia in the prone position.

There are occasions when induction of anesthesia takes place after positioning in the prone position. Very obese patients may position themselves on the operating table in the prone position to minimize the risk of injury to both the patient and the operating room personnel assisting with the transfer.[28] Patients with unstable spinal fractures can be carefully log-rolled into position, gross neurologic function ascertained by way of a predetermined set of hand signals, and then the patient anesthetized. This provides a much more reliable test of cord integrity in regard to motor function than is provided by somatosensory evoked potential (SSEP) monitoring in the asleep patient. However, it is important to remember that neurologic deficits may still occur as a result of positioning despite such care-ful management.[29] Whether positioning occurs before or after induction of anes-thesia, the airway may be controlled prior to prone positioning. Either blind nasal passage, oral passage, or fiberoptically as-sisted intubation may be chosen depend-ing on the individual situation.

When turning the anesthetized patient to the prone position, adequate numbers of personnel must be recruited to ensure patient safety. The anesthesia care pro-vider should typically take charge of the head and airway and direct the position-ing efforts. Both arms should be kept straight and close to the patient's sides to avoid hyperextension injury to the shoul-der. For the short duration of the turn it-self, it may be necessary to temporarily disconnect monitoring lines and the breathing circuit to prevent their acci-dental disruption or extubation. Monitor-ing should be resumed as soon as possible after adequate ventilation is confirmed.

All bony prominences should be pad-ded, as well as any potential contacts be-tween the patient and metal supports. Surfaces intended to provide substantial weight bearing (i.e., chest, iliac crests, knees) should be kept free of wrinkles or excessively textured coverings, as these may contribute to skin breakdown.

While exceedingly rare, the potential for venous air embolism during spinal surgery in the prone position does exist. A recent report of three such cases noted that the gravitational gradient between the right side of the heart and the vertebra may be as great as 15 cm.[6] A positioning device that allows the abdomen to hang free and the lower extremities to be de-pendent may further increase the poten-tial for entrainment of air by increasing the likelihood of negative caval pres-sures. Other factors implicated by Albin et al[6] were a contracted blood volume and inadequate intravascular volume replace-ment.

Beach Chair Position

The beach chair position or shoulder po-sition, as the name implies, is used pri-marily to provide surgical access to the shoulder joint. With the patient in this se-mirecumbent position, the shoulder is ac-cessible from both the anterior and pos-terior approach and the upper extremity is freely movable throughout the usual anatomic range of motion.

To achieve the beach chair position, the operating table is first flexed at the level of the hip, bringing both the head and feet toward a more upright position. The foot section of the table is then low-ered to provide flexion at the level of the knees. This maneuver decreases the ten-sion on the muscular components of the posterior aspect of the lower extremities as well as the sciatic nerve. The back sec-tion of the table is then brought to a more vertical position while at the same time the entire table is placed in an approxi-mate 10 to 20 degree Trendelenburg po-sition. This increases the degree of hip flexion, and brings the patient's torso to a more vertical position while keeping the lower extremities close to heart level. This fulfills surgical requirements for ac-cess while minimizing the tendency for peripheral venous pooling (Fig. 5-14).

The patient is then shifted laterally on the table toward the edge so that the op-erative shoulder is free of the mattress. Care must be taken to see that the pa-tient's hips, head, and neck remain firmly supported by the operating table. A strong retaining strap should be placed across the patient's hips to prevent fur-ther lateral movement.

A pad is placed between the patient's scapulae to bring the operative shoulder forward and free of the mattress. This tends to cause the neck to extend, and extra padding is usually required to re-gain a more neutral head position.[3] The head should not be excessively rotated away from the surgical field as this creates

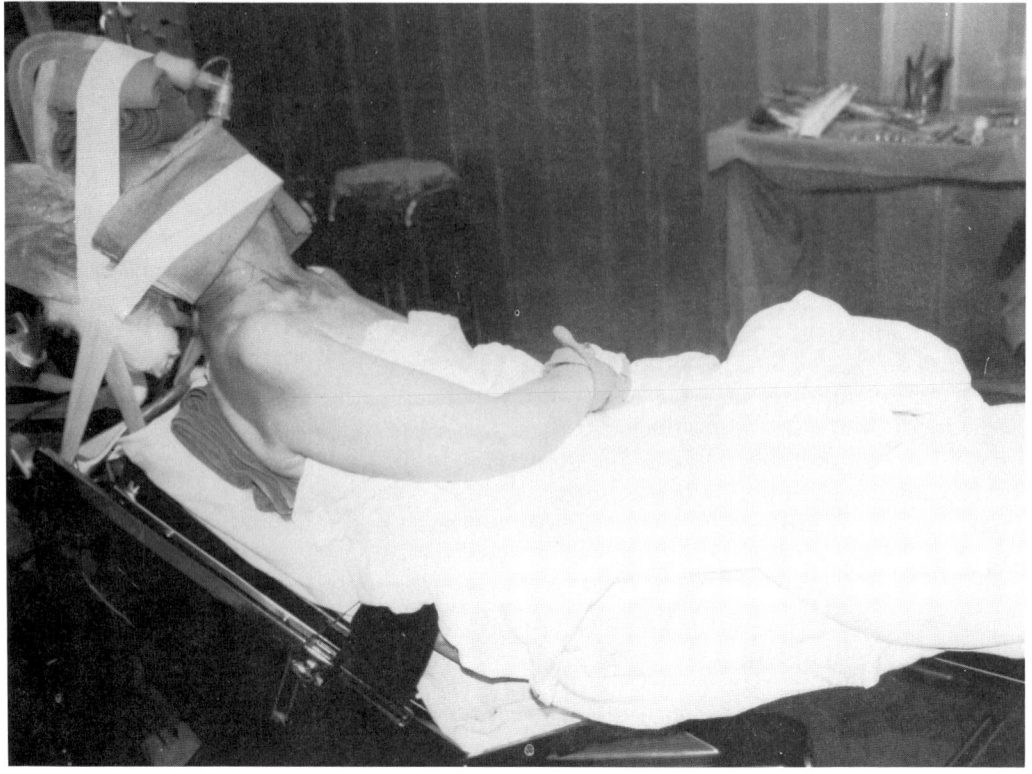

Fig. 5-14. Lateral view of upright shoulder position.

the potential for stretch injury to the brachial plexus, particularly during surgical manipulation of the upper extremity. The head should be secured in such a manner as to provide airway security and to minimize the chances of it being pulled off of the table during the surgical procedure. Once the surgical drapes are in place, access to the patient's face and airway are quite limited, so that extra care at this stage of the procedure to ensure airway security is warranted. We usually do so by fashioning a snug but not compressive "sling" for the head using towelling and adhesive tape. One band crosses the forehead and another is secured along the angle of the jaw. If a forehead strap is used alone, when the patient is pulled laterally during the procedure, the head may actually slip out from beneath a single strap. Care must be taken to see that no pressure is applied to the eyes or ears, and all airway connections should be tightened and reinforced with tape (Fig. 5-15).

If regional anesthesia is being used, we do not utilize such a restraint for the head as this would be extremely restrictive for the awake patient.

The nonoperative arm may be secured on an arm board. However, if a surgical assistant is to stand on that side, the arm board may be in the way. Alternatively, the arm may be placed across the patient's abdomen with adequate padding around the elbow to prevent ulnar nerve compression.

To minimize venous pooling in the lower extremities with assumption of the head-elevated shoulder position, the legs

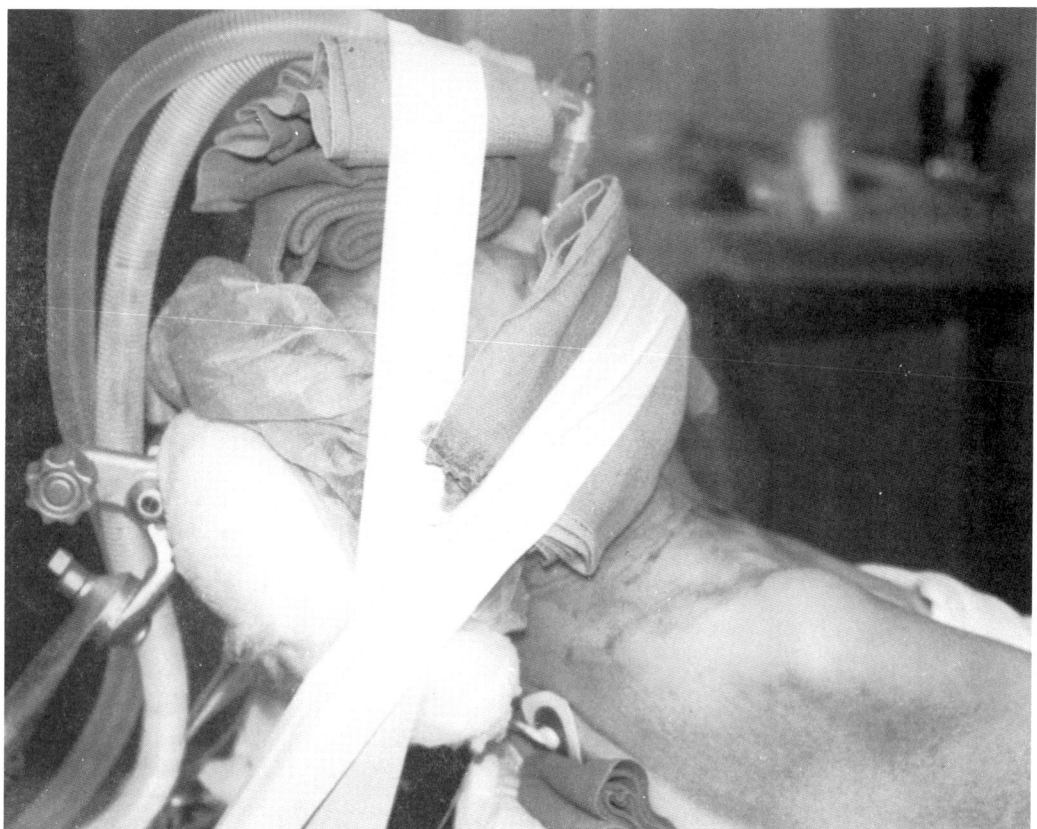

Fig. 5-15. Securing the head for the upright shoulder position.

should be wrapped or elastic stockings worn. A pillow placed beneath the knees provides extra padding and protection. Additional padding placed beneath the ankles decreases the weight bearing by the heels and avoids skin loss due to compression.

A theoretical concern whenever the operative site is above the level of the heart is the potential for venous air embolism. Practically speaking, this has not been a problem in patients undergoing shoulder surgery. Speculation as to why this may be so is just that. However, it might be prudent to take precautions and monitor for the occurrence of venous air embolism in patients with a known right-to-left shunt.

Fracture Table Positioning

Repairs of hip and femur fractures frequently necessitate the use of an orthopedic fracture table. Although quite intimidating at first glance, it is possible to master its use with some experience (Fig. 5-16).

The fracture table consists primarily of a body section that supports the head and thorax, a sacral plate with a vertical perineal post on which the pelvis rests, and adjustable foot plates to which the feet are anchored.

One advantage of this table is its ability to maintain traction on the fractured extremity. This allows manipulation of the fracture site to achieve a closed reduction and then fixation. The second advantage

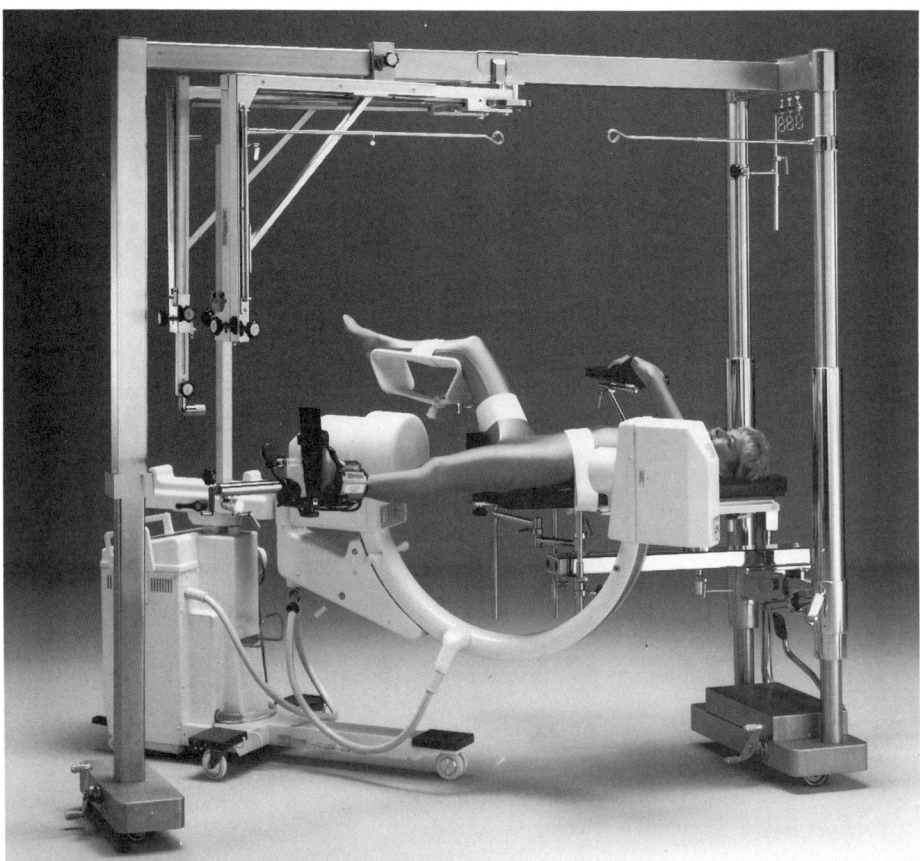

Fig. 5-16. The fracture table allows unobstructed access for closed reduction and pinning of hip and lower extremity fractures with the aid of fluoroscopic guidance. (Courtesy of Midmark Corporation, Versailles, OH.)

is access to the fracture site in several planes for fluoroscopic/radiographic examination and evaluation.

Because these patients present with painful fractures and are usually in traction devices when they arrive in the operating suite, the process of inducing anesthesia and positioning them on the fracture table requires some advance planning and communication.

Manipulation of the affected extremity can be quite painful and induction of

anesthesia is usually accomplished before the patient is moved from the hospital bed to the fracture table. Use of the fracture table is not a contraindication to regional anesthesia. With adequate sedation and continued traction on the fractured extremity the patient may be turned laterally in the hospital bed for performance of a spinal or epidural block. The nonfractured leg should be in the dependent position. It may be necessary to use a paramedian approach for these blocks as many of the patients with fractured hips are quite elderly and optimal positioning is difficult under the circumstances. Consideration should be given to using an isobaric injectate when administering a spinal anesthetic to a patient to be placed on the fracture table. The considerable amount of movement and jostling required to properly position the patient on the table can adversely affect the level of anesthesia achieved with either hyper- or hypobaric agents.

Many practitioners prefer to simply induce general anesthesia and then transfer the anesthetized, intubated patient to the fracture table.

Regardless of the anesthetic choice, it is important to maintain traction on the affected extremity throughout the period of transfer and positioning. If possible, the perineal post should be removed prior to the transfer. This avoids the need to lift the patient over the post, which can place considerable strain on those assisting in the move. Once the thorax and head are firmly supported on the top portion of the table, the patient should be shifted toward the perineal post until the pelvis is snug against it. Male genitalia should be free from compression by the post to avoid injury. There are several reports of pudendal nerve injuries associated with use of the fracture table and attributed to excessive compression by the perineal post.[30]

Once the patient is properly positioned against the well-padded perineal post, the foot is attached to the foot plate or holder and sufficient traction applied to optimize distraction and alignment of the fracture site. This is accomplished by the surgical team, usually with the aid of fluoroscopy (Fig. 5-17).

The unaffected limb can be similarly anchored to a foot plate and abducted to allow x-ray access to the surgical site. Alternatively the unaffected limb may be flexed at both the hip and knee and placed in an elevated leg holder, which is then abducted, similar to the lithotomy position.

Compartment syndromes developing as a result of ischemia due to overly compressive leg wraps in the elevated position, and intraoperative hypotension have been reported in patients on whom leg holders were used for the lithotomy position.[31,32] The potential for development of compartment syndrome may exist with use of the fracture table leg holder as well.

The arm ipsilateral to the fractured extremity must be kept clear of interference with radiographic access to the fracture site. The arm may be secured across the patient's abdomen with sufficient padding at the elbow to prevent ulnar nerve compression. Alternatively, the arm may be placed in an aerial sling fashioned on an ether screen. The danger with this method is the potential for brachial plexus injury when the arm is overly abducted and the plexus is stretched over the pectoralis muscle and clavicle. If this technique is used, the shoulder must be kept in a neutral position and the pectoralis muscle palpated to ensure its laxity. These areas should be re-examined frequently and adjustments made as needed throughout the surgical procedure.[14]

The contralateral arm may be placed on an arm board with precautions as noted earlier in this chapter.

The fracture table may also be used with the patient in the lateral decubitus position for femoral intramedullary rod placement (Fig. 5-18). In this position the fractured limb is uppermost and a tibial or femoral traction pin attached to the fracture table rather than the foot holder is used to maintain traction. The upper body rests on the back support with the dependent iliac crest resting on the well-padded lower edge of this section. As

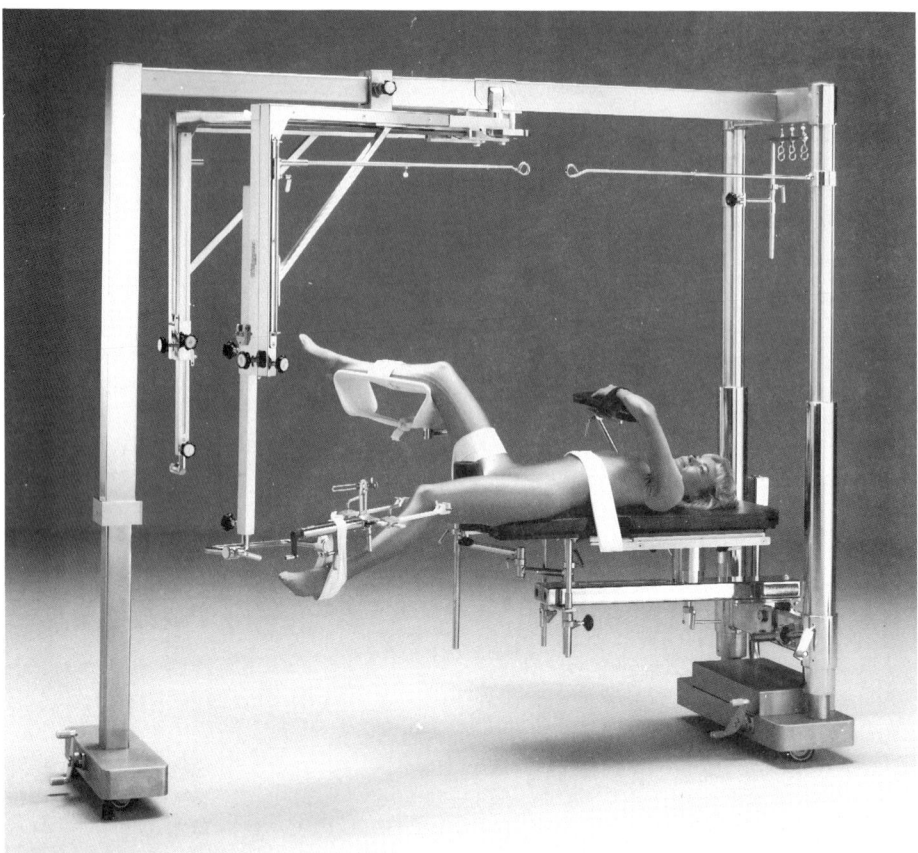

Fig. 5-17. Proper positioning of the patient on the fracture table is essential to surgical success. Care must be taken to avoid excess stretch of the brachial plexus when positioning the arm on the overarm board or when suspending it from an ether screen. When properly placed, there should be no tension on the pectoralis muscle. (Courtesy of Midmark Corporation, Versailles, OH.)

with the traditional lateral decubitus position discussed earlier, the arms can be placed on a two-tiered arm board or some similar arrangement, and the use of a chest roll is advocated to maintain vascular integrity in the dependent arm. The head should be supported to maintain alignment with the axial skeleton.

The pelvis is stabilized by a well-padded radiolucent C-shaped device that is placed between the thighs and curves ventrally to the anterior superior iliac crest. As with the perineal post used in

the supine position, care must be taken to avoid compression of male genitalia and compression of the pudendal nerve.[33] The dependent leg is placed in a well-padded leg holder.

Positioning patients properly on the fracture table is usually of more direct concern to the orthopedic surgeon than is achieving certain other positions. If done improperly, not only does the patient run the risk of injury, but it may make the surgical procedure impossible. Positioning to achieve proper reduction of the frac-

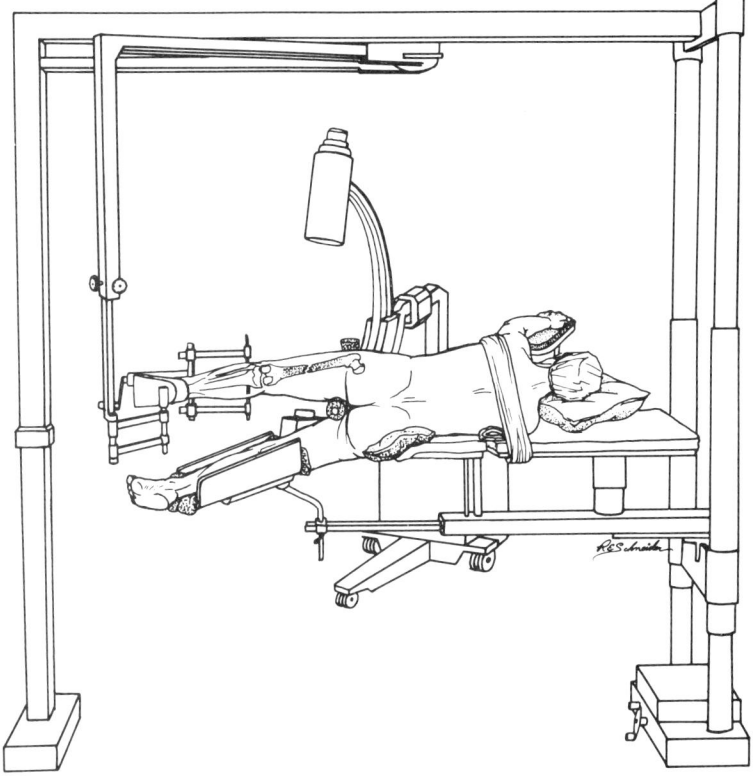

Fig. 5-18. Lateral position on the fracture table. (From Day,[57] with permission.)

ture and alignment of the pieces may take more time than the surgical procedure itself.

MONITORING

Intraoperative monitoring for most patients having orthopedic surgery is rarely any different than what is routinely provided elsewhere in the surgical suite. Adherence to the ASA Standards for Basic Intra-Operative Monitoring is recommended[34] (Table 5-3).

Patients presenting for orthopedic surgery cover a wide range of clinical practice and varying degrees of pathology, including such diverse conditions as the infant with a congenital deformity, the healthy young athlete with a sports-related injury, the middle-aged rheumatoid needing joint replacement, the elderly invalid with a fractured hip, and the traumatized victim of a motor vehicle accident. Each of these patients and clinical scenarios must be evaluated on an individual basis with regard to monitoring needs. Factors influencing monitoring decisions include underlying patient pathology (e.g., cardiovascular disease, history of cerebrovascular accidents, and bronchospasm), surgical procedure planned, predicted duration of that procedure, potential for blood loss or major fluid shifts, position of the patient during surgery, and planned anesthetic technique.

Table 5-3. ASA Standards for Basic Intra-operative Monitoring

Qualified anesthesia personnel present at all times

Oxygenation
    Analysis of inspired gases
    Quantitative method of analyzing patient blood oxygenation (i.e., pulse oximetry)

Ventilation
    Adequacy
        Chest excursion
        Observation of reservoir bag
        Auscultation of breath sounds
        Analysis of expired gases to deter-mine end-tidal carbon dioxide
        Disconnect alarm with mechanical ventilation

Circulation
    Continuous display of electrocardiogram
    Determination of heart rate and blood pressure every 5 minutes
    At least one:
        Palpation of pulse, auscultation of heart sounds, intra-arterial pres-sure, tracing, ultrasound peripheral pulse monitor, pulse plethysmog-raphy or oximetry

Body temperature

(Modified from the ASA Directory of Members,[34] with permission.)

Regional anesthesia techniques are applicable to many orthopedic surgical procedures. With regional anesthesia one has the added advantage of being able to communicate directly with the patient to ascertain level of comfort, adequacy of anesthesia, and mental status. However, this does not replace the need for basic vital sign monitoring, including assessment of adequacy of ventilation. This is particularly of concern when intravenous sedation is also administered. Pulse oximetry is helpful in this setting but if oxygen is being insufflated, a drop in arterial oxygen saturation may be delayed considerably while excessive carbon dioxide tensions rise or go unrecognized. With the patient in the lateral position, it may be difficult to use a precordial stethoscope. We have found it useful to place an extension from the mass spectrometer just inside the close-fitting oxygen mask to document carbon dioxide fluctuations with each respiratory effort.

Arterial Cannulation

Indwelling arterial cannulae are useful in any situation for which frequent sampling of blood is anticipated for determination of arterial blood gas levels, glucose, hemoglobin or hematocrit, electrolytes, or coagulation parameters. Morbidity from the single puncture and catheter placement is thought to be considerably less than multiple punctures of the same site during a lengthy orthopedic procedure. Major tumor resections, revisions of total joints, and spinal instrumentation are all associated with the potential for significant blood loss and fluid shifts. If deliberate hypotension is to be part of the anesthetic management, an indwelling arterial catheter should be routine.

Limb or digit replantation and reconstruction procedures can require many hours to complete, and while not as dramatic as some of the previously mentioned cases, blood loss is insidious and potentially as great. Direct arterial pressure monitoring is quite useful in this setting to assess changes in blood volume and to help ensure adequacy of perfusion in newly created microvascular anastomoses.

No invasive procedure is without morbidity. In one study of almost 1,700 patients undergoing arterial cannulation, 25 percent experienced partial or complete radial artery occlusion after decannulation. However, no ischemic damage to the hand or disability occurred in any of those patients.[35] In another series of 1,000 patients there were only two cases of significant occlusion seen. An embolectomy was performed for one and a radial artery reconstruction was done for the other. Neither patient suffered permanent sequelae.[36] Duration of cannulation (greater than 3 days) is thought by some to be a significant factor for diminution of flow.[36,37] Risk can be minimized by using a small-gauge Teflon cannula, removing it as soon as possible, and using good aseptic technique.[36,37]

Central Venous Pressure Catheters

Monitoring of central venous pressure (CVP) can be valuable during surgical cases in which potential for blood loss or fluid shifts is quite high. While intraoperative changes in positioning may affect the significance of the absolute number, following the trend of monitored values can provide insight into adequacy of intravascular volume and need for volume replacement. When this knowledge is combined with urine output measurements, arterial pressure, and hematocrit, the practitioner can make well-informed decisions about the necessity for volume replacement, blood transfusion, or vasopressors.

Patients with wound infections or chronic osteomyelitis and trauma victims who require multiple surgical procedures for debridement may benefit from the placement of a central venous line for intravascular access and long-term administration of antibiotics and nutritional supplementation.

Precordial Doppler

While rare, there are now several reported cases of major venous air embolism (VAE) occurring during spinal instrumentation and/or laminectomy in the prone position.[5,6] Only one of these cases used a precordial Doppler to detect VAE. When the Doppler was activated, 4 cc of air was aspirated from the CVP line. Attempted aspiration of air from the CVP line was negative in all the other cases. Whether the timing of the aspiration was not coincident with the occurrence of the air embolus or the CVP catheters were not properly positioned to capture the air is unclear. Furthermore, it is uncertain whether air emboli in the prone patient behave as reported in the more extensively studied upright patient.[38]

Albin et al[6] believed that the type of positioning used to achieve the prone posture contributed significantly to the occurrence of VAE. The use of a device that allows the abdomen to hang free and in which the lower extremities are dependent may amplify the gravitational gradient that already exists between the surgical field and the heart by further decreasing caval pressures. They believe that in association with a contracted blood volume or inadequate fluid replacement, these factors may increase the likelihood of VAE.[6]

While the CVP may not always be effective for aspirating air in the prone position, the information it provides regarding volume status may allow the practitioner to avoid the complication of VAE by more accurately replacing intravascular fluid volume.

Because of the rarity of the occurrence of VAE in the prone patient, the decision to add a precordial Doppler to the intraoperative monitoring is left to the individual practitioner.

Pulmonary Artery Catheter

The decision to place a pulmonary artery catheter for intraoperative monitoring should be dictated by the condition of the patient. There is not, to my knowledge, any orthopedic surgical procedure that requires routine placement of a pulmonary artery catheter. Certainly a history of congestive heart failure, compromised cardiac function, a recent myocardial infarction, or unstable angina would influence the anesthesia practitioner to strongly consider the utility of a pulmonary artery catheter. Again, however, the decision should be made on an individual case-by-case basis.[39]

Temperature

Hypothermia is a frequent observation in surgical patients on arrival in the postanesthesia recovery unit.[40] Orthopedic surgical patients may be at particular risk in operating rooms that utilize laminar flow because of the rapid turnover of room air and "wind chill" that is created. Operating room temperatures are frequently set low to keep operating personnel more comfortable beneath hoods and other barrier devices used in the name of infection control. Major regional anesthetics (i.e., spinal and epidural) induce a sympathetic blockade, which increases blood flow to the skin, thereby increasing radiant heat loss and the likelihood of hypothermia, while general anesthesia inhibits central thermoregulation.[40,41]

Patients with limited cardiac and/or pulmonary reserve may not be able to tolerate or provide for the up to 400 percent increase in oxygen demand that can accompany shivering in response to decreased body temperature.[42] The success of microvascular surgery may be compromised if the patient should peripherally vasoconstrict in response to a cold environment and diminish blood flow through newly created anastomoses. Peripheral vasoconstriction may also shift blood volume centrally and contribute to underestimation of fluid needs.[42] Hypo-

thermia can lead to coagulation abnormalities as well as interfere with interpretation of monitoring such as SSEPs and pulse oximetry.[43,44] Therefore, precautions should be taken to prevent the loss of heat, including keeping the patient covered, using active or passive in-line gas humidifiers, and maintaining an appropriately warm room temperature. The Bair Hugger (Augustine Medical Products, Inc., Eden Prairie, MN), a forced-air warming device, has been shown to be an effective and efficient means of preventing hypothermia in surgical patients, as well as re-warming patients who have become hypothermic.[45–47]

Although less likely, hyperthermia may also be seen. Possible causes include active infection and/or septicemia, small children undergoing minor or peripheral surgery beneath multiple layers of surgical drapes, transfusion reaction, and malignant hyperthermia. Careful evaluation, including appropriate laboratory testing, may be needed to differentiate potentially life-threatening causes from those with a more benign course.

Neurophysiologic Monitoring

Although usually associated with spine and neurologic surgery, neurophysiologic monitoring has a number of applications in orthopedic surgery as well. The purpose of this effort is to provide early detection of potentially reversible neurologic injury with the goal of preserving function.

SSEPs are used most frequently during spinal instrumentation procedures, and in many instances have eliminated the need for an intraoperative "wake-up test" in these patients.[48,49] False-negative examinations do, however, occur, particularly when there is a selective insult to motor pathways not directly monitored by standard evoked potential techniques.[50]

Stimulation is applied to major peripheral nerves (peroneal or tibial in the leg, and median or ulnar in the arm) and recorded centrally by surface electrodes on the scalp, neck, or esophagus; or peripherally proximal to the stimulus input. Signal averaging is then done to filter out artifact from other sources of electrical energy, movement, and electromyographic activity.

Intraoperative use of SSEPs is complicated by the type and depth of anesthetic, body temperature, blood pressure, and other physiologic variables.[48,49] Signal amplitude reduction is directly related to depth of anesthesia. Inhalational anesthetics have the greatest potential in this regard.[51] A reduction of mean arterial pressure to 70 mmHg or less has been associated with a decreased amplitude as well.[48]

A significant change in intraoperative SSEPs is defined as a consistent increase in latency (2.0 ms greater than baseline) and amplitude reduction (50 percent less than baseline) at both the neck and scalp recording sites with an intact peripheral response.[44]

At the Mayo Clinic, over a 3-year period, 351 patients underwent spine surgery with SSEP monitoring. Of these, 6 had significant changes in SSEPs intraoperatively. Three were reversed within 5 to 10 minutes after surgical intervention and exhibited no permanent neurologic deficits postoperatively. One patient developed a permanent neurologic deficit despite surgical removal of spinal instrumentation. Two patients reversed spontaneously after 15 minutes, one of whom had a persistent L5 radiculopathy postoperatively. Of the 345 remaining patients who did not experience an intraoperative change in SSEPs, 2 had postoperative deficits consistent with anterior spinal artery syndrome, and 7 had persistent lumbar radiculopathies.[44]

When a significant change is identified, efforts to reverse it must be taken by both the surgical and anesthesia personnel involved. Surgical causes such as excessive spinal distraction, trauma, and hematoma must be ruled out. Discontinuation of inhalational agents and correction of hypotension, hypoxemia, hypocarbia, and anemia can help to improve spinal cord blood flow, and may contribute to the restoration of SSEPs and avoid postoperative neurologic deficit.

It is important to remember that vascular compromise to the peripheral nerves may also result in loss of SSEP signals. In one case at our institution, a sudden loss of the SSEP signal from the tibial nerve 6 hours into an anterior spinal fusion was found to be secondary to occlusion of the common iliac artery to that same leg. The signal returned (albeit diminished) once restoration of flow through a Dacron interposition graft was accomplished. SSEPs returned to baseline 1 week postoperatively.

SSEPs are also used for intraoperative diagnosis of brachial plexus avulsions. The surgeon selectively stimulates the nerve roots and the response is recorded over the contralateral scalp. Confirming the presence or absence of axonal continuity then helps to direct the efforts of the surgical team to those areas with the best chance for recovery.[52]

Electromyography is frequently monitored along with SSEPs during spinal instrumentation and/or fusion procedures. Fine wire electrodes are placed directly into the muscles and patients are monitored for neurotonic discharges. These discharges occur in response to mechanical or metabolic irritation of the nerves innervating the muscle and alert the surgeon of undue stretch or dissection in the vicinity of the nerve.[52]

Electromyography may also be monitored during total hip arthroplasty if the surgeon is concerned about the potential for sciatic nerve injury with leg length-ening and during shoulder repair for recurrent anterior dislocation with the potential for injury to the musculocutaneous and axillary nerves.

Compound muscle action potentials and nerve action potentials may also be used intraoperatively to stimulate and localize lesions of peripheral nerves and guide the surgeons as to the most appropriate procedure (e.g., ulnar transposition vs. cubital tunnel release).[53] Precise preoperative localization of lesions is not always possible with less invasive modalities because of technical difficulties and anatomic variability.

To summarize, proper positioning of patients for orthopedic surgery is essential for a successful outcome, both from an anesthetic and an orthopedic standpoint, although it is often slighted or taken for granted. If improperly positioned, patients are placed at risk for the development of permanent disabling sequalae. Careful attention to detail is needed to ensure the safety and integrity of the surgical patient. The anesthesia practitioner should be aware of the physical limitations of the patient, the optimal surgical position, and its physiologic and anatomic consequences. Communication between the patient, surgeon, and anesthesia personnel is crucial to establish an acceptable position to meet the individual needs of all parties involved.

Many orthopedic positions and a number of specialty procedures necessitate special monitoring in excess of the minimal standards because of inaccessibility to the patient, the duration of the procedure, or the degree of physiologic trespass engendered. The anesthesia practitioner must be able to anticipate when a particular procedure or position will warrant extra monitoring. The patient's medical condition must also be considered when planning for intraoperative monitoring needs.

Providing anesthesia services for or-

thopedic surgical cases can be both challenging and rewarding. To do so safely, anesthesia practitioners must familiarize themselves with the types of procedures performed as well as the positioning and monitoring implications.

REFERENCES

1. Dhunér K-G: Nerve injuries following operations: a survey of cases occurring during a six-year period. Anesthesiology 11:289, 1950
2. Parks BJ: Postoperative peripheral neuropathies. Surgery 74:348, 1973
3. Mitterschiffthaler G, Theiner A, Posch G: Lesion of the brachial plexus, caused by wrong positioning during surgery. Anasth Internsivther Notfallmed 22:177, 1987
4. Spiess BD, Sloan MS, McCarthy RJ et al: The incidence of venous air embolism during total hip arthroplasty. J Clin Anesth 1:25, 1988
5. Lang SA, Duncan PG, Dupuis PR: Fatal air embolism in an adolescent with Duchenne muscular dystrophy during Harrington instrumentation. Anesth Analg 69:132, 1989
6. Albin MS, Ritter RR, Pruett CE, Kalff K: Venous air embolism during lumbar laminectomy in the prone position: report of three cases. Anesth Analg 73:346, 1991
7. Smith JW, Pellicci PM, Sharrock N et al: Complications after total hip replacement. The contralateral limb. J Bone Joint Surg [Am] 71:528, 1989
8. Aschoff A, Steiner-Milz H, Steiner H-H: Lower limb compartment syndrome following lumbar discectomy in the knee-chest position. Neurosurg Rev 13:155, 1990
9. Keim HA, Weinstein JD: Acute renal failure—a complication of spine fusion in the tuck position. J Bone Joint Surg [Am] 52:1248, 1970
10. Smith BL: Physiologic changes in the normal conscious human subject on changing from the erect to the supine position. p. 13. In Martin TJ (ed): Positioning in Anes-

thesia and Surgery, 2nd Ed. WB Saunders, Philadelphia, 1987

11. Brown EM, Elman DS: Postoperative backache. Anesth Analg 40:683, 1961

12. Patel KD, Henschel EO: Postoperative alopecia. Anesth Analg 59:311, 1980

13. Po BT, Hansen HR: Iatrogenic brachial plexus injury: a survey of the literature and of pertinent cases. Anesth Analg 48:915, 1969

14. Covington JW: The role of posture in anesthesia. Clin Anesth 3:24, 1968

15. Jackson L, Keats AS: Mechanism of brachial plexus palsy following anesthesia. Anesthesiology 26:190, 1965

16. Wright IS: The neurovascular syndrome produced by hyperabduction of the arms. Am Heart J 29:1, 1945

17. Lincoln JR, Sawyer HP: Complications related to body positions during surgical procedures. Anesthesiology 22:800, 1961

18. Britt BA, Gordon RA: Peripheral nerve injuries associated with anaesthesia. Can Anaesth Soc J 11:514, 1964

19. Hovagim AR, Backus WW, Manecke G et al: Pulse oximetry and patient positioning: a report of eight cases. Anesthesiology 71:454, 1989

20. Jaffe TB, McLeskey CH: Position-induced Horner's syndrome. Anesthesiology 56:49, 1982

21. Walkup HE, Murphy JD: Retinal ischemia with unilateral blindness—a complication occurring during pulmonary resection in the prone position. J Thorac Surg 23:174, 1952

22. Mankowitz E: Blood pressure measurement during lateral tilt. Anaesthesia 34:84, 1979

23. Lawson NW: The lateral decubitus position. Anesthesiologic considerations. p. 155. In Martin TJ (ed): Positioning in Anesthesia and Surgery. 2nd Ed. WB Saunders, Philadelphia, 1987

24. Welborn SG: Unusual positions. Urology: anesthesiologic considerations. p. 249. In Martin TJ (ed): Positioning in Anesthesia and Surgery. 2nd Ed. WB Saunders, Philadelphia, 1987

25. Martin TJ: The prone position. Anesthesiologic considerations. p. 191. In Martin TJ (ed): Positioning in Anesthesia and Surgery. 2nd Ed. WB Saunders, Philadelphia, 1987

26. Skeehan TM, Hensley FA Jr: Axillary artery compression and the prone position. Anesth Analg 65:318, 1986

27. Winter R, Munro M: Lingual and buccal nerve neuropathy in a patient in the prone position. A case report. Anesthesiology 71:452, 1989

28. Swerdlow BN, Brodsky JB, Butcher MD: Placement of a morbidly obese patient in the prone position. Anesthesiology 68:657, 1988

29. Deem S, Shapiro HM, Marshall LF: Quadriplegia in a patient with cervical spondylosis after thoracolumbar surgery in the prone position. Anesthesiology 75:527, 1991

30. Hofmann A, Jones RE, Schoenvogel R: Pudendal-nerve neurapraxia as a result of traction on the fracture table. J Bone Joint Surg [Am] 64:136, 1982

31. Adler LM, Loughlin JS, Morin CJ, Haning RV Jr: Bilateral compartment syndrome after a long gynecologic operation in the lithotomy position. Am J Obstet Gynecol 162:1271, 1990

32. Lydon JC, Spielman FJ: Bilateral compartment syndrome following prolonged surgery in the lithotomy position. Anesthesiology 60:236, 1984

33. Lindenbaum SD, Fleming LL, Smith DW: Pudendal-nerve palsies associated with closed intramedullary femoral fixation. J Bone Joint Surg [Am] 64:934, 1982

34. American Society of Anesthesiologists, Directory of Members. American Society of Anesthesiologists, Park Ridge, IL, 1991, p. 670.

35. Slogoff S, Keats AS, Arlund C: On the safety of radial artery cannulation. Anesthesiology 59:42, 1983

36. Mandel MA, Dauchot PJ: Radial artery cannulation in 1,000 patients: precautions and complications. J Hand Surg 2:482, 1977

37. Bedford RF: Long-term radial artery cannulation: effects on subsequent vessel function. Crit Care Med 6:64, 1978

38. Black S, Cucchiara RF: Tumor surgery. p. 285. In Cucchiara RF, Michenfelder JD (eds): Clinical Neuroanesthesia. Churchill Livingstone, New York, 1990

39. Spackman TN, Rorie DK: Monitoring during cardiovascular surgery. p. 81. In Tarhan S (ed): Cardiovascular Anesthesia and Postoperative Care. 2nd Ed. Year Book Medical Publishers, Chicago, 1989

40. Vaughan MS, Vaughan RW, Cork RC: Postoperative hypothermia in adults: relationship of age, anesthesia, and shivering to rewarming. Anesth Analg 60:746, 1981

41. Sten R, Sessler DI: The thermoregulatory threshold is inversely proportional to isoflurane concentration. Anesthesiology 72:822, 1990

42. Flacke JW, Flacke WE: Inadvertent hypothermia: frequent, insidious, and often serious. Semin Anesth 2:183, 1983

43. Bunker JP: Coagulation during hypothermia in man. Biol Med 97:199, 1958

44. Harper CM, Daube JR: Surgical monitoring with evoked potentials; the Mayo Clinc experience. p. 275. In Desmedt JE (ed): Neuromonitoring in Surgery. Elsevier Science Publishers, New York, 1989

45. Hynson JM, Sessler DI: Comparison of intraoperative warming devices. Anesth Analg 72:S118, 1991

46. Sessler DI, Moayeri A: Skin-surface warming: heat flux and central temperature. Anesthesiology 73:218, 1990

47. Lennon RL, Hosking MP, Conover MA, Perkins WJ: Evaluation of a forced-air system for warming hypothermic postoperative patients. Anesth Analg 70:424, 1990

48. Daube JR, Harper CM, Litchy WJ, Sharbrough FW: Intraoperative monitoring. p. 739. In Daly DD, Pedley TA (eds): Current Practice of Clinical Electroencephalography. 2nd Ed. Raven Press, New York, 1990

49. Grundy BL: Intraoperative monitoring of sensory-evoked potentials. Anesthesiology 58:72, 1983

50. Ginsburg HH, Shetter AG, Raudzens PA: Postoperative paraplegia with preserved intraoperative somatosensory evoked potentials. J Neurosurg 63:296, 1985

51. Pathak KS, Ammadio M, Kalamchi A et al: Effects of halothane, enflurane, and isoflurane on somatosensory evoked potentials during nitrous oxide anesthesia. Anesthesiology 66:753, 1987

52. Daube JR, Harper CM: Surgical monitoring of cranial and peripheral nerves. p. 115. In Desmedt JE (ed): Neuromonitoring in Surgery. Elsevier Science Publishers, New York, 1989

53. Kline DG, Hackett ER, Happel LH: Surgery for lesions of the brachial plexus. Arch Neurol 43:170, 1986

54. Kropp KA: Unusual positions. Urology: surgical aspects. p. 241. In Martin TJ (ed): Positioning in Anesthesia and Surgery. 2nd Ed. WB Saunders, Philadelphia, 1987

55. Singh I: The prone position. p. 181. In Martin TJ (ed): Positioning in Anesthesia and Surgery. 2nd Ed. WB Saunders, Philadelphia, 1987

56. Reid SA, Grundy BL: The head-elevated positions. Surgical aspects: the neurosurgical skull clamp. p. 71. In Martin TJ (ed): Positioning in Anesthesia and Surgery. 2nd Ed. WB Saunders, Philadelphia, 1987

57. Day LJ: Unusual positions. Orthopedics: surgical aspects. p. 223. In Martin TJ (ed): Positioning in Anesthesia and Surgery. 2nd Ed. WB Saunders, Philadelphia, 1987

6

The Pediatric Patient: Regional Anesthesia

Denise J. Wedel

Pediatric patients make up a significant portion of the orthopedic surgical list in a hospital serving all age groups. Children can present with a variety of orthopedic surgical problems. Congenital deformities such as club foot, hip dysplasia, and finger syndactyly present in infancy, while fractures of the forearm are usually seen in the older, school-age child. Other surgical problems include infections or malignancies affecting bone or joints and spinal deformities associated with an underlying muscle disorder. Traumatic orthopedic injuries, which are usually caused by motor vehicle accidents, can be associated with multiple injuries involving other organ systems. There are increasing numbers of surgical procedures for sports-related injuries in children.

Basic guidelines concerning anesthetic management of the pediatric patient are discussed in depth in textbooks dedicated to that subject. The recommendations concerning appropriate monitoring, fluid management, general anesthetic induction and maintenance techniques, and special considerations in the pediatric patient such as choice of anesthesia circuits, maintenance of body temperature, and airway considerations are equally valid in the orthopedic pediatric population. This chapter, therefore, concentrates on the use of regional anesthesia in the child undergoing orthopedic surgery.

The application of regional anesthetic techniques to the pediatric population has been met with increasing enthusiasm by parents, surgeons, and anesthesia care providers.[1-3] Such techniques are uniquely adaptable to the pediatric orthopedic population. The surgical procedure often involves a single extremity, an ideal situation for regional anesthesia. Management of postoperative factors such as surgical pain, adequate blood flow to the surgical site, and early ambulation and hospital discharge are desirable endpoints obtained with regional anesthesia. From a technical standpoint, regional anesthetic procedures are often easier to perform in children than in adults because of the relative lack of subcutaneous tissue. This allows easy palpation of bony and vascular landmarks and improved spread of local anesthetics.

INDICATIONS AND CITED ADVANTAGES

Many of the advantages cited for pediatric regional anesthesia are similar to those reported in the adult population

129

Table 6-1. Advantages of Pediatric
Regional Anesthesia

Postoperative pain control
Earlier ambulation and hospital discharge
Decreased postoperative nausea and vomiting
Postoperative sympathectomy
Avoidance of upper airway manipulation
Technical ease of block placement
Ready acceptance by parents
Neonates: decreased respiratory complications
Avoidance of general anesthesia
    Family history of malignant hyperthermia
    Chronic pulmonary disease
    Cardiac disease
    Neuromuscular disease
    Full stomach

(Table 6-1). For example, improved pain control and a decreased incidence of nausea and vomiting in the postoperative period, earlier ambulation, and shorter hospital stays are advantages shared by both age groups. However, specific benefits from the effects of neural blockade, with or without a concomitant light general anesthetic, can be observed in children. These include the avoidance of upper airway complications, and in the high-risk neonatal population, a decrease in the respiratory complications that have been reported following general anesthesia.[4,5] Specifically, in the orthopedic surgical pediatric patient undergoing microvascular procedures such as replanting limbs or digits, the continuation of regional anesthesia techniques into the postoperative period can provide added benefits related to the establishment and maintenance of sympathetic blockade with the associated increase in blood flow.

Regional anesthesia is also useful when general anesthetics are relatively contraindicated or associated with increased morbidity such as in patients with cardiac, neuromuscular,[6] or chronic pulmonary disease,[7] or a family history of malignant hyperthermia.[8]

CITED DISADVANTAGES

Concerns expressed about performing regional block techniques in children probably reflect a lack of familiarity with the neuroanatomy and local anesthetic pharmacology as it relates to this population by physicians and other medical care providers. They may also reflect a projection of adult fears concerning needles and associated complications. Specific disadvantages cited have included medicolegal concerns, lack of patient cooperation, requirement for heavy sedation and attendant risks of airway complications, apprehension experienced by children relating to the loss of sensation and movement, and lack of parental acceptance. However, when examined closely, these disadvantages are largely theoretical and are best managed by thoughtful preoperative preparation and flexibility in the anesthesia care provider's approach to the individual child.

PREOPERATIVE PREPARATION AND MANAGEMENT OF SEDATION

Medicolegal concerns with pediatric neural blockade are no different from those associated with general anesthesia. Parental permission must be obtained following a frank discussion of the advantages and risks of each proposed procedure. Parental acceptance of regional anesthesia is usually quite high, an observation that is not surprising considering the postoperative benefits that are being offered.

The preoperative visit plays an important role in creating a trusting relationship with both the parent and child, and will aid the anesthesia care provider in determining the best approach to the block. This approach will vary according to the age, level of anxiety when separated from the parent, and previous surgical experience, among other factors. During the preoperative visit the child and parent should be instructed in the details of neural blockade during the intra- and postoperative period, particularly if prolonged sensory and motor block are anticipated. Most children are primarily afraid of the unknown, and will welcome and accept understandable explanations of potentially frightening events. However, if the physician–patient relationship and trust are disrupted, the child may become very uncooperative and distressed, even requiring abandonment of the proposed technique. It is important to recall that children often tend to view new experiences without an extensive overlay of life experience, and therefore interpret events according to their own internal standards. For example, an adult patient may accept that par-

esthesias are not truly painful when you explain that they are stimulations of the nerve similar to those experienced when the "funny bone" is accidentally hit. However, a child will usually interpret all noxious or unexpected stimuli as painful, and may lose trust in an adult who tries to mask such discomforts by calling them by another name.

The choice of preoperative and preblock sedation is often a critical factor in patient satisfaction and acceptance of regional anesthesia. Appropriate sedation can vary from none, in rare instances, to light general anesthesia for the very young or anxious child (Table 6-2). Intranasal[9] or oral midazolam is effective when administered preoperatively to allay anxieties and allow intravenous access to be established. Oral midazolam is bitter, but this taste can be partly masked with Hershey's Strawberry Syrup. A suitable anxiolytic/sedative dose of midazolam (5 mg/ml) in syrup is 0.5 mg/kg with sedation occurring in about 20 minutes.

Table 6-2. Agents Used in Premedication and Intraoperative Sedation

Drug	Dose (mg/kg)	Route	Onset Time (min)	Advantages/Disadvantages
Ketamine	1–2	IV	<5	Rapid onset, reliable; ↑ secretions (give atropine), may cause apnea (IV), blunts airway responses, sterile abscess (IM)
Fentanyl	0.001–0.005	IV	<5	Rapid, reliable; IV route threatening and painful
Midazolam	0.01–0.03	IV	<5	Reliable sedation; unpleasant taste (IN and PO) (PO mix with syrup), absorption can be delayed (PR)
	0.05–0.1	IM	5–10	
	0.1–0.2	IN	15–30	
	0.5–0.6	PO	15–30	
	1–3	PR	10	
Methohexital	25–30	PR	5–10	± painful; onset unreliable, hiccups
Chloral hydrate	30–100	PO, PR	30–60	Sedation, unpleasant taste, slow onset

IV, intravenous; IM, intramuscular; PO, oral; PR, rectal; IN, intranasal.
(Modified from Yaster & Maxwell,[1] with permission.)

If the child can be encouraged to hold the syrup in the mouth, onset is more rapid because of the mucosal absorption. A number of other alternatives such as intramuscular ketamine or midazolam, rectal methohexital, and mask inhalational agents can be used. Intravenous administration of the standard sedative agents can also be used to provide appropriate conditions for placement of the regional anesthetic as well as ensuring adequate sedation during surgery.

GENERAL CONSIDERATIONS

Anatomic Differences

As mentioned above, regional anesthetic techniques are often technically simpler to perform in children. Small children tend to have less overlying subcutaneous fat, allowing easy palpation of landmarks, and their nerves are smaller and thinner, permitting better diffusion of the local anesthetic. However, neonatal nerves are not fully myelinated, therefore lower concentrations of local anesthetic are required for neural blockade. Fascial and ligamentous structures in children are thinner and easier to penetrate. Use of a blunt-beveled needle for peripheral nerve blocks is helpful in recognizing these structures and can aid in accurate block placement.[10]

Anatomy of the structures involved in central neuraxial blockade also differs in children. Both the spinal cord and the dural sac extend lower in the spinal canal in infants and achieve the adult position at about 1 year of age (Fig. 6-1). The neonatal spinal cord can extend as far as L3 and the dural sac to S3, compared to the adult positions at L1 and S1, respectively.[11,12] Because of these anatomic considerations, it is preferable to perform spinal anesthesia in small children below L3. At this level, the subarachnoid space is encountered at 10 to 15 mm below the skin. Infants and children weighing less than 15 kg have a relatively higher total volume of spinal fluid (4 ml/kg compared to 2 ml/kg in adults[13]) and may require relatively higher milligram per kilogram doses of local anesthetic to achieve adequate subarachnoid blockade. Epidural fat in small children has a gelatinous, spongy appearance with distinct individual fat globules as compared with the densely packed adult epidural fat. The spread of epidural local anesthetic is therefore greater in children.[14] Because of the smaller size of nerve roots, complete blockade of the larger L5 and S1 roots is usually attained in children. At the level of the lower lumbar spine, the epidural space is located only 10 to 18 mm below the skin, so care must be taken to avoid dural puncture, particularly if adult-sized equipment is utilized.[15] It should be noted that the hemodynamic responses to sympathetic blockade induced by spinal and epidural anesthesia in children are blunted, and hypotension is uncommon even with extensive sensory blockade.[16–20]

Selection of Materials and Techniques

Block Selection

The selection of a specific block technique will depend on several factors that should be carefully evaluated in the preoperative period. These include (1) the age and physical status of the child; (2) the proposed surgical site as well as possible additional sites (e.g., bone graft harvest); (3) the position required for surgery; (4) anticipated fluid shifts; (5) the duration of the procedure; (6) the degree of pain anticipated in the postoperative period; (7) the type of surgical dressing

BIRTH ADULT

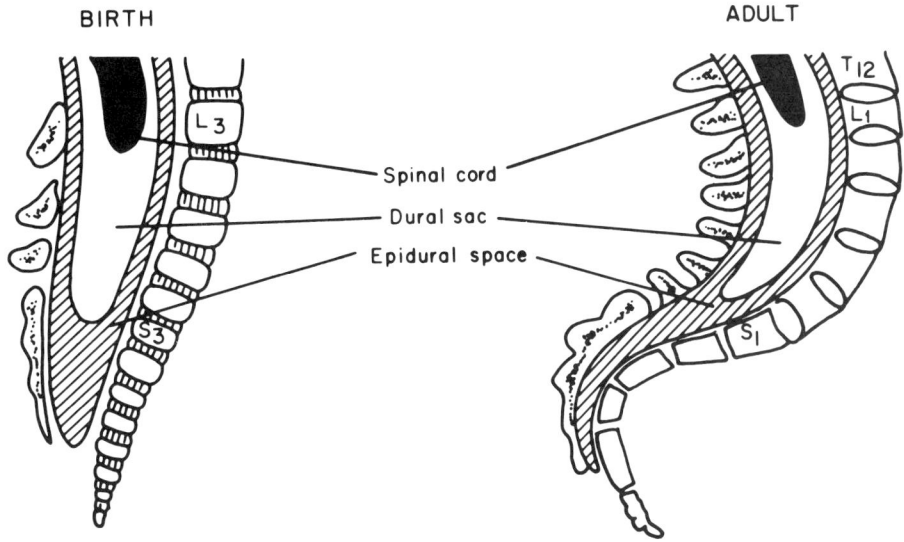

Fig. 6-1. Age-related differences in the length of the spinal cord and dural sac are demonstrated. The spinal cord (solid black) extends as low as L3 in the newborn, assuming the adult position of L1 at about 1 year of age. The dural sac (clear) extends as low as S3 in the newborn, also achieving the adult position of S1 at about 1 year of age. The epidural space is represented by the crosshatched area.

or cast planned; and (8) the experience of the anesthesia care provider. The type of nerve block, choice of local anesthetic agent and additives, and plan for postoperative pain management should be tailored to suit these variables.

Block Technique

Appropriate monitoring should be instituted prior to beginning the nerve block. Resuscitation drugs and equipment, including appropriately sized masks, endotracheal tubes, and laryngoscopes, should be present in the regional anesthesia induction area.

Special needles designed for pediatric regional anesthesia offer some advantages because of their shorter length, smaller gauge, and blunt bevel. Insulated needles, designed for use with a nerve stimulator in locating peripheral nerves, may be useful for blockade in heavily sedated patients. Limiting the variety of

needles and other equipment used in pediatric regional anesthesia will help the practitioner develop a "feel" for the tissue elasticity and relative anatomic location of neural structures.

Safety Measures

Prevention of complications starts in the preoperative period with careful patient selection, and continues in the intraoperative period. During placement of the block, several measures can be taken to decrease the risk of neural and local anesthetic complications. Paresthesia techniques for location of peripheral nerves are rarely appropriate in children because of their perception of paresthesias as noxious stimuli and the presence of heavy sedation, which might mask inadvertent intraneural injection. The excellent spread of local anesthetic in children and relative sensitivity of the smaller nerves to these agents results in a high rate of successful blockade whatever technique is used. As mentioned earlier, a nerve stimulator can be used to locate peripheral nerves by stimulating a motor response. However, equally good results are seen with "sheath" or perivascular techniques in smaller children.[10]

Precautions taken during the injection of the local anesthetic to decrease the risk of toxicity are listed below:

1. Calculate the appropriate local anesthetic dose on a body weight basis and then recheck the calculations.
2. Add epinephrine in concentrations of 1:200,000 to all local solutions unless the block is at an anatomic site supplied by terminal arteries (penis, digits, etc.).
3. Following negative aspiration, inject a test dose (0.5 to 3 ml) and observe for signs of intravascular epinephrine or local anesthetic toxicity (hypertension, tachycardia, central nervous system excitement) for 1 to 2 minutes before proceeding with further injection. In the case of epidural injection, signs of intrathecal placement (development of spinal anesthesia) should also be monitored.
4. The remainder of the calculated local anesthetic dose should be injected slowly and incrementally.
5. Frequent aspiration for blood or cerebrospinal fluid during injection will verify that the needle or catheter has not become misplaced.

The use of a test dose containing epinephrine in pediatric epidural blocks is controversial. A study by Desparmet et al[21] reported that in halothane-anesthetized children undergoing epidural anesthesia, intravascularly injected test doses containing 5 µg/ml of epinephrine did not reliably result in a positive response (more than 10 beats/min increase in heart rate). In the same report, pretreatment with atropine improved the reliability of the epinephrine-containing test dose. Conditions that may interfere with interpretation of the test dose include the presence of light general anesthesia, positioning of the patient, intubation, premedication with vagolytic agents, and patient age. Careful patient assessment and frequent gentle aspiration prior to injection of local anesthetic should be used in addition to the test dose in small children to avoid toxicity from inadvertent intravascular injection.

Assessment of Blockade

Determination of whether a regional block technique has resulted in surgical anesthesia can be challenging in the pediatric patient, particularly if the child is heavily sedated or receiving light general anesthesia. Application of noxious stimuli, such as a pinch or needle stick in the area of anticipated blockade, may result in a withdrawal response if *no* neural blockade is present or if blockade is inadequate. However, variable degrees of sensory block may be difficult to determine prior to surgical intervention. The practitioner should therefore be prepared to deepen the level of sedation or anesthesia immediately if the child reacts to skin incision. The awake or lightly sedated pediatric patient presents a more difficult challenge. The anesthesia care provider must be careful to maintain the patient's confidence, and not transmit personal anxieties concerning the efficacy of the block to the child. It is essential to avoid applying noxious stimuli to potentially unblocked areas. The use of an alcohol-drenched sponge to assess areas of blockade is usually well tolerated by the patient while giving an accurate assessment of the extent of sensory blockade. Even young children can verbalize "wet" or "dry" and "nothing." If motor blockade is present, the child should be reassured that this is an excellent sign of the block's efficacy. However, it is equally important to remind the patient that the motor and sensory block will resolve following the surgical procedure, and to reinforce the advantages of postoperative pain relief associated with the lack of sensation.

PHARMACOLOGY AND PHARMACOKINETICS OF LOCAL ANESTHETICS

The recommendations for safe maximum doses of local anesthetics in children are in general referenced to studies in adults with a dose per weight calculation (Table 6-3). Many of the factors that affect serum concentrations of local anesthetic agents in children are similar to those in adults. These include the site of administration, speed of injection, total dosage, addition of vasoconstrictors, local anesthetic pharmacologic profile, and underlying medical conditions or other physiologic factors that affect drug availability and metabolism. Few studies specifically address local anesthetic pharmacodynamics and pharmacokinetics in

the pediatric population, but some differences have been noted.

Metabolism of both ester and amide local anesthetics is theoretically decreased in neonates. Ester-type agents are metabolized by plasma cholinesterase. Plasma levels of this enzyme are depressed to half the normal adult levels in infants up to 6 months of age.[22] The amides are metabolized by the liver and bound to plasma proteins. Neonates up to 3 months of age have immature metabolic degradation pathways and reduced liver flow, resulting in increased amounts of amide anesthetic agents excreted unchanged in the urine.[23,24] Furthermore, neonates and young infants have lower levels of albumin and α_1 acid glycoproteins,[25] which are the proteins essential for drug binding.[26] This leads to increased plasma concentrations of free drug, which may be associated with an increase in toxicity. However, a possible protective factor in this age group is the relatively larger volume of distribution at steady state, which may result in lowered plasma drug levels.[27] The metabolism of the intermediate-duration amide, prilo-

Table 6-3. Recommended Local Anesthetic Agents and Maximum Dosages (mg/ml) for Pediatric Regional Anesthesia

Drug (concentration)	Spinal	Caudal/Epidural/Peripheral[b]	Duration (hr)
Tetracaine (0.1%)	0.2–0.6[a]		1.5–3.0
Lidocaine (5%)	1–2.5		1.0–1.5
Lidocaine (1–1.5%)	—	4–7 (IV regional: 3–5)	0.8–2.0
Mepivacaine (1–1.5%)	—	5–7	1.0–2.5
Prilocaine (1–1.5%)	—	5–7	—
Chloroprocaine (2%)	—	7–10	0.5–1.0
Bupivacaine (0.125–0.25%)	—	2–3	2.5–12.0
Bupivacaine (0.5–0.75%)	0.3–0.4		1.0–2.5

[a] Minimum dosage for child <10 kg is 1–2 mg.
[b] Upper limits are appropriate with the addition of epinephrine to the solution.

caine, is associated with the development of methemoglobinemia in adults. Infants have decreased levels of methemoglobin reductase, and fetal hemoglobin is oxidized more readily than adult,[28] resulting in a greater susceptibility to developing this complication. For these reasons, use of this agent is contraindicated in infants.

In both children and adults, rapidity of vascular absorption of local anesthetics is partially dependent on the site of injection. In general, absorption and blood level will vary according to the vascularity of the site. The resulting order from highest absorption and blood levels to lowest is as follows: topical tracheal spray, interpleural, intercostal, caudal, epidural, brachial plexus, single peripheral nerve block, and subcutaneous injection.[29] The increases in peak blood concentrations that are greater than expected in children following intercostal, topical, caudal, and interpleural blocks are probably secondary to the relatively higher cardiac output in this population.[27,29,30]

Toxicity from local anesthetic agents is rarely observed in children, possibly because of effects of heavy sedation or general anesthesia, both of which raise seizure thresholds.[31,32] The hypothesis that children are less sensitive to local anesthetic toxicity when compared to adults is not supported in the animal model.[33] Other causes of drug reactions during neural blockade, such as epinephrine reaction, oversedation, local anesthetic allergy, and vasovagal responses, should also be ruled out when an adverse effect is encountered. The treatment of local anesthetic toxicity in the pediatric population follows the same basic principles recommended for adults. Control of the airway with adequate oxygenation, cardiovascular support, and treatment of seizure activity is essential to ensure a good outcome.

SPECIFIC BLOCK TECHNIQUES

Blocks of the Central Neuraxis

Subarachnoid Blockade

The first reported use of spinal anesthesia in children and infants was in 1909.[34] The technique's popularity declined in the mid-1950s when interest in regional anesthesia waned with the advent of improved, noninflammable and nontoxic inhalational agents. However, in the 1980s a resurgence of interest took place, particularly in high-risk infants,[4,5] and has continued into the present.[35]

Indications/Complications   Subarachnoid blocks can be used in the pediatric orthopedic population for any orthopedic surgical procedure involving the lower extremities. The main advantages of spinal anesthesia are twofold: (1) cerebrospinal fluid (CSF) provides a definite marker during performance of the block, resulting in a high success rate; and (2) the small dose of local anesthetic required decreases the risk of toxicity. These features make this a particularly useful technique in children with significant pulmonary impairment (e.g., advanced cystic fibrosis or muscular dystrophy). It is also useful in patients in whom intubation and mechanical ventilation associated with general anesthesia may result in postoperative problems (e.g., in the ex-premature neonate). The major complication associated with this technique is post-dural puncture headache (PDPH). This risk proportionately increases with decreasing patient age from the geriatric era, but few data are available for infants and neonates. Caudal or epidural anesthesia may be preferable in cases in which the advantages of spinal anesthesia are not clear. Should PDPH occur, treatment with an epidural blood patch can be performed in children.[36]

This technique is associated with a high success rate[37] in adults.

Techniques Older children and adolescents are positioned in a similar fashion to adult patients undergoing spinal blockade. Infants can be held in the sitting or lateral position with the back maximally flexed. However, the infant's neck must remain extended, as several studies have reported significant hypoxemia secondary to airway obstruction with neck flexion.[38,39] Using aseptic technique and appropriate sedation, a small-gauge spinal needle of appropriate length is inserted through an interspinous ligament below L3 in the midline. When CSF is encountered, the chosen local anesthetic is injected. Specialized 1-in. (25-mm), 25-gauge styletted spinal needles are commercially available for use in neonates and infants. Some authors recommend the use of 22-gauge spinal needles because the brisk flow of CSF aids in determination of proper needle placement.[1] Unstyletted needles are not recommended because of the reported risk of introducing a plug of epidermis into the spinal canal, resulting in the rare complication of epidermoid tumor.[40] In older children, 25- to 27-gauge pencil-point needles may be advantageous in the prevention of PDPH, but data are not yet available.

Agents and Dosage Tetracaine and lidocaine are the two agents most commonly reported for spinal anesthesia in infants.[4,5,41] Spinal dosages in the infant are higher than expected because of their relatively increased CSF volume compared to adults. The recommended minimum dose of hyperbaric tetracaine is 1 to 2 mg, with a calculated dose on a weight basis of 0.5 to 0.6 mg/kg for children under 10 kg.[1] Isobaric bupivacaine has also been used for spinal anesthesia in infants.[42] In older children, as in adults, isobaric solutions such as 0.5 or

0.75 percent bupivacaine offer adequate sensory levels for lower extremity procedures. However, little has been published concerning recommended intrathecal dosages of these agents in the pediatric population.

Caudal Anesthesia

Multiple reports support the safety, simplicity and efficacy of caudal anesthesia in the pediatric population.[19,29,43-50] These blocks provide excellent intraoperative and postoperative analgesia and may reduce the risk of reflex laryngeal spasm and the need for endotracheal intubation.

Indications/Complications Caudal blocks can be used in the pediatric orthopedic population alone or in combination with light general anesthesia for procedures involving the lower extremities.

Reported complications, other than failure due to incorrect needle placement, are rare. Potential problems include (1) intravascular or intraosseous injection resulting in systemic toxicity; (2) dural puncture and intrathecal injection; (3) hypotension; (4) urinary retention; and (5) penetration of viscera.[51] Adequate knowledge of the anatomy of the sacral area and meticulous block technique can prevent most complications and result in a high rate of successful blockade.

Technique Small children are placed in the lateral position with the knees and hips flexed, the upper leg drawn up further than the lower. Alternatively, adolescents and older children can be blocked in the prone position, which may be advantageous when the presence of subcutaneous fat interferes with palpation of the bony landmarks in the lateral position. The semiprone position can be used in all ages. Whichever position is chosen, an experienced individual should manage the airway and control the level of sedation. Appropriate monitoring is essential for the safe performance of caudal blocks as with all regional anesthetic techniques.

The sacral hiatus is easily palpated above the coccyx, between the sacral cornua. Following standard aseptic technique a short (1- to 2-in.), preferably short-beveled, 22- to 25-gauge needle is inserted at a 45- to 60-degree angle to the skin. As the needle passes through the sacrococcygeal ligament, which overlies the sacral hiatus, a characteristic "pop" is felt. The needle bevel should face anteriorly to avoid piercing the anterior wall of the sacrum, which can result in bleeding. Once the needle has entered the caudal canal, the angle can be decreased 15 degrees and the needle advanced 2 to 3 mm. Advancement of the needle beyond this depth is not necessary and increases the risk of dural puncture and vascular injection. Once the needle is in place, careful and repeated aspiration for blood and CSF is performed prior to and during injection of local anesthetic. There should be no resistance to injection. Incorrect needle placement may result in subcutaneous injection of part or all of the local anesthetic. This can be detected by palpating the tissue overlying the sacrum above the needle insertion site. If tissue swelling occurs, the needle should be removed and the block repeated.

If needle placement is unsuccessful after two or three attempts, a suggested alternate route is intervertebral injection at the level of the S2-S3 interspace below the posterior superior iliac spine.[52] This site may also be preferable for catheter placement because of the lower risk of stool and urine contamination. The theoretically increased risk of dural puncture at this higher level was not observed in this study. If a continuous technique is desired, a catheter can be placed through a variety of thin-walled needles available commercially. Microcatheters can be placed through smaller-gauge needles, possibly decreasing the risk of bleeding complications. However, they are more likely to kink following placement, and it is difficult or impossible to aspirate blood or CSF through them. If commercial catheter kits are unavailable, a standard intravenous catheter (20 or 22 gauge) can be advanced off the metal cannula and used for continuous or intermittent caudal injection.

Agents and Dosage One of the advantages of caudal anesthesia in small children (younger than 8 years of age) is the linear relationship between volume of local anesthetic injected and height of sensory blockade. This relationship has been demonstrated with radiopaque dye and local anesthetic in the clinical setting.[14,53,54] Similar findings have been shown with the injection of dye in an autopsy study.[55] Various formulas to calculate dosage of local anesthetics for pediatric caudal anesthesia have been based on the patient's weight,[56,57] age,[14] and height.[58] However, the simplest and most clinically applicable recommendations take advantage of the consistent volume/height of blockade relationship. For example, Armitage recommends a dosage of 0.5 ml/kg for a sacral level of blockade, 1 ml/kg for a lower thoracic sensory level, and 1.25 ml/kg to achieve a block to the midthoracic region.[56] The maximum safe dosage of agent should always be calculated to avoid toxicity. This precaution is especially important in older children, in whom local anesthetic volumes calculated on a weight basis may easily exceed recommended total dosages if adult concentrations are used. Caudal blocks are usually performed in children to provide analgesia during surgery and pain relief in the postoperative period. Therefore, high concentrations of local anesthetic are usually unnecessary. Blood levels following caudal injection of 3 ml/kg of 0.25

percent, bupivacaine in children under 12 years of age ranged from 1.2 to 1.4 μg/dl, which are well below the limits of toxicity in the adult population.[29]

The duration of analgesia following caudal blockade is dependent on a number of factors, including the chosen drug, total dosage, patient age, surgical site, and presence of vasoconstrictors.[59,60] If the block is performed solely for postoperative pain relief, concentrations of bupivacaine ranging from 0.125 to 0.25 percent have been shown to provide some degree of postoperative analgesia, with decreased motor block associated with the lower concentrations.[61,62] If the block is performed at the beginning of a surgical procedure that lasts more than 2 hours, the caudal can be repeated at the completion of surgery with half of the original volume of local anesthetic to prolong pain relief. As described earlier, a catheter can be placed in the caudal epidural space for continuous analgesia in the postoperative period. However, because of the increased risk of contamination in the sacral area as well as the early ambulation encouraged in the pediatric orthopedic patient following surgery, single-shot techniques are often preferable. The use of epidural narcotics added to the epidural local anesthetic is gaining popularity in the pediatric population.[63-69] Complications related to this technique are similar to those reported in adults, and include urinary retention, delayed respiratory depression, itching, and nausea. Appropriate postoperative monitoring of the patient's respiratory status is necessary. A key factor in the education of the pediatric nursing service is the importance of safety precautions if intrathecal opioids are administered.

Lumbar Epidural Blockade

Indications/Complications Epidural anesthesia in the pediatric population was first reported by Sievers[70] in 1936,

with a subsequent enthusiastic report of 77 cases in 1954.[71] In smaller children this technique has not been championed as enthusiastically as caudal anesthesia for a number of reasons. As described above, caudal anesthesia in children under 8 years of age is a safe, simple technique with a reliable correlation between local anesthetic volume and sensory level. In small children, lumbar epidural blocks carry a higher risk of dural puncture and possible cord damage if an interspace above L3-L4 is chosen for needle placement. These risks are largely related to the use of adult-sized equipment in the pediatric population. As needles specifically designed for pediatric blocks become available commercially, the technical aspects of epidural blockade should improve.

In older children and adolescents, lumbar epidural anesthesia provides excellent anesthesia for orthopedic surgical procedures on the lower extremities. When combined with sedation or light general anesthesia, this technique has been shown to decrease the endocrine response to surgical stress,[72] and is satisfactory to both patient and surgeon. One of the major advantages of epidural anesthesia is the opportunity to provide postoperative pain control. This can be accomplished by continuous infusions of low-concentration local anesthetic alone or in combination with narcotics. Patients who are treated with continuous passive motion devices following knee surgery benefit from the muscle relaxation and pain relief resulting from epidural bupivacaine infusions.[73] The risk of local anesthetic toxicity with this technique is minimal, even when the catheter is left in place for several days.[74]

Technique As discussed under General Considerations, the spinal cord extends as low as L3 in infants, therefore needle placement for epidural blockade in small children is best performed below this level. The depth of the epidural space beneath the skin increases with age. In small children it lies only 10 to 18 mm below the skin surface.[15] Ligamentous and other tissues are softer and thinner in children, requiring meticulous attention to technique during needle placement. The technique of needle and catheter placement in older children and adolescents is similar to that in adults. Loss of resistance with air or saline should be used to identify the epidural space. However, epidural injection of large amounts of either substance may result in a patchy block because of mechanical interference of nerve blockade or dilution of the local anesthetic.[75-78]

Agents and Dosage   Recommendations regarding local anesthetic dosages for epidural anesthesia are similar to those for caudal anesthesia.[79] Addition of epinephrine to the solution results in a prolonged duration of blockade, conferring a protective effect against local anesthetic toxicity as well.[60] Other safety measures include incremental injection, frequent aspiration during injection, and determination of the maximum safe drug dosage.

Blocks of the Upper Extremity

Intravenous (Bier) Block

Indications/Complications   Intravenous (Bier) regional anesthesia is effective in providing anesthesia for upper extremity surgery distal to a tourniquet. This technique, described by Bier[80] in 1908, is well-tolerated by the pediatric population, requiring minimal cooperation and resulting in excellent anesthesia and motor blockade.[81-84] The duration of anesthesia is determined by the safe tolerance of the inflated tourniquet, approximately 60 to 90 minutes. Reported complications are rare with this technique in

children. They include inadequate block, tourniquet pain requiring general anesthesia, neurologic damage and compartment syndrome secondary to excessive tourniquet pressures, thrombophlebitis, and local anesthetic toxicity. The latter problem is usually related to early or accidental tourniquet deflation or local anesthetic overdosage. It can be readily prevented by meticulous management of the tourniquet and calculation of safe maximum drug doses. The use of the long-acting local anesthetic bupivacaine for intravenous blocks has resulted in several deaths as a result of local anesthetic toxicity following tourniquet release.[85] For this reason, bupivacaine is not recommended for Bier block anesthesia.

Relative contraindications to intravenous regional anesthesia include lack of patient cooperation, sickle cell disease, septicemia, inability to apply a tourniquet because of arm immobility or other causes, and a projected surgical duration of longer than 90 minutes.

Technique   Intravenous regional blocks are easy to perform in children and have a high success rate. Appropriate premedication will vary according to the anxiety of the individual patient. Intravenous access must be secured in a nonsurgical site prior to proceeding with the injection of intravenous local anesthetic for the regional blockade of the surgical site. This access ensures the early and appropriate treatment of any complications that might occur as well as allowing incremental sedation during the surgical procedure. An appropriately sized pneumatic tourniquet (diameter should cover no more than one-third of the upper arm) is placed over surgical cotton on the operative arm. A double tourniquet can be used, and will provide the anesthesia care provider with the option of inflating the distal tourniquet when the patient complains of pain from the proximal tourniquet. However, in smaller children, double tourniquets are often too large for the upper extremity. In these cases it is safer to use an appropriately sized single tourniquet, particularly for short-duration cases such as alignment and casting of a forearm fracture. An intravenous needle (22- or 20-gauge Teflon or butterfly) is placed as near as possible to the surgical site.

Exsanguination of the limb can often be quite painful, especially if the surgical lesion is due to trauma. If the patient will tolerate it, wrapping the elevated extremity tightly with an elastic bandage, starting from the distal finger tips and proceeding to the level of the tourniquet, is the most effective method of exsanguination. If a bloodless field is not necessary for surgical exposure (e.g., in the case of closed forearm reduction and pinning), other methods of exsanguination can be used (e.g., elevation of the hand for 2 to 3 minutes or the use of a trauma splint inflated to above systolic pressure) that will be adequate and less painful.

Once the arm is exsanguinated, the proximal tourniquet is inflated to a pressure of 250 to 350 mmHg (an appropriate pressure can be calculated by adding 150 to the patient's systolic pressure). The calculated dose of local anesthetic is then injected slowly through the intravenous cannula on the surgical side. Onset of anesthesia is rapid and motor block is adequate for skeletal manipulations. Anesthesia is preceded by a mottled white appearance of the superficial tissues of the upper extremity. The tourniquet can be safely deflated after 20 minutes. There are some data that suggest that cyclic deflation and reinflation results in a decrease in arterial local anesthetic drug levels and a decreased risk of toxicity.[86]

Agents and Dosage   Both lidocaine and prilocaine, in concentrations of 0.5 percent, have been recommended for intravenous regional anesthesia. Recom-

mended maximum doses range from 3 to 5 mg/kg. Bupivacaine should not be used because of the risk of toxicity and death. 2-Chloroprocaine has been associated with thrombophlebitis when injected intravascularly, although new formulations that have decreased levels of the additive bisulfite may be better tolerated.

Brachial Plexus Blockade: Axillary Approach

Indications   The axillary approach to the brachial plexus is a technique that is readily adaptable to the pediatric population.[87–89] This form of anesthesia is excellent for orthopedic surgical procedures performed at or below the elbow. Anatomically, the brachial plexus is very superficial in children because of their relative lack of subcutaneous fat. Diffusion of local anesthetic is rapid, and the smaller size of the nerves enhances blockade even when lower concentrations of local anesthetic are used. These factors combine to make the axillary approach to the brachial plexus a highly successful form of neural blockade in the pediatric patient.[10]

Complications/Contraindications   Complications are rare, and include arterial puncture, local anesthetic toxicity, peripheral nerve injury, and failed block. Contraindications to this technique include surgical lesions that prohibit abduction of the arm, as well as the usual contraindications cited in adults such as local infection, local anesthetic allergy, and progressive neurologic lesions.

Technique   The block is performed as described for the adult population. Most children will require moderate to heavy sedation during placement of the block and subsequent surgery. The superficial position of the brachial plexus in the axilla of a child is the most important anatomic difference from the adult patient. A number of techniques can be used for the axillary approach. The elicitation of paresthesias may be tolerated by the older child, but in general, the pediatric patient equates paresthesias with pain, and will not accept this technique well. A nerve stimulator can be used to elicit motor responses, allowing accurate needle placement in the heavily sedated patient. However, sheath blocks are also very effective in this population and require minimal extra equipment and personnel. The commercially available 1-in., short-beveled, 25-gauge pediatric nerve block needle is ideal for this block. The length is appropriate for children under 12 years of age, and the blunt bevel allows the anesthesia care provider to readily feel the "click" as the sheath is entered. Distal pressure should be maintained during injection of the local anesthetic solution in order to facilitate proximal spread, resulting in a higher incidence of blockade of the musculocutaneous and axillary nerves. Transarterial approaches can also be used in children, although there is a theoretical risk of vascular compression due to hematoma formation following vascular puncture. Injection in more than one site, as is often recommended for adult patients undergoing axillary blockade, is not necessary in the pediatric population, and may result in injection of excessive volumes of local anesthetic.

Agents and Dosage   Maximum local anesthetic dosages should always be calculated on a body weight basis. The addition of epinephrine to the solution provides several benefits, including (1) prolongation of the block; (2) enhanced motor blockade; (3) shorter onset of blockade; and (4) provision of an intravascular "marker" during injection of the local anesthetic. Lower concentrations of local anesthetic solutions can be used in children (e.g., 0.25 percent bupivacaine, 1 percent lidocaine) because of the en-

hanced block and the addition of heavy sedation or light general anesthesia during surgery. This factor also decreases the risk of local anesthetic toxicity. Absorption of axillary doses of bupivacaine (2 mg/kg and 3 mg/kg) has been shown to be rapid, but venous plasma concentrations were well below toxic levels with both doses.[90] Table 6-4 gives recommended volumes of anesthetic solutions for peripheral block procedures.

Brachial Plexus Blockade: Supraclavicular Approach

The supraclavicular approach to the brachial plexus is rarely used in the pediatric population because of the risk of pneumothorax. However, the anatomy is more clearly defined in children, which aids in correct needle placement. This approach is best suited to surgical procedures of the proximal arm and elbow.[91] The traditional technique of supraclavicular blockade involving location of the first rib with the needle point is not recommended in the pediatric population. A perivascular approach, with needle placement at the lower end of the interscalene groove, is technically easier and has a decreased risk of pulmonary complications. The subclavian artery can usually be easily palpated in children, and serves as a reliable landmark. A short-beveled needle, no more than 1 in. in length, should be used. Use of an adult-sized needle for this block is the most likely cause of pneumothorax. As with the axillary technique, a nerve stimulator can be used to aid in needle placement, or a sheath technique can be employed. The needle should be directed caudad and slightly medial at a level within the interscalene groove about 1 to 2 cm above the site where the subclavian artery is palpated. A "click" will be palpated as the needle passes through the fascial sheath surrounding the brachial plexus if a blunt needle is used. Alternatively, stimulation of the

Table 6-4. Recommended Volumes of Anesthetic Solution for Peripheral Blocks

Site of Block	Recommended Volume of Anesthetic Solution According to the Weight of Children				Total Volume (ml/kg)
	<20 kg	20–29 kg	30–45 kg	>45 kg	
Supraclavicular/ interscalene block	0.5–1 ml/kg	15–20 ml	20–22.5 ml	22.5–25 ml	0.25
Axillary block	0.3–0.6 ml/kg	10–15 ml	13–18 ml	18–20 ml	0.33
Femoral nerve block	0.5 ml/kg	10–12.5 ml	12.5–15 ml	15–17.5 ml	0.30
Sciatic nerve block	0.5 ml/kg	10–12.5 ml	12.5–15 ml	15–17.5 ml	0.15–0.2

motor nerves of the upper extremity will be visible as a muscle twitch if a nerve stimulator is employed. This block requires lower volumes of local anesthetic than the axillary approach because of the close anatomic orientation of the brachial plexus at the level of the clavicle.

Brachial Plexus Blockade: Interscalene Approach

Interscalene block can be successfully performed in children at the level of the cricoid cartilage (C6) using a sheath technique, as described for the supraclavicular block. The interscalene approach is rarely indicated in the pediatric population, as it is most useful for shoulder procedures, which are rarely performed in this age group. The interscalene approach does not reliably block the lower branches of the brachial plexus (C8–T1), which makes it a poor choice for hand or forearm surgery. Complications are rare, but potentially severe, and include intravascular injection and epidural or intrathecal block. Phrenic nerve block usually occurs, but is only significant if respiratory mechanics are marginal.

Other Peripheral Nerve Blocks

Blocks of the radial, ulnar, and median nerves at the wrist are easy to perform in children and carry minimal risk. These blocks require very small volumes of local anesthetic (0.5 to 1 ml) and can be performed prior to surgery or at the end of the procedure to provide pain relief in the postoperative period. However, the ease and safety of the axillary approach to the brachial plexus in children decreases the need for more peripheral blocks, which have a theoretical risk of nerve injury.

Blocks of the Lower Extremity

Femoral Nerve Block and Lateral Femoral Cutaneous Nerve Block

Indications/Complications   Femoral and lateral femoral cutaneous blocks of the lower extremity have been recommended in pediatric patients for intraoperative anesthesia and postoperative pain control. Suitable surgical procedures involving the thigh and femur include manipulation and reduction of femoral fractures, harvest of split-thickness skin grafts, and muscle biopsies from the upper leg.[8,92–94] They are especially well-suited to pain management of fractures of the femur, where adequate blockade allows transportation of the child for radiographic and other diagnostic procedures without narcotic-induced obtundation of the airway or interference with physical examination for signs of other traumatic injuries. These blocks are simple to perform, and are rarely associated with complications in this population. Theoretical problems include intravascular injection of local anesthetic, nerve injury, and prolonged block interfering with ambulation.

Technique Anatomic landmarks and needle placement are the same as in adults (see Ch. 12). Pediatric patients have minimal subcutaneous tissue in the area of these blocks; therefore the nerves are quite superficial compared to adults. A line drawn between the anterior superior iliac crest and the pubic tubercle represents the course of the inguinal ligament. The femoral nerve can be blocked just lateral to the femoral artery at a point 1 to 1.5 cm below the ligament. If a blunt-beveled needle is used, two "clicks" will be felt as the needle passes through the fascia lata and the fascia iliaca. Since the femoral artery lies between these two fascial structures, placing the needle by eliciting maximum arterial pulsations in the hub may be misleading and result in inadequate blockade. Distal pressure should be maintained during injection of the local anesthetic to facilitate proximal spread. A nerve stimulator can also be used for accurate needle placement; however, the sheath technique is very effective in children.

The lateral cutaneous nerve of the thigh can be blocked just medial to the anterior superior iliac spine, where it lies in a fascial canal as it passes under the inguinal ligament. Alternatively the needle can be inserted 1 to 2 cm medial and caudad to the anterior superior iliac spine and local anesthetic injected above and below the fascia lata in a fanwise fashion both medially and laterally. This nerve supplies only skin sensation to the lateral thigh, so dilute concentrations of local anesthetic are effective and provide increased safety.

Agents and Dosages Assuming that direct intravascular injection does not occur, the femoral and lateral femoral cutaneous nerves lie in an area of relatively low vascularity. As always, the maximum drug dosage should be calculated prior to blockade, and the addition of epinephrine to the solution decreases the vascular uptake. The use of bupivacaine for these blocks has been shown to be safe in children, and is associated with prolonged analgesia in the postoperative period.[95]

Sciatic Nerve Block

Indications Blockade of the sciatic nerve results in anesthesia of the foot and is rarely indicated by itself. When combined with femoral nerve block, it provides long-duration anesthesia and analgesia of the lower extremity below the knee. For surgery at or above the knee, blockade of the obturator and lateral femoral cutaneous nerve of the thigh would also be required. Blockade of the sciatic nerve using an anterior approach has been advocated for postoperative analgesia in children undergoing surgery of the foot.[95] This technique was associated with reliable pain relief and was reported to be simple to perform and without significant complications. The sciatic nerve can also be blocked at the level of the popliteal fossa where it divides into the common peroneal and tibial nerves. This technique has also been reported to provide good analgesia in children.[96] Finally, the terminal branches of the sciatic nerve can be blocked at the ankle with low volumes of local anesthetic. This simple technique, usually in conjunction with heavy sedation or light general anesthesia, can provide excellent intraoperative anesthesia and reliable postoperative analgesia with minimal effect on postoperative early ambulation.

Complications   Complications are rare with blockade of the sciatic nerve. Theoretically, intravascular injection and nerve injury can occur; however, the most common problem is inadequate anesthesia.

Technique   The anatomy and techniques for blockade of the sciatic nerve are similar to that in adults (see Ch. 12). A modification of the anterior approach to the sciatic nerve using a loss of resistance technique with air to detect the movement of the needle from the muscle compartment to the neurovascular sheath containing the sciatic nerve has been reported in children.[96] The cited advantage of this modification is the reliable location of the sciatic nerve in children of varying sizes. A nerve stimulator and insulated needle are also helpful in accurate needle positioning and allow appropriate sedation to be administered during block placement. The blockade of the sciatic nerve in the popliteal fossa is performed with the patient in the prone position. For smaller children, heavy sedation will be required. Induction of general anesthesia and tracheal intubation will ensure a secure airway during positioning and block placement. Again, a nerve stimulator is a useful aid in this approach.

Agents and Dosage   The sciatic nerve is located in an anatomic area with low vascular uptake. Therefore, relatively large volumes of local anesthetic can be safely injected. However, motor block is usually not required, hence lower concentrations are appropriate. The addition of epinephrine shortens onset of blockade and prolongs the duration.

Ankle Blocks
Blockade of the peripheral branches of the sciatic (posterior tibial, superficial peroneal, deep peroneal, and sural nerves) and femoral (saphenous nerve) nerves at the ankle is described in Chapter 12. These blocks are simple to perform, require low volumes of local anesthetic, have minimal complications, and provide good postoperative analgesia with minimal effect on ambulation. Since this technique requires three to five needle sticks, most children will require sedation for block placement. The resulting anesthesia is suitable for any procedure below the ankle in which either a tourniquet is not required or a forefoot tourniquet can be applied.

In conclusion, regional anesthesia can be successfully applied to the pediatric orthopedic patient population. These techniques provide excellent intraoperative anesthesia along with the important benefit of postoperative pain relief. A variety of safe, short-acting sedatives can be used to facilitate block placement while diminishing anxiety and discomfort for the patient. Heavy sedation or light general anesthesia, with or without tracheal intubation, is also appropriate for management of children in the operating room. The level of sedation or anesthesia required will depend on the individual child's temperament, past surgical experience, planned surgical procedure, adequacy of blockade, and the experience and comfort level of the surgeon and anesthesia care provider. A number of anatomic factors actually simplify block techniques in the pediatric population. These include a smaller nerve diameter allowing enhanced and earlier neural blockade and the absence of overlying subcutaneous tissue (in most children). The technical aspects of neural blockade differ little from those applied in adults, although knowledge of anatomic and pharmacologic differences is imperative before embarking on regional anesthesia in this population. Perhaps the most critical safety factor involves meticulous calculation of maximum drug dosages in order to choose safe local anesthetic volumes. Calculation of drug dosages based on an "eyeball" estimate according to the child's proportion of an adult size is inaccurate and unsafe. The proven effectiveness of lower concentrations of the local anesthetic agents in children gives an added margin of safety. With appropriate enthusiasm, tempered by meticulous technique, experience, and knowledge, the anesthesia care provider can use regional anesthetic techniques in the pediatric population to improve the quality of care and minimize the trauma of surgery and hospitalization.

REFERENCES

1. Yaster M, Maxwell LG: Pediatric regional anesthesia. Anesthesiology 70:324, 1989
2. Brown TCK, Schulte-Steinberg O: Neural blockade for pediatric surgery. p. 669. In Cousins MJ, Bridenbaugh PO (eds): Neural Blockade. JB Lippincott, Philadelphia, 1988
3. Dalens B: Regional anesthesia in children. Anesth Analg 68:654, 1989
4. Abajian JC, Melish RWP, Brown AF et al: Spinal anesthesia for surgery in the high-risk infant. Anesth Analg 63:359, 1984
5. Harnik EV, Goy GR, Potolicchio S et al: Spinal anesthesia in premature infants recovering from respiratory distress syndrome. Anesthesiology 64:95, 1986
6. Rosen KR, Broadman LM: Anaesthesia for diagnostic muscle biopsy in an infant with Pompe's disease. Can Anaesth Soc J 33:790, 1986
7. Meignier M, Souron R, Le Neel JC: Postoperative dorsal epidural analgesia in the child with respiratory disabilities. Anesthesiology 59:473, 1983
8. Berkowitz A, Rosenberg H: Femoral nerve block with mepivacaine for muscle biopsy in malignant hyperthermia patients. Anesthesiology 62:651, 1985
9. Wahlberg EJ, Wills RJ, Eckhert J: Plasma concentrations of midazolam in children following intranasal administration. Anesthesiology 74:233, 1991
10. Wedel DJ, Krohn JS, Hall JA: Brachial plexus anesthesia in pediatric patients. Mayo Clin Proc 66:583, 1991
11. Elze C: Centrales Nervensystem. In Braus H (ed): Anatomie des Menschen. Springer-Verlag, Berlin, 1932
12. O'Rahilly R, Meyer DB: The timing and sequence of events in the development of the human vertebral column during the embryonic period proper. Anat Embryol 157:167, 1979
13. Gouveia MA: Raquianestesia para pacientes pediatricos—experiencia pessoal em 50 casos. Rev Bras Anest 20:501, 1970
14. Schulte-Steinberg O, Rahlfs VW: Spread of extradural analgesia following caudal injection in children—a statistic study. Br J Anaesth 49:1027, 1977
15. Desparment J: Equipment for paediatric epidurals. Anaesthesia 41:337, 1986
16. Dohi S, Naito H, Takahashi T: Age related changes in blood pressure and duration of motor block in spinal anaesthesia. Anesthesiology 50:319, 1979
17. Delleur MM, Murat I, Saint-Maurice C: Hemodynamic changes during lumbar epidural anesthesia in children. Anesthesiology 65:A426, 1986
18. Berkowitz S, Greene BA: Spinal anesthesia in children: report based on 350 patients under 13 years of age. Anesthesiology 12:376, 1977
19. Melman E, Pennelas J, Maruffo J: Regional anesthesia in children. Anesth Analg 54:387, 1975
20. Parnes DI, Tsibuljkin EK, Gordeev VI et al: Hemodynamics and respiration in the postoperative peridural blockade in children. Vestn Khir 106:110, 1971
21. Desparmet J, Mateo J, Ecoffey C, Mazoit X: Efficacy of an epidural test dose in children anesthetized with halothane. Anesthesiology 72:249, 1990
22. Zsigmond EK, Downs JR: Plasma cholinesterase activity in newborns and infants. Can Anaesth Soc J 18:278, 1971
23. Mihaly GW, Moore RG, Thomas J et al: The pharmacokinetics and metabolism of the anilide local anasthetics in neonates. I. Lignocaine. Eur J Clin Pharmacol 13:143, 1978

24. Meffin P, Long GJ, Thomas J: Clearance and metabolism of mepivicaine in the human neonate. Clin Pharmacol Ther 14:218, 1973
25. LeDez KM, Swartz J, Strong A et al: The effect of age on the serum concentration of alpha-1 acid glycoprotein in newborns, infants and children. Anesthesiology 65:A421, 1986
26. Morselli PL, Franco-Morselli R, Borsi L: Clinical pharmacokinetics in newborns and infants. Age related differences and therapeutic implications. Clin Pharmacokinet 5:485, 1980
27. Tucker GT, Mather LE: Clinical pharmacokinetics of local anesthetics. Clin Pharmacokinet 4:241, 1979
28. Feig SA: Methemoglobinemia. p. 278. In Nathan DG, Oski FA (eds): Hematology of Infancy and Childhood. WB Saunders, Philadelphia, 1974
29. Eyres RL, Bishop W, Oppenheim RC, Brown TCK: Plasma bupivacaine concentrations in children during caudal epidural anesthesia. Anaesth Intensive Care 11:20, 1983
30. Rothstein P, Arthur GR, Feldman HS et al: Bupivacaine for intercostal nerve blocks in children: blood concentrations and pharmacokinetics. Anesth Analg 65:625, 1986
31. Eyres RL, Brown TCK, Hastings C: Plasma level of bupivacaine during convulsions. Anaesth Intensive Care 14:385, 1983
32. deJong RJ, Heavner JE: Diazepam prevents local anesthetic seizures. Anesthesiology 34:523, 1979
33. Morishima HO, Pederson H, Finster M et al: Toxicity of lidocaine in adult, newborn, and fetal sheep. Anesthesiology 55:57, 1981
34. Gray HT: A study of spinal anaesthesia in children and infants. From a series of 200 cases. Lancet 1:913, 1909
35. Welborn LG, Rice LJ, Hannallah RS et al: Postoperative apnea in former preterm infants: prospective comparison of spinal and general anesthesia. Anesthesiology 72:838, 1990
36. Purtock RV, Buhl JL, Abram SE: Epidural blood patch in a 9-year-old boy. Reg Anesth 9:154, 1984
37. Abouleish E, de la Vega S, Blendinger I, Tio T-O: Long-term follow-up of epidural blood patch. Anesth Analg 54(4):459, 1975
38. Weisman LE, Merenstein GB, Steenbarger JR: The effect of lumbar puncture position in sick neonates. Am J Dis Child 137:1077, 1983
39. Gleason CA, Martin RJ, Anderson JV et al: Optimal position for a spinal tap in preterm infants. Pediatrics 71:31, 1983
40. Batnitzky S, Keucher TR, Mealey J, Campbell RL: Iatrogenic intraspinal epidermoid tumors. JAMA 237:148, 1977
41. Blaise GA, Roy WL: Spinal anaesthesia for minor paediatric surgery. Can Anaesth Soc J 33:227, 1986
42. Mahe V, Ecoffey C: Spinal anesthesia with isobaric bupivacaine in infants. Anesthesiology 68:601, 1988
43. Arthur DS, McNicol LR: Local anesthetic techniques in paediatric surgery. Br J Anaesth 58:760, 1986
44. Hannallah RS, Broadman LM, Belman AB et al: Comparison of caudal and ilioinguinal/iliohypogastric nerve blocks for control of post-orchiopexy pain in pediatric ambulatory surgery. Anesthesiology 66:832, 1987
45. Jensen BH: Caudal block for postoperative pain relief in children after genital operations. A comparison between bupivacaine and morphine. Acta Anaesthesiol Scand 25:373, 1981
46. Spear RM, Desparmet JM, Maxwell LG: Caudal anesthesia in the awake, high-risk infant. Anesthesiology 69:407, 1988
47. Ecoffey C, Desparmet J, Maury M et al: Bupivacaine in children: pharmacokinetics following caudal anesthesia. Anesthesiology 63:A465, 1985
48. Ecoffey C, Desparmet J, Maury M et al: Pharmacokinetics of lignocaine in children following caudal anesthesia. Br J Anaesth 56:1399, 1984
49. McGowan RG: Caudal analgesia in children (500 cases for procedures below the diaphragm). Anaesthesia 37:806, 1982
50. Dalens B, Hasnaoui A: Caudal anesthesia in pediatric surgery: success rate and adverse effects in 750 consecutive patients. Anesth Analg 68:83, 1989
51. Dawkins CJM: An analysis of the com-

plications of extradural and caudal block. Anaesthesia 24:554, 1969

52. Busoni P, Sarti A: Sacral intervertebral epidural block. Anesthesiology 67:993, 1987

53. Schulte-Steinberg O: Caudal Anaesthesie bei Kindern und die Ausbreitung von 0.25% iger Bupivacaine Lösung. Anaesthetist 21:94, 1972

54. Schulte-Steinberg O: Zum gegenwaartigen Stand der kaudalen Epiduralanaesthesie in Kindersalter. Anaesthesiol Reanim 6:323, 1981

55. Brown TCK, Fisk GC: Anaesthesia for Children. Blackwell Scientific Publishers, Oxford, 1979, p 258.

56. Takasaki M, Dohi S, Kawabata Y, Kahashi T: Dosage of lidocaine for caudal anesthesia in infants and children. Anesthesiology 47:527, 1977

57. Armitage EN: Caudal block in children. Anaesthesia 34:396, 1979

58. Spiegel P: Caudal anesthesia in pediatric surgery: a preliminary report. Anesth Analg 41:218, 1962

59. Warner MA, Kunkel SE, Offord KO et al: The effects of age, epinephrine, and operative site on duration of caudal analgesia in pediatric patients. Anesth Analg 66:995, 1987

60. Murat I, Delleur MM, Saint-Maurice C: The effects of age and the addition of adrenalin to bupivacaine for continuous lumbar epidural anesthesia in children. Anesthesiology 65:A428, 1986

61. Wolf AR, Valley RD, Fear DW et al: Bupivacaine for caudal analgesia in infants and children: the optimal effective concentration. Anesthesiology 69:102, 1988

62. Gunter JB, Dunn CM, Bennie JB et al: Optimum concentration of bupivacaine for combined caudal-general anesthesia in children. Anesthesiology 75:57, 1991

63. Shapiro LA, Jedeiken RJ, Shaler D, Hoffman S: Epidural morphine analgesia in children. Anesthesiology 61:210, 1984

64. Rosen K, Rosen D, Bank E: Caudal morphine for post-op pain control in children undergoing cardiac procedures. Anesthesiology 67:A510, 1987

65. Jenson PJ, Siem-Jorgensen P, Nielsen TB et al: Epidural morphine by the caudal route for postoperative pain relief. Acta Anaesthesiol Scand 26:511, 1982

66. Krane EJ, Tyler DC, Jacobson LE: The dose response of caudal morphine in children. Anesthesiology 71:48, 1989

67. Krane EJ, Jacobson LE, Lynn AM et al: Caudal morphine for postoperative analgesia in children: a comparison with caudal bupivacaine and intravenous morphine. Anesth Analg 66:647, 1987

68. Attia J, Ecoffey C, Sandouk P et al: Epidural morphine in children: pharmacokinetics and CO_2 sensitivity. Anesthesiology 70:418, 1989

69. Krane EJ: Delayed respiratory depression in a child after caudal epidural morphine. Anesth Analg 67:79, 1988

70. Sievers R: Peridural Anaesthesie zur Cystoscopie biem Kind. Arch Klin Chir 185:359, 1936

71. Ruston FG: Epidural anaesthesia in infants and children. Can Anaesth Soc J 1:37, 1954

72. Murat I, Walker J, Esteve C et al: Effect of lumbar epidural anaesthesia on plasma cortisol levels in children. Can J Anaesth 35:20, 1988

73. Pettine KA, Wedel DJ, Cabanela ME, Weeks JL: The use of epidural bupivacaine following total knee arthroplasty. Orthop Rev 18(8):894, 1989

74. Denson DD, Raj PP, Finnsson RA et al: Continuous perineural infusion of bupivacaine for prolonged analgesia: pharmacokinetic considerations. Int J Clin Pharmacol Ther Toxicol 21:591, 1983

75. Dalens B, Bazin JE, Haberer JP: Epidural air bubbles as a cause of incomplete analgesia during epidural anesthesia. Anesth Analg 66:679, 1987

76. Philip BK: Effect of epidural air injection on catheter complications. Reg Anaesth 10:21, 1985

77. Phillip BK: Relative risks of epidural air injection in children and adults (letter). Anesth Analg 67:600, 1988

78. Miguel R, Morse S, Murtagh R: Epidural air associated with multiradicular syndrome. Anesth Analg 73:92, 1991

79. Ecoffey C, Dubousset AM, Samii K: Lumbar and thoracic epidural anesthesia for urologic and upper abdominal surgery in

infants and children. Anesthesiology 65: 87, 1986

80. Bier A: Über einen neuen Weg Lokalanaesthesie an den Gliedmassen zu Erzeugen. Verh Dtsch Ges Chir 37(2):204, 1908

81. Gingrich TF: Intravenous regional anesthesia of the upper extremity in children. JAMA 200:135, 1967

82. Carrell ED, Eyring EJ: Intravenous regional anesthesia for childhood fractures. J Trauma 11:301, 1971

83. Fitzgerald B: Intravenous regional anaesthesia in children. Br J Anaesth 48:485, 1976

84. Rudzinski JP: Pediatric application of intravenous regional anesthesia. Reg Anesth 8:69, 1983

85. Heath ML: Deaths after intravenous regional anesthesia (letter). Br Med J 285:913, 1982

86. Sukhani R, Garcia CJ, Munhall RJ et al: Lidocaine disposition following intravenous regional anesthesia with different tourniquet deflation techniques. Anesth Analg 68:633, 1989

87. Eriksson E: Axillary brachial plexus anaesthesia in children with Citanest. Acta Anaesthesiol Scand 16:291, 1965

88. Ross D, Williams DO: Combined axillary plexus block and basal sedation for cardiac catheterization in young children. Br Heart J 32:195, 1970

89. Niesel HC, Rodriguez P, Wilsmann I: Regional analgesia of the upper extremity in children. Anaesthesist 23:178, 1974

90. Campbell RJ, Ilett KF, Dusci L: Plasma bupivacaine concentrations after axillary block in children. Anaesth Intensive Care 14:343, 1986

91. Leak WD, Winchell SW: Regional anesthesia in pediatric patients: review of clinical experience. Reg Anaesth 7:64, 1982

92. McNicol LR: Lower limb blocks for children. Anaesthesia 41:27, 1986

93. Grossbard GD, Love BR: Femoral nerve block: a simple and safe method of instant analgesia for femoral shaft fractures in children. Aust NZ J Surg 49:592, 1979

94. Ronchi L, Rosenbaum D, Athouel A, Lemaitre JL et al: Femoral nerve blockade in children using bupivacaine. Anesthesiology 70:622, 1989

95. McNicol LR: Sciatic nerve block for children. Anaesthesia 40:410, 1985

96. Kempthorne PM, Brown TCK: Nerve blocks around the knee in children. Anaesth Intensive Care 12:14, 1984

7

The Geriatric Patient

Edward P. Didier

The exact point of transition from being adult to being geriatric is not important to the anesthetic management of the growing number of older candidates for orthopedic surgical correction, repair, or reconstruction. However, societal, ethical, physiologic, pharmacologic, pathologic, and personality matters could and should affect anesthesia planning for the older patient. This chapter deals with these anesthesia-related considerations in elderly patients.

GENERAL CONSIDERATIONS

In our everyday existence chronologic age is important in many societal, civic, and religious aspects of our life. Our age in years has an impact on our eligibility for various religious rites; application for driver's license; right to vote and hold office; entering school, military service, saloons, and cinemas; and joining service clubs and associations. "Retirement age" has been identified by many institutions and industries and accepted by a large portion of the population, even though recently declared to be legally unenforceable. Chronologic age has much lesser significance in the health care aspects of

our lives except for the inappropriate use of this number in formulating administrative caveats, guidelines, and regulations.[1,2]

More important to the anesthesia provider than the chronologic age of a patient is the functional integrity of important organ systems and the pathogeny. There is no direct relationship between longevity and pathologic change, and it is not appropriate to identify old age as a disease. On the other hand, the longer one lives, the greater is the opportunity for disease process to begin and progress.

Although it is not clear what effect the passing of time has on organs in the absence of disease, it is obvious that disease, disability, and infirmity are seen with increasing frequency as people age. There are probably genetic, environmental, lifestyle, and fortuitous elements in the four broad categories of adverse progression.[3]

First, there are degenerative changes (physiolysis), usually having long latent periods, which may be the result of indolent disease processes, environmental exposure to substances of low toxicity but pernicious action, or chronic wear and tear from active living. Depending on the site and nature of these degenerative changes, other organ systems may become involved secondarily. For example, chronic exposure to tobacco smoke may cause pulmonary emphysema, which in turn may cause cardiac dysfunction, which may ultimately result in other organ system derangement. Osteoporosis can result in respiratory compromise by means of skeletal deformity causing restrictive lung disease and pulmonary hypertension.

Next in consideration are the problems related to malignant transformation. Although there is a cancer for every age group, the longer one lives, the greater is the chance of developing malignancy. The orthopedist's role in management of primary and metastatic bone cancer can present significant challenges to the anesthesia team in any age group but in older patients who have had the time to develop other medical problems, the task becomes even more complex.

The immunologic basis of many diseases is receiving increasing attention. The role of the immune system in malignancy, infection, and collagen, and in endocrine, metabolic, cardiopulmonary, digestive, hematopoietic, skeletal, and even psychiatric diseases is being studied as a possible key to origin, management, and prevention. It is unlikely, however, that the impact of the remarkable progression of immunologic knowledge will significantly alter the practice of orthopedic surgeons during this generation, although there is increasing interest in the immunologic factors involved in prosthesis retention and fracture healing. Yet it has already notably affected the practice of anesthesia, particularly in the areas of toxicity of anesthetic drugs on patients and personnel, blood transfusion, and pharmacodynamics.

Finally the mechanical effects of years of impact, abrasion, radiation, and vibration may result in bone and joint problems, calluses, cataracts, aches, pains, stiffness, and many other of the inconveniences of the elderly. Sometimes it is that old back problem that causes pain when it rains or when a bed is too hard or too soft, but is not accompanied by overt pathology. As stated by the late Maurice Chevalier, "Growing old is not necessarily fun, but it's better than the alternative."

PREOPERATIVE CONSIDERATIONS

Literally translated, the word orthopedic means "straight child," making the term *geriatric orthopedics* an oxymoron. Even so, the older population is well represented on the orthopedic surgical schedule, and the proportion is likely to increase as life expectancy increases.[4] The technical aspects of surgical procedures differ little in elderly patients. Anesthesia management and postoperative care, however, are considerably more demanding and complex.

The objectives of surgery are to:

1. Restore or improve function
2. Remove malignant or diseased tissue
3. Control pain
4. Control hemorrhage or infection

The objective of anesthesia and postoperative care is to make the surgical objectives possible—with safety and comfort. With the complex problems often seen in the elderly, these objectives often require a team approach, involving surgeon, anesthesia care team, postoperative care staff, patient family, clergy, and family doctor. Considerations beyond diagnosis become more important when making surgical decisions about old people. The availability of a "good" operation for the problem and a surgeon who can perform the procedure is not necessarily a mandate to proceed. There are other considerations.

First, does the patient have concomitant disease that would increase the likelihood of an unfavorable outcome to a prohibitive degree? The old saying about the operation being a success but the body (heart, lungs, kidneys, liver, etc.) being unable to stand the anesthesia needs to be considered in the decision to recommend surgery. Although we have available effective means of preventing, monitoring, managing, or countering adverse effects and complications, it is important that we know beforehand what the problems are likely to be and how much increased risk they impose. A thorough medical evaluation is particularly important in older patients in the consideration of options.[5-9]

Next, is there another method or approach to managing the problem that might be more acceptable to patient and family? Often there are simpler surgical options or even medical regimens that may accomplish limited goals at much less risk and expense. Complex reconstructive surgery to restore ambulation in a patient with disabling cardiac or pulmonary disease is probably not justifiable if there are alternatives.

Also, one must decide if the proposed surgery will result in an improved lifestyle for the patient. Older people often have developed or retained an avid interest in some activity such as golf, bowling, tennis, bird watching, or whatever, and will seek a resolution to the disability that has prevented their engaging in the chosen pursuit. Is it likely that the operation will enable the patient to return to that favorite activity? If there is a substantial chance that it will not, is the patient still interested in trying?

ETHICAL CONSIDERATIONS

There is a temptation among anesthesia providers to allow others to deal with ethical issues, based most likely on the premise that the administration of anesthesia is not optional, is usually only incidentally related to the surgical outcome, and is so complex as to be beyond the capacity of the patient to fully understand. The formulation of an anesthesia plan, the skillful management of the procedure and an appropriate postanesthesia recovery program are certainly the responsibility of the anesthesia team, but there are responsibilities and considerations beyond these in which participation is imperative.

Under the realm of "informed consent," there are many subtle issues that must be resolved. Some of these issues apply to surgical patients of any age, but others are unique to the older population. Remember, informed consent is really a binary matter—one is what the patient or guardian thinks they consented to, the other is what you think they consented to. Here are some things to consider.

Is the patient intellectually intact such that a reasonable understanding and acceptance of surgical and anesthesia consequence is possible? This is often very difficult to determine. During a painstaking and comprehensive review of the procedure, its risks, goals, consequences, and hazards, the patient may appear to understand and even ask appropriate questions. Later one may find that very little substance of the discussion was retained. Older people come with very different backgrounds and have had many years to solidify their personalities. At one extreme there are those who seem to have experienced everything and are still indifferent, unimpressed, or bored by it all, and at the other are those who have experienced everything and have firm opinions regarding their status. There are some who are used to being cared for and have become habitually compliant, and some who have always done for themselves and are suspicious and antagonistic toward those who would take over decision making for them, particularly if the usurpers are "youngsters."[10] Senility and dementia are not necessarily threshold conditions to be determined by a sensitive and selective test as either present or absent. The truth is that there may be no such thing as "informed" consent, and our only recourse is to be as honest and complete in our presentation as possible, and to record in the chart a summary of what was said, what questions were asked, and how the patient responded.

If there are uncertainties about the patient's understanding and the validity of consent, the usual approach is to deal with relatives—one hopes close relatives—or someone with either legal guardianship or durable power of attorney. This can either be straightforward or, rarely, an element of great complexity. If there are many relatives directly involved, or even some involved indirectly, who cannot agree on the recommended course, one must proceed with extreme caution and with authorative legal advice. When a single or group of relatives refuse permission, cooperation, or dialogue, there is the possibility of requesting guardianship by the court. This is an extreme situation and used mostly in invasive care of minors when parents are obstinate or unwilling to accept sound medical advice. It is rarely resorted to in adults, but there is precedent.

What can one do in the face of obdurate and unreasonable demands on the part of the patient or representative that are deemed to be inconsistent with proper surgical, anesthesia, or medical practice? Obviously as a physician, you do not have to and should not agree to do something that you consider wrong or improper. Probably the most commonly encountered caveat is that imposed by Jehovah's Witness patients who will not agree to blood transfusion under any circumstances. Under some conditions this imposes an impossible constraint on proper

management and if you are of this opinion, there are three alternatives. One, you may disassociate yourself from the case. In some practice situations where you are the sole qualified practitioner, this may expose you to the risk of being charged with abandonment. Second you may agree to this condition and hope that you can get by with blood substitutes. You must then be prepared to allow a patient under your care to die from blood loss, possibly resulting in painful scrutiny and review by your peers. The third approach is my preference, and has been acceptable in my practice for many years. This consists of explaining to the patient that you have respect for the teachings of the religion, that you will use only acceptable modalities of volume replacement unless, in your opinion, death is imminent and certain without transfusion, at which time you will invoke your personal commandment, "Thou shalt not kill," and do what is necessary. You must explain that in the rare instance that this situation should arise, there would be no opportunity for the patient to reconsider while anesthetized; it would not be the patient's choice, so you would have to resort to the dictates of your conscience and administer lifesaving transfusions. So far, my patients have either accepted this condition or remained silent, which in either case, I have exhaustively entered on the anesthesia record. The risk here is being charged with battery. I find this an acceptable hazard.

There are many examples of unreasonable demands from patients and relatives, which must be dealt with before the fact. Some of the demands from my experience are worth citing as examples. One patient insisted on having her total hip arthroplasty done under local anesthesia. I explained to her that it would be inconsistent with our usual practice, that the amount of anesthetic solution would likely exceed the toxic limit, and she might be subjected to needless suffering. It turned out that what she feared was insensibility and loss of control, so we accomplished the procedure, after thorough discussion, with a subarachnoid block. Another request from a patient's family was that, for religious reasons, in the event of death, I should place a metal rod through the patient's heart before moving the remains from the operating room. I explained that in this unlikely event we would undertake cardiopulmonary resuscitation and we would use a stainless steel needle for intracardiac drug injection, which would be equivalent to using the metal rod. This was acceptable to the family. Documentation of these requests from patient and family and the response they receive is the major management tool in avoiding problems after the fact.

Once the decision to proceed with surgery is made, it is important that all members of the care team have reached consensus. Not infrequently the anesthesia personnel will become involved only after the patient agrees to surgery. Ordinarily this presents no problem, but occasionally there will be a difference of opinion regarding objectives, management, and feasibility. Should this happen, it would be inappropriate for the anesthesia provider to "go along" without an open discussion with the surgeon to share concerns and reach a compromise.

Probably the most frequent problem arises over timing. If the need to start the operation before laboratory testing and other preoperative concerns have been addressed is not apparent to everyone, the problem must be resolved to the satisfaction of all before starting. This, of course, is the case in all types of surgery, but when the risk is greater, as in geriatric surgery, so is the need for consensus— and confidence among the members of the team. In the event of less than optimal outcome, solidarity among all those involved is a valuable asset.

Another problem in this area has to do with the patient who has been properly designated as "do not resuscitate" who needs a surgical procedure. It is not improper to consider palliative surgical procedures such as tracheotomy, stabilization of painful pathologic fractures, and other operations intended to ease pain or facilitate nursing care, or to surgically intervene in acute pathologic events not directly related to the primary disease. The dilemma is whether to suspend the "do not resuscitate" status while the patient is in the operating room and during the postoperative period. In my view, the acceptance of the patient as a candidate for anesthesia and surgery constitutes a temporary revision in the "do not resuscitate" status, and allows the care team to apply the usual standards of response to emergencies for surgical patients. Accepting that anesthesia and surgery have inherent risks regardless of the patient's physical status, it seems logical to accept the usual standards of care for the patient during anesthesia and during the perioperative period, particularly when the need for resuscitation is not related to the patient's primary disease, but rather to the intervention. Under these circumstances, it is most important to discuss these matters with the patient, family, and medical/surgical personnel prior to the undertaking and note the details of the discussion in the medical record.[11-14]

A related problem may be perceived with the increasing number of patients who have agreed to a set of stipulations regarding their medical care should they become incapable of making a decision, the so-called living will. Often these stipulations are specific and preclude the use of mechanical ventilation, parenteral nutrition, renal dialysis, and other options generally available. Occasionally the stipulations will be vague and imprecise, and merely exclude the use of "heroic measures" to prolong life. Surgical intervention, as previously discussed, is unlikely to be specifically excluded, that is, it is not to be identified as a heroic measure. Once the decision to undertake a surgical procedure is made and described, it must be accepted by the patient and family that there may be a need to suspend the stipulations, or at least to interpret them differently, during the perioperative period. The intent here is to allow the surgical team the freedom to provide the usual standard of care for any anesthesia- or surgery-related problem, without being hampered by unrelated preordained constraints. As one might expect, the difficulty arises when the complication does not respond to management and treatment in the usual time frame. Now, one is faced with a derivative of the original intent of the living will and a reinterpretation of the stipulations. By agreeing to surgery did the patient actually add a codicil to the living will? Not really. The stipulations of the living will still apply to the new situation, but the proscription of certain treatment modalities should be excluded when they are part of the *usual* management during the operative and postoperative period. For example, the use of mechanical ventilation for a limited time during postoperative recovery is quite common, and should not be denied because of its mention in another context.[15,16]

There is an almost endless variety of these types of problems that may arise among surgical patients. Among the elderly, they can be particularly troublesome because of the complexities associated with concurrent diseases, possible intellectual impairment, and less certain outcome. It is important that these issues be addressed prior to the operative procedure, consensus reached, and the details carefully recorded in the medical record. Acute trauma surgery in the older patient often makes this process impossible or incomplete, but even so, requires

thorough documentation of whatever negotiations were made. Further considerations of this matter appear later.

ANESTHESIA CONSIDERATIONS

Elsewhere in this book are chapters devoted to specific elements in orthopedic anesthesia. In this section some aspects of anesthesia management as they apply to older patients are examined and some considerations in modifying our practice to accommodate the altered physiology seen in the geriatric population are reviewed.

Risk

The risk of unfavored outcome in anesthesia and surgery increases with age. Multiple studies have established this to be the case, and the statistical and demographic evidence is convincing. Few studies, however, have addressed the specific causes of this finding, other than the increased incidence of concurrent diseases in this population. Earlier in this chapter, I cautioned against equating aging with disease. Even though there is a predictable degradation in organ performance with advancing age, this is not thought to be a significant risk factor in the absence of disease. The risk of surgery and anesthesia, then, is related to the presence of disease or disorder in specific organ systems and is clearly related to the degree of involvement and the number of organ systems involved[17–19] (Table 7-1).

There have been attempts to predict the maximal age achievable by human beings. The idea that it is possible to predict a maximal age on the basis of age-related, non-disease-related, decrement in cellular population and function is in-

Table 7-1. Aging Changes That Increase Risk

Cardiovascular
    Coronary artery disease
    Cardiomyopathy
    Peripheral vascular disease
Pulmonary
    Obstructive lung disease (smoking)
    Restrictive lung disease
    Weak cough
    Chronic bronchitis (pollution)
Renal
    Decreased glomular filtration rate
    Delayed response to excretion of salt load
Immunity
    Decreased antibody levels
    Multiple antigen exposure
Nutrition
    Obesity
    Cachexia
    Malabsorption
Homeostasis
    Thermoregulation compromise
    Anemia and clotting abnormalities
    Osteoporosis

triguing. Unfortunately, it is an unrealistic hope, since there is not a linear decrement in function in any individual, nor is it consistent in any population.[20,21] The belief that there is a maximal possible age beyond which survival becomes an anomaly has no place in deciding the advisability of surgical treatment of a given problem because there are so many exceptions. The real basis for assessing risk is based on physical status, which, in turn, is based on the presence and extent of disease.

Drug Sensitivity

There are practical consequences to age-related alterations in response to drugs that are important considerations in anesthesia management. In general, there can be expected a slower uptake and distribution related to decreased perfusion, an increased sensitivity related to a shrinking of the "compartment" to which the drug is distributed, and a prolongation of effect related to the higher concentration in the "compartment" and prolonged metabolic processing or renal excretion. As a rule this attenuated response calls for the use of smaller doses, longer periods between doses, and prolonged observation during the recovery period.

The concentration of volatile anesthetic agents should be decreased in elderly patients. This may be related to the above factors, plus the possibility of a decrease in neuron density or even a decrease in cerebral metabolism.[22–24] Recovery is also predictably slower, and is a factor to consider in managing anesthesia for outpatient surgery among older people (Table 7-2).

Muscle relaxants can be expected to have a greater duration of action, particularly those dependent on renal excretion.[25] Succinylcholine, used for endotracheal intubation, may be somewhat prolonged in action because of the decrease in plasma cholinesterase in older people. Since the dosage, onset, and duration of action are usually not evaluated with great precision during induction, this seldom is of any clinical importance. Atracurium and vecuronium seem to be exceptions to the above cautions because of their different clearance pathways. The effects of reversal drugs such as neostigmine may be slow in onset in older patients,[26] and there may be an increased incidence of cardiac arrhythmias.

Opiates in general have a more intense and prolonged effect in the aged, particularly in regard to their depressant effects. The analgesic effects are also probably greater, but there are few studies to quantitate this commonly assumed response.[27] This is of particular importance in administering these drugs in the post-

Table 7-2.   Pharmacokinetic Effects of Physiologic Changes in the Aged

Physiologic Change	Pharmacokinetic Effect
Increased circulation time	Delayed onset, prolonged effect
Decreased cardiac output	Changes in distribution
Decreased lean body mass	
Decreased body water	
Increased body fat	
Decreased serum albumin	Reduced binding
Decreased liver 　Mass 　Blood flow 　Enzyme activity	Reduced metabolism, detoxification
Decreased renal 　Mass 　Glomerular filtration rate 　Tubular secretion	Impaired elimination
Decreased metabolic rate	Delayed elimination

(From Miller,[44] with permission.)

operative period, when monitoring and observation may not be as intensive as while the patient is in the operating room.

The same considerations regarding sensitivity and duration probably apply to the pharmacodynamics and kinetics of local anesthetic agents. One should be aware of this when the regional anesthetic technique involves administering amounts of agent that approach the recommended safe limits. It is of lesser importance in epidural or spinal anesthesia, where the major consideration is the size of the space into which the injection is made and dosage is well below the maximum allowable. There is a tendency for an increased spread of anesthetic effect from a given dose in epidural administration in the elderly, so volume should be reduced.[28]

Induction agents such as sodium thiopental, methohexital, etomidate, and propofol similarly require downward adjustment in dosage, and can be expected to have a longer duration in the elderly. Diazepam, one of the most widely prescribed tranquilizers and a popular premedication agent, has been clearly shown to have an extremely prolonged half-life in older people, and for this reason is being replaced in favor of midazolam in the operating room and perioperative period.

Adverse Drug Interactions

Older patients take more prescription medicines and over-the-counter drugs than do younger people. This increases the possibility of adverse interaction, which is often unexpected and difficult to recognize. Some examples of this unexpected interaction are (1) the coagulation abnormality from aspirin use increasing the effect of postoperative antiembolic medication, (2) the blunting of the effect of vasopressors by certain antihypertensive medications, (3) electrolyte abnormalities exacerbated by diuretic medications, and (4) disturbance of postoperative bowel function due to perioperative withdrawal of habitual laxative use. There are numerous other possibilities associated with the actual or perceived need to withhold usual medications during the perioperative period. β-blockers, certain antihypertensive agents, chronic steroid use, glaucoma medication, thyroid replacement, insulin, bronchodilators, and anticoagulants are some of the common prescription medications that may require specific orders to adjust or maintain dosage when the elderly patient comes to surgery.[28,29]

A number of proprietary medications and substances routinely used by patients may also influence the actions of anesthesia-related drugs. Alcohol use is quite common among older people, and may cause a variety of symptoms of a vague and puzzling nature during a forced withdrawal period. Chronic caffeine intoxication from excessive coffee or tea ingestion has been reported to result in central nervous system and autonomic disturbances after sudden cessation. Aspirin, as previously mentioned, can exaggerate the response to anticoagulant therapy. Chronic nicotine poisoning, from smoking, chewing, or sniffing tobacco, can be related to a variety of autonomic and central nervous system symptoms when it is suddenly withdrawn from one who is addicted. In addition, some of these substances, when chronically present in sufficient levels, can interfere with or adversely affect the actions of adjuvant anesthetic drugs that have a similar or opposing pharmacologic effect.

Outpatient Surgery

There is a growing trend to perform surgery on outpatients to reduce cost of hospitalization. Often, this option induces an added risk in older patients, who require longer recovery periods, may be confused after the physical effects of anesthetics wear off, and may require more nursing care to assist with their routine functions, such as eating, elimination, and ambulation.[30]

When outpatient care is mandated, it is vital that a capable family member or friend be available to accompany and care for the older outpatient for as long as necessary for complete recovery. The selection of anesthetic agents as well as type of anesthesia must also be based on the need to enable the patient to safely leave the hospital in a matter of hours rather than days (see Ch. 11).

Emergency Surgery

One of the most severe challenges to the skill of the anesthesia team is the management of the geriatric patient who needs emergency surgery. There is insufficient time for the usual history and physical examination, and the more emergent the situation is, the less medical information there is available. Starting with such a disadvantage, things tend to get worse.

Many older victims of trauma have preexisting conditions that complicate the management of their injuries. Osteoporosis, muscle wasting, coagulation disorders, and skeletal abnormalities often result in a greater amount of harm for the same amount of trauma than in a younger person. Inasmuch as older patients heal more slowly than younger patients, the need for prolonged care is more likely, and prolonged immobility is poorly tolerated by patients who have systemic disorders, cardiac disease, renal or hepatic abnormalities, and other maladies common to senior citizens. One of the objectives of trauma management in older patients, then, is early mobility.

Occasionally, the need for immediate surgery is driven to some extent by the convenience of the surgical team. As a rule this is not an acceptable reason for taking short cuts in information-gathering, medical workup, and informed consent. The desire of the resident surgeon to get on with the case so it can be done personally, or the need for the surgeon to get the surgery started "right now" so as not to interfere with other commitments, is not appropriate. Since the possibility of things going astray is greater in older patients, and greater again when some options are denied by the need to save a life or preserve a limb, it is well to anticipate one's testimony in response to a plaintiff's attorney regarding the need to rush to the operating room.

Gastric Aspiration

Aspiration pneumonia is a well-known and serious complication of anesthesia. Aspiration of gastric material is more likely in a poorly prepared patient or one who has recently ingested food, another risk factor in emergency surgery. The possibility of aspiration is greater in older patients even when properly prepared for surgery by withholding food and liquid intake. Because of longer retention in the digestive tract and relaxation of the upper esophageal sphincter common to older people, there is additional risk of this unfortunate event. Along with this relaxation with aging, there is also an increased incidence of esophageal diverticulum formation, and the possibility of the diverticulum retaining food for long periods of time. When this diverticulum disgorges its contents during induction of anesthesia or prior to tracheal intubation, it can have the same consequences as aspiration of food from the stomach, without the additional acid insult. Although diverticuli can be silent and asymptomatic, the patient usually knows about its presence and it may be seen on the chest x-ray. Achalasia is almost always known to be present by the patient and ordinarily does not surprise the well-prepared anesthesia provider. Whenever there is any doubt, appropriate maneuvers to minimize the risk of aspiration should be taken.

As with most other maladies, aspiration pneumonia is a more serious complication in older patients, who may well have pre-existing diseases that complicate their recovery further. The mortality from aspiration pneumonia increases with the acidity, quantity of aspirate, and degree of fecal contamination. Treatment is uncertain, prolonged, and expensive. In older people, even with survival, aspiration pneumonia may result in chronic pulmonary disability. It is better prevented than treated, and prevention starts with awareness of the possibility on the part of the anesthesia care team.[31,32]

Temperature Regulation

Thermoregulation becomes less reactive and precise among the elderly, and can be further compromised by anesthetic and adjuvant drugs. Although current standards of practice mandate temperature monitoring as part of the assessment system during anesthesia, the common association seems to be linked to the possibility of malignant hyperthermia, which is possible but quite rare in the elderly. Failure to heed the temperature reading during anesthesia can have serious sequelae. Heat loss can occur during regional as well as general anesthesia. Shivering, unless obtunded by drugs, can provide an additional clue during regional anesthesia, but is usually not seen with general anesthesia until emergence.

Since the comfort of heavily clothed operating room personnel usually drives the setting of the thermostat, it is usually necessary to replace heat lost by the patient by one or more of the usual means: use of additional blankets on the nonoperative area of the patient's body, including the head; use of air-driven warming blankets; heating inspired gases; and use of heated pads and mattresses. All of these methods are more or less effective, but they all must be monitored carefully to prevent overheating or burns to the integument and monitoring of temperature must continue throughout the recovery period.[33]

Positioning

Part of the aging process seems to be the insidious loss of flexibility of joints, often accelerated by degenerative disease. There is an associated loss of muscle tone, which gives the flesh a somewhat dough-like texture. When positioning these patients on the operating table, particularly when they are anesthetized, it is necessary to prevent joint movement beyond the usual limits, even though the relationship of the parts may appear to be within normal configuration. By exceeding the patient's normal limits, one can cause significant postoperative discomfort in nonsurgical areas. The shoulder, hip, and back are frequent areas of patient complaint, and neck and knee complaints are fairly common. Using care and support of these areas while transferring the patient to and from the operating table is the best way to avoid these problems.

Of similar importance is the need to ensure adequate circulation to the extremities after the desired position is achieved. Ischemia of the extremities because of impingement of the arterial supply by excessive flexion or extension is more likely in older patients because of degradation of arterial tone, arteriosclerosis, or bony spurs or concretions. Obstruction of venous return is also a possibility, and if it occurs, is often hidden from view during long surgical procedures.

Peripheral nerve compression is more likely for several reasons, some stated above. In addition, the softer, less dense nature of tissues allows modest pressure on a nerve to have more frequent adverse effects than in younger patients, who have more muscle mass and better tissue tone.[34]

Delirium and Dementia

Several carefully controlled studies have shown that general and regional anesthesia do not, per se, cause a prolonged decrement in intellect or orientation.[35–38] During the perioperative period, however, many commonly used drugs can cause temporary problems with orientation and mentation. In aged patients, their effects last longer, and smaller amounts are required to exceed the desired effect in both degree and duration. The older patient may appear to be delirious or agitated because of over- or improper medication, and this occasionally results in additional depressant medicines being administered, which usually further prolongs the difficulty and may seriously interfere with recovery. When there is any doubt, it is better to stop all questionable medications and start over. When patient-controlled analgesia is used, the program must be carefully assessed in the elderly to prevent overmedication.

It is not rare for an aged patient to recover from the physical effects of anesthesia but show an apparent change in intellect, recall, and orientation that becomes permanent.[39] There is no sound explanation of this phenomenon on a physiologic basis, but there is a consensus that the problem may be more apparent than real. Oftentimes a spouse, child, or companion will recall, after the fact, that the patient was getting more forgetful and vague for some period before the operation.[40] Under normal, everyday, nonstressful, routine living, these changes are easily dealt with or ignored by the family, but after a major event such as anesthesia and surgery, they come into more acute focus because of the unfamiliar environment and people. I am not aware of the reverse of this sequence taking place in the perioperative period— that is, anesthesia and surgery does not ever improve function in a delirious or demented patient. However, acute confusional states can sometimes be associated with use of anticholinergic drugs, depression, previous stroke, infections, and perioperative hypotension. Since an acute confusional state contributes to postoperative morbidity, the treatable causes should be addressed.[41]

Hematologic Problems

Not infrequently older patients have experienced multiple surgical procedures that required blood replacement. Some of these patients present with multiple and exotic antibodies that cause difficulties with the crossmatch. Because of this and several other factors, predeposit of autologous blood is gaining favor among surgical patients, and when possible, provides a distinct advantage for all concerned. Also, intraoperative and postoperative collection of shed blood for processing and reinfusion is gaining favor and has obvious benefits.

Older patients also are more prone to postoperative blood clots and emboli, probably on the basis of generally poorer circulation, among other factors.[42] Appropriate use of early ambulation, pressure stockings, or automated pneumatic massage devices, along with meticulous postoperative use of anticoagulants, are an important part of care for the elderly.

FINANCIAL CONSIDERATIONS

The problem of rapidly increasing expenditure for health care in the United States is getting great media attention, to the point where only the most indifferent or preoccupied citizens are not concerned. Medicaid, Medicare, and health insurance purveyors are in near panic over the increasing costs, and their response is predictable, if not proper: raise premiums, increase exclusions, or both. In the case of federal or state providers the problem is addressed by limiting doctor fees, hospital charges, and eligibility.

Younger people are often covered by some form of health insurance, provided by their employer with or without some degree of personal contribution, or by some form of privately obtained insurance, but many older people depend on Medicare, often with some form of privately financed supplementary policy. In either instance the actuarial problems multiply as health care resources are sought in ever-increasing quantities by a growing group of patients. Currently, 10 to 15 percent of the U.S. Gross National Product is identified as health care costs, an enormous amount of money, requiring a prodigious amount of administering, record-keeping, allotting, paying, and receiving. Administrative costs will soon take 15 percent of health care dollars, and these dollars will not pay for a single surgical procedure, diagnostic test, or hospital room. Thirty-seven million citizens of all ages have no insurance and are, for varying reasons, ineligible or unable to buy any health care coverage.[43]

At the present time, the system of health care providers has accommodated to the enforced stipulations imposed by third-party payers and government agencies. With the imposition of restraints on payment to hospitals and doctors based on diagnostic-related groups started for Medicare patients in 1983, and the requirement for preadmission approval for these patients, we are probably seeing the first lurch toward rationing health care. The aged population, many of whom are dependent on Medicare, are likely to be the first victims of cost containments. Since there is a practical limit to requiring outpatient status for specific surgical interventions, the next logical step will undoubtedly be the identification of an upper age limit for eligibility for various procedures. This is already the practice in other countries where the government provides access and support for all health care.

When and if this becomes the case in the United States, only the well-to-do will be candidates for elective reconstructive surgery, cardiac bypass surgery, and other procedures commonly done in older patient populations. As the numbers of rule-makers, administrators, enforcers, and accountants increases, the proportion of health care money actually used to provide health care will decrease. The purveyors of this service will be regulated along with the constraints on choice of medication and procedures. Eventually, the health-related professions will become a less desirable career choice and quality will decline.

These dire predictions are not inevitable, but they seem likely at the present time. No matter how much more efficient the system becomes, it is unlikely to keep up with the increasing demand for the good life in spite of age, disease, self-abuse, and neglect. Those most likely to be affected first and worst will be our geriatric population. Next, it will be the capable and dedicated providers, who will be constrained from using expensive drugs, diagnostic tests, and procedures, resulting in frustration, anger, and maybe even despair.

In my view, it is the responsibility of the health-related professions to intervene in this downward spiral in providing quality and quantity of care, by active participation in the decision-making process regarding costs, availability, distribution, and nature of medical care. The systems in place now are not working satisfactorily. I recall from my laboratory days a commonly accepted belief that when an experiment was going bad, attempts to fix it just made it worse. Perhaps we should start over with qualified people building a new system instead of politicians trying to patch up a sinking ship. It is our responsibility to involve ourselves in the process individually and through participation in our societies, and political parties, and associations.

REFERENCES

1. National Center for Health Statistics: Health, United States, 1983. (PHS) 83:1232. U.S. Government Printing Office, Washington, DC, 1983
2. Kane RA, Kane RL: Assessing the Elderly: A Practical Guide to Measurement. Lexington Books, Lexington, MA, 1981
3. Rowe JW, Rahn RL: Human aging: usual and successful. Science 237:143, 1987
4. Levit KR, Lazenby H, Waldo D: National health expenditures, 1984. Health Care Finan Rev 7:1, 1985
5. Galazka SS: Preoperative evaluation of the elderly surgical patient. J Fam Pract 27(6):622, 1985
6. Vaz FG, Seymour DG: A prospective study of elderly general surgical patients: preoperative medical problems. Age Ageing 18:309, 1989
7. Johnson JC: Surgical assessment of the elderly. Geriatrics 43(suppl):83, 1988
8. Keating HJ: Preoperative considerations in the geriatric patient. Med Clin North Am 71:569, 1987
9. Seymour DG, Vaz FG: Aspects of surgery in the elderly: preoperative medical assessment. Br J Hosp Med 37:102, 1987
10. Pankratz L, Lofoed L: The assessment and treatment of geezers. JAMA 259:1228, 1988
11. Daly MP: The medical evaluation of the elderly preoperative patient. Prim Care 16:361, 1989
12. Guidelines for the appropriate use of do-not-resuscitate orders. JAMA 265:1868, 1989
13. Truog RD: "Do-not-resuscitate" orders during anesthesia and surgery. Anesthesiology 74:606, 1991
14. Martin RL, Soifer BE, Stevens WC: Ethical issues in anesthesia: management of the do-not-resuscitate patient. Anesth Analg 73:221, 1991
15. Lazaroff AE, Orr WF: Living wills and other advanced directives. Clin Geriatr Med 2:3, 1986
16. Klein JE: Right-to-die issues in Minnesota. Minn Med 74:33, 1991
17. Pedersen T, Eliasen K, Hendriksen E: A

prospective study of mortality associated with anesthesia and surgery: risk indicators of mortality in hospital. Acta Anaesthesiol Scand 34:176, 1990

18. Cohen M, Duncan PG, Tate RB: Does anesthesia contribute to operative mortality? JAMA 260:2859, 1988
19. Manning FC: Preoperative evaluation of the elderly patient. Am Fam Phys 39:123, 1988
20. Olshansky SJ, Carnes BA, Cassel C: In search of Methuselah: estimating the upper limits to human longevity. Science 250:634, 1990
21. Jones RM: Anesthesia and old age, editorial. Anaesthesia 44:377, 1989
22. Katz SM, Fagraeus L: Anesthetic considerations in geriatric patients. Clin Geriatr Med 6:499, 1990
23. Ward RM, Hutton P: Factors modifying the use of anesthetic drugs in the elderly. Br Med Bull 46:156, 1990
24. Dwyer R, Fec JPH, Clarke RSJ: End tidal concentrations of halothane and isoflurane during induction of anaesthesia in young and elderly patients. Br J Anaesth 64:36, 1990
25. Matteo RS, McDaniel DD, Brothertone WP, Diaz J: Pharmacokinetics of tubocurarine in the aged. Anesthesiology 57(suppl):A271, 1982
26. Sheref SE: Pattern of CNS recovery following reversal of neuromuscular blockade. Br J Anaesth 57:188, 1985
27. Sear JW, Hand CW, Moore RA: Studies on morphine disposition: plasma concentrations of morphine and its metabolites in anesthetized middle-aged and elderly surgical patients. J Clin Anesth 1:164, 1989
28. Ogilvie RI, Ruedy J: Adverse drug reactions during hospitalization. Can Med Assoc J 97:1450, 1967
29. Hurwitz N: Predisposing factors in adverse reactions to drugs. Br Med J 1:536, 1969
30. Lichtiger M: Management of the geriatric outpatient. Prob Anesth 3(4):620, 1989
31. Coombs DW: Aspiration pneumonia pro-

phylaxis. (Editorial) Anesth Analg 62:1055, 1983
32. White PF: Anesthetic techniques for the elderly outpatient. Int Anesthesiol Clin 26:105, 1988
33. Yam PCI, Carli F: Maintenance of body temperature in elderly patients who have joint replacement. Anaesthesia 45:563, 1990
34. Martin JT: Positioning in Anesthesia and Surgery. WB Saunders, Philadelphia, 1987, p. 303.
35. Jones MJT, Piggott SE, Vaughan RS et al: Cognitive and functional competence after anesthesia in patients aged over 60: controlled trial of general and regional anesthesia for elective hip or knee replacement. Br Med J 300:1683, 1990
36. Chung FF, Chung A, Meier RH: Comparison of perioperative mental function after general anesthesia and spinal anesthesia with intravenous sedation. Can J Anaesth 36:382, 1989
37. Chung F, Seyone C, Dyck B et al: Age-related cognitive recovery after general anesthesia. Anesth Analg 72:217, 1990
38. Nielson WR, Gelb AW, Casey JE et al: Long-term cognitive and social sequelae of general vs regional anesthesia during arthroplasty in the elderly. Anesthesiology 73:1103, 1990
39. Carter M: Effects of anesthesia on mental performance in the elderly. Nurs Times 85:40, 1989
40. Pousada L, Leipzig RM: Rapid bedside assessment of postoperative confusion in older patients. Geriatrics 45:59, 1990
41. Gustafson Y, Berggren D, Brännström B et al: Acute confusional status in elderly patients treated for femoral neck fracture. J Am Geriatr Soc 36:525, 1988
42. Müller R, Mušikić P: Hemorheology in surgery—a review. Angiology 38:581, 1987
43. USA Today. Special Report. March 11, 1991
44. Miller R: Anesthesia for the aged: some pharmacokinetic and pharmacodynamic considerations. Mt Sinai J Med 54(4):305, 1987

8

Spinal Surgery

Terese T. Horlocker

SPINAL CORD BLOOD FLOW AND AUTOREGULATION

The vascular supply of the spinal cord is quite complex in both its origin and pattern of flow in and around the cord. Surgical manipulation and instrumentation, direct trauma, individual anatomic variations, and anesthetic agents and techniques all may affect spinal cord blood flow and autoregulation. It is important to apply the principles of neuronal protection during spinal cord surgery to prevent cord ischemia and preserve function.

The spinal cord is supplied with arterial blood by one anterior and two posterolateral vessels that run the length of the cord and by segmental radicular arteries that enter the vertebral foramina and reach the spinal cord by way of the nerve roots. Individual variation exists in the number of radicular arteries, their origin, and their route to the spinal cord.

Anterior Spinal Artery

The anterior spinal artery arises from the terminal segments of each vertebral artery, which then join to form a single vessel and descend in the median fissure of the spinal cord (Fig. 8-1). A series of six to eight anterior radicular arteries from the vertebral, thyrocervical, costocervical, intercostal, and iliac vessels supply the anterior spinal artery at various levels along the length of the spinal cord. The largest of these radicular arteries is the radicularis magna (artery of Adamkiewicz), which supplies the anterior spinal artery in the thoracolumbar region of the spinal cord. Its origin is between T9 and T12 in 60 percent, between T5 and T8 in 14 percent, and below L1 in 26 percent of cases.[1] The radicularis magna may be responsible for one-quarter to one-half of the blood supply of the spinal cord.

In the upper and midcervical portions of the cord, the flow in the anterior spinal arteries is caudad, but because of the great variations in arterial anatomy, the direction is uncertain in other areas. Presumably, because the radicularis magna is a major source of blood supply to the thoracic cord, the flow there is cephalad. The relatively large distances between the radicular vessels place "watershed" areas of the cord at risk for ischemia, particularly in the upper thoracic and lower lumber regions. Anterior spinal artery ischemia results in loss of motor function and pain and temperature sensation since the anterior two-thirds of the cord is supplied by the anterior spinal artery. Dorsal column functions are spared.

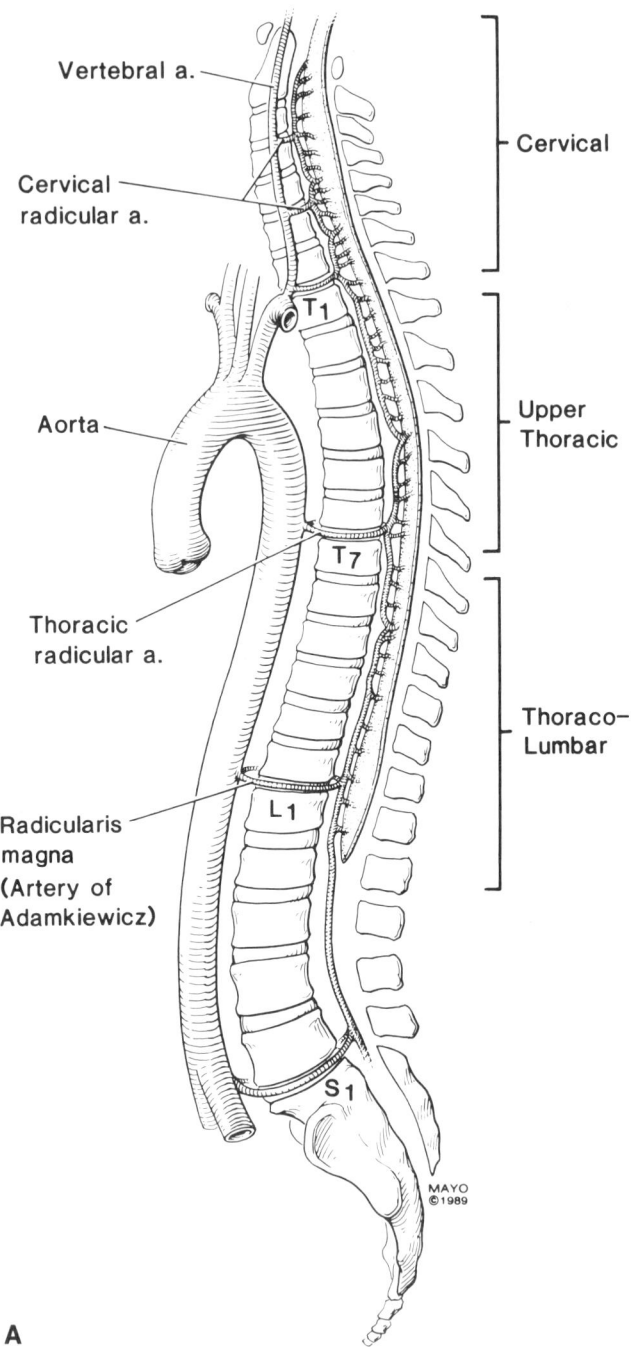

Fig. 8-1. Blood supply of the spinal cord. Anterior spinal artery. (**A**) Vertical distribution. Radicular arteries are variable in location but are shown here at T1, T7, L1, and S1. Although all radicular arteries contribute to nutritive blood flow, the greatest proportion of flow is from the radicularis magna (artery of Adamkiewicz). (*Figure continues.*)

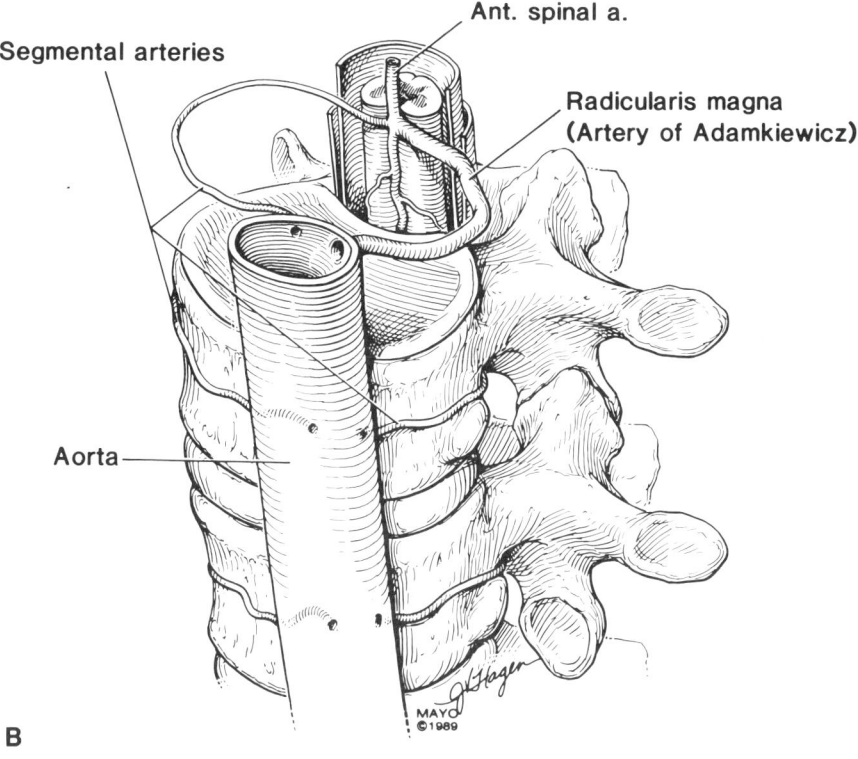

B

Fig. 8-1 (*Continued*). (**B**) Segmental blood supply at the level of the radicularis magna, which is between T9 and T12 in 60 percent of cases. (From Horlocker et al,[78] with permission.)

Posterior Spinal Arteries

The paired posterior spinal arteries arise from the posterior inferior cerebellar arteries to descend along the posterolateral aspect of the cord. They receive contributions from 25 to 40 posterior radicular arteries. The posterior spinal arteries supply only the dorsal columns. Because they are widely anastomosed, injury to one of them will not necessarily result in cord ischemia.

Blood flow to the spinal cord is approximately 40 percent of cerebral blood flow, with the cervical and lumbosacral regions receiving twice that of the thoracic area.[2] Spinal cord blood flow parallels that of cerebral blood flow in both autoregulation and chemical regulation.[2,3] Spinal cord blood flow autoregulates between mean arterial pressures of 60 and 150 mmHg. Outside this range, flow is pressure dependent.[4] Ischemia may occur if spinal cord perfusion pressure is maintained below autoregulatory limits. Likewise, spinal cord blood flow responds to arterial oxygen and carbon dioxide tensions in the same manner as cerebral blood flow.[5] Hypocapnia decreases flow, while hypercapnia and hypoxia result in vasodilation and increased flow. Autoregulation may be affected by trauma, surgery, and anesthetics, emphasizing the need to consider spinal cord perfusion pressure in patients undergoing spinal surgery.

SPINAL CORD INJURIES

Spinal cord injury occurs at a rate of 11,000 new cases per year. Approximately one-half of these are at the cervical level.[6] Traffic accidents are the leading cause, accounting for 30 to 50 percent of all injuries. Other mechanisms include diving accidents, sports, and falls. Spinal cord injuries typically occur to men in their mid-twenties. The mortality is nearly 50 percent because of associated injuries.[7]

Most patients who have sustained injury to the spinal cord have had a fracture or dislocation of the spinal column; however, not all individuals who have had an injury to the spinal column have sustained injury to the spinal cord. Nonetheless *all* patients with injury to the spine need continued and careful observation to prevent further injury. Ten percent of quadriplegic patients become so after the accident while receiving medical care.[8]

Cervical Spine Injuries

The cervical spine is particularly vulnerable to injury because of its extreme mobility. Its great range of rotation, flexion, and extension all lead to mechanical instability. The site and nature of damage to the cervical spinal cord are determined by the direction of impact, position of the head relative to the thorax, and mechanism of injury. Associated skeletal and soft tissue changes are often present with cervical trauma. Facial and skull lacerations are useful in localizing the site of injury and direction of applied forces at impact.

Axis fractures are strongly correlated with head and other cervical spine injuries (40 and 18 percent, respectively) (Fig. 8-2).[9] A flexion injury may cause the head to move or slide forward. Because the atlas is firmly attached to the occipital condyles, the subluxation will occur between the atlas and axis. As the axis is carried forward, its weakest point, the dens, becomes dislocated anteriorly. The cord is frequently spared because of the relatively large size of the bony canal. In extreme extension injuries, the dens may be dislocated posteriorly. In this situation, neurologic deficits range from minimal to respiratory insufficiency and death.

Flexion injury is the most common injury to the cervical spine and is typically caused by a blow to the occiput. If the force is adequate, there will be interruption of posterior ligaments and dislocation of facet joints. Depending on the degree of flexion and amount of force applied, a burst fracture may occur. A posterior fragment of the fractured vertebral body may also be forced into the vertebral canal. Flexion injuries produce the most severe spinal cord trauma. The neurologic deficit is immediate. Patients usually show loss of all spinal cord modalities except joint position sense and deep touch (dorsal column functions), which are spared.

Extension injuries occur during a fall or rear-end automobile collision in which the head is forced backward. Older people have an increase in cervical lordosis and spondylosis and are therefore more prone to injuries of this type. Sufficient force will cause rupture of the anterior longitudinal ligament. Radiologic findings may be minimal, but in patients with previous compromise of the spinal canal, only slight displacement may produce significant neurologic deficits. Hyperextension of the cervical spine produces the central cervical spine syndrome. The central gray area of the cord, which is supplied by the anterior spinal artery, is compromised, while the periphery of the cord, supplied by the circumferential arteries, is spared. This lesion is characterized by quadriparesis, affecting upper extremities more than lower, with possible sparing of the sensory modalities and bowel and bladder function.

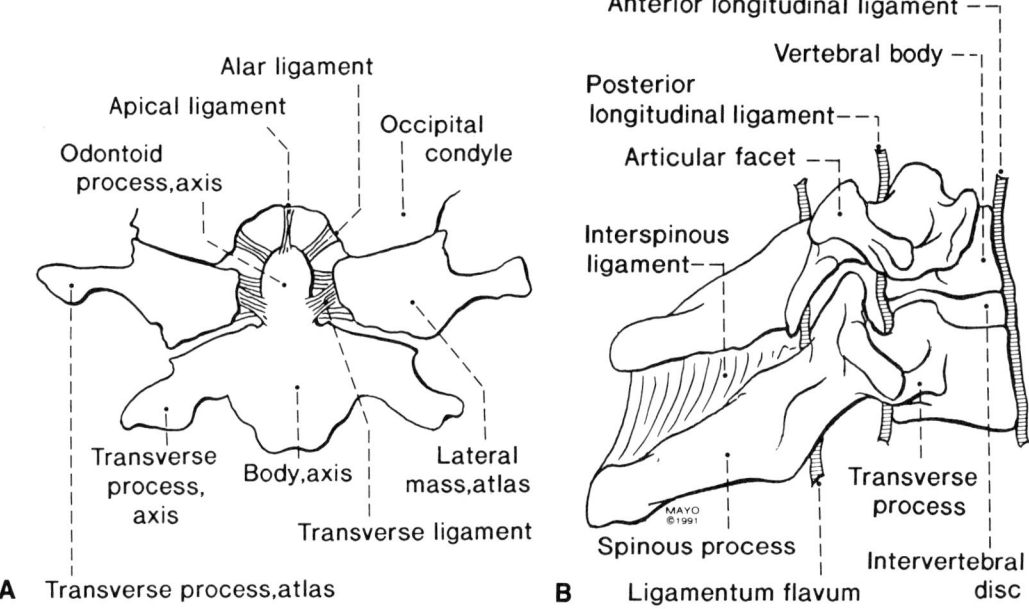

Fig. 8-2. Cervical spine anatomy. (**A**) Occipitoatlantoaxial complex. Coronal section, anterior arch of atlas removed. The occipitoatlantoaxial unit supports the head, allows the necessary range of motion of the head and neck, and protects the spinal cord. (**B**) Lower cervical spine. Lateral view. Structures contributing to cervical stability include anterior and posterior ligaments, intervertebral disc, facet joints, and the interspinous and supraspinous ligaments. (From Crosby & Lui,[79] with permission.)

Thoracic and Lumbar Spine Injuries

The four vertebrae that comprise the thoracolumbar junction—T11, T12, L1, and L2—constitute a vulnerable site for fracture dislocations. Thoracic vertebrae above this level are stabilized by rib and intercostal attachments, while the lower lumbar vertebrae are resistant to trauma because of their larger vertebral body size and heavy ligamentous reinforcement.

Flexion rotation is the most common mechanism of fracture dislocation of the thoracolumbar spine. Flexion forces in combination with thoracic rotation in one direction and pelvic rotation in the opposite direction cause a fracture of the T12-L1 facet joint. This fracture dislocation is unstable and usually the patient sustains severe neurologic injury.

An axial burst fracture is produced when a force is applied perpendicular to the axis of the spine. The vertebral disc is forced into the interior of the vertebral body, pushing fragments anteriorly, posteriorly, and laterally. Neurologic injury occurs when a portion of the vertebral body protrudes into the neural canal. These fractures are stable if the posterior elements are intact.

Pure flexion injuries to the lumbar spine produce a compression fracture of the vertebral body without dislocation or fracture of the posterior elements. This type of fracture is usually stable and does not cause neural compromise.

Physical Examination

The examination of a person with a suspected spinal cord injury begins with a rapid assessment for possible injury to other systems. Cervical injuries are frequently associated with head injury, thoracic fractures with pulmonary and cardiovascular injury, and lumbar fractures with abdominal and long bone injuries. The patient should be examined immediately for signs of respiratory insufficiency, airway obstruction, rib fractures, and facial trauma. It is important not to overlook chest wall injuries, flail chest, or pneumothorax. Location of pain over spinous processes and surrounding soft tissue is useful in determining the level of injury. Bruises over the head and neck, shoulder, or buttock will indicate the possible mechanism of injury. The abdomen should be evaluated for intra-abdominal injury and bleeding as well as paralytic ileus.

Serial neurologic examination is necessary to assess function of the spinal cord above the level of the fracture. Motor function may be studied by observing the respiratory mechanics and the position assumed by the extremities. The fifth cervical segment is perhaps the most important in providing clinical evidence of cervical spinal injury. This segment controls motor function of the deltoid, biceps, brachialis, and brachioradialis muscles. If these muscles are flaccid the fifth cervical nerve is involved and there will be partial diaphragmatic paralysis. A complete lesion at the fourth cervical segment is not compatible with survival unless artificial respiration is initiated. The absence of intercostal breathing suggests a cervical or high thoracic injury, while the presence of both intercostal and diaphragmatic breathing represents an injury below the midthoracic spine.

Examination of the lower extremities and perineum documents cauda equina root function. Motor function to the iliopsoas, quadriceps, hamstrings, and anterior and posterior tibialis muscles is supplied by the lumbar roots. When paralysis is present, careful sensory examination may show that a lesion is incomplete. Sensation in the perineal area indicates sacral sparing. Deep tendon reflexes are usually present with an incomplete lesion but may be absent during the period of spinal shock.

Early Management

During transport, the patient should be moved on a spine board with the neck immobilized to prevent further injury. Anteroposterior and lateral radiographs of the spine should be made at the time of initial evaluation. The use of portable radiologic equipment will minimize patient movement and handling. Computed tomography may be necessary to diagnose an injury with equivocal radiographic findings.

Tracheal Intubation

Airway management is critical in patients with cervical spinal cord injury. The most common cause of death with acute cervical spinal cord injury is respiratory failure. All patients with severe trauma or head injuries should be assumed to have an unstable cervical fracture until proven otherwise radiographically. The neck should be stabilized by manual traction applied by someone other than the intubator, and in specific cases, skull tongs or halo traction should be applied. Fiberoptic intubation of an awake patient may be performed after the oropharynx and larynx are topically anesthetized. Blind nasotracheal intubation can be used when spontaneous respirations are present and there is no evidence of facial or basal skull fractures. In a truly emergent situation, oral intubation with direct laryngoscopy is the usual approach. The trachea should be intubated with minimum flexion or extension of the neck. Intravenous lidocaine may be administered to attenuate laryngeal reflexes. The use of muscle relaxants to facilitate relaxation is controversial. The paraspinal muscle spasm that occurs after cervical fracture serves to immobilize the cervical spine. Succinylcholine may transiently increase intracranial pressure and produces relaxation of the paraspinal muscles, which may displace the fracture and traumatize the cord. If succinylcholine is used, the patient should not be transferred until muscle tone is restored.

Nonoperative Management

Treatment is based on the presence or absence of neurologic function and the radiographic evaluation of vertebral displacement and instability. Skeletal traction accomplished by placement of a halo or skull tongs is an effective method of reducing a cervical fracture. Thoracolumbar dislocation may be treated with bedrest, bracing, or casting. Postural reduction with bedrest is the most popular method of nonoperative treatment in lower spine trauma.

Operative Management

If the patient has gross displacement that cannot be reduced by nonoperative methods, surgical reduction with internal fixation must be performed. Prompt reduction not only corrects mechanical deformation but may improve spinal cord blood supply and reverse ischemia.

Cervical spine fractures are most often surgically treated by anterior open reduction and fusion. The surgical incision approximates the anterior border of the sternocleidomastoid muscle. Lateral retraction of the carotid artery may endanger blood flow to the brain particularly in the elderly patient. Sloan reported a case in which carotid retraction during cervical fusion produced alteration in the somatosensory evoked potentials consistent with ischemia. The waveforms returned to baseline upon retractor removal.[10] Retraction of the esophagus and trachea medially may cause pharyngeal laceration, laryngeal edema, and recurrent laryngeal nerve paralysis. Cerebrospinal fluid leaks and trauma to the vertebral artery have also been reported. Not all cervical spine fractures may be approached anteriorly. Fractures of the dens and C2-C3 fractures are relatively inaccessible by this approach. Injuries that compromise the vertebral canal posteriorly with penetrating or impinging bone fragments require laminectomy for decompression. A posterior cervical approach with the patient in the prone position is used. Thoracolumbar fracture dislocations are also typically approached posteriorly. Once correct alignment has been achieved, the spine must be stabilized by a method of internal fixation such as Harrington rods. The patient is kept immobilized at bedrest for 8 to 12 weeks postoperatively. Surgical treatment is independent of neurologic function. Patients who are paraplegic are managed the same as those with no neurologic deficits.

Respiratory Considerations

Ventilatory impairment increases with the higher level of spinal injury. The neurologic examination is crucial for determining the level of injury and anticipating complications. A high cervical lesion that includes the diaphragmatic segments (C3–C5) will result in respiratory failure, and death will occur unless artificial pulmonary ventilation is utilized. Lesions between C5 and T7 will cause significant alterations in respiratory function owing to the loss of abdominal and intercostal support. The indrawing of flaccid thoracic muscles during inspiration produces paradoxical respirations, resulting in a vital capacity reduction of 60 percent. Inability to cough and effectively clear secretions results in atelectasis and infection. Paralytic ileus and gastric distension increase abdominal pressure, further compromising diaphragmatic excursion. This effect can be reduced by placement of a nasogastric tube to suction. It is also important not to overlook associated injuries such as pneumothorax or flail chest. The incidence of pulmonary embolism is increased as a result of decreased muscle tone venodilatation.

Cardiovascular Considerations

During spinal shock there is loss of sympathetic vascular tone below the injury. If the cardioaccelerator fibers (T1–T4) are damaged, bradycardia results. The unopposed vagal tone may lead to asystole with tracheal suctioning or laryngoscopy. Atropine will attenuate the vagal effects. Accompanying hemorrhagic shock may not produce a compensatory tachycardia; the rate may remain at 40 to 60 beats/min. The tendency to treat hypotension with fluids during spinal shock and the inability of the cardiovascular system to compensate in response to fluid loading leads to the development of pulmonary edema. Pulmonary artery catheter placement is recommended for fluid management in a patient with a high cervical lesion.[7] Autonomic instability should be treated with direct-acting vasoconstrictors, vasodilators, and positive and negative chronotropic drugs as needed. Indirect sympathetic agonists or antagonists should be avoided because of their unpredictability.

Maintaining Spinal cord Integrity

Spinal shock occurs acutely and results in complete cessation of spinal cord functions below the level of the lesion. This results in flaccid paralysis, loss of visceral and somatic sensation, and paralytic ileus. Vasopressor reflexes are also lost. Spinal shock may persist from a few days to 3 months. Even with severe spinal cord injury some degree of cord function may gradually return, although this is unpredictable. Generally the patients who recover the most function are those who show rapid early improvement in their neurologic deficits.

Patients with unstable spines who are not quadriplegic or paraplegic may become so during positioning for surgery. The period of greatest risk is associated with turning the patient prone. Safe positioning may be performed by utilizing a Foster frame rotating bed or by manufacturing an anterior thoracic body mold and rolling the patient prone while in the shell. When appropriate, line placement, intubation, and positioning can be performed while the patient is awake with general anesthesia induced only after voluntary upper and lower extremity movement is confirmed.

All patients with spinal cord trauma should be considered to have compromised cords, and an important component of anesthetic management is the preservation of spinal cord blood flow. Blood pressure and intravascular volume should be maintained within normal levels to ensure adequate spinal cord perfusion pressure. Sustained hypotension may worsen neurologic deficits. Hyperventilation should be avoided since hypocarbia decreases spinal cord blood flow. Neurophysiologic monitoring, such as the utilization of somatosensory evoked potentials (SSEPs), assists in prompt diagnosis of neurologic change and early intervention in situations of potential neurologic ischemia. Anesthetic considerations in the presence of SSEP monitoring are described in detail below (see under Scoliosis). The wake-up test may also be used to confirm neurologic dysfunction in the presence of SSEP changes.

Electrolyte Abnormalities

Patients with motor deficits from spinal cord injuries may develop hyperkalemia after administration of succinylcholine. The amount of potassium released depends on the degree of paralysis. It is usually safe to administer succinylcholine for the first 48 hours. After that time, the muscle cell membranes become supersensitive to depolarizing muscle relaxants. The increases in serum potassium levels are maximal between 4 weeks and 5 months after spinal injury.[11] Serum potassium levels may increase from normal to as high as 14 mEq/L, causing ventricular fibrillation or cardiac arrest. Therefore, succinylcholine should be avoided in all spinal cord-injured patients after 48 hours. There are no contraindications to the nondepolarizing agents.

Hypercalcemia results from flaccid paralysis and immobilization, predisposing the patient to ventricular arrhythmias. In addition, the mobilization of bone calcium content may lead to osteoporosis, pathologic fractures, and renal calculi.

Temperature Control

Disruption of the sympathetic pathways carrying temperature sensation and subsequent loss of vasoconstriction below the level of injury cause spinal cord-injured patients to be poikilothermic. Maintenance of normal temperature can be achieved by applying exog-

enous heat to the skin, increasing ambient air temperature, warming intravenous fluids, and humidifying gases.

Autonomic Hyperreflexia

After recovery from spinal shock, 85 percent of patients will exhibit autonomic hyperreflexia when there has been complete cord transection above T5. The syndrome can also occur with injuries at lower levels and is characterized by severe paroxysmal hypertension with bradycardia, arrhythmias, and cutaneous vasoconstriction below and vasodilation above the level of the injury. The episode is typically precipitated by distention of a viscus (bladder or rectum), but can be induced by any noxious stimulus. The lack of supraspinal inhibition allows the sympathetic outflow below the lesion to react to the stimulus unopposed. If untreated, the hypertensive crisis may progress to seizures, intracranial hemorrhage, or myocardial infarction. If autonomic hyperreflexia occurs, it should be treated by removal of the stimulus, deepening anesthesia, and administration of direct-acting vasodilators.

Renal Considerations

Renal failure is a major cause of death in spinal cord-injured patients. Recurrent urinary tract infections, pyelonephritis, and hypercalcemia and renal calculi resulting from immobilization lead to chronic renal failure. Renal amyloidosis is associated with paraplegia. Renal function should be carefully assessed preoperatively and drugs excreted by the kidney such as muscle relaxants and some antibiotics used cautiously.

SCOLIOSIS

Scoliosis is a deformity of the spine resulting in lateral curvature and rotation of the vertebrae and also deformity of the rib cage (Fig. 8-3). On the concave side of the curve, the discs and vertebral bodies become wedge-shaped, the posterior angles of the ribs are shallow, and the vertebrae and spinous processes rotate toward the concavity. On the convex side of the curvature, the ribs are pulled back, making the posterior angle more acute. Thoracic and lumbar regions are the most frequent sites of the primary curvature.[12]

Patients with scoliosis may also develop kyphosis, or posterior rotation of the spine. Kyphoscoliosis is rare and is usually a congenital abnormality. These patients may require kyphectomy and anterior fusion in addition to posterior fusion to achieve spinal stability.[13]

The severity of the scoliosis is defined by the angle of scoliosis, or the Cobb angle (Fig. 8-4). The larger the angle, the more severe the scoliosis. It is generally agreed that nonoperative treatment, such as application of a Milwaukee brace, should be used in patients with a small curvature and in children who have not achieved skeletal maturity. Surgical correction is performed for deformities with a Cobb angle over 50 degrees.[14] Improved methods of internal fixation have resulted in a trend toward earlier surgery.[15]

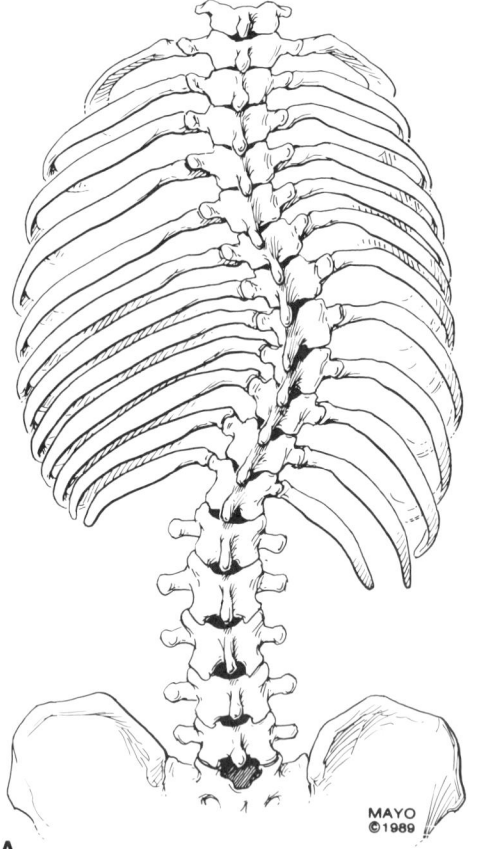

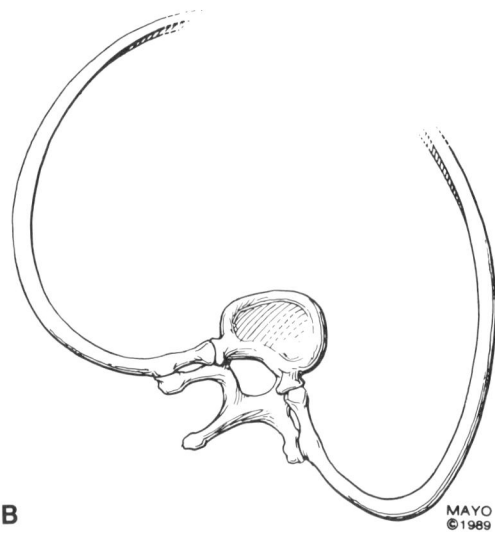

Fig. 8-3. Deformity of the vertebrae and rib cage in scoliosis. (**A**) Primary curvature occurs most frequently in the thoracic and lumbar regions. The vertebral bodies are wedge-shaped and the posterior angles of the ribs are shallow on the side of concavity. (**B**) On the convex side, the rib angles are more acute. (From Horlocker et al,[78] with permission.)

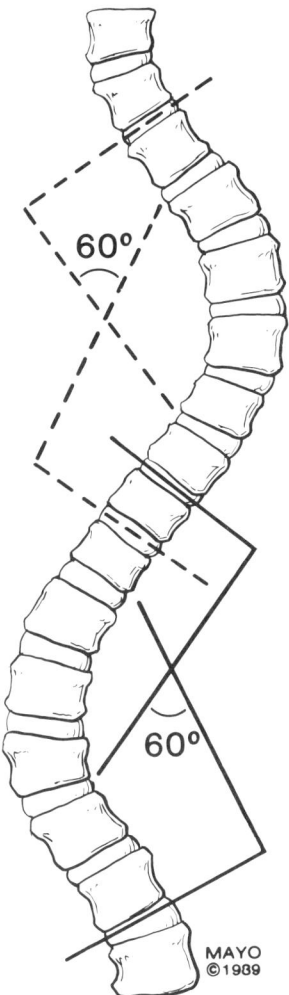

Fig. 8-4. Angle of scoliosis (Cobb angle). Lines are drawn parallel to the vertebral bodies at the lowest and highest borders of the curve. Perpendicular lines are drawn to these lines and the angles are measured at the point of intersection. The angle of curvature consists of the cephalad and caudad angles. (From Horlocker et al,[78] with permission.)

Classification of Scoliosis

In 1973, the Scoliosis Research Society identified multiple etiologies in the development of scoliosis[16] (Table 8-1). As a result of the eradication of poliomyelitis, the incidence of scoliosis predominantly reflects the incidence of idiopathic scoliosis, which represents 75 to 90 percent of cases. The incidence is 4 per 1,000 girls and 0.3 per 1,000 boys, with an overall incidence of 1.8 per 1,000.[17] The remaining 10 to 25 percent of cases are associated with neuromuscular diseases; congenital abnormalities, including congenital heart disease; trauma; and mesenchymal disorders. A diagnosis of scoliosis in a patient should therefore include a family history and physical examination, with particular attention to the respiratory, cardiac, and neuromuscular systems.

Idiopathic Scoliosis

Idiopathic scoliosis, the most common type of scoliosis, has three well-defined periods of onset: infantile (0 to 4 years), juvenile (4 to 9 years), and adolescent (10 years to maturity). It is generally thought that the higher the curve and the earlier the onset, the worse the prognosis; however, 50 percent of infantile scoliosis cases resolve spontaneously.

Infantile scoliosis can be classified as resolving or progressive. Male infants more frequently have progressive curves and a higher incidence of kyphosis. In one survey of 14 patients, the mean angle of scoliosis was 130 degrees and three patients died of cardiac or respiratory failure.[18] Resolving infantile scoliosis does not usually increase beyond 30 degrees and seldom requires treatment.[16]

Adolescent idiopathic scoliosis is most common. Ninety percent of patients are girls and 90 percent of the curves are right sided and thoracic in origin.[19] Typically 7 to 10 vertebrae are involved and curve progression occurs rapidly. At skeletal maturity, two-thirds of patients will have a Cobb angle greater than 70 degrees and will require surgical correction. Curve progression may continue even after skeletal maturity. The average increase in the curve is 30 degrees.

Table 8-1. Classification of Spinal Deformities

I. Idiopathic
  A. Infantile (3 years of age or younger)
    1. Resolving
    2. Progressive
  B. Juvenile (4 to 9 years of age)
  C. Adolescent (10 years of age or older)
II. Neuromuscular
  A. Neuropathic
    1. Upper motor neuron lesion
      a. Cerebral palsy
      b. Spinocerebellar disease
        (1) Friedrich's
        (2) Charcot-Marie-Tooth
        (3) Roussy-Lévy
      c. Syringomyelia
      d. Spinal cord tumor
      e. Spinal cord trauma
      f. Other
    2. Lower motor neuron lesion
      a. Poliomyelitis
      b. Other viral myelitis
      c. Traumatic
      d. Spinal muscular atrophy
        (1) Werdnig-Hoffmann
        (2) Kugelberg-Welander
      e. Myelomeningocele (paralytic)
    3. Dysautonomia (Riley-Day)
    4. Other
  B. Myopathic
    1. Arthrogryposis
    2. Muscular dystrophy
      a. Duchenne (pseudohypertrophic)
      b. Limb-girdle
      c. Facioscapulohumeral
    3. Fiber type disproportion
    4. Congenital hypotonia
    5. Myotonia dystrophica
    6. Other
III. Congenital
  A. Congenital scoliosis
    1. Failure of formation
      a. Wedge
      b. Hemivertebra
    2. Failure of segmentation
      a. Unilateral bar
      b. Bilateral ("fusion")
    3. Mixed
  B. Congenital kyphosis
    1. Failure of formation
    2. Failure of segmentation
    3. Mixed
  C. Congenital lordosis
  D. Associated with neural tissue defect
    1. Myeomeningocele
    2. Meningocele
    3. Spinal dysraphism
      a. Diastematomyelia
      b. Other

IV. Neurofibromatosis
V. Mesenchymal
  A. Marfan's disease
  B. Homocystinuria
  C. Ehlers–Danlos disease
VI. Traumatic
  A. Fracture or dislocation (nonparalytic)
  B. Postirradiation
  C. Postlaminectomy
  D. Other
VII. Soft tissue contractures
  A. Burn
  B. Other
VIII. Osteochondrodystrophies
  A. Achondroplasia
  B. Spondyloepiphyseal dysplasia
  C. Diastrophic dwarfism
  D. Mucopolysaccharidosis
IX. Scheuermann's disease
X. Infection
  A. Tuberculosis
  B. Bacterial
  C. Fungal
  D. Parasitic
  E. Other
XI. Tumor
  A. Benign
  B. Malignant
XII. Rheumatoid disease
  A. Juvenile rheumatoid
  B. Adult rheumatoid
  C. Marie-Strümpell
XIII. Metabolic
  A. Rickets
  B. Juvenile osteoporosis
  C. Osteogenesis imperfecta
XIV. Related to lumbosacral area
  A. Spondylolisthesis
  B. Spondylolysis
  C. Other congenital anomaly
  D. Other
XV. Thoracogenic
  A. Postempyema
  B. Post-thoracoplasty
  C. Post-thoracotomy
  D. Other
XVI. Hysterical
XVII. Functional
  A. Postural
  B. Secondary to short leg
  C. Other

(Modified from Goldstein & Waugh,[16] with permission.)

Idiopathic scoliosis appears to be genetically inherited in adolescent scoliosis, with an autosomal-dominant mode of inheritance with reduced penetrance. The pattern has not been defined in infantile scoliosis. Although most patients with idiopathic scoliosis have no other associated anomalies, 7 percent of patients also have mental retardation, congenital heart defects, and other limb defects.[17]

Scoliosis Associated with Neuromuscular Disease

Neuropathic and myopathic scolioses are spinal curvatures caused by disease or anomalous function or development of nervous tissue or muscle. Poliomyelitis was once the leading cause of neuromuscular scoliosis. Degeneration of anterior horn cells in the spinal cord results in muscle weakness. Involvement of respiratory muscles leads to decreased force of inspiration and expiration, impaired cough, and atelectasis. Bulbar involvement impairs swallowing, predisposing the patient to aspiration and pneumonia. These patients often need aggressive preoperative pulmonary therapy. Residual effects of muscle relaxants and narcotics may cause respiratory failure postoperatively because of the limited respiratory reserve.

Patients with myelomeningocele undergoing scoliosis repair require careful positioning to avoid vertebral fractures. These patients have a high incidence of kyphosis and often require kyphectomy, including ligation of the nonfunctioning spinal cord. Ligation of the cord can lead to increases in intracranial pressure as well as the effects of sympathectomy due to cord transection. Patients with an intraventricular shunt must have shunt patency confirmed preoperatively. Profuse blood loss may occur because of scar tissue from previous repair as well as the proximity of the epidural plexus.

Neurofibromatosis, or von Recklinghausen's disease, consists of irregular pigmented areas in the skin (café au lait spots) and multiple neurofibromas. There is a large spectrum of neuroskeletal abnormalities in patients with von Recklinghausen's disease. Skeletal deformities, including bone cysts and scoliosis, are found in 30 to 50 percent of patients. Neurofibromas arise within nerve trunks and may be located anywhere on or in the body. Most neurofibromas are asymptomatic; however, when they occur in fixed nonexpandable spaces, they may cause neural ischemia. The most clinically significant neurofibromas are those that occur in the intervertebral canal, where they may compress spinal roots or the spinal cord, or in the posterior fossa, where they may compromise the acoustic nerve or medulla. There is an association between neurofibromatosis and meningiomas or gliomas. In addition, 1 percent of these patients will develop pheochromocytomas.

Cerebral palsy is a nonprogressive central motor deficit resulting from hypoxic events occurring in the prenatal or perinatal periods. Physical and intellectual disabilities are variable and may make communication difficult, resulting in poor patient cooperation. The accompanying spastic diplegia or quadriplegia may cause scoliosis, particularly in nonambulatory patients. Patients with more severe forms may have a pseudobulbar palsy, which predisposes to swallowing difficulties and aspiration. Spasticity and rigidity lead to abnormal limb positions and contractures that interfere with positioning and placement of monitoring lines.

Friedreich's ataxia is a progressive disease of the spinal cord and cerebellum that can be associated with scoliosis. Onset is usually in late childhood and survival beyond early adult life is rare. Involvement of the spinocerebellar pathways, pyramidal tract, peripheral nerves, and dorsal columns results in gait disturbance, tremor, impairment of position sense, and in some patients, optic atrophy. Degeneration and necrosis of cardiac muscle fibers may also occur. Progressive muscle weakness involves the respiratory muscles and leads to respiratory failure.

Muscular dystrophy is the general designation of a group of chronic progressive disorders of skeletal musculature leading to weakness, atrophy, contracture, and disability. Most of these disorders are hereditary. Duchenne muscular dystrophy, an X-linked trait, is the most common form of muscular dystrophy. Patients are usually asymptomatic until 3 to 5 years of age, by which time enough muscle mass has been lost to impair function. The presenting signs typically include difficulty ascending stairs or rising from the floor, reflecting involvement of the proximal muscles in the lower extremities. By 9 years of age, 45 percent of patients are unable to ambulate independently, leading to the development of scoliosis. Death occurs before age 20 in 75 percent of patients as a result of respiratory or cardiac failure.[20] Pulmonary complications frequently occur in the advanced stages of muscular dystrophy. Respiratory muscle weakness with resultant alveolar hypoventilation, atelectasis, and decreased ability to clear secretions predisposes these patients to cor pulmonale, aspiration, and pneumonia. Postoperatively they require aggressive pulmonary therapy to mobilize and remove secretions and prevent respiratory infections.

Cardiac involvement is present in over 80 percent of patients with Duchenne muscular dystrophy. These children may have electrocardiographic evidence of the disease when clinically asymptomatic because of their restricted activity level. The most common electrocardiographic findings of cardiomyopathy are tall precordial R waves, deep precordial Q waves, bundle branch block, P-R interval prolongation, and ST segment elevation or depression. Cardiac arrhythmias may be precipitated by changes in vagal or sympathetic tone, inhalational agents, hypercapnia, or succinylcholine.[21]

Succinylcholine is contraindicated in patients with Duchenne or other muscular dystrophy.[22] The increase in muscle membrane permeability may lead to acute hyperkalemia and cardiac arrest after administration of succinylcholine. In addition, a sustained contraction in response to succinylcholine may produce difficulty in ventilation and intubation and extensive rhabdomyolysis. Subsequent myoglobinuria, an indicator of muscle trauma from prolonged contraction, may cause acute tubular necrosis and renal failure.

Patients with muscular dystrophy may be at increased risk for developing malignant hyperthermia.[23] Although an elevated resting creatine phosphokinase level is often present in these patients, it is not a reliable predictive factor for malignant hyperthermia. A nontriggering anesthetic is recommended for these patients, including avoidance of depolarizing muscle relaxants and potent volatile agents. They should be observed for clinical evidence of malignant hyperthermia such as hypercapnia, tachycardia, respiratory and metabolic acidosis, ventricular dysrhythmias, and an increase in body temperature. Should malignant hyperthermia be suspected, any volatile anesthetic agents should be discontinued and appropriate supportive measures initiated. Intravenous dantrolene should be administered.

In addition to the possible complications from administration of succinylcholine, these patients are also sensitive to the residual effects of nondepolarizing muscle relaxants. Paradoxically, when physical inactivity causes significant disuse atrophy of normal muscle groups, there can be resistance to nondepolarizing agents from the increased number of embryonic receptors present at the neuromuscular junction. Because of these uncertainties, a nerve stimulator should be used to guide doses of nondepolarizing muscle relaxants.

Respiratory Function

Idiopathic Scoliosis

Scoliosis has profound effects on the respiratory and cardiovascular systems (Fig. 8-5). In patients with untreated scoliosis, death usually occurs by age 45. Cor pulmonale or respiratory failure accounts for 60 percent of deaths.

The abnormal chest wall and mechanical disadvantage of intercostal muscles result in a restrictive pattern of pulmonary disease that is manifested by decreases in total lung capacity and vital capacity. In one group of patients, the vital capacity was reduced to 60 percent of predicted, while the total lung capacity and functional residual capacity were 70 and 80 percent of predicted, respectively. The lung volumes and total compliance of the respiratory system are inversely related to the angle of curvature.[24] Patients with idiopathic scoliosis rarely show respiratory impairment with curves less than 65 degrees. However, curves of less than 30 degrees may be associated with severe respiratory compromise in patients with neuromuscular-associated scoliosis.[25] Tachypnea and small tidal volumes reduce the work of breathing but increase dead space ventilation and alveolar hypoventilation.[26] Alveolar development will be arrested if marked scoliosis is present before age 8.[24]

Vital capacity appears to be a reliable prognostic indicator of perioperative respiratory reserve. If vital capacity exceeds 70 percent of predicted, respiratory reserve should be adequate. Postoperative ventilation will most likely be required for patients with a vital capacity less than 40 percent of predicted.[13] While the long-term effect of scoliosis repair is to halt the decline in respiratory function, pulmonary function acutely deteriorates immediately postoperatively. Vital capac-

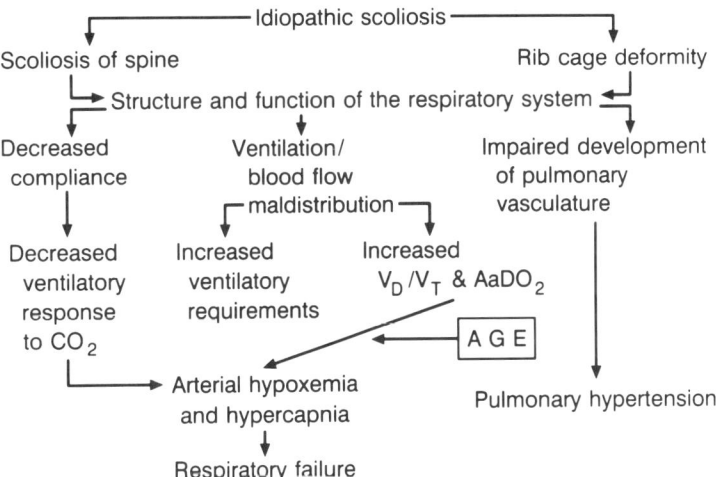

Fig. 8-5. Factors in idiopathic scoliosis that contribute to respiratory function abnormalities and failure. V_D/V_T, dead space/tidal volume ration; $AaDo_2$, alveolar-arterial oxygen gradient. (From Kafer,[80] with permission.)

ity decreases by 40 percent and the alveolar–arterial oxygen gradient increases by 50 percent.[27] These changes may require 7 to 10 days to resolve. Significant improvement in respiratory function is unlikely and rarely exceeds a 10 percent increase in vital capacity 1 year postoperatively.[13] Occasionally surgical correction may result in a permanent decrease in pulmonary function.[28]

The primary abnormality in gas exchange is ventilation/perfusion maldistribution, which contributes to hypoxemia. The most common arterial blood gas abnormality is a reduced oxygen tension with a normal carbon dioxide tension.[24] Deterioration of the mechanical properties of the lung results in further ventilation/perfusion maldistribution, increased ventilatory requirements, and eventually respiratory failure. Hypercapnia develops with increasing age as compensatory mechanisms fail. Prolonged hypoxia, hypercapnia, and pulmonary vascular constriction may result in irreversible pulmonary vascular changes and pulmonary hypertension.

In summary, the thoracic cage and vertebral deformities of scoliosis lead to reduced lung volumes, ventilation/perfusion abnormalities, reduced chest wall compliance, and increased pulmonary vascular resistance. The hypoxemia resulting from these functional abnormalities causes increased ventilatory requirements. Initially, these compensatory mechanisms are adequate, but the progression of skeletal deformities and age-associated deterioration in arterial blood gas levels eventually lead to hypercapnia, respiratory failure, and ultimately death.

Scoliosis Associated With Neuromuscular Disease

In general, the prognosis of scoliosis caused by neuromuscular disease is worse than that of idiopathic scoliosis. The respiratory function of these patients is compromised not only by the skeletal abnormalities of scoliosis but also by abnormalities of the central respiratory control system, impairment of protective airway mechanisms, and loss of respiratory muscle function from denervation or myopathy. These patients frequently need postoperative ventilatory support.

Weakness of respiratory musculature produces a further decrease in total lung capacity, vital capacity, and functional residual capacity. Reduction of inspiratory and expiratory forces leads to ineffective cough, atelectasis, and pneumonia. Involvement of the pharyngeal and laryngeal musculature may result in poor airway control mechanisms and aspiration. Bilateral diaphragmatic paralysis is associated with a reduction in vital capacity to 30 to 65 percent of predicted in the upright position and 15 to 30 percent of predicted in the supine position.[12]

Central nervous system involvement may cause an impaired ventilatory response to carbon dioxide, impaired automatic control of ventilation, and infrequent sighs. Patients may also exhibit an increased sensitivity to muscle relaxants and narcotics and need to be observed carefully for signs of respiratory insufficiency.

Cardiovascular Function

Thoracic scoliosis may result in cardiac failure. At autopsy, these patients exhibit right ventricular hypertrophy and hypertensive pulmonary vascular changes. The skeletal deformities contribute to the elevated pulmonary vascular resistance in several ways. The rib-cage compression of the lung impairs normal development of the pulmonary vascular bed and also causes alveolar collapse. This forces blood to flow through extra-alveolar vessels, which have increased resistance. Prolonged alveolar hypoxia due to hypoventilation and ventilation/perfusion mismatch eventually causes irreversible vasoconstriction and pulmonary hypertension.

Increases in right heart pressures and cor pulmonale are not only features of untreated progressive scoliosis. In a recent echocardiographic study of asymptomatic adolescents with idiopathic scoliosis, Primiano[29] noted increases in pulmonary vascular resistance that were independent of severity of scoliosis. These results suggest that cardiopulmonary abnormalities develop parallel to rather than in response to the structural changes. Electrocardiographic evidence of pulmonary hypertension and right atrial enlargement (P wave greater than 2.5 mm, R greater than S in V_1 and V_2) is late in appearance and unreliable. An echocardiogram appears to be a more sensitive preoperative screen than the electrocardiogram if findings or physical examination are suspicious. Echocardiography should also be performed in all patients with an apical murmur to determine the presence of mitral valve prolapse, which is present in 25 percent of patients with idiopathic scoliosis.

Children with congenital heart disease have an increased incidence of scoliosis. Scoliosis is especially associated with co-arctation and cyanotic heart disease, suggesting a common embryonic insult. The high incidence of mitral valve prolapse in patients with scoliosis may signify a generalized soft tissue collagen defect.[30] Children with congenital cardiac anomalies may have complex patterns of blood flow that require special anesthetic considerations to maintain oxygenation and cardiac output. Even after definitive repair, residual cardiac disease may be present and shunting may occur if hemodynamic and acid-base stability is not maintained. Patients with congenital cardiac disease and mitral valve prolapse are at increased risk for infective endocardi-

tis and should receive antibiotic prophylaxis perioperatively.

Preoperative Assessment

The primary aim of preoperative evaluation of patients with scoliosis is to detect the presence and extent of cardiac or pulmonary compromise. Respiratory reserve is assessed by exercise tolerance, vital capacity, and arterial blood gas tensions. In spite of the additional functional abnormalities in patients with co-existing neuromuscular disease, such as loss of abdominal muscle function and impairment of cough, the preoperative respiratory evaluation is the same as for any other respiratory disease. A history of exercise intolerance, hypercapnia, or respiratory failure indicates poor respiratory reserve and increases the likelihood of postoperative assisted ventilation. Polycythemia suggests the presence of chronic hypoxia. Pulmonary function testing should include measurement of the vital capacity (seated and supine), forced expiratory volume, and total lung capacity. Although the vital capacity is a reliable prognostic indicator of respiratory flow reserve, it does not assess brain stem regulation of respiration and the potential for postoperative respiratory insufficiency. The chest x-ray and physical examination will diagnose acute, treatable pulmonary processes. Patients with severe pulmonary disease may require hospital admission preoperatively for chest physiotherapy, bronchodilators, and treatment of respiratory infections. A history of cardiac failure or a click murmur heard on examination should be further evaluated with an echocardiogram. Further cardiac studies are performed as indicated to optimize cardiovascular status preoperatively.

A brief neurologic examination is also performed at the time of the preoperative evaluation. At this time, it is important to discuss the wake-up test with the patient, emphasizing the role of the wake-up in diagnosing and minimizing neurologic sequelae. The patient also should be reassured that little pain will be felt and that it will not be an unpleasant experience. Finally, cervical mobility and upper airway anatomy are evaluated to discover any potential airway or positioning difficulties and the need for fiberoptic intubation.

Patients should also be encouraged to participate in preoperative autologous blood donation. Collection is typically initiated 4 weeks preoperatively, allowing 4 to 7 days between donations. Usually 4 or more units of blood can be collected over this period of time and stored as a liquid at 4°C. A donation period greater than 4 weeks can be used for patients with greater transfusion requirements (such as a combined anterior-posterior fusion) or those whose cardiac status or hemoglobin level would not tolerate short intervals between blood donations. Blood collected over a more prolonged period must be stored as frozen red blood cells until surgery. Since frozen red blood cells must be transfused within 24 hours of thawing, it is important to thaw only those units that will be needed intraoperatively.

Autologous blood donation may not be feasible in young children, patients in poor overall medical condition, or those who weigh less than 100 pounds. In these situations, directed donors may be available from the family members who have a blood type compatible with the patient. Directed donation units are screened for hepatitis and human immunodeficiency virus (HIV) in the same manner as other homologous blood. The use of directed donation units has increased because of patient demand; however, these units have not proven to have a lower infectious risk than that of the general donor population.

Anesthetic Management

Anesthetic considerations in orthopedic surgery for scoliosis include management of a patient in the prone position, hypothermia secondary to a long procedure with an extensive exposed area, and replacement of blood and fluid losses, which may be extensive. Recently, attention has been focused on the maintenance of spinal cord integrity, the prevention and treatment of venous air embolism, and reduction of blood loss through hypotensive anesthetic techniques.

Usual monitors include electrocardiogram, blood pressure cuff, pulse oximeter, core temperature probe, and esophageal stethoscope for monitoring breath and heart sounds. An indwelling urinary catheter is used to monitor urine output, while a nasogastric tube is placed to decompress the stomach until resolution of perioperative ileus. A capnograph is useful for assessing adequacy of ventilation as well as detecting air embolus and malignant hyperthermia. Two large-bore intravenous catheters are placed. The radial artery is cannulated for direct blood pressure measurement and assessment of blood gases. A central venous catheter is helpful in evaluating blood and fluid management and can be used to aspirate air should venous air embolism occur. Patients with evidence of pulmonary hypertension or severe co-existent cardiovascular or pulmonary disease may require a pulmonary artery catheter, measurement of pulmonary artery and wedge pressures, and determination of serial cardiac outputs. Since the surgical wound is higher than the heart, a precordial Doppler may be used to detect venous air embolism.

Minimal premedication is administered if the wake-up test will be used. Anesthesia is induced with thiopental (5 mg/kg), fentanyl (2 μg/kg), and pancuronium (0.1 mg/kg) unless intubation difficulties are anticipated. In some cases, fiberoptic intubation is required.

After induction and establishment of vascular access are completed, the patient is positioned for surgery. The prone position is used for the posterior approach. Pressure points should be carefully padded. An orthopedic frame can be used to free the chest and abdomen. Thoracic pressure hinders effective ventilation, while abdominal pressure causes engorgement of the vertebral venous plexus and excessive bleeding. Lateral or semilateral positioning is used when the spine is approached anteriorly. After positioning, exposed body surfaces are wrapped or a Bair hugger (a forced-air warming device) is applied to minimize heat loss. Other methods to maintain normothermia include humidifying inhaled gases and heating intravenous fluids.

A nitrous oxide–narcotic-relaxant technique supplemented as necessary by volatile anesthetics is most commonly used for maintenance of anesthesia. The use of low concentrations of inhalational anesthetics will help maintain normotension, reduce total narcotic requirements, and still allow satisfactory interpretation of SSEPs. Narcotics may be administered by either bolus or continuous infusion. A loading dose of fentanyl 2.5 μg/kg followed by an infusion of 1.5 to 2.5 μg/kg/h or intermittent boluses of 50 to 100 μg every 20 to 30 minutes will usually provide adequate analgesia. Alternatively, an initial dose of morphine 250 μg/kg may be injected followed by 5- to 10-mg boluses every 30 to 40 minutes or a continuous infusion of 150 to 250 μg/kg/h. Continuous infusion may reduce total narcotic requirement by over 50 percent and results in a smoother and more rapidly achievable wake-up test.[31] Excessive narcotic administration, which is more likely to occur with the intermittent bolus technique, may lead to prolonged ventilatory support and delay in postoperative neurologic evaluation. An additional advantage of the continuous narcotic infusion technique is the elimination of bolus-induced variations in SSEPs, making it easier to interpret SSEP changes that occur during surgical manipulation. Neuromuscular blockade is monitored with a nerve stimulator, preferably at the wrist. Electrodes placed for electromyographic monitoring can also be used to monitor twitch height. Supplemental doses of muscle relaxants are given based on twitch monitoring to prevent overdosage and enable reversal during the wake-up test.

Surgical Approach and Positioning

Posterior Approach

Posterior spinal fusion is the most commonly used procedure to halt progression of spinal curvature when conservative measures have failed. Instrumentation developed by Harrington[32] in the 1960s provides internal distraction and stability; however, prolonged casting for 6 to 18 months after surgery may be required to achieve spinal fusion. Luque[33] introduced segmental spinal instrumentation, a technique that distributes correctional forces throughout the instrumented area of the spine by wiring each vertebra in the scoliotic curve. This results in better correction of the curvature, reduced bone and implant failure, and earlier mobilization (often eliminating the need for postoperative casts or other orthopedic appliances).[33,34] However, the increased instrumentation associated with sublaminar segmental wire placement produces longer operative times, increased blood loss, and perhaps a higher incidence of neurologic sequelae (5 to 7 percent) compared to conventional Harrington instrumentation (1 to 2 percent).

Modifications of surgical technique and experience have steadily decreased this complication.[35] After the instrumentation is completed, bone chips from the posterior iliac crest or elsewhere are placed longitudinally over the prepared site of fusion.

In correct prone positioning for thoracolumbar spine surgery, the head is turned, the neck is slightly flexed, and the arms are anteriorly flexed and abducted to reduce tension on the brachial plexus (Fig. 8-6). If only one arm is abducted, the head should be laterally rotated toward the ipsilateral arm to prevent stretch injury to the brachial plexus. Since rotation of the neck in patients with cervical spondylosis may alter cerebrovertebral circulation and compromise the spinal cord, patients should be evaluated for neck pain or neurologic symptoms with neck rotation preoperatively.[36] The chest and iliac crest are supported by chest rolls or other supports to leave the abdomen free. This allows diaphragmatic excursions and reduces paravertebral venous congestion. Breasts should be positioned medially to avoid traumatic injury. The dependent ear and eye should be checked frequently during surgery to avoid injury and ischemia. Pressure on the globe can result in retinal damage, especially in patients with glaucoma. Eyes should be taped closed to avoid corneal abrasion, which occurs in the dependent eye with a frequency of 0.17 percent.[37] Use of ophthalmic lubricants has no documented effect on the incidence of corneal abrasion. Necrosis of the dependent ear cartilage may occur if the pinna is doubled back on itself.

Anterior Approach

The anterior approach for correction of kyphosis and scoliosis has gained popularity over the last 10 years. Anteriorly placed instrumentation such as the Dwyer screw and cable apparatus is used when posterior elements of the spine are deficient or when there is a significant degree of lordosis requiring correction. This technique offers the advantage of a limited fusion area, a compression fusion, and less blood loss compared to the Harrington apparatus. A major disadvantage to the Dwyer apparatus is the risk of damage to the spinal cord during vertebral body screw placement, particularly in the thoracic spine, because of the relatively small size of the vertebral bodies and the

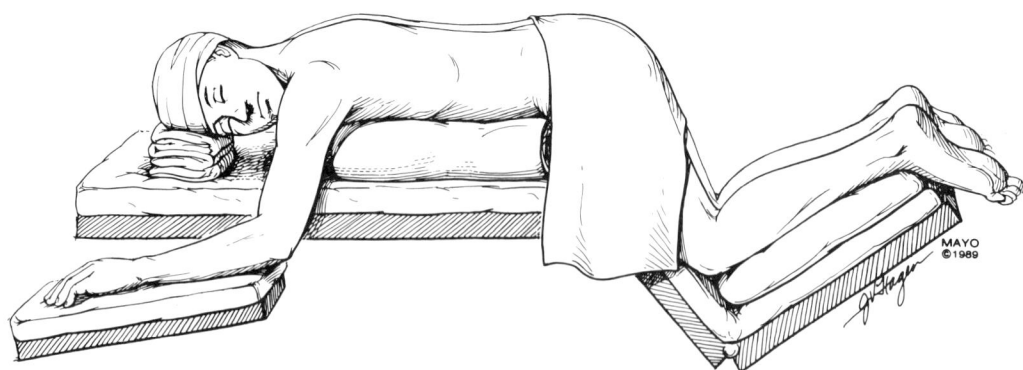

Fig. 8-6. Prone position. The head is turned with the dependent ear and eye protected from pressure. Chest rolls are in place, the arms are brought forward without hyperextension, and the knees are flexed. (From Horlocker et al,[78] with permission.)

large number of segmental spinal arteries that require ligation.[19] Fusion is usually accomplished with bank bone rather than autologous bone.

The anterior approach to the spine is achieved with the patient in the lateral position, usually with the convexity of the curve uppermost, although some surgeons always prefer to approach the thoracolumbar region from the left regardless of the convexity to avoid the liver and the inferior vena cava.[19] Positioning of patients in the lateral position is discussed in detail in Chapter 5. The vertebrae in the lumbar region can be exposed by a single flank incision, while those in the lower thoracic and lumbar area may be visualized by removing the tenth rib and dividing the diaphragm to enter the abdominal cavity. This incision will allow exposure from T9 to the pelvis. Removal of the sixth rib in addition to the tenth will increase upper thoracic exposure.[38] Wound closure requires pleural repair and reattachment of the diaphragm. The thoracoabdominal approach for anterior fusion may be associated with more postoperative respiratory insufficiency than conventional posterior fusion because of lung and diaphragmatic manipulation during scoliosis correction.

Combined Anterior and Posterior Fusion

Patients with unstable spines or those with severe primary curvatures may require both anterior and posterior instrumentation and/or fusion. Frequently the anterior procedure is accomplished first and is followed by secondary Harrington rod instrumentation 2 weeks later. This approach allows slightly greater distractive forces to be applied when the Harrington rod is introduced, with less risk of damage to the spinal cord since the spine has been partially stabilized and corrected by the initial anterior procedure.[38] Anterior fusion followed by immediate posterior fusion is occasionally performed when the area to be fused is small and the primary curvature is below the diaphragm.

Blood Loss

Most blood loss in spinal instrumentation and fusion occurs with decortication, is proportional to the number of vertebral levels decorticated, and usually necessitates perioperative transfusions. Complications associated with homologous blood transfusions include acquired immunodeficiency syndrome (AIDS), hepatitis, transfusion reactions, and isoimmunization. The use of autologous blood reduces these risks; the use of preoperative autologous donations has been previously discussed. Blood loss and transfusion requirements may also be reduced through the use of positioning, intraoperative blood salvage, induced hypotension, and intraoperative hemodilution, although reported results are inconsistent.[31,39–41]

Patient positioning should minimize epidural venous engorgement by freeing the abdomen. Positive end-expiratory pressure is avoided to promote venous return. Subcutaneous infiltration of 1:500,000 epinephrine prior to skin incision may also decrease blood loss. Preoperative donation of autologous blood or infusion of a large volume of crystalloid before surgical incision to reduce the hematocrit to 25 to 28 percent decreases blood viscosity and enhances organ blood flow. Normovolemic hemodilution combined with induced hypotension and autotransfusion can decrease or eliminate the need for homologous transfusion.[40]

Moderate induced hypotension (reduction of systolic pressure 20 mmHg from baseline or lowering mean arterial pressure to 65 mmHg in the normotensive patient) has been shown to decrease blood loss, reduce transfusion requirements by 50 percent, and shorten operating times.[40,42] However, induced hypotension is not without risk and has also been reported to cause cord ischemia and neurologic deficit.[43,44] Factors associated with increased risk of spinal cord damage include preoperative hypertension, hypocapnia, intraoperative mean arterial pressure of less than 60 mmHg, rapid decrease in blood pressure, and anemia.[45] Patients with severe deformity, congenital scoliosis, or kyphosis may have an abnormal pattern of spinal cord blood supply, which is more easily compromised during surgical distraction or compression. The purported benefits of deliberate hypotension must be weighed against the potential risk of acute neurologic complications.

The various agents used to induce hypotension in scoliosis surgery include trimethaphan, nitroglycerin, sodium nitroprusside, halothane, enflurane, and isoflurane.[46] The volatile agents provide anesthesia as well as hypotension. Enflurane and isoflurane have less myocardial depressant effects, decrease systemic vascular resistance to a greater extent, and are less arrhythmogenic than halothane.[47] However, all volatile anesthetics produce a dose-dependent deterioration of SSEP waveforms. Sodium nitroprusside produces a reliable decrease in blood pressure and at least initially increases spinal cord blood flow, but may be associated with tolerance, tachyphylaxis, toxicity, and rebound hypertension.[48] Nitroglycerin maintains or increases spinal cord blood flow, but may be ineffective in achieving target blood pressure.[47,49] Pretreatment with a β-blocker such as propranol (0.06 mg/kg) or an angiotensin-converting enzyme inhibitor can prevent rebound hypertension and reflex tachycardia and reduce dose requirements and toxicity for intravenous hypotensive agents.[50]

Hypotension should be induced prior to surgical incision to prevent hemodilution and excess fluid administration. Blood pressure is slowly decreased to achieve a mean arterial pressure of 60 to 70 mmHg or systolic blood pressure 20 to 30 mmHg less than preoperative systolic values.[40,46] Upon completion of the surgical procedure, blood pressure is allowed to gradually recover to prevent reactionary hemorrhage.

Several catastrophic events may occur during spine surgery. The large amount of exposed bone and the elevated location of the surgical incision relative to the cardiac level predispose to venous air embolism. The actual incidence of venous air embolism in scoliosis surgery is unknown; however, two cases have been reported in the literature, one of which was fatal.[51,52] The presenting sign in both cases was unexplained hypotension. A decrease in end-tidal carbon dioxide and an increase in end-tidal nitrogen was also noted on mass spectrometry. In neither patient was air present on aspiration of the central venous pressure catheter. In one patient, a large amount of air was discovered in the heart and pulmonary vessels on autopsy. The anesthesia care provider, therefore, should be aware of the possibilities of venous air embolism since prompt diagnosis and treatment will increase patient survival. Should venous air embolism be suspected, the wound should be flooded with saline, nitrous oxide discontinued, and vasopressors administered. Massive embolism may necessitate turning the patient supine and initiating cardiopulmonary resuscitation.

Another rare complication during spine surgery is trauma to the aorta, vena cava, or iliac vessels. Unexplained hypotension or signs of hypovolemia without obvious blood loss should alert the anesthesia care provider to this possibility.[53] In addition, hemothorax or pneumothorax, manifested by hypoxia or a change in pulmonary compliance, may occur during procedures involving the thoracic spine.

Spinal Cord Monitoring

Paraplegia is one of the most feared complications of spinal surgery. In a series of 33,250 patients compiled by the Scoliosis Research Society for 1971 to 1979, the incidence of neurologic injuries was 1.2 percent, with partial or complete paraplegia occurring in one-half of these.[54] Only a small number of spinal cord injuries are the result of direct surgical trauma. Most neurologic damage is believed to be due to distraction of the spinal cord by instrumentation, disruption of arterial blood supply, or compression due to hematoma formation. Patients with severe deformity, congenital scoliosis, kyphosis, or preoperative neurologic deficit are at increased risk for spinal cord injury during scoliosis surgery. When patients awaken paraplegic, neurologic recovery is unlikely; however, immediate removal of instrumentation will improve prognosis. It is therefore essential that any intraoperative compromise of spinal cord function be detected as early as possible and reversed immediately. The two methods developed to accomplish this are the wake-up test and SSEP monitoring.

The wake-up test, first described by Vauzelle,[55] consists of the intraoperative awakening of patients after completion of spinal instrumentation. The patients are informed of this procedure preoperatively and reassured they will feel minimal pain and will be quickly reanesthetized after they have moved their hands and feet. Ideally the surgeon should notify the anesthesia care provider 30 to 45 minutes in advance so that bolus administration of muscle relaxant and narcotic can be avoided immediately prior to awakening the patient. During this period of time, the volatile anesthetic is discontinued and the patient is allowed to gradually awaken. Narcotic infusion may be continued until 5 minutes before wake-up.[31] Awakening is accomplished by withdrawing the nitrous oxide and ventilating the patient by hand. Sealing the wound with wet packs has also been advocated to minimize the occurrence of venous air embolism with spontaneous deep inspiration.[54] No attempt is made to fully reverse muscle relaxation, ideally leaving the patient partially paralyzed but able to make limited but detectable movements of the hands and feet. The patient is addressed by first name and is asked to move both hands, and after a positive response, both feet. Patients will usually respond within 5 minutes.[31,54,56] If the patient moves neither hands nor feet, naloxone is administered in 20-μg increments until a proper patient response is elicited. Narcotic antagonists are rarely required with continuous narcotic infusion, however, narcotics given as boluses frequently require reversal at time of awakening.[31] If there is satisfactory movement of the hands, but not the feet, nitrous oxide is reinstituted, the distraction on the rod is released one notch, and the wake-up test repeated. If movement still does not occur, other causes of paraplegia such as hematoma must be considered. Increasing the blood pressure and blood volume may be attempted in order to increase spinal cord perfusion. Throughout the test, the patient is continuously reassured, and upon satisfactory completion of the test, administration of nitrous oxide is resumed and diazepam 0.15 mg/kg administered. Surgical manipulation should recommence only when the patient no longer responds to commands. Recall of the event occurs in 0 to 20 percent of patients and is only rarely viewed as unpleasant.[31,54]

To date there have been no false-negative wake-up results; no patient who was neurologically intact when awakened intraoperatively had a neurologic deficit upon completion of the procedure. However, Diaz[57] reported a case involving a 16-year old boy with presumed idiopathic scoliosis who had a negative wake-up test intraoperatively and normal motor function immediately postoperatively. The patient developed a flaccid quadriplegia over the next 12 hours from a previously undiagnosed syrinx that had been extended by the scoliosis correction. This case cannot be truly called a false-negative wake up test since the patient initially awakened neurologically intact, and subsequent deterioration of his neural function was not directly caused by spinal instrumentation. Thus, intraoperative awakening has proved very valuable in the early recognition of neurologic deficits in patients undergoing surgical correction of scoliosis. This technique does not require complex electrical equipment or technical expertise for interpretation. The wake-up test is obviously not a continuous monitor; it is only done at intervals. Certain hazards of the wake-up test do exist and include recall, pain, air embolism, rod dislocation, and accidental extubation or removal of intravenous and arterial lines. In addition, the wake-up test requires patient cooperation and may be difficult to perform on young children or mentally deficient individuals.

An adjunct or alternative to the wake-up test is the monitoring of SSEPs. Spinal cord function is continuously monitored by measuring the cortical or subcortical response to a repetitive peripheral sensory stimulus. Most often an electrical pulse is delivered to major peripheral nerves such as the median nerve at the wrist and the posterior tibial nerve at the ankle. Cortical potentials are recorded from the scalp, while subcortical potentials can be recorded from the epidural space, spine, interspinous ligaments, or

cervical vertebrae. Somatosensory stimulation of peripheral nerves follows the dorsal column pathways of proprioception and vibration. These sensory pathways are supplied by the posterior spinal artery, leaving the motor pathway, which is supplied by the anterior spinal artery, unmonitored. Therefore, the potential exists for postoperative paraplegia in a patient with preserved intraoperative SSEP monitoring.

A number of variables are known to alter SSEP waveforms. In addition to neural injury, the amplitude and latency of cortical but not subcortical SSEPs are altered by hypercarbia, hypoxia, hypotension, and hypothermia.[43,58] Of interest to the anesthesia care provider are the effects of anesthetics on SSEPs. As previously described, all the volatile anesthetics produce a dose-related decrease in the amplitude and an increase in the latency of cortical SSEPs, but have very little effect on subcortical SSEP recordings.[59] The difficulty in interpretation of SSEP waveforms in the presence of volatile anesthetics has led some anesthesia care providers to avoid volatile anesthetics completely during SSEP monitoring.[60] However, more recent studies have shown that effective SSEP recording can be accomplished with 0.75 MAC (minimum alveolar concentration) halothane and 1.0 MAC enflurane or isoflurane (each with 60 percent nitrous oxide).[61] Greater concentrations of volatile agents can be used in the absence of nitrous oxide since nitrous oxide itself decreases the amplitude of SSEPs. Narcotics increase the latency of cortical SSEP, but amplitude is generally unaffected. It appears that SSEPs can be effectively monitored even with high-dose narcotic technique.[62]

Several techniques may be used to improve SSEP monitoring in the presence of volatile anesthetics. Concomitant recording of posterior tibial and median nerve potentials allows the use of the median response as a control. Systemic events would equally affect both median and posterior tibial responses, while the posterior tibial waveform alone would be affected by spinal instrumentation. The use of an epidural recording electrode (subcortical monitoring) placed above the level of surgery will produce waveforms generally unaffected by volatile anesthetics, hypoxia, hypercarbia, and hypothermia in contrast to cortical evoked potentials.

Acute alterations in SSEP amplitude or latency signify spinal cord compromise and may be the result of direct trauma, ischemia, compression, or hematoma. A deepening of the anesthetic can also cause similar changes and must be ruled out as the source. Should changes occur, it is recommended that surgery stop, blood pressure be returned to normal or 20 percent above normal, and volatile agents decreased or discontinued.[43] Arterial blood gases may be drawn to rule out a metabolic derangement. If the waveform does not return to normal, the surgeon should release distraction on the cord. A wake-up test is often performed at this time to corroborate the high incidence of false-positive SSEPs or to definitely exclude neurologic deficits.[63] To date, no studies comparing the sensitivity of intraoperative wake-up with SSEP monitoring have been conducted. It is of critical importance, however, to note that postoperative paraplegia has occurred in at least one patient with preserved SSEP monitoring intraoperatively.[63]

Postoperative Care

Most posterior spinal fusion patients can be extubated immediately after the operation if preoperative vital capacity values were acceptable. Residual narcotic or muscle relaxant may lead to hypoventilation or apnea, especially in patients with an associated neuromuscular disease. Postoperative pneumothorax may be present. Aggressive postoperative pulmonary care, including incentive spirometry, is necessary to avoid atelectasis and pneumonia.

Continued hemorrhage is another concern in the postoperative period. Careful monitoring of systemic and central venous pressures, urine output, and wound drainage is essential. Neurologic status must also be monitored closely for deterioration.

In summary, anesthetic management of scoliotic patients involves a thorough preoperative evaluation of the patient's cardiac, pulmonary, and neurologic function. Intraoperative attention to temperature control, blood loss, positioning, and spinal cord integrity is essential. Continued attention to pulmonary status, neurologic function, and blood loss define postoperative concerns.

DEGENERATIVE VERTEBRAL COLUMN DISEASE

Spinal stenosis, spondylosis, and spondylolisthesis are all forms of degenerative vertebral column disease. It is not unusual for more than one of these degenerative changes in the spine to occur concomitantly, leading to a more rapid progression of neurologic symptoms and the need for surgical intervention.

Spinal Stenosis

Spinal stenosis may be best defined as an inadequate space for the neural contents of the spinal canal; it most commonly occurs in the lumbar spine. Patients with baseline narrowing of the spinal canal are more susceptible to the effects of trauma and aging than individuals with more available reserve space. In these patients, a major neurologic deficit may occur with only a minor injury. Fracture dislocation, disc extrusion, hyperextension (which allows nerve roots to relax and thicken and at the same time decreases space within the spinal canal), and facet hypertrophy all contribute to neural compression and ischemia. The typical presentation of uncomplicated spinal stenosis includes a long history of low back pain and dysesthesias exacerbated by walking. Symptoms disappear with sitting or lying down. Activity is usually discontinued prior to the development of weakness because of pain and numbness, so many patients do not complain of motor deficits and only rarely show a specific sensory deficit on examination. However, in 30 percent of patients, spinal stenosis is complicated by a herniated disc, and loss of motor sensation and reflexes may be evident.[64] Changes in the anteroposterior diameter of the spinal canal and compression of neural structures are best identified by a combination of computed tomography or magnetic resonance imaging and myelography. Stenosis is rarely encountered at the L5-S1 interspace and is more frequently seen at the L3-L4 and L4-L5 levels. Multilevel stenosis is a common finding.[65] The aim of surgery is decompression with an increase in available space. Laminectomies are performed at the levels identified by myelography preoperatively. Usually two or more levels require decompression. No stabilization or instrumentation of the spine is required for spinal stenosis.

Spondylosis

Degenerative disc disease, or spondylosis, results from progressive desiccation of the nucleus pulposus. A fracture of the annulus fibrosus allows nuclear herniation. Reactive osteophytes and continued spondylosis result in neurologic sequelae when either the spinal cord or nerve root is impinged.[66] The initial pain accompanying a herniated disc is due to stretching of the posterior longitudinal ligament of the spine, associated nerve root compression, muscle spasm, and facet inflammation. Untreated radiculopathy may progress to numbness, weakness, and hyporeflexia in the corresponding nerve root distribution. Disc herniation usually occurs laterally, compressing nerve roots as they leave the canal. Most commonly the C5-C6 and C6-C7 discs in the cervical area and L4-L5 and L5-S1 discs in the lumbar area are affected. The ratio of lumbar to cervical disc disease is 6:1.[67] More than one-half of patients report a history of trauma preceding onset of symptoms even though the basic etiology is a degenerative process. Myelography is useful in supporting physical findings. The typical appearance is a filling defect corresponding to the involved interspace with lack of definition of the root pouches. Initial treatment is immobilization and bedrest. Surgery is considered only if conservative measures are ineffective. Signs of spinal cord compression with or without root symptoms are indications for laminectomy.

Spondylolisthesis

Spondylolisthesis is defined as a slipping forward of one vertebra on the vertebra beneath. Degenerative spondylolisthesis is caused by long-standing intersegmental instability. The facets and annulus fibrosis at the level of slip show severe degeneration. While this disease does occur in the cervical spine, it is most common in the lumbar spine. The L4-L5 interspace is involved 6 to 9 times more often than any other level; with the L3-

L4 and L5-S1 interspaces following in that order.[68] The incidence increases with age and occurs 4 times more frequently in women. The initial complaint is back pain or back and leg pain. Many patients experience pain on walking but characteristically find relief by lying down—the classic symptoms of spinal stenosis. A comparison of supine and standing lateral radiographs will allow assessment of the instability and slip present, which is exacerbated by an erect posture. Treatment depends on symptoms. Spinal stenosis, which is the condition that usually causes the patient to seek medical attention, is also the condition that makes surgical treatment necessary. Posterior fusion with iliac crest bone grafting is the most common surgical procedure for spondylolisthesis. Occasionally a reduction with instrumentation of the listhetic vertebra may be required with slips of greater than 50 percent.[69]

Positioning

Cervical laminectomy is performed in the prone, lateral, or sitting position, while thoracolumbar laminectomy is usually performed prone. Considerations for positioning a prone patient have been previously discussed. Patients undergoing cervical laminectomy should be assessed preoperatively for cervical range of motion and the presence of neurologic symptoms during flexion, extension, or rotation. Only positions that do not produce pain or paresthesias should be used during induction, intubation, and surgery. Awake fiberoptic intubation may be necessary in patients with severely limited cervical movement. Anterior disc resection in the supine position may distort the trachea and compromise carotid blood flow secondary to retractor placement. Inaccessibility of the airway during cervical laminectomy may result in endotracheal tube disconnection or obstruction. The endotracheal tube should be well secured and closely monitored intraoperatively.

The use of the sitting position for cervical laminectomy has become increasingly popular. Blood flows away from the site of operation, producing a clear operative field and better surgical exposure. In this position, the patient sits with head, arms, and chest supported. The legs are flexed and elevated to increase venous return. Hypotension can be minimized by gradual attainment of the sitting position, especially in the elderly, and by aggressive fluid and vasopressor therapy.[70] The patient must be carefully positioned and dependent areas padded to prevent compression injuries to nerves and skin. Flexion at the knee reduces tension on the sciatic nerve. Cervical flexion may obstruct venous return and cause swelling of the face and tongue. Extreme cervical flexion may obstruct the airway. There is a report of postoperative triparesis presumed to have occurred as a result of extreme cervical flexion.[71]

A disadvantage of the sitting position is the increased occurrence of venous air embolism. While the incidence of venous air embolism in sitting posterior fossa cases is 40 percent, the incidence is only 5 to 25 percent in sitting cervical spine procedures. This decreased incidence may alter the need for a central venous pressure catheter. If attempted placement of a right atrial catheter in the sitting cervical patients is unsuccessful, it is reasonable to proceed with the case. The use of capnography, mass spectrometry, and precordial Doppler should be routine for such cases as they are noninvasive yet effective in detecting venous air embolism. Venous air embolism can occur in all positions associated with laminectomies since the wound is above cardiac level. Incidences of venous air embolism (defined by aspiration of air through a central venous catheter) in patients undergoing neurosurgical procedures in the sitting, supine, prone, and lateral positions are 25, 18, 10, and 8 percent, respectively.[72]

Anesthetic Management

Both general and regional anesthesia can be safely administered for lower thoracic and lumbar surgery. Some anesthesia care providers and surgeons prefer the use of spinal anesthesia; typically, a hypobaric solution is employed. If the myelogram is done just before surgery, the spinal anesthetic may be administered through the same needle after the contrast medium is removed. Advocates of regional anesthesia maintain that this type of anesthesia reduces blood loss and improves operating conditions by shrinking epidural veins. If a regional technique is used, a local anesthetic of sufficient duration must be selected. Should surgery last longer than the regional block, conversion to general anesthesia will be difficult. Most spinal surgery, however, is performed under general endotracheal anesthesia. General anesthesia is preferred for essentially all thoracic and cervical procedures because of the high spinal level that would be required with a regional technique. In addition, general anesthesia ensures airway access, is associated with greater patient acceptance, and can be used for lengthy operations. Succinylcholine should be avoided if there are progressive neurologic deficits because of the possible hyperkalemic response.

EPIDURAL AND SPINAL ANESTHESIA AFTER MAJOR SPINAL SURGERY

Previous spinal surgery has been considered to represent a relative contraindication to the use of regional anesthesia. Many of these patients experience chronic back pain and are reluctant to undergo epidural and spinal anesthesia, fearing exacerbation of their preexisting back complaints. Several postoperative anatomic changes make needle or catheter placement more difficult and complicated after major spinal surgery. Degenerative changes such as spondylolisthesis occur in the spine below the level of fusion, increasing the potential for spinal cord ischemia and neurologic complications with regional anesthesia. In a study of 48 patients with chronic low back pain after spinal fusion, 8 showed significant spinal stenosis on computed tomography and required surgical decompression.[73] The ligamentum flavum may be injured during surgery, resulting in adhesions within or obliteration of the epidural space. Spread of epidural local anesthetic may be affected by adhesions, producing an incomplete or "patchy" block. Obliteration of the epidural space may increase the incidence of dural puncture and make subsequent epidural blood patch placement impossible. Finally, needle placement in an area of the spine that has undergone bone grafting and fusion is not possible with either midline or lateral approaches; needle insertion can be accomplished only at unfused segments.

The guidelines for epidural anesthesia after spinal surgery are unclear. Daley[74] reviewed the charts of 18 patients with previous Harrington rod instrumentation who underwent 21 attempts at epidural anesthesia for obstetric analgesia. Continuous lumbar epidural anesthesia was successfully established in 20 of 21 attempts; however, only 10 were performed easily on the first attempt. The remaining 11 patients required excessive amounts of local anesthetics and/or complained of a patchy block. There was no correlation between the level of surgery and the ease of insertion or quality of epidural anesthesia.

There were no complications except for low back pain in two patients with multiple attempts at catheter placement. Crosby[75] studied nine parturients with previous Harrington rod instrumentation who underwent epidural anesthesia for analgesia during labor and delivery. Five of the nine catheters were successfully placed on the first attempt. Four of the nine were complicated and involved multiple attempts prior to successful insertion, traumatic catheter placement requiring a second insertion, inadequate epidural analgesia with subsequent dural puncture on a repeated attempt, or an inability to locate the epidural space despite attempts at two levels. Seven of the nine patients obtained satisfactory analgesia. There were no adverse sequelae related to the epidural insertion. Hubbert[76] described attempted epidural anesthesia in 17 patients with Harrington rod instrumentation. Four of five patients with fusions terminating above L3-L4 had successful epidural placement. However, in 12 patients with fusions extending to L5-S1 interspace, 6 attempts were unsuccessful, 5 required multiple attempts, and 1 patient had a dural puncture after multiple attempts prior to success, at epidural placement. A false loss of resistance was reported to have occurred frequently. Howard[77] reported a case in which a 31-year-old woman with Harrington rod instrumentation to L3 received an epidural at the L4-L5 level for induction of labor. Bupivacaine 0.125 percent was administered as a 5-ml bolus with subsequent infusion at 10 ml/h. Forty minutes later the patient had a sensory level of C3. The authors suspected subdural catheterization. No studies have reported on the complications and quality of spinal anesthesia in patients with previous spinal surgery. However, one would suspect that while needle placement may be more difficult or traumatic in these patients, the spread of local anesthetic within the subarachnoid space and quality of block would not be affected. A spinal anesthetic may be more desirable after spinal surgery since the technique is not dependent on a subjective loss of resistance, but instead has a definite endpoint: the presence of cerebrospinal fluid. In addition, a smaller needle may produce less trauma and reduce the incidence of postoperative low back pain.

In summary, epidural anesthesia may be successfully performed in patients with previous spinal surgery; however, successful catheter placement will be possible on the first attempt in only 50 percent of patients even with an experienced anesthesiologist. While adequate epidural anesthesia is eventually produced in 40 to 95 percent of patients, there appears to be a higher incidence of traumatic needle placement, inadvertent dural puncture, and unsuccessful epidural needle or catheter placement, especially if spinal fusion extends to L5-S1.[74–76] Spinal anesthesia may produce a more reliable block and cause less trauma than epidural anesthesia, although this has not been studied. The presence of postoperative spinal stenosis or other degenerative changes in the spine and/or pre-existing neurologic symptoms may preclude the use of regional anesthesia in these patients.

REFERENCES

1. Messick JM, Newberg LA, Nugent M, Faust RJ: Principles of neuroanesthesia for the nonneurosurgical patient with CNS pathophysiology. Anesth Analg 64:143, 1985
2. Marcus ML, Heistad DD, Ehrhardt JC, Abboud FM: Regulation of total and regional spinal cord blood flow. Circ Res 41:128, 1977

3. Hickey R, Albin MS, Bunegin B, Gelineau J: Autoregulation of spinal cord blood flow: is the cord a microcosm of the brain? Stroke 17:1183, 1986

4. Griffiths IR: Spinal cord blood flow in dogs: the effect of blood pressure. J Neurol Neurosurg Psychiatry 36:914, 1973

5. Griffiths IR: Spinal cord flow in dogs. 2. The effect of the blood gases. J Neurol Neurosurg Psychiatry 36:42, 1973

6. Ransohoff J, Bendo AA, Giffin JP et al: Mechanisms of injury and treatment of acute spinal cord trauma. p. 361. In Cottrell JE, Turndorf H (eds): Anesthesia and Neurosurgery. CV Mosby, St. Louis, 1980

7. Albin MS: Resuscitation of the spinal cord. Crit Care Med 6:270, 1978

8. Rogers WA: Fractures and dislocations of the cervical spine. An end-result study. J Bone Joint Surg [Am] 39:341, 1957

9. Hadley MN, Browner C, Sonntag VKH: Axis fractures: a comprehensive review of management and treatment of 107 cases. Neurosurgery 17:281, 1985

10. Sloan TB, Ronai AK, Koht A: Reversible loss of somatosensory evoked potentials during anterior cervical spinal fusion. Anesth Analg 65:96, 1986

11. Cooperman LH: Succinylcholine-induced hyperkalemia in neuromuscular disease. JAMA 213:1867, 1970

12. Kafer ER: Respiratory and cardiovascular functions in scoliosis and the principles of anesthesia management. Anesthesiology 52:339, 1980

13. Gibbons PA, Lee IS: Scoliosis and anesthesia. Int Anesthesiol Clin 23:149, 1985

14. Youngman PME, Edgar MA: Posterior spinal fusion and instrumentation in the treatment in adolescent idiopathic scoliosis. Ann R Coll Surg 67:313, 1985

15. McMaster MJ: Management of scoliosis. J R Soc Med 75:685, 1982

16. Goldstein LA, Waugh TR: Classification and terminology of scoliosis. Clin Orthop 93:10, 1973

17. Wynne-Davies R: Familial (idiopathic) scoliosis: a family survey. J Bone Joint Surg [Br] 50:24, 1968

18. Scott JC, Morgan TH: The natural history and prognosis for infantile idiopathic scoliosis. J Bone Joint Surg [Br] 37:400, 1955

19. Waugh TR, Riseborough E: Scoliosis. p. 177. In Ruge D, Wiltse LL (eds): Spinal Disorders Diagnosis and Treatment. Lea & Febiger, Philadelphia, 1977

20. Siegel IM: Diagnosis, management, and orthopaedic treatment of muscular dystrophy. AAOS Instr Course Lect 30:3, 1981

21. Seay AR, Ziter FA, Thompson JA: Cardiac arrest during induction of anesthesia in Duchenne muscular dystrophy. J Pediatr 93:88, 1978

22. Gronert GA, Theye RA: Pathophysiology of hyperkalemia induced by succinylcholine. Anesthesiology 43:89, 1975

23. Cobham IG, Davis HS: Anesthesia for muscular dystrophy patients. Anesth Analg 43:22, 1964

24. Kafer ER: Idiopathic scoliosis: mechanical properties of the respiratory system and ventilatory response to carbon dioxide. J Clin Invest 55:1153, 1975

25. Smyth RJ, Chapman KR, Wright TA et al: Pulmonary function in adolescents with mild idiopathic scoliosis. Thorax 39:901, 1984

26. Kafer ER: Idiopathic scoliosis: gas exchange and the age-dependence of arterial blood gases. J Clin Invest 58:825, 1976

27. Lin HY, Nash CL, Herndon CH, Anderson NB: The effect of corrective surgery on pulmonary function in scoliosis. J Bone Joint Surg [Am] 56:1173, 1974

28. Baydur A, Swank SM, Stiles CM, Sassoon CSH: Respiratory mechanics in anesthetized young patients with kyphoscoliosis: immediate and delayed effects of corrective spinal surgery. Chest 97:1157, 1990

29. Primiano FP, Nussbaum E, Hirschfeld SS et al: Early echocardiographic and pulmonary function findings in idiopathic scoliosis. J Pediatr Ortho 3:475, 1983

30. Hirschfeld SS, Rudner C, Nash CL et al: The incidence of mitral valve prolapse in adolescent scoliosis and thoracic hypokyphosis. Pediatrics 40:451, 1982

31. Pathak KS, Brown RH, Nash CL, Cascorbi HF: Continuous opioid infusion for scoliosis fusion surgery. Anesth Analg 62:841, 1983

32. Harrington PR: Treatment of scoliosis. Correction and internal fixation by spine

instrumentation. J Bone Joint Surg [Am] 44:591, 1962

33. Luque ER: Segmental spinal instrumentation for correction of scoliosis. Clin Orthop 163:192, 1982

34. Thompson GH, Wilber RG, Shaffer JW et al: Segmental spinal instrumentation in idiopathic scoliosis. A preliminary report. Spine 10:623, 1985

35. MacEwen GD, Bunnell WP, Sviram K: Acute neurologic complications in the treatment of scoliosis. J Bone Joint Surg [Am] 57:404, 1975

36. Schmidek H, Smith D: Anterior cervical disc excision in cervical spondylosis. p. 1327. In Schmidek H (ed): Operative Neurosurgical Techniques: Indications, Methods, and Results. Vol. 2. Harcourt Brace Jovanovich, New York, 1988

37. Cucchiara RF, Black S: Corneal abrasion during anesthesia and surgery. Anesthesiology 69:978, 1988

38. Jenkins DHR, Weeks RD, Yau ACMC, Du RR (eds): Thoracolumbar approach T10-L1 (anterior and anterolateral) for single-body or limited interbody fusions. p. 35. In Manual of Spinal Surgery. Butterworths, Boston, 1981

39. Lennon RL, Hosking MP, Gray JR et al: The effects of intraoperative blood salvage and induced hypotension on transfusion requirements during spinal surgical procedures. Mayo Clin Proc 62:1090, 1987

40. Mandel RJ, Brown MD, McCollough NC et al: Hypotensive anesthesia and autotransfusion in spinal surgery. Clin Orthop 154:27, 1981

41. Brodsky JW, Dickson JH, Erwin WD, Rossi CD: Hypotensive anesthesia for scoliosis surgery in Jehovah's Witnesses. Spine 16:304, 1991

42. McNeil JW, DeWald RL, Kuo KN et al: Controlled hypotensive anesthesia in scoliosis surgery. J Bone Joint Surg [Am] 56:1167, 1974

43. Grundy BL, Nash CL, Brown RH: Arterial pressure manipulation alters spinal cord function during correction of scoliosis. Anesthesiology 34:249, 1981

44. Grundy BL, Nash CL, Brown RH: Deliberate hypotension for spinal fusion: prospective randomized study with evoked potential monitoring. Can Anaesth Soc J 29:452, 1982

45. Lindop MJ: Complications and morbidity of controlled hypotension. Br J Anaesth 47:799, 1975

46. Patel NJ, Patel BS, Paskin S, Laufer S: Induced moderate hypotensive anesthesia for spinal fusion and Harrington-rod instrumentation. J Bone Join Surg [Am] 67:1384, 1985

47. Yaster M, Simmons RS, Tole VT et al: A comparison of nitroglycerin and nitroprusside for inducing hypotension in children: a double blind study. Anesthesiology 65:174, 1986

48. Fahmy NR, Mossad B, Milad M: Spinal cord blood flow during induced hypotension: comparison of nitroprusside and trimethaphan. Anesthesiology 53:87, 1980

49. Spargo PM, Tait AR, Knight PR et al: Effect of nitroglycerin induced hypotension on canine spinal cord blood flows. Br J Anaesth 59:640, 1987

50. Porter SS, Asher M, Fox DK: Comparison of intravenous nitroprusside, nitroprusside-captopril and nitroglycerin for deliberate hypotension during posterior spine fusion in adults. J Clin Anesth 1:87, 1988

51. Lang SA, Duncan PG, Dupius PR: Fatal air embolism in an adolescent with Duchenne muscular dystrophy during Harrington instrumentation. Anesth Analg 69:132, 1989

52. Frankel AS, Holzman RS: Air embolism during posterior spinal fusion. Can J Anaesth 35:511, 1988

53. Thiagarajah S: Anesthetic management of spinal surgery. p. 587. In Frost EAM (ed): Anesthesiology Clinics of North America. Vol. 5. WB Saunders, Philadelphia, 1987

54. Dorgan JC, Abbott TR, Bentley G: Intraoperative awakening to monitor spinal cord function during scoliosis surgery. J Bone Joint Surg [Br] 66:716, 1984

55. Vauzelle C, Stagnara P, Jouvinroux P: Functional monitoring of spinal cord activity during spinal surgery. Clin Orthop 93:173, 1973

56. Jones ET, Matthews LS, Hensinger RN: The wake-up technique as a dual protector of spinal cord function during spine fusion. Clin Orthop 168:113, 1982

57. Diaz JH, Lockhart CH: Postoperative quadriplegia after spinal fusion for scoliosis with intraoperative awakening. Anesth Analg 66:1039, 1987

58. Stejskal L, Travnicek V, Sourek K, Kredba J: Somatosensory evoked potentials in deep hypothermia. Appl Neurophysiol 43:1, 1980

59. Jones SJ, Edgar MA, Ransford AO, Thomas NP: A system for the electrophysical monitoring of the spinal cord during operations for scoliosis. J Bone Joint Surg [Br] 65:134, 1983

60. Grundy BL: Intraoperative monitoring of sensory evoked potentials. Anesthesiology 58:72, 1983

61. Pathak KS, Ammadio M, Kalamchi A et al: Effects of halothane, enflurane, and isoflurane on somatosensory evoked potentials during nitrous oxide anesthesia. Anesthesiology 66:753, 1987

62. Grundy BL, Brown RH, Berilla JA: Fentanyl alters somatosensory cortical evoked potentials. Anesth Analg 59:544, 1980

63. Ginsburg HH, Shetter AG, Raudzens PA: Postoperative paraplegia with preserved intraoperative somatosensory evoked potentials. J Neurosurg 63:296, 1985

64. Ruge D: Spondylosis. p. 312. In Ruge D, Wiltse LL (eds): Spinal Disorders Diagnosis and Treatment. Lea & Febiger, Philadelphia, 1977

65. Epstein NE, Epstein JA: Lumbar spinal stenosis. p. 149. In Camins MB, O'Leary PF (eds): The Lumbar Spine. Raven Press, New York, 1987

66. Hudson A, Berry H, Mayfield F: Chronic injuries of peripheral nerves by entrapment. p. 2430. In Youmans FR (ed): Neurological Surgery, A Comprehensive Guide to the Diagnosis and Management of Neurosurgical Problems. Vol. 4. WB Saunders, Philadelphia, 1982

67. Murphey F, Simmons JCH, Brunson B: Ruptured cervical discs 1939–1972. Clin Neurosurg 20:9, 1973

68. Wiltse LL: Spondylolisthesis and its treatment; fusion with and without reduction.

p. 193. In Ruge D, Wiltse LL (eds): Spinal Disorders Diagnosis and Treatment. Lea & Febiger, Philadelphia, 1977

69. Neuwirth MG: Spondylolysis and spondylolisthesis in children and adults. p. 251. In Camins MB, O'Leary PF (eds): The Lumbar Spine. Raven Press, New York, 1987

70. Cucchiara RF: Safety of the sitting position. Anesthesiology 61:790, 1984

71. Young ML, Smith DS, Murtagh F et al: Comparison of surgical and anesthetic complications in neurosurgical patients experiencing venous air embolism in the sitting position. Neurosurgery 18:157, 1986

72. Albin MS, Chang JL, Babinski M et al: Intracardiac catheters in neurosurgical anesthesia. Anesthesiology 50:67, 1979

73. Laasonen EM, Soini J: Low-back pain after lumbar fusion: surgical and computed tomographic analysis. Spine 14:210, 1989

74. Daley MD, Morningstar BA, Rolbin SH et al: Epidural anesthesia for obstetrics after spinal surgery. Reg Anesth 15:280, 1990

75. Crosby ET, Halpern SH: Obstetric epidural anaesthesia in patients with Harrington instrumentation. Can J Anaesth 36:693, 1989

76. Hubbert CH: Epidural anesthesia in patients with spinal fusion. Anesth Analg 64:843, 1985

77. Howard R: Subdural catheterization and opiate administration in a patient with Harrington rods. Can J Anaesth 37:712, 1990

78. Horlocker TT, Cucchiara RF, Ebersold MJ: Vertebral column and spinal cord surgery. p. 325. In Cucchiara RF, Michenfelder JD (eds): Clinical Neuroanesthesia. Churchill Livingstone, New York, 1990

79. Crosby ET, Lui A: The adult cervical spine: implications for airway management. Can J Anaesth 37:77, 1990

80. Kafer ER: Respiratory and cardiovascular functions in scoliosis. Bull Eur Physiopathol Respir 13:299, 1977

9

Orthopedic Tumors

Steven H. Rose

Orthopedic tumors span a spectrum from benign lesions with little potential for growth to aggressive malignancies requiring radical surgical approaches. Similarly, the patients in whom they occur range from those in vigorous good health to those who are severely ill. Virtually every organ system can be compromised, and it is important to carefully evaluate these patients preoperatively to determine their fitness for surgery and detect the presence of conditions that could alter their anesthetic management. Disorders of metabolic, cardiac, pulmonary, renal, hepatic, hematologic, and neurologic function may be caused by either the disease or its treatment and are important to address.

This chapter considers classification of orthopedic tumors, their treatment, and the anesthetic implications of both.

PRIMARY BONE TUMORS

Benign

Enchondroma

Enchondromas are one of the most common benign lesions of bone. They are most often seen in the bones of the hands or feet, although the humerus and femur are also common sites. They may be dis-covered incidentally, after pathologic fracture, or as part of the workup in a patient complaining of pain after relatively minor trauma. Simple removal (often through curettage and iliac crest bone grafting) is usually curative. Histologic examination shows essentially normal-appearing cartilage.

Chondroblastoma

Chondroblastomas are relatively rare lesions that occur in the epiphyses of young adults. More than half occur in the proximal humerus, distal femur, or proximal tibia. Patients typically present with complaints of pain, often involving a joint (since the lesions generally border a joint). They are usually treated by curettage and subsequent packing of the cavity with bone chips. This treatment is curative in about 65 percent of the cases, with about 35 percent experiencing local recurrence.

Osteoid Osteoma

Osteoid osteomas are reactive lesions of unknown cause. They occur most frequently in the lower extremities, with about 60 percent of the cases involving the tibia or femur. They appear to be osteolytic lesions surrounded by dense reactive periosteal bone radiographically. The lesions are typically painful and may require excision for that reason. If pain is minimal or absent, treatment may not be necessary as the lesions generally resolve without treatment over several years.

Osteoblastoma

Osteoblastomas (giant osteoid osteomas) are benign, usually lytic, osteoblastic tumors that are not surrounded by dense reactive periosteal bone. Forty percent involve the sacrum or the spine but they may occur in any bone. Patients frequently present with pain, swelling, or fracture. Treatment is by curettage and bone grafting or radiotherapy, and is usually successful. It is important to differentiate these tumors from osteosarcomas, which have a much poorer prognosis.

Giant Cell Tumor

Giant cell tumors (osteoclastomas) are eccentrically placed lesions of bone. About half are located at the knee. The distal radius is the second most common site. Patients often present with pain or joint symptoms. Treatment depends on the stage of the lesion. At least half are successfully managed by thorough curettage alone, but stage three lesions often require en bloc resection. Malignant degeneration is a concern, especially after recurrence.

Chondromyxoid Fibroma

Chondromyxoid fibromas are rare tumors characterized by the presence of multinucleated giant cells. The tibia is most often affected. Patients usually present with pain or swelling. Treatment is generally curettage or en bloc resection and is usually successful, although a few do locally recur.

Aneurysmal Bone Cyst

Aneurysmal bone cysts are uncommon vascular lesions of bone characteristically located in the spine or long bones. Patients generally present with pain, a mass, or pathologic fractures. The cyst is usually filled with blood and tissue elements. The most common treatment is radical curettage and bone grafting, and may in some cases be facilitated by preoperative arterial embolization.

Unicameral Bone Cyst

Unicameral bone cysts are childhood lesions. They are most commonly located in the proximal humerus, tibia, or femur adjacent to the epiphyseal plate, and may become quite large. They may require no treatment (degenerating spontaneously) but the presence of an impending or actual pathologic fracture may warrant intervention. Injection of steroids into the cyst may be successful,[1] or curettage and bone grafting may be undertaken. Unfortunately, the recurrence rate is high after either procedure.

Osteochondroma

Osteochondromas are the most common primary benign bone tumors (representing about 40 percent of cases). They are relatively large lesions usually situated near joints, the elbow and knee being most common. The lesions are probably in part a growth abnormality and consist of abnormal bone with a cartilaginous covering. Patients may present with a mass, pain, or joint problems secondary to impingement of the mass upon soft tissues. Symptomatic patients may be treated by excision of the mass. By puberty, growth of the lesion ends.

Fibrous Dysplasia

Fibrous dysplasia is a benign developmental condition characterized by slow-growing lesions that start in early childhood. The lesions may be large and may weaken the bone, resulting in pathologic fractures. Surgical treatment consists of curettage and bone grafting. The lesions may be highly vascular and have the potential for considerable hemorrhage.

They are self-limited and growth stops or the lesions resolve when the patient reaches adulthood. The triad of fibrous dysplasia, café au lait skin lesions, and early sexual development (due to endocrinopathy) comprises Albright syndrome.

Nonossifying Fibroma

Nonossifying fibromas are the most common benign tumors of children and the most common cause of childhood pathologic fractures. Although fibrous cortical defects have been found in 35 percent of young children on radiographic survey,[2] most disappear by age 11.[3] Patients may present with pathologic fractures. Surgical treatment, when necessary, usually consists of curettage of the lesions and bone grafting.

Malignant

Chordoma

Chordomas are relatively rare tumors of bone, representing 3 to 4 percent of primary bone tumors.[4] They are thought to be derived from notochordal tissue remnants. The tumors are generally located along the central neuraxis and are more common in adults than children. They are slow-growing malignancies that often become symptomatic by compression of adjacent tissues. The only possibility for cure is radical surgical resection, although limited surgery and radiotherapy may offer palliation of symptoms. Early diagnosis and treatment offers the greatest chance for recovery but the tumor is still often lethal.

Osteogenic Sarcoma

Osteogenic sarcomas are a diverse group of tumors that collectively comprise the most common primary malignant tumors of bone. They occur most frequently in the long bones of the lower extremities, and are particularly common in the distal femur. Patients usually present with complaints of progressive pain, swelling, or pathologic fracture. The primary tumor spreads locally, invading surrounding tissues, and metastatic spread, most often to the lungs, is common. Unfortunately, metastatic disease is often present before the primary tumor is recognized. The presence of metastatic disease greatly worsens the prognosis as in its absence amputation may be curative. Chemotherapy is the primary treatment for metastatic disease[5] and laboratory methods for assessing the tumor's response to antineoplastic drugs may be beneficial.[6]

Osteosarcoma variants include multifocal osteosarcoma (an aggressive rapidly progressive tumor), telangiectatic or hemorrhagic osteosarcoma (a purely lytic or destructive lesion), parosteal or periosteal sarcoma (located on the bone surface and associated with a better prognosis), radiation-induced osteosarcoma, and sarcomatous degeneration of Paget's disease.

Chondrosarcoma

Chondrosarcomas are malignant lesions derived from cartilaginous tissue. They occur most often in older patients (especially when compared to osteosarcomas) and are commonly located in the pelvis, ribs, and proximal femur. Chondrosarcomas vary widely in character, from slow-growing lesions unlikely to metastasize to highly aggressive lesions. The presenting complaint in patients with chondrosarcomas is usually pain.

Treatment depends on the stage of the lesion. Primary disease can often be eliminated by surgical treatment and the prognosis for "cure" (as evidenced by 10-year survival) is almost 70 percent after wide excision of the lesion or amputation.[7] Unfortunately, the central locations of many chondrosarcomas necessitate relatively radical surgery. Limb-sparing surgery holds promise but there is considerable justified concern about recurrence.

Fibrosarcoma

Fibrosarcomas are malignant lesions of bone that include fibroblasts and intercellular collagen. They occur most commonly in young adults, who typically present with pain or pathologic fractures. More than half of the lesions are located in the femur, tibia, or pelvis. The nature of the lesions ranges from slow growing to highly aggressive. Metastases are hematogenously spread and usually lodge in the lungs. Treatment depends on the grade and stage of the lesions. Surgical resection of primary tumors is effective, and radiotherapy and chemotherapy are used in patients with high-grade lesions or metastatic disease.

Malignant Fibrous Histiocytoma

Malignant fibrous histiocytomas are tumors that previously would have been classified as high-grade or pleomorphic fibrosarcomas. They are more common in soft tissues than in bone and are characterized by poorly differentiated spindle cells and tumor histiocytes. The presenting complaint is usually pain and pathologic fractures are unusual. They occur across a wide age range and are most commonly located in the femur. Although metastatic spread is hematogenous and often involves the lung, it may be spread through lymph as well. Consequently, at the time of surgery lymph node dissection is often undertaken, and if positive lymph nodes are identified adjuvant chemotherapy or radiotherapy may be indicated. Despite total surgical removal of the primary tumor and adjuvant therapy, the prognosis of patients with this tumor is poor.

Adamantinoma

Adamantinomas are rare malignant tumors that occur almost exclusively in the tibia. The most common presenting clinical complaint is pain in the lower leg and radiographically a cystic pattern connected by sclerotic regions is seen. They occur within a broad age range and are usually treated by surgical excision or amputation. Limb salvage techniques have been undertaken and early complete removal of the tumor is generally curative.

OTHER MUSCULOSKELETAL TUMORS

Benign

Chondroma

Chondromas are benign lesions most often located in the hands and feet. They are generally painless and managed by simple excision. Fortunately, soft tissue cartilaginous tumors are almost always benign.[8] It may be difficult to histologically differentiate these lesions from low-grade chondrosarcomas.

Synovial Chondromatosis

Synovial chondromatosis is a condition in which multiple cartilaginous loose bodies are present within a joint, usually the knee. Symptomatic lesions may be treated surgically but the disease is often self-limited.

Neurilemmoma

Neurilemmomas (schwannomas) are benign lesions of nerve tissue that originate from Schwann cells or other supporting neural tissues. They are most commonly located in the forearm but may be widely distributed. Treatment consists of tumor resection, sparing the nerve when possible. Malignant degeneration is rare.

Glomus Tumor

Glomus tumors are painful lesions most commonly located under a fingernail, although they may affect the foot as well.

They develop from the neuromyoarterial glomus, which is richly provided with nerve fibers. They may cause considerable pain. Treatment is by simple excision.

Ganglion Cyst
Ganglion cysts are relatively common cystic structures that often occur in the wrist or foot. Treatment may involve aspiration of the cyst or excision.

Hereditary Multiple Osteocartilaginous Exostosis
Hereditary multiple osteocartilaginous exostosis is a genetic disorder of multiple exostotic lesions transmitted in an autosomal-dominant fashion. Lesions are usually excised only if they are symptomatic, deforming, painful, or suspicious for malignant degeneration.

Hemangiomas of Skeletal Muscle
Hemangiomas of skeletal muscle occur relatively often and are thought to originate from embryotic tissue. Pain, often of long duration, is the usual presenting complaint. Treatment is usually surgical excision.

Desmoid Tumors/ Fibromatosis
Desmoid tumors or fibromatoses are tumors of fibrous origin. There are several types and they occur in several locations. The main therapeutic modality is wide surgical excision but they tend to recur locally.

Lipomas
Lipomas are relatively common benign tumors that most often occur in adults. The typical presentation is a painless mass that has often been present for a long time. Treatment is usually surgical excision. Careful assessment is necessary to avoid misdiagnosis of a more aggressive lesion.

Malignant

Lymphoma of Bone
Although bone is often affected by generalized lymphoma it is unusual to have non-Hodgkin's lymphoma in bone alone. It generally occurs in adults and is more common in men than women. The pelvis, proximal femur, ribs, and distal femur are most commonly affected.[8] The presenting complaints are usually pain and swelling or pathologic fracture. If the disease is isolated, radiotherapy may be indicated as the tumor is quite radiosensitive. If metastatic or systemic disease is present, combined therapy (chemotherapy and radiotherapy) is the usual treatment. Surgery is generally not indicated except as necessary to manage pathologic fractures. Five-year survival is reportedly about 44 percent.[9]

Myeloma
Myeloma is a plasma cell malignancy that is occasionally solitary but is more often multiple. The presenting complaint is usually pain or pathologic fracture and the diagnosis is established by demonstrating osteolytic lesions, an increase in the number of plasma cells, M-type proteins in plasma or urine, or Bence Jones proteins. Solitary lesions are generally treated with radiotherapy or, on occasion, surgical resection. Multiple disease is managed with selective radiotherapy and chemotherapy. Pathologic fractures are usually treated with open reduction and internal fixation, sometimes accompanied by postoperative irradiation. Median survival has been reported to be about 3 years.[10]

Histiocytosis
The histiocytoses are lesions derived from primitive histiocytes. The malignant form, seen most often in children, is also known as Letterer-Siwe disease and is associated with a poor prognosis. Hand-

Schüller-Christian disease is multicentric, may involve other organ systems, and has an intermediate prognosis. Eosinophilic granuloma, a localized form of the disease, has a better prognosis and lesions usually heal after curettage and bone grafting.

Ewing's Sarcoma

Ewing's sarcomas are malignant diseases derived from primitive mesenchyme that occur in children more commonly than in adults. They are most often located in the femur and pelvis, although they may occur in virtually any bone. The presenting complaints are usually pain and swelling. Metastatic spread commonly affects the lungs and bone. The lesions are generally radiosensitive, and radiotherapy, chemotherapy, and surgery have all been used therapeutically. Using these approaches, 5-year survival is about 60 percent.

Malignant Vascular Tumors of Bone

A variety of extremely rare malignant vascular tumors of bone have been reported. They range from tumors of borderline malignancy to highly aggressive lesions. Of greatest significance are high-grade (III and IV) hemangioendotheliomas (angiosarcomas). Multimodal therapy (chemotherapy, radiotherapy, and surgery) are important therapeutic modalities. Selective arterial embolization should be seriously considered before biopsy or resection to decrease the risk of potentially massive blood loss.

Metastatic Bone Disease

Metastatic lesions are the most common malignant neoplasms of bone by a wide margin. The most frequent sources are breast, prostate, kidney, thyroid, and lung carcinomas. Metastatic lesions are generally blood-borne and are common in the spine, pelvis, femur, rib, and skull. The

presenting complaint is often severe pain or pathologic fracture. Abnormal laboratory values (such as increased alkaline phosphatase) may also be signs of metastatic disease of bone. Treatment depends on the type and stage of the primary malignancy. A combination of operative fixation of current or impending pathologic fracture, radiotherapy, chemotherapy, or other palliative approaches may be indicated. Blood loss may be massive during surgical resection, especially with metastatic hypernephroma.

Rhabdomyosarcoma

Rhabdomyosarcomas are highly malignant tumors of striated muscle. They occur most commonly in children and young adults. Multiagent chemotherapy, limited surgery, and radiotherapy have been used in concert to improve survival as clinical or subclinical metastases are often present before medical attention is sought. A multidisciplinary approach is optimal to establish the pathologic diagnosis, the stage of the tumor, and the therapeutic approach.

Liposarcoma

Liposarcomas are the second most common soft tissue sarcomas in adults. The usual presenting complaint is of a mass that may or may not be painful. Four types of lesions may occur. The most common is myxoid liposarcoma, which is a highly vascular tumor. It usually is slow growing and is often treated by surgical resection. Round cell and pleiomorphic liposarcomas are more aggressive and are usually managed by amputation. Well-differentiated liposarcomas are slow growing and are often treated by resection alone.

Synovial Sarcoma

Synovial sarcomas are malignant lesions of synovial origin that occur most frequently in young adults. They are most commonly located in the lower extremities. Treatment often requires amputation and may include lymph node dissection. Radiation is often prescribed as adjuvant therapy.

Squamous Cell Sarcoma

Squamous cell sarcomas are usually slow growing malignancies of the hand. Treatment is generally wide local excision and careful postoperative surveillance for recurrence.

Paget's Sarcoma

Sarcomatous degeneration may rarely occur in patients with Paget's disease. Those with polyostotic disease are at highest risk. Amputation with adjuvant therapy (usually chemotherapy) is the most common treatment, but the prognosis remains poor.

CHEMOTHERAPY

Unfortunately, surgical resection of malignant tumors is not always possible. Metastatic spread to virtually any tissue in the body may have occurred before the diagnosis of the primary tumor is established. Tumors may also be multifocal or poorly accessible, making a surgical approach impractical. Fortunately, advances have increased the efficacy and decreased the toxicity of cancer chemotherapy as the sole or adjuvant treatment for malignant disease.

Cancer is characterized by uncontrolled growth of mutated cells that often undergo rapid division. Most cancer chemotherapy drugs act by influencing the action of enzymes involved in DNA synthesis. They are designed to be toxic to rapidly dividing malignant cells but have minimal toxic effects on normal cell lines. Accordingly, normal cells that have high turnover rates (such as bone marrow,

gastrointestinal mucosa, and hair follicles) are quite susceptible to toxicity, accounting for the common predictable clinical adverse effects (bone marrow suppression, increased susceptibility to infection, thrombocytopenia, leukopenia, anemia, nausea, vomiting, diarrhea, gastrointestinal mucosal ulceration, and alopecia) (Table 9-1).

Cancer chemotherapy drugs are usually classified as alkylating agents, antimetabolites, antibiotics, vinca (plant) alkaloids, enzymes, and random synthetics (Table 9-2).

Alkylating Agents

Alkylating agents comprise the largest class of anticancer drugs. Their therapeutic action is via alkylation of nucleic acids, principally DNA. Side effects include bone marrow suppression (which is the dose-limiting factor), gastrointestinal mucosal damage, increased skin pigmentation, pulmonary fibrosis, alopecia, central nervous system excitation, and uric acid nephropathy. Inhibition of plasma cholinesterase has also been reported, which may prolong the action of succinylcholine.[11] The prolongation that occurs, however, may not be clinically significant.[12]

Nitrogen Mustards

Commonly used nitrogen mustards include mechlorethamine, cyclophosphamide, melphalan, and chlorambucil. Mechlorethamine was the first anticancer drug introduced to clinical medicine. It is a rapid-acting agent administered intravenously and is a potent vesicant. It is currently most often used as part of the chemotherapeutic approach to Hodgkin's lymphoma. Myelosuppression (leukopenia and thrombocytopenia) is the usual dose-limiting factor. Maximal myelosuppression occurs 1 to 2 weeks after administration of the drug. The accompa-

Table 9-1. Classification of Chemotherapeutic

	Immuno-suppression	Thrombo-cytopenia	Leukopenia	Anemia
Alkylating drugs				
Nitrogen mustards				
Mechlorethamine	+	+ + +	+ + +	
Cyclophosphamide	+ + + +	+	+ +	+
Melphalan	+	+ +	+ +	+ +
Chlorambucil	+	+ +	+ +	+ +
Alkyl sulfonates				
Busulfan	+	+ + +	+ + +	+ + +
Nitrosoureas				
Carmustine		+ +	+ +	+ +
Lomustine		+ + +	+ + +	+ +
Semustine		+ +	+ +	+ +
Streptozocin		+	+	+
Antimetabolites				
Folic acid analogs				
Methotrexate	+ + +	+ + +	+ + +	+ + +
Purine analogs				
Mercaptopurine	+ + +	+ +	+ +	+ +
Azathioprine	+ + + +		+ + +	
Thioguanine	+ + +	+	+ +	+ +
Pyrimidine analogs				
Fluorouracil	+ + + +	+ + +	+ + +	+ + +
Cytarabine	+ + +	+ + +	+ + +	
Antibiotics				
Dactinomycin	+	+ + +	+ + +	+ + +
Daunorubicin	+	+ +	+ + +	+ +
Doxorubicin		+	+ + +	+ +
Bleomycin		+	+	+
Mithramycin	+	+ + + +	+ + + +	+ + +
Mitomycin		+ + +	+ + + +	+ + +
Vinca Alkaloids				
Vinblastine	+ +	+	+ + +	+
Vincristine	+ +	+	+ +	+
Enzymes				
Asparaginase	+ +	+	+	+
Synthetics				
Cisplatin	+	+ +	+ +	+ +
Hydroxyurea	+	+ +	+ + +	+ +
Procarbazine	+	+ + +	+ + +	+ +
Mitotane				
Hormones				
Corticosteroids	+ + +		+ + +	
Progestins				
Estrogens/Androgens				

+, minimal; + +, mild; + + +, moderate; + + + +, marked.
(Data from Selvin[15] and McCammon.[42])

Drugs and Their Associated Side Effects

Cardiac Toxicity	Pulmonary Toxicity	Renal Toxicity	Hepatic Toxicity	Nervous System Toxicity	Stomatitis	Plasma Cholinesterase Inhibition
	+			+ +		+ +
		+	+		+	+ +
	+					+
	+		+	+		+
	+ +	+ +			+	+
	+	+			+	
			+		+	
			+		+	
		+ + +	+ + +			
	+	+ +	+		+ + +	
		+ +	+ + +	+ + +		+
		+ +	+ +	+ +		+
		+ + +	+ + +	+ + +		+
				+	+ + +	
	+		+		+	
					+ + +	
+ + +					+ +	
+ + +			+		+ +	
	+ + +				+ + +	
		+ +	+ +	+	+ + +	
+	+			+		
				+	+	
		+		+ +		
		+	+ + +	+	+	
+		+ + + +		+ +		
				+	+	
				+	+	

Table 9-2. Classification of the Anticancer Drugs[a]

Alkylating agents
    Nitrogen mustards
        Mechlorethamine (Mustargen, HN_2, nitrogen mustard)
        Cyclophosphamide (Cytoxan)
        Chlorambucil (Leukeran)
        Melphalan (Alkeran, L-PAM, L-phenylalanine mustard)
    Alkyl sulfonates: busulfan (Myleran)
    Nitrosoureas
        Carmustine BCNS, BiCNU)
        Lomustine (CCU, CeeNU)
        Semustine (Methyl-CCNU)
        Streptozocin (Zanosar) streptozotocin
    Ethylenimines: thiotepa
    Triazenes: decarbazine (DTIC)
Antimetabolites
    Folic acid analogs: methotrexate (Folex, Mexate)
    Purine analogs
        Thioguanine (6TG, 6-thioguanine)
        Mercaptopurine (6MP, purinethol)
    Pyrimidine analogs
        Cytarabine (cytosine arabinoside, Cytosar, ara-C)
        Fluorouracil (5-FU, 5-fluorouracil)
Antibiotics
    Anthracyclines
        Doxorubicin (Adriamycin)
        Daunorubicin (daunomycin)
    Bleomycins: bleomycin (Blenoxane)
    Mitomycin (Mitomycin C, Mutamycin)
    Dactonomycin (Actinomycin-D, Cosmegen)
    Plicamycin (mithramycin, Mithracin)
Vinca alkaloids
    Vincristine (Oncovin)
    Vinblastine (Velban)
Enzymes: L-Asparaginase (Elspar)
Hormones
    Corticsteroids
    Estrogens/antiestrogens
        Tamoxifen (Nolvadex)
        Estramustine (Emcyt)
    Androgens/antiandrogens
    Progestins
    LHRH antagonists
        Buserelin
        Leuprolide
Miscellaneous
    Hydroxyurea (Hydrea)
    Procarbazine (N-methylhydrazine, Matulane, Natulan)
    Mitotane (o,p'-DDD, Lysodren)
    Hexamethylmelamine (HMM)
    Cisplatin (cis-platinum II; CDDP)
    Etoposide (VP-16-213)
Monoclonal antibodies

[a] Proprietary and other names are given in parentheses.
(Modified from Sikic,[43] with permission.)

nying immunosuppression may activate latent herpes zoster infections.

Cyclophosphamide, one of the most commonly used antineoplastic agents, is useful in the treatment of a broad spectrum of cancers. It is commonly used in Burkitt's and other lymphomas, breast cancer, ovarian cancer, oat-cell cancer, and sarcomas. The dose-limiting factor is myelosuppression, principally leukopenia, as severe thrombocytopenia is less common than with other nitrogen mustards. Other side effects include cystitis, nausea and vomiting, pulmonary fibrosis, and hepatotoxicity.

Melphalan, another nitrogen mustard, is derived from mechlorethamine. It is primarily used as palliative therapy for multiple myeloma and cancers of the ovary and breast. It causes more prolonged myelosuppression than other drugs in its class and has been associated with pulmonary toxicity.

Chlorambucil is an aromatic derivative of mechlorethamine. It is slow acting and is often used to treat chronic lymphocytic leukemia and primary macroglobulinemia. It may also be used to treat myeloma and cancers of the breast or ovary. Its toxicity is similar to that of other drugs in its class.

Alkyl Sulfonates

Busulfan is an alkylating agent most commonly used for palliative treatment of chronic granulocytic leukemia. It is also useful in the treatment of "blast crises" (as chronic granulocytic leukemia becomes acute). Major side effects include granulocytopenia, thrombocytopenia, gynecomastia, and pulmonary fibrosis.

Nitrosureas

Nitrosureas act by alkylation and carboxylation of nucleic acids and proteins and are effective against a wide spectrum of cancers. They are particularly useful in the treatment of meningeal leukemias

and brain tumors as their lipophilicity facilitates transfer across the blood–brain barrier. Myelosuppression (which is typically delayed for 4 to 5 weeks) is the dose-limiting factor in carmustine, lomustine, and semustine administration. Streptozocin, which is derived from the organism *Streptomyces acromogenes*, is most useful in treating pancreatic islet cell carcinoma and carcinoid disease.[13] Serious hepatic and renal toxicity may be seen in about two-thirds of the patients who receive this drug.[14] Hyperglycemia may also be caused by a toxic effect of streptozocin on pancreatic islet cell function.[15]

Ethylenimines

Thiotepa is an ethylenimine that is presently used mainly as an intravesicular agent to treat cancer of the bladder. Nausea and myelosuppression are the main side effects.

Triazenes

Dacarbazine is commonly used in the treatment of metastatic melanoma and is one of the drugs useful against sarcomas. Nausea, leukopenia, and thrombocytopenia are the main side effects.

Antimetabolites

Antimetabolites include analogs of folic acid, purines, and pyrimidines, and act via substitution of the analog for a naturally occurring metabolite important in cell synthesis. They primarily affect rapidly proliferating cells such as those of the bone marrow and gastrointestinal tract.

Folic Acid Analogs

Methotrexate, an antagonist of folic acid and the first antineoplastic chemotherapeutic agent shown to "cure" a solid tumor (choriocarcinoma), acts by inhibiting the binding of folic acid and dihydrofolate reductase.[16] Its principal toxicity is myelosuppression (leukopenia and thrombocytopenia). Gastrointestinal toxicity and severe renal disease are potentially troublesome side effects. It is also useful in the treatment of osteogenic sarcomas.

Purine Analogs

Thioguanine is an analog of guanine useful in the treatment of acute granulocytic leukemia. Myelosuppression is the most common serious side effect associated with its use, although liver toxicity has also been reported. Mercaptopurine is an analog of hypoxanthine used in the treatment of leukemia. Its major toxicities include myelosuppression and severe liver failure. Azathioprine, a derivative of 6-mercaptopurine, is most often used as an immunosuppressive agent.

Pyrimidine Analogs

Cytarabine is an analog of cytidine and deoxycytidine useful in the treatment of acute myelogenous leukemia. The chief side effect associated with its use is severe myelosuppression.

Fluorouracil is a pyrimidine analog that requires enzymatic activation. It is useful in the treatment of gastrointestinal and breast cancers, among others. Its side effects include myelosuppression, gastrointestinal toxicity, and (rarely) ataxia.

Antibiotics

Antineoplastic antibiotics are products of soil fungi that interfere with DNA or RNA synthesis.[17]

Anthracyclines

Doxorubicin and daunorubicin are anthracycline antibiotics. Doxorubicin is useful in the treatment of a broad spectrum of cancers. Daunorubicin is most often used to treat acute leukemias. The clinical value of both agents has been limited by dose-related irreversible cardiomyopathy[15,18–20] and myelosuppression. Previous radiotherapy or treatment with cyclophosphamide increases the risk of cardiomyopathy.[21]

Bleomycin

Bleomycin is active against a broad spectrum of malignant disease, including testicular carcinoma and several lymphomas. It is not usually limited by myelosuppression but mucocutaneous side effects are common[22] and severe pulmonary toxicity is a significant concern. About 5 to 10 percent of patients receiving bleomycin develop pulmonary toxicity, which may result in severe pulmonary fibrosis and respiratory failure. The risk of pulmonary toxicity increases with total dose (especially over 300 U) and with increased patient age.[22–24] It may also be potentiated by radiotherapy.[25,26] Pulmonary side effects are usually, but not always, reversible. The role of an increased inspired oxygen concentration during anesthesia is controversial as is the decision to administer colloids instead of crystalloids.[27–33]

Mitomycin

Mitomycin is an antibiotic that impairs DNA synthesis of some utility in the palliative treatment of stomach, pancreatic, colon, breast, and cervical carcinomas. Its principal toxicity is myelosuppression. A syndrome of hemolytic anemia, thrombocytopenia, and renal failure has also been described.[34]

Dactinomycin

Dactinomycin is a useful agent in patients with Ewing's sarcoma, rhabdomyosarcoma, gestational choriocarcinoma, testicular cancer, lymphoma, melanoma, and a variety of other sarcomas. Its main side effects are severe nausea, vomiting, and myelosuppression.

Plicamycin

Plicamycin is a highly toxic agent useful in the treatment of embryonal tumors of the testis. It is toxic to the bone marrow, liver, and kidneys and is associated with hemorrhagic diatheses.

Vinca (Plant) Alkaloids

Vinblastine and vincristine are clinically useful antineoplastic drugs derived from the periwinkle plant. Their mechanism of action is via disruption of microtubular function in cells undergoing division. Clinical uses of the drugs include treatment of acute lymphoblastic leukemia, lymphomas, Ewing's sarcoma, rhabdomyosarcoma, and others. Vinblastine is particularly efficacious in treating patients with testicular cancer. The major toxic side effect of vincristine is neurotoxicity that is generally manifest as a sensorimotor neuropathy. Generalized weakness and autonomic dysfunction may occur as well. Neurotoxicity occurs more rarely with vinblastine and the usual dose-limiting factor of this drug is severe leukopenia.

Enzymes

L-asparaginase is an enzyme that is especially efficacious in the treatment of acute lymphocytic leukemia. Its mechanism of action is catalyzation of the hydrolysis of L-asparagine to aspartic acid and ammonia. Side effects are allergic phenomena, including anaphylactic shock, as well as hepatic, renal, pancreatic, central nervous system, and coagulative disorders.

Hormones

Hormones have been known to influence the growth of malignant tumors for some time. They may be stimulatory (such as androgens in patients with prostatic cancer) or inhibitory (such as antiendocrine therapy in some types of breast cancer). Commonly used classes of drugs include corticosteroids, luteinizing hormone-releasing hormone (LHRH) antagonists, estrogens, antiestrogens, progestins, androgens, and antiandrogens. A general advantage of hormonal therapy is its decreased toxicity when compared with other antineoplastic chemotherapy.

Miscellaneous/Synthetics

Mitotane

Mitotane is derived from the insecticide DDT and selectively destroys cells of the adrenal cortex, decreasing levels of circulating corticosteroids. It is used to treat adrenocortical cancer. Major side effects include nausea and sedation. Steroids must be given before a major stress to avoid an addisonian crisis.

Cisplatin

Cisplatin is a platinum-containing compound used principally in the treatment of testicular and ovarian cancer. Its mechanism of action involves disruption of the DNA helix and inhibition of DNA synthesis. Major side effects include severe renal toxicity, severe nausea, and ototoxicity.

Hydroxyurea

Hydroxyurea is a derivative of urea used in the treatment of chronic granulocytic leukemia. Its mechanism of action is interference with DNA synthesis via inhibition of the enzyme ribonucleoside diphosphate reductase. Major toxicity is related to bone marrow dysfunction.

Procarbazine

Procarbazine was developed as a monoamine oxidase (MAO) inhibitor and was found to have antineoplastic activity. Its mechanism of action is through interference with DNA syntheses and it is most useful in the treatment of Hodgkin's disease. Side effects include nausea, leukopenia, and thrombocytopenia. It is a weak MAO inhibitor and anesthesia should be managed accordingly. If vasopressors are needed, decreased doses of direct-acting sympathomimetics are recommended. Narcotics (especially meperidine) have also been associated with significant adverse effects.

RADIOTHERAPY

Radiotherapy is used as the sole or adjuvant therapy in some patients with radiosensitive orthopedic tumors. It may be delivered as external beam radiation (projecting the radiation source from outside the body to the desired site) or delivered systemically. Brachytherapy is also an option. It involves placement of the radiation source within the body by any of a variety of techniques. The radiation dose and the site at which it is delivered determines the biologic response and toxicity (Table 9-3). Whole-body irradiation may result in nausea and vomiting, bone marrow suppression (and therefore the risk of hemorrhage or infection), electrolyte disorders, and central nervous system dysfunction of various degrees. Patients presenting for surgery after radiotherapy should be managed with an awareness of possible immunocompromise (employing meticulous aseptic technique and in some instances administering prophylactic antibiotics). Radiotherapy can also affect the upper airway (edema and possible upper airway obstruction), lung (pneumonitis and fibrosis), heart (dysrhythmias, decreased contractility, and pericarditis), kidney (radiation nephritis), liver (radiation hepatitis), adrenal and thyroid glands (adrenal insufficiency and hypothyroidism), and major vessels (atherosclerosis). Central nervous system function may be impaired and radiation enteritis can affect gastrointestinal and genitourinary function through its effects on mucous membranes.

Radiotherapy has been shown to increase the toxicity of volatile anesthetics in experimental animals[35] and may alter the response to some intravenous drugs used commonly in anesthesia. It may prolong the effects of barbiturates,[36] prolong the effect of succinylcholine,[37] and increase the likelihood of local anesthetic toxicity.[38]

ANESTHETIC MANAGEMENT

Careful preoperative evaluation of patients with orthopedic tumors is the foundation of their anesthetic care. Communication between the anesthesia care provider, surgeon, oncologist, and other members of the medical care team ensure a coordinated approach to the management of these patients. A thorough medical evaluation should be undertaken before surgery, with emphasis on the relevant pathologic effects of the disease and its therapy. Virtually any organ system can be compromised.

Hematologic Abnormalities

Hematologic abnormalities are common in patients with orthopedic malignancies. Since myelosuppression is a common side effect of radiotherapy and chemotherapy, careful evaluation of hematologic function is warranted. Anemia, polycythemia, thrombocytopenia, coagulopathies, and hypercoagulability may occur and require therapy. In patients in

Table 9-3. Toxicity of Radiotherapy

Site	Approximate Dose (Rads)[a]	Toxicity
Larynx	6,500	Edema, cartilage necrosis
Lung	2,000	Pneumonitis
	3,000	Pulmonary fibrosis
Heart	4,000	Pancarditis, pericarditis
	5,000	Pericardial stricture or effusion, cardiomyopathy
Liver	2,500	Hepatitis
	3,500	Liver failure, ascites
		Biliary tract stricture
Kidney	2,000	Nephritis, hypertension
	<2,000	Chronic nephrosclerosis
Pituitary	4,500	Hypopituitarism
Thyroid	4,500	Hypothyroidism
Adrenal	<6,000	Hypoadrenalism
Brain	4,500	Cerebritis
		Somnolence syndrome
	5,500	Brain necrosis
Spinal cord	4,500	Lhermitte's syndrome
	5,000	Transverse myelitis
Bone, cartilage	6,000	Necrosis, fracture
Bone marrow	2,000	Marrow hypoplasia, leukopenia, thrombocytopenia, immunodeficiency

[a] Minimal dose that will result in a significant complication within a normal tissue in 1 to 3 percent of patients within a 5-year period after treatment.
(Modified from Cheng & Kay,[44] with permission.)

whom considerable blood loss is likely, the availability of appropriate blood and blood products should be ensured. Baseline tests of coagulation are indicated in patients who are likely to have coagulation defects. Autologous predeposit and intraoperative blood salvage (in patients with benign disease) should be considered. Preoperative arterial embolization should be considered in patients with highly vascular lesions.

Endocrinologic Abnormalities

Endocrinologic abnormalities may occur as paraneoplastic phenomena, as a result of direct tumor invasion, or iatro-genically from steroid or other pharmacologic interventions. Adrenal insufficiency is a concern, particularly in patients undergoing surgical stress. Electrolyte disorders are common and include hypercalcemia (by direct invasion of bone or ectopic hormone production), hyperuricemia, and hyponatremia. The syndrome of inappropriate antidiuretic hormone (SIADH) may occur secondary to ectopic elaboration of antidiuretic hormone or in response to chemotherapy.

Nephrotoxicity

Nephrotoxicity may be caused by chemotherapy, hyperuricemia, or immunologic mechanisms. In patients with hyperuricemia, allopurinal, hydration, and alkalinization of the urine may be indicated. Careful consideration of fluid and electrolyte replacement is necessary and monitoring perioperative urine output is important.

Cardiac Toxicity

Cardiac toxicity is an important concern in patients who have received chemotherapeutic regimens including Adriamycin, daunorubicin, doxorubicin, and cisplatin. Severe and often fatal cardiomyopathy occurs in a small percentage of patients[39]; therefore cardiac function should be investigated preoperatively in patients receiving these drugs.[40] A variety of electrocardiographic changes, including serious dysrhythmias, have been reported as well. Careful selection of anesthetic agents and hemodynamic monitoring consistent with the scope of the operative procedure and the patient's baseline cardiac performance is recommended.

Pulmonary Dysfunction

Pulmonary dysfunction may be caused by many antineoplastic chemotherapeutic agents, including alkylating agents, methotrexate, cytarabine, mitomycin C, carmustine, and bleomycin.[41] Considerable controversy exists regarding the anesthetic management of patients receiving bleomycin. Some have advocated limiting inspired oxygen concentrations as much as possible and administering colloids rather than crystalloids to patients being treated with bleomycin, but results have not been consistent.[28-30] It seems prudent to carefully monitor oxygen saturation and use the lowest fraction of inspired oxygen consistent with adequate oxygen delivery to the tissues.

Immunologic Abnormalities

Immunosuppression is a common side effect of chemotherapy and radiotherapy. Meticulous aseptic technique is mandatory during invasive procedures to prevent potentially catastrophic infections.

Hepatic Toxicity

Hepatic toxicity from chemotherapy may occur and is most often associated with the antimetabolites. There are clear implications of decreased hepatic function regarding anesthesia. The choice and dose of anesthetic agents and adjuvant drugs may be altered if hepatic function is significantly decreased.

Neurologic Dysfunction

Central neurologic dysfunction can be caused by cerebral metastases, metabolic disorders, radiotherapy, or chemotherapy. Peripheral neuropathies have been reported in patients receiving cisplatin, mechlorethamine, vincristine, and other chemotherapeutic agents. An awareness of the possibility of peripheral neuropathy as a side effect of drug therapy is important to consider before performance of regional anesthesia. Baseline mental status should be assessed preoperatively to determine if any deficit noted postoperatively was pre-existent.

Miscellaneous Effects

Anticholinesterase effects have been reported in association with alkylating agents. Inhibition of MAO has been reported after administration of procarbazine.

MONITORING

Basic monitoring that is rapidly becoming a national standard should be utilized in any patient undergoing general or major regional anesthesia (see Ch. 5). Use of additional monitoring depends on the magnitude of the surgery and the physical status of the patient. Direct arterial pressure monitoring is often indicated and carries a relatively small risk of complications. It is particularly useful when patient positioning complicates or precludes access for arterial cannulation intraoperatively. In major tumor resections, frequent blood gas analyses are indicated to assess respiratory parameters and the adequacy of perfusion (as indicated by acid-base analysis). Central venous pressure monitoring or pulmonary artery cannulation may be useful in patients when significant blood loss is anticipated or cardiopulmonary disease necessitates careful monitoring of volume status and cardiovascular performance. The possibility of air embolism should be considered, and if it is a significant risk precordial Doppler ultrasonic monitoring, capnography, or mass spectroscopy (preferably patient-dedicated), and the placement of a multiorifice central venous catheter (with confirmation of proper positioning) is recommended. Transesophageal echocardiography is another extremely sensitive monitor for air embolism that may be useful. If muscle relaxants are administered, assessment of neuromuscular blockade by electrical nerve stimulation is recommended. Evoked potential monitoring (such as somatosensory evoked potential monitoring) may be indicated if the anticipated procedure jeopardizes the integrity of the spinal cord or other neural elements. Monitoring for spinal surgery is discussed in more detail in Chapter 8.

POSITIONING

Positioning patients for orthopedic tumor surgery can be challenging, particularly in patients undergoing radical surgical procedures. The same fundamental principles regarding patient positioning that apply to any patient should be adhered to. Ideally the patient should be positioned for maximal surgical exposure with minimal physiologic consequences and no risk of position-related injury (due to trauma, pressure, or stretch). To achieve these goals, some patients may require more than one approach, necessitating repeated positioning, preparation, and draping. A compromise may be required between the desire for maximal surgical exposure and concern about injury or physiologic compromise. Particular care should be used in patients whose disease predisposes them to pathologic fracture. In this group of patients even trivial trauma may result in injury. Communication between all members of the surgical team is extremely important. Patient positioning is covered in more depth in Chapter 5.

BLOOD LOSS

Some types of orthopedic tumor surgery are commonly associated with massive blood loss. The type of lesion, surgical approach, and status of coagulation are all important variables to consider preoperatively. Lesions associated with major hemorrhage include metastatic disease from hypernephroma, lung and thyroid carcinomas, malignant vascular tumors of bone, aneurysmal bone cysts, and fibrodysplasia. Radical resections (such as hemipelvectomy) may also bleed massively and rapidly. Communication between the surgeon, anesthesia care provider, and blood bank personnel facilitates appropriate transfusion of blood and blood products. Ideally, tests of coagulation should be rapidly available to guide transfusion therapy. Transfusion therapy is addressed in detail in Chapter 2.

In situations where massive bleeding is a concern, direct arterial pressure monitoring, central venous or pulmonary artery pressure monitoring, and adequate venous access are recommended. Placement of several large-bore intravenous cannulas enable rapid transfusion. Appropriate warming devices and pressure infusion systems should be available.

CHOICE OF ANESTHETIC

Although some practitioners advocate only general anesthesia for patients with possible malignancies, regional anesthesia with appropriate sedation should be considered as an anesthetic option. The combination of regional and general anesthesia in a "balanced" technique also deserves consideration and may offer advantages for postoperative pain relief. The role of regional anesthesia as prophylaxis against phantom limb pain, reflex sympathetic dystrophy, and other chronic pain problems is of clinical interest and holds promise. Central neural blockade should probably be avoided in patients with coagulopathy or brain metastases, but to arbitrarily avoid regional techniques in all patients with orthopedic tumors is not warranted.

In summary, clinical management of patients with orthopedic tumors is optimized by a team approach involving physicians from several specialities. A carefully considered integrated anesthetic plan that addresses preoperative preparation, intraoperative management (including anesthetic choice, monitoring,

adequate vascular access, and positioning), and provision of postoperative analgesia facilitates the best possible clinical outcome.

REFERENCES

1. Scaglietti O, Marchetti PG, Bartolozzi P: The effects of methylprednisolone acetate in the treatment of bone cysts. J Bone Joint Surg [Br] 61:200, 1979
2. Caffey J: On fibrous defects in cortical walls of growing tubular bones: their radiologic appearance, structure, prevalence, natural course, and diagnostic significance. Adv Pediatr 7:13, 1955
3. Selby S: Metaphyseal cortical defects in the tubular bones of growing children. J Bone Joint Surg [Am] 43:395, 1961
4. Dahlin DC, MacCarty CS: Chordoma: study of 59 cases. Cancer 5:1170, 1952
5. Link M, Goorin A, Miser A et al: The effect of adjuvant chemotherapy on relapse-free survival in patients with osteosarcoma of the extremity. N Engl J Med 314:1600, 1986
6. Rosen G, Caparros B, Huvos AG et al: Preoperative chemotherapy for osteogenic sarcoma. Cancer 49:1221, 1982
7. Henderson ED, Dahlin DC: Chondrosarcoma of bone: a study of two hundred and eighty-eight cases. J Bone Joint Surg [Am] 45:1450, 1963
8. Dahlin DC, Salvador AH: Cartilaginous tumors of the soft tissues of the hands and feet. Mayo Clin Proc 49:721, 1974
9. Dahlin DC: Bone Tumors: General Aspects and Data on 6,221 Cases. 3rd Ed. Charles C Thomas, Springfield, IL, 1978, p. 173
10. McIntyre OR: Current concepts in cancer: multiple myeloma. N Engl J Med 301:193, 1979
11. Chung F: Cancer, chemotherapy, and anesthesia. Can Anaesth Soc J 29:364, 1982
12. Dillmann JB: Safe use of succinylcholine during repeated anesthetics in a patient

treated with cyclophosphamide. Anesth Analg 66:351, 1987

13. Schein P, Kahn R, Gorden P et al: Streptozotocin for malignant insulinomas and carcinoid tumor. Arch Intern Med 132:555, 1973

14. Broder LE, Carter SK: Pancreatic islet cell carcinoma. II. Results of therapy with streptozotocin in 52 patients. Ann Intern Med 79:108, 1973

15. Selvin BF: Cancer chemotherapy: implications for the anesthesiologist. Anesth Analg 60:425, 1981

16. Jolivet J, Cowan KH, Curt GA et al: The pharmacology and clinical use of methotrexate. N Engl J Med 309:1094, 1983

17. Umezawa H: Principles of antitumor antibiotic therapy. p. 817. In Holland JF, Frei E (eds): Cancer Medicine. Lee & Febiger, Philadelphia, 1973

18. Ainger LE, Bushore J, Johnson WW et al: Daunomycin—a cardiotoxic agent. J Natl Med Assoc 63:261, 1971

19. Minow RA, Gottlieb JA, Freireich EJ: Electrocardiogram QRS voltage changes in adriamycin cardiomyopathy. Proc Am Assoc Cancer Res 16:87, 1975

20. Lefrak EA, Pitha J, Rosenheim S et al: Adriamycin (NSC-123127) cardiomyopathy. Cancer Chemother Rep 6:203, 1975

21. Bristow MR, Billingham ME, Mason JW, Daniels JR: Clinical spectrum of anthracycline antibiotic cardiotoxicity. Cancer Treat Rep 62:873, 1978

22. Blum RH, Carter SK, Agre KA: A clinical review of bleomycin—a new antineoplastic agent. CA 31:903, 1973

23. Cooper JAD Jr, White DA, Matthay RA: Drug-induced pulmonary disease. Part 1. Cytotoxic drugs. Am Rev Respir Dis 133:321, 1986

24. Scheulen ME: Reduction of pulmonary toxicity. Cancer Treat Rev 14:231, 1987

25. Samuels ML, Johnson DE, Holoye PY, Lanzotti VJ: Large-dose bleomycin therapy and pulmonary toxicity: a possible role of prior radiotherapy. JAMA 235:1117, 1976

26. Catane R, Schwade JG, Turrisi AT III et al: Pulmonary toxicity after radiation and bleomycin: a review. Int J Radiat Oncol Biol Phys 4:1513, 1979

27. Goldiner PL, Carlon G, Cvitkovic E et al: Factors influencing postoperative morbidity and mortality in patients treated with bleomycin. Br Med J 1:1664, 1978

28. Douglas MJ, Coppin CML: Bleomycin and subsequent anaesthesia: a retrospective study at Vancouver General Hospital. Can Anaesth Soc J 27:449, 1980

29. LaMantia KR, Glick JH, Marshall BE: Supplemental oxygen does not cause respiratory failure in bleomycin-treated surgical patients. Anesthesiology 60:65, 1984

30. Matalon S, Harper WV, Nickerson PA, Olszowka J: Intravenous bleomycin does not alter the toxic effects of hyperoxia in rabbits. Anesthesiology 64:614, 1986

31. Bauer KA, Skarin AT, Balikian JP et al: Pulmonary complications associated with combination chemotherapy programs containing bleomycin. Am J Med 74:557, 1983

32. Toledo CH, Ross WE, Hood CI, Block ER: Potentiation of bleomycin toxicity by oxygen. Cancer Treat Rep 66:359, 1982

33. Ingrassia TS III, Ryu JH, Trastek VF, Rosenow EC III: Oxygen-exacerbated bleomycin pulmonary toxicity. Mayo Clin Proc 66:173, 1991

34. Cantrell JE, Phillips TM, Schein PS: Carcinoma-associated hemolytic-uremic syndrome: a complication of mitomycin C chemotherapy. J Clin Oncol 3:723, 1985

35. Zauder HL, Orkin LR: Effect of radiation on response to anesthetic agents. NY State J Med 63:1943, 1963

36. Yam KM, Dubois KP: Effects of x-irradiation of the hexobarbital-metabolizing enzyme system of rat liver. Radiation Res 31:315, 1967

37. Iwatzuki, Yokosawa: Tokoku J Exper Med 71:79, 1959; quoted in Belfrage P, Schildt B: Increased sensitivity to the muscle-relaxing effect of succinylcholine in irradiated rabbits. Acta Anesth Scand 11:65, 1967

38. Young MT, Parsons SAA, Mezistrono J, Morris LE: Effects of anesthesia in irradiated animals. Anesthesiology 23:74, 1962

39. Gottlieb JA, Lefrak EA, O'Bryan RM et al: Fatal adriamycin cardiomyopathy (CMY): prevention by dose limitation. Proc Am Assoc Cancer Res 14:88, 1973

40. Gottdiener JS, Mathisen DJ, Borer JS et al: Doxorubicin cardiotoxicity: assessment of late left ventricular dysfunction by radionuclide cineangiography. Ann Intern Med 94:430, 1981

41. Goldiner PL, Schweizer O: The hazards of anesthesia and surgery in bleomycin-treated patients. Semin Oncol 6:121, 1979

42. McCammon RL: Cancer. p. 631. In Stoelting RK, Dierdorf SF (eds): Anesthesia and Co-Existing Disease. Churchill Livingstone, New York, 1983

43. Sikic BI: Antineoplastic agents. p. 797. In Craig CR, Stitzel RE (eds): Modern Pharmacology. 2nd Ed. Little Brown, Boston, 1982

44. Cheng EY, Kay J: Manual of Anesthesia and the Medically Compromised Patient. JB Lippincott, Philadelphia, 1990, p. 499

10

Microvascular Surgery

Beth A. Elliott

Since the introduction of the operating microscope in the early 1960s, microvascular and microsurgical techniques have played an increasing role in many surgical specialities. The initial application to replantation of severed digits and extremities has now been expanded to include plastic and reconstructive surgery, neurosurgery, urology, otolaryngology, gynecology and infertility, and ophthalmology.[1]

The increased precision and definition that the operating microscope allows has made possible the treatment of conditions that were previously incurable. Limb salvage, digital replantation, and repair of tissue defects with free-flap procedures are now commonplace in today's operating suite. Patients who might previously have faced amputation or severe disfigurement and dysfunction may now have a chance for partial, if not full, recovery from an aesthetic as well as a functional standpoint.

Microvascular surgery can be subdivided into two categories: *replantation*, defined as reattachment of a body part that has been completely severed with no remaining attachment to the patient, and *revascularization*, the re-establishment of blood flow through a complete or incompletely severed body part. Primary anastomoses of the native vessels or a vein graft interposition may be necessary to re-establish perfusion.

Patients presenting for replantation and/or revascularization are generally victims of trauma. The mechanism of injury and extent of the trauma to the surrounding tissues are major determinants of success with replantation. Success is greatest with clean "guillotine"-type amputations of the thumb, multiple digits, or the hand that occurred at the transmetacarpal level, wrist, or forearm, or in a child,[2,3] almost any body part.

Poor candidates for replantation are those with severe crush, avulsion, or mangled soft tissue injuries, amputation at multiple levels (e.g., finger, hand, and forearm), patients with atherosclerotic vessels, or those with warm ischemia time of greater than 10 hours. Patients with single-digit amputation proximal to the insertion of the flexor digitorum superficialis tendon are also generally considered to be poor candidates for replantation.[2] The sensory impairment and stiffness of the replanted single digit are significantly more debilitating than a single-digit amputation. Conversely, even a stiff replanted thumb may prove quite functional; therefore every effort is made to salvage the severed thumb.[4]

In children less than 5 years of age, the vessels may be too small to allow adequate reanastomosis, even with the aid of the operating microscope.[5]

217

Success of replantation attempts diminishes after 10 hours postinjury even with appropriate cooling of the amputated part, and is inversely proportional to the muscle mass involved (i.e., the more proximal the amputation, the greater amount of muscle involved, and the lower the survival rate).[2]

The vast majority of replantation surgery involves the upper extremity. Even with a fair amount of impairment, the functional result of replantation in the upper extremity is far superior to any currently available prosthesis. Conversely, the delayed rehabilitation associated with replantation attempts of the lower extremity may not compare favorably to the many acceptable prosthetic devices available.[6]

SURGICAL CONSIDERATIONS

Replantation

The initial focus of the surgical team is directed towards debridement of the wound and identification and tagging of neurovascular structures in both the stump and the amputated part. It is not uncommon for the amputated part to precede the patient to the operating room for this task. In almost all cases, a total or near-total reconstruction of the affected limb or digits is done to minimize the secondary procedures required. Bony stabilization and flexor tendon repairs are done first in most replantation procedures to provide a stable foundation for the neurovascular repairs to follow. Arterial anastomoses are performed prior to venous repair to achieve blood flow to the amputated part as early as possible and to flush out metabolic breakdown products. In a severely traumatized limb, it may be necessary to use vein grafts as arterial substitutes to ensure adequate vessel length. Fascicular neurorrhaphies, or nerve repairs, are typically performed once arterial inflow has been reestablished. Following extensor tendon repairs, attention is directed toward establishment of a more definitive venous outflow. With larger amputated parts, it may be necessary to perform prophylactic fasciotomies to relieve elevated compartmental pressures due to edema formation.

Free-Tissue Transfer

Free-tissue transfer or free-flap procedures involve the en-block transfer of tissue with an intact vascular pedicle from the donor site to a remote location, where blood flow is re-established by microvascular anastomosis to vessels in the new site. This technique is used to provide vascularized tissue for reconstruction of defects resulting from trauma, infection, or tumor resection. In addition to filling dead space, the vascularized free flap enhances blood flow to the surrounding tissues, improving the milieu for healing from the standpoint of increased oxygen tension, but also by allowing better access to the damaged site for immunologic defense mechanisms as well as antibiotics.[6]

The choice of donor site is determined primarily by the tissues required for the planned reconstruction. Other factors include concomitant injury, previous surgical procedures, and cosmetic result. Vascularized free flaps may be composed of a single tissue, such as a skin flap or latissimus dorsi muscle, or may be a composite of several tissues, including bone, muscle, and skin. Free-flap donor sites are chosen based on the presence of a dominant, easily identifiable vascular supply.

For skin coverage only, the groin flap, utilizing the superficial circumflex or epigastric vessels, may be used. The latissimus dorsi flap can provide both vascularized muscle and skin. A long pedicle (up to 10 cm) and the relatively large diameter of the thoracodorsal vessels on which this flap is based make it a popular donor tissue site.

When a vascularized bone flap is required, there are basically two choices. For bony defects of less than 12 cm, a flap based on the deep circumflex artery can be used for reconstruction. In addition to bone from the ilium, a composite flap including skin and muscle can be created. For bony defects of greater than 12 cm, a vascularized free fibular graft is needed. The advantage of a vascularized over a traditional nonvascularized bone graft is the ability of the former to remodel, produce callus, and meet the applied stress in the reconstructed site during patient mobilization.[6]

Whereas replantation and revascularization are, by necessity, performed on an acute emergent basis, free-flap transfers are rarely performed for an acute injury. When the injury is grossly contaminated, extensive debridement followed by a somewhat delayed reconstruction is preferable. As the scope of microvascular surgery has evolved and more experience has been gained, success rates are improving. Free-flap transfers are being used at an earlier stage and on a more elective basis, rather than being withheld as a last-ditch effort.[7] Generally speaking, free-flap transfers to the upper extremity fare better than those to the lower extremity, and reconstruction of defects following tumor resection fare better than those following osteomyelitis.[8–10] Early failures are usually related to vascular phenomena and ischemia, and later failures are usually secondary to infection.[9] Other contributing factors leading to failure of a microvascular surgical procedure are technical difficulties at the time of the surgery, diseased vessels, vasospasm, hypotension, edema, hematoma, and as

Table 10-1.   Contributing Factors Leading to Failure of Replantation

---

Acute vascular events: arterial or venous thrombosis, vasospasm
Technical difficulties at the time of surgery
Chronic peripheral vascular disease
Hypotension
Edema
Hematoma
Hypothermia
Prolonged warm ischemia time
Infection
Nicotine, ?caffeine

---

mentioned earlier in this chapter, ischemia time prior to reperfusion. Recognition of the role that these factors play has led to the development of many different protocols for the perioperative management of these patients (Table 10-1).

PREOPERATIVE EVALUATION

Patients who are victims of trauma must first be evaluated and treated for potentially life-threatening injuries. Fluid resuscitation and control of hemorrhage in the critically injured patient must take precedence over replantation/revascularization concerns. A thorough investigation of associated injuries must be accomplished in the preoperative period as well. Loss of a hand or extremity becomes secondary if, in the rush to replantation, a cervical spine injury or splenic rupture goes unrecognized (Table 10-2).

Patients presenting for elective surgery allow a more leisurely preoperative evaluation. A complete medical history and physical examination should be obtained in all patients prior to being subjected to the rigors of a lengthy microvascular procedure and anesthetic.

Table 10-2. Anesthetic Considerations for Microvascular Surgery

---

Preoperatively
    Control of hemorrhage
    Fluid resuscitation
    Associated trauma
    Anesthetic planning: regional vs. general, multiple surgical sites, duration of surgery
Intraoperatively
    Positioning: special precautions against pressure needs
    Monitoring: insidious blood loss
    Maintenance of adequate blood flow through vascular anastomoses
        Perfusion pressure
        Blood viscosity
        Vascular cross-sectional area
Postoperatively
    Pain management
    Disposition: intensive care unit vs. ward nursing care

Patients who smoke tobacco or use other products containing nicotine are urged to discontinue this practice preoperatively. Some consider the continued use of these products a relative contradiction for microvascular surgery. Nicotine has been implicated in both the laboratory and clinical settings for placing microvascular anastomoses at risk for failure.[11,12] Some centers also restrict the use of substances containing caffeine or other xanthines, while others do not. Caffeine has a direct peripheral vasodilating effect but also produces a vasoconstrictive effect as a result of medullary stimulation.[13]

POSITIONING

Microvascular surgery is meticulous and time-consuming work. It is not unusual for these procedures to last for 10 to 16 hours or longer. The patient must lie still, usually in the same position, for the duration of the procedure. Careful attention must be paid to the details of positioning these patients, and extra padding (either jelly pads or egg crate mattresses) used to protect the skin from developing pressure necrosis. Awake patients are able to periodically move or shift their weight to alleviate the problem, but patients heavily sedated or under general anesthesia are unable to do so. The anesthesia care provider should take responsibility to periodically reposition the patient's head and other extremities within reach and if possible, gently massage the skin areas of weight-bearing surfaces such as the occiput, forehead, and heels to increase circulation.

MONITORING

Monitoring used during microsurgical procedures should be tailored to meet the needs of the individual patient. Routine monitoring should include electrocardiogram, blood pressure, temperature, pulse oximetry, and auscultation of the heart and lungs.

It can be quite helpful for the intraoperative management of these patients to periodically check hemoglobin and hematocrit values. Blood loss during these cases can be significant, more so for free-flap procedures than digital replant procedures, because of the limited ability to use tourniquets. Typically the blood loss that does occur is insidious, occurring over hours and seeping into surgical drapes. Unrecognized blood loss and third-space shifting of intravascular fluid must be anticipated. Maintaining an adequate intravascular volume and hematocrit are essential to the success of the procedure. An indwelling arterial catheter allows for easy sampling as well as provides valuable beat-to-beat hemodynamic information.

Establishing adequate intravenous access is crucial for these cases. Access to the patient may be quite limited once the surgical procedure is underway. A central venous catheter may, on occasion, be indicated because of lack of peripheral access, as well as for following the volume status of the patient.

Because of the lengthy nature of microvascular surgery, an indwelling urinary catheter is routinely placed. Measurement of urine output is valuable in assessing intravascular volume and managing fluid replacement therapy, and it avoids the potential problems associated with overdistention of the bladder.

DETERMINANTS OF FLOW

Maintenance of flow through the microvascular anastomoses is one of the primary goals in the anesthetic management of these cases. The Poiseuille–Hagan formula (below), which defines the flow of newtonian fluids through rigid tubes, has been applied to describe the flow of blood through the vascular system.

$$Flow = (P_A - P_B) \times \frac{\pi}{8} \times \frac{1}{\eta} \times \frac{r^4}{L}$$

Although this application is somewhat flawed (i.e., blood is not a newtonian fluid and the vascular system is hardly a rigid structure), there are some basic concepts that are useful to bear in mind. Simply stated, it reveals that flow is directly related to changes in perfusion pressure and cross-sectional area, and inversely related to the viscosity of the fluid.[14] Understanding these simple physiologic concepts has proven useful clinically. Intraoperatively, if flow is impaired into a free flap, steps can be taken to improve it by increasing the perfusion pressure, relieving vasospasm by adding a vasodila-

tor, or decreasing the viscosity of the intravascular fluid.

Perfusion Pressure

Consideration of perfusion pressure needs should begin preoperatively. The patient's fluid status should be assessed. A patient presenting for an emergent reimplant may have suffered significant blood loss prior to arrival in the operating suite. This problem should be addressed before induction of anesthesia.

In many intraoperative scenarios, a fall in perfusion pressure or arterial blood pressure might be treated with the administration of a vasopressor. With microvascular procedures, agents that produce vasoconstriction are not necessarily contraindicated, but they should be reserved for use after other measures have failed.

Increasing the intravascular volume with the infusion of either crystalloid or colloid may increase systemic blood pressure sufficiently to reverse hypoperfusion of a free-flap or digital replant. Overzealous infusion of crystalloid solutions can reduce the intravascular colloidal pressure, leading to the development of edema throughout the body and in the flap as well. Edema may exert sufficient external hydrostatic pressure to significantly reduce perfusion to the very area in which one is attempting to improve flow.[15] The anesthesia care provider must keep a close eye on fluid replacement with these potential problems in mind. Communication with the surgeon may be beneficial in assessing the degree of edema formation present[16] and blood volume lost.

Colloid solutions such as albumin and hetastarch (a synthetic colloid solution derived from corn) are equieffective volume expanders, and can be given without the risk of disease transmission associated with the infusion of red blood cells or plasma.[17-19] Because of concerns about interference with coagulation parameters when given in large volumes, it is recommended that the total hetastarch volume be limited to no greater than 20 ml/kg/24 hr.[20-23]

Viscosity

As the hematocrit increases, the viscosity of the blood increases as well. Capillary flow is slowed and red blood cells may clump together in three-dimensional formations known as *rouleaux*, which further reduces flow. Low-molecular-weight dextran, a synthetic colloid solution, will break up these rouleaux formations, making it a useful adjunct during microvascular procedures.[14] In addition to breaking up rouleaux, low-molecular-weight dextran-40 is thought to enhance fibrinolysis, and some studies have demonstrated an antiplatelet effect as well (although this is disputed).[24] Dextran is also valuable as a volume expander. Because of the concern about negative effects on coagulation, not all centers use dextran routinely during microvascular surgery, but reserve it for situations in which the patency of the vascular anastomoses is in question.[25]

As mentioned earlier, blood loss in these cases is slow and insidious. Frequent determination of hematocrit may be of more use than the usual methods of assessing blood loss such as observation of surgical drapes. Many centers will deliberately allow the hematocrit to drift down to 30 percent while replacing blood loss with colloid or crystalloid. This practice minimizes the need for transfusion and maximizes acceptable hemodilution from an oxygen-carrying capacity and viscosity standpoint.[14,16,26]

It should be remembered, however, that hemodilution to a hematocrit of 30

percent may not be tolerated equally by all patients, and may pose an unacceptable risk for patients with cardiovascular, cerebrovascular, or renal disease.

The advent of intraoperative red blood cell salvage using the Cell Saver device has dramatically reduced the number of homologous units transfused in these cases. Patients presenting for elective reconstruction procedures should be encouraged to predonate units of their own blood to minimize their exposure to homologous blood products.

Vascular Cross-Sectional Area

Many factors may impact on the vascular cross-sectional area. These include choice of anesthetic technique and agents, use of direct-acting vasodilating or vasoconstricting agents, level of sympathetic tone and endogenous catecholamines, and temperature. Major contributing factors are outlined below. The skilled practitioner can use this knowledge to manipulate the vascular tone to the advantage of the surgeon, and can make a significant contribution toward a successful outcome for the patient (Table 10-3).

Temperature

Body temperature is a major determinant of peripheral blood flow. It has long been recognized that temperature regulation is impaired in the anesthetized patient. This fact, combined with the typically long duration of most microsurgical procedures and the infusion of room-temperature intravenous solutions and refrigerated blood, predisposes these patients to hypothermia. The consequences of this are myriad: peripheral vasoconstriction, sympathetic stimulation, shivering, increased oxygen demand, a leftward shift of the oxygen–hemoglobin dissociation curve, and impaired coagulation.[27] Cold may also lead to a potentially misleading

Table 10-3. Factors Affecting Vascular Cross-Sectional Area

Choice of anesthetic
    Regional anesthesia: local sympathectomy, vasodilation
    General anesthesia: systemic vasodilation
Vasoactive agents
    Topically applied vasodilating agents: local anesthetics, papaverine, α-adrenergic blocking agents
    Systemic vasodilators: nitroprusside, ganglionic blocking agents, α-adrenergic blocking agents, β-adrenergic agonists
    Endogenous and exogenous catecholamines or vasoconstricting agents
Pain
    Unrelieved pain: sympathetic stimulation and vasoconstriction
Temperature
    Hypothermia: sympathetic stimulation, vasoconstriction
Underlying level of sympathetic tone

increase in hematocrit, increased aggregation of red blood cells, and increased plasma and whole blood viscosity.[14] The direct vasoconstrictive effect of cold has been reported in denervated tissue as well.[14]

Consequently, it is extremely important to prevent the development of hypothermia. Intravenous infusion solutions should be warmed to body temperature, inspired anesthetic gases (if any) should be heated and humidified, and the operating suite should be kept no cooler than 21°C.[26–28] Traditional water-filled warming blankets are ineffective in preventing hypothermia in adult patients or children with over 0.5 m² body surface area.[29] Until recently, the only effective means to actively warm a patient was to heat and humidify inspired gases.[30] However, the introduction of the Bair Hugger (a forced-air warming device) has added another very effective method to prevent and treat hypothermia in the surgical patient.[31,32] Advantages of this device are that it can be used for patients having regional as well as general anesthesia, it is not necessary to cover the entire patient, and the risk of burns, leaks, or electrical shock are either nonexistent or minimal.

Pain

Pain control, both intra- and postoperatively, is an important consideration in the care of patients undergoing microsurgical procedures. Unrelieved, pain can result in significant sympathetic stimulation. The resultant vasoconstriction is a result of neuronal discharge as well as a release of endogenous catecholamines. The anesthetic plan must take this into account, regardless of the technique chosen.

Potent inhalational anesthetics will blunt the sympathetic response to pain that occurs intraoperatively. However, once these agents have dissipated, the anesthesia care provider must be prepared to respond to the need for adequate pain control. The inclusion of narcotics in the anesthetic plan is recommended to avoid severe pain on emergence from anesthesia and reduce the intraoperative requirement for potent inhalational anesthetics, with their associated hemodynamic effects.

If a single-shot regional anesthetic technique is used, the anesthesia practitioner must ascertain that the proposed surgical procedure can be accomplished within the expected duration of the local anesthetic chosen. Should the local anesthetic become ineffective during the surgical procedure, preparations should be made to administer some other means of intraoperative pain relief or induce general anesthesia. Consideration should be given to this eventuality whenever regional anesthesia is prescribed.

Continuous regional anesthetic techniques are gaining in popularity among anesthesia as well as surgical providers.[14,25,26,33,34] Not only are these techniques effective in providing intraoperative pain relief, but they may be continued for several days postoperatively for control of pain and provision of sympathetic blockade and concomitant vasodilatation. Continuous infusions of local anesthetics may be used for pain relief in both upper and lower extremities. Infusions of local anesthetics may be limited in application when multiple surgical sites are required. Excellent pain relief for multiple surgical sites can, however, be achieved with the infusion of epidural narcotics. The use of epidural narcotics may be restricted in some practices because of the potential for respiratory depression. It should be remembered that epidural narcotics do not provide the peripheral vasodilation and sympathetic block associated with local anesthetics. A combined infusion of local anesthetic and narcotic can provide excellent pain relief as well as a sympathetic block.

Pharmacologic Manipulation of the Microcirculation

Despite years of investigation, researchers have yet to identify a reliable and effective means of preventing and treating vasospasm and thrombosis in microvascular anastomoses. A number of agents have been used with varying rates of success. What may work quite well in one model may be totally ineffective in another.

Topically applied agents such as lidocaine and bupivacaine (both local anesthetic agents that produce direct relaxation of smooth muscle), papaverine (a smooth-muscle relaxant), and chlorpromazine (an α-adrenergic blocking agent) are commonly used at the time of surgery with good success. These agents, while being quite diverse in nature, are very effective in relieving vasospasm.[24,35] Their use is limited to intraoperative use because of the need for topical application.

Regional anesthetic techniques (i.e., brachial plexus, stellate ganglion, epidural, and lumbar sympathetic blocks) are very effective in providing sympathetic blockade to proximal vessels of an extremity, but are not effective in preventing vasospasm in the denervated tissues of the replanted part due to direct surgical stimulation.[25,26] These techniques are frequently used in the clinical setting in the hope that improving overall delivery of blood flow to an extremity will improve blood flow through the free flap or replant. Intravenous regional application of guanethidine (a ganglionic blocking agent) has been shown to increase the survival of skin flaps both in the laboratory as well as the clinical setting.[28,36] While this technique may prove helpful in the postoperative period, it is of limited utility in the operating suite.

All the potent inhalational anesthetic agents are vasodilators of the peripheral circulation to varying degrees. Isoflurane in particular can increase blood flow through skin and muscle 200 to 300 percent at normal anesthetic concentrations, and will decrease systemic vascular resistance by 50 percent at 1.9 MAC (minimum alveolar concentration).[37] Isoflurane is the preferred vasodilating agent in some practices.[26] The use of isoflurane or any other inhalational anesthetic agent is usually limited to the operating room.

Some authors have advocated the use of direct-acting vasodilating agents such as sodium nitroprusside.[38] Its preferential dilation of the arterial circulation and ease of rapid titration are cited as advantages. Trimethaphan (a ganglionic blocking agent), hydralazine (an α-adrenergic blocking agent), and phenoxybenzamine (an α-adrenergic blocking agent) have also been advocated for use in the operating suite for their systemic vasodilating properties. However, these drugs are not effective in preventing vasospasm due to direct surgical stimulation.[26] Varying degrees of hypotension may be produced by these drugs, depending on the underlying sympathetic tone and intravascular volume. Regardless of which, if any, of these agents is used, care must be taken to maintain adequate perfusion pressure.

Isoxuprine (a β-adrenergic receptor agonist) has been used in the past with varying success for the salvage of failing skin flaps, and relief of vasospasm in digital replants.[39–42] Current therapeutic regimens for salvage of a tenuous microvascular anastomosis include use of intra-arterial fibrinolytic agents such as streptokinase and urokinase, papaverine, heparin, low-molecular-weight dextran, and chlorpromazine.[43,44]

THE ANESTHETIC PLAN

When choosing an anesthetic plan for a microvascular procedure, there are certain concepts that should be kept in mind, and questions that must be answered:

1. The procedure may be quite lengthy. Will the patient tolerate the intended position for this period, particularly if a regional anesthetic is planned?
2. The procedure may involve more than one operative site. Are the patient and the surgeon willing to accept that a regional anesthetic may need to be supplemented with either local anesthetic infiltration by the surgeon or a brief general anesthetic?
3. Are there associated injuries? Will they need to be addressed during this visit to the operating room? Will more than one surgical service be involved during the case?
4. What other concurrent illnesses or conditions may the patient have that might preclude a particular type of anesthesia (e.g., language barrier, psychiatric disease, pediatric patient, neurologic disease, infection or injury at the intended site of local anesthetic injection)?
5. What is the nature of the planned procedure? Will there be special positioning needs?
6. Where will the patient be sent postoperatively? Is intensive care unit care warranted?
7. Regardless of anesthetic choice, conditions that promote vasospasm or vasoconstriction (e.g., pain, hypotension, hypothermia) must be avoided.
8. Have appropriate arrangements been made for replacement of blood products or cell salvage?

A preoperative discussion with the surgeon involved should help to clarify some of the above questions. To effectively plan an anesthetic for a microvascular procedure, communication with the surgical service is essential. Once the needs of the surgeon have been established, the needs of the patient must also be taken into consideration. This does not mean that the needs of the surgeon necessarily take precedence over those of the patient, but it is difficult, if not impossible, to intelligently discuss the various anesthetic options and attendant risks without first understanding what the scope of the surgery will be.

It is necessary to discuss with patients their medical history and previous anesthetic history, and to address any concerns and apprehensions about anesthesia. Not infrequently, patients arriving for surgery have pre-existing ideas as to what type of anesthetic they prefer. Unless there is a compelling medical reason to use or avoid a particular form of anesthesia, it is wise to consider the patient's wishes. Either way, a kind and considerate manner is key to winning the patient's respect and cooperation.

OPERATING ROOM SET-UP

Once the anesthetic plan has been decided and discussed with the patient, final preparation of the operating room must be attended to. The room temperature should be increased to 21°C or higher, and equipment for maintenance of patient temperature (heated humidifier, Bair Hugger, etc.) brought to the room if not already present. Proper orientation and padding of the operating table should be confirmed with the operating room staff. Appropriate intravenous fluids should be set up and the availability of colloidal volume expanders ensured. Arterial and central venous monitoring capability should be arranged, if indicated.

The blood bank should be contacted to ensure availability of blood. Vasodilating agents, heparin, dextran, narcotics, and other pharmacologic agents that may be required should be readily available. The usual check of anesthesia equipment (anesthesia machine, laryngoscope, endotracheal tube, oxygen reserves, etc.) should be performed.

REGIONAL VERSUS GENERAL ANESTHESIA

Despite years of experience with providing anesthesia for microvascular surgery, the optimal anesthetic technique has yet to be determined with any great certainty. Advocates of both regional and general anesthesia can be found, while a combined technique is favored by many practitioners. As with any type of surgical procedure, the anesthetic plan for microvascular procedures *must* be tailored to meet the needs of the individual patient. Strict adherence to rigid protocols ignores the multiplicity of associated illness and limitations in this increasingly heterogeneous population. Within reason, patient preference should be considered in the decision regarding use of regional versus general anesthesia.

Regional Anesthesia

In the past, regional anesthetic techniques were limited in their application because of their "one-shot" nature and the relatively short duration of available local anesthetics. However, with the introduction of techniques using indwelling catheters, regional anesthesia can be continued, not only for the duration of the surgery, but for several days postoperatively as well. Indwelling epidural catheters have been used for some time for lower extremity surgery and brachial plexus catheters are gaining popularity for upper extremity procedures.[16,25,26,34] Indwelling brachial plexus catheters have been placed using the classic approaches at the interscalene, supraclavicular, and axillary levels. There are several described techniques. One technique involves first filling the fibrous sheath surrounding the neurovascular structures with local anesthetic or saline and then "popping" through the distended sheath with a needle through which a catheter is directed.[44] Another technique localizes the plexus with an electrical nerve stimulator and a sheathed needle. Once the appropriate motor response is elicited, the sheath is then advanced into the perineural space. This sheath may be used for the continuous infusion, or a longer catheter may be threaded through it to be left in place.[45]

Either way, the catheter should be firmly secured to ensure its continued function. Indwelling catheters are not only useful for long surgical procedures, but they can be left in place for several days postoperatively for pain control.[46] Typically, the concentration of local anesthetic infused postoperatively is sufficient for sympathetic and sensory block. Motor block or "surgical" anesthetic levels are not the goal with these infusions. Epidural infusions may be composed of local anesthetic alone, (usually 0.125 to 0.25 percent bupivacaine) or may also contain low concentrations of narcotic (0.1 percent bupivacaine + 5 μg fentanyl/ml). Infusions for continuous brachial plexus blockade are local anesthetics alone, typically 0.125 to 0.25 percent bupivacaine.

In addition to the sensory and motor blockade that allows surgery to proceed on awake patients, the sympathetic blockade that regional anesthesia provides is also useful because of the vasodilation that results. Vasodilation makes for easier identification and anastomosis of very small vessels (as small as 1 mm) and maximizes blood flow into the affected extremity. When a regional anesthetic technique is used for microvascular surgery, it is recommended that epinephrine not be included in the local anesthetic solution because of concern about systemic absorption and the resultant vasoconstriction.[47] Small doses of epinephrine, such as would be included in a test dose, should not present a significant problem and can be a valuable means of determining whether a catheter has been inadvertently placed in a vascular structure.

Some concern has been raised about the possibility of a "steal" phenomenon occurring with regional anesthetic techniques that produce sympathetic blockade for an entire extremity.[48] Theoretically, vasodilation secondary to sympathetic blockade affect only those vessels that are innervated, and not those in the replanted part. Clinically, this has not been a major concern, but if suspected, a more distal block might be of some benefit. Surgically placed catheters adjacent to peripheral nerves have been used for continuous infusion of local anesthetics in an attempt to limit the potential vascular bed for vasodilation and to provide pain relief postoperatively.[15]

By anesthetizing only the extremity that includes the surgical field, rather than the entire patient (as with a general anesthetic), cardiorespiratory trespass is minimized, and the potential for airway mishaps and cardiovascular depression is decreased. Because of this, patients with a full stomach or difficult airway are excellent candidates for regional anesthetic techniques.

Failed Blocks

Whenever a regional anesthetic is planned, it is appropriate to alert the patient that the blocks are occasionally inadequate, even in experienced hands. At the time of this disclosure one should also assure patients that they will not experience pain. By allotting adequate time for performance of the block and also to permit sufficient time for it to "set up," the chances of failure are diminished. Many times, particularly with upper extremity procedures, if a block appears "spotty," the operating surgeon may be able to supplement with local injections and avoid the need for general anesthesia. Again, communication with the surgical team is important.

Not infrequently, a patient may confuse retained proprioception with nociception. Whenever a patient complains of pain with stimulation, an effort should be taken to determine the exact nature of that pain. Is it sharp and easily localized to the exact area of stimulation? Is the complaint appropriate to the level of stimulus? Is there evidence of a motor block? With the exception of blocks using etidocaine, it is highly unlikely that the sensory fibers have been spared in the presence of a profound motor block. Gentle reassurance and appropriate sedation can go a long way toward salvaging a "failed" block under certain circumstances. One must, however, be honest in the assessment of these situations. Sedation should not be used as a substitute for general anesthesia when, in fact, the block is inadequate to permit the surgery to proceed.

Outpatients

Because of the increasing applications of the operating microscope, many microsurgical procedures may be sufficiently brief and limited in scope to permit the patient to be cared for as an outpatient.[49] In those situations, an indwelling catheter may not be necessary, and care should be taken to match the duration of the local anesthetic used to the expected duration of the procedure. Many practitioners may wish to examine the patient's neurologic status prior to discharge from the outpatient area. If the neural blockade is still quite dense, this examination will be of no use and may delay discharge.

Inpatients

For longer procedures such as replants, residual blockade the day of surgery is of little consequence, and it can be to the patient's advantage to continue to have a dense level of blockade. Many of these longer procedures may warrant a continuous catheter technique to provide sufficient duration of blockade and postoperative pain management. If a single-shot technique is used for one of these longer procedures, preparations should be made in the event that the block becomes ineffective before the surgery is completed.

Tourniquet Pain

Tourniquet pain can be difficult during long procedures under regional anesthesia. Most often, as time wears on, the patient will become restless and begin to complain of arm or leg pain but may not be able to localize it. Once it has begun, typically 60 to 90 minutes after inflation of the tourniquet, little can be done to relieve it short of releasing the tourniquet pressure for a period of time or providing supplemental general anesthesia. This problem should be dealt with promptly, as any movement by the patient will be greatly exaggerated to those looking through the operating microscope, and may jeopardize the outcome of the surgery. Despite much investigation, the exact mechanism of tourniquet pain has yet to be elucidated. Evidence does suggest that more is involved than simple tissue ischemia and anaerobic metabolism.[50] It should be remembered that tourniquet pain is not limited to patients under regional anesthesia. Patients under general anesthesia often develop resistant hypertension at about the same stage of their procedures, believed to be secondary to tourniquet pain.[51]

General Anesthesia

General anesthesia is chosen for microvascular procedures for a variety of reasons. Most commonly cited is that the anesthesia care provider can reliably maintain general anesthesia for the duration of the surgery despite the long time course of the procedure. There are no "failed" general anesthetics. The patient is unaware of the passing of time and any discomfort from having spent prolonged periods in one position. The likelihood of the patient moving during critical aspects of the surgery is diminished, unless the level of anesthesia is light enough to cause the patient to buck, cough, or strain on the endotracheal tube. General anesthesia permits the practitioner to maintain a controlled airway, adequate oxygen delivery, and ventilation. With the patient completely asleep, it may be technically more convenient to place invasive monitoring lines and to obtain a more accurate measure of body temperature.

As mentioned earlier, all of the inhalational agents are potent vasodilators of the peripheral circulation. Advocates of general anesthesia cite this as an added benefit, particularly when confronted with very small caliber vessels for revascularization. Disadvantages of systemic vasodilation are the potential for hypotension in the marginally volume-repleted or cardiac-compromised patient and the acceleration of heat loss from the body, leading to postoperative shivering and vasoconstriction. To avoid the sympathetically mediated response to pain on awakening from a general anesthetic, it is necessary to also administer sufficient narcotics or other pain relievers to ensure adequate control of pain in the immediate postoperative period.

In an emergent situation, as many of these cases are, patients must be assumed to have a full stomach. If a general anesthetic is planned, precautions must be taken to minimize the risk of aspiration of gastric contents. Either an awake intubation or a "rapid-sequence" induction/intubation including cricoid pressure can be incorporated into the anesthetic management of these patients, depending on the needs of the patient and the skill of the practitioner.

Combined Regional and General Anesthesia

In many cases, neither regional nor general anesthesia is ideal for a given situation. A combined technique can provide the beneficial effects of each, while minimizing the negatives. A regional anesthetic can provide excellent pain relief during the period prior to induction of general anesthesia as well as for the post-operative period. Inclusion of a regional anesthetic will permit the use of less inhalational agent intraoperatively and potentially reduce the chance of significant hemodynamic perturbation. On the other hand, addition of an inhalational agent to a regional anesthetic permits the placement and tolerance of an endotracheal tube, providing a controlled airway, and thereby avoiding the worry of an inadequate block or the need for heavy sedation in a patient with a full stomach. It also increases patients' tolerance of long procedures and progressively uncomfortable positions.

In summary, regardless of what type of anesthetic plan—regional, general, or combined—is devised, there are certain tenets that must be followed. Survival of the patient must come first and foremost before any consideration is given to replantation or revascularization of traumatized extremities. Once this has been reasonably ensured, maintenance of blood flow through the new anastomosis or free flap must be considered a prime directive. This is best achieved by maintaining a normal body temperature, adequately replacing fluids and blood as needed to maintain perfusion pressure, adequate pain control, and maximizing blood flow to the extremity involved through systemic vasodilation or neural blockade. Communication with the surgical services involved is necessary to plan and institute an anesthetic technique that will meet the needs of the patient as well as the surgeon, and to coordinate plans for postoperative pain management.

REFERENCES

1. O'Brien BMcC: The role of microsurgery in modern surgery. Ann Plast Surg 24:258, 1990

2. Beatty ME, Smith AA: Hand and microvascular surgery. Evolution to present practice. J Fla Med Assoc 76:592, 1989

3. Horowitz JH, Nichter LS, Kenney JG, Morgan RF: Lawnmower injuries in children: lower extremity reconstruction. J Trauma 25:1138, 1985

4. Buncke HJ, Alpert BS, Johnson-Giebink R: Digital replantation. Surg Clin North Am 61:383, 1981

5. O'Brien BMcC: Microvascular surgery of the upper extremity. J Hand Surg 10:982, 1985

6. Townsend PLG: Microvascular surgery of the lower limb. Br J Hosp Med, November 1985, p. 277

7. Irons GB, Wood MB, Schmitt EH: Experience with one hundred consecutive free flaps. Ann Plast Surg 18:17, 1987

8. Wood MB, Cooney WP, Irons GB: Skeletal reconstruction by vascularized bone transfer: indications and results. Mayo Clin Proc 60:729, 1985

9. Wood MB, Cooney WP, Irons GB: Lower extremity salvage and reconstruction by free-tissue transfer. Analysis of results. Clin Orthop 201:151, 1985

10. Wood MB: Upper extremity reconstruction by vascularized bone transfers: results and complications. J Hand Surg 12A:422, 1987

11. Yaffe B, Cushin BJ, Strauch B: Effect of cigarette smoking on experimental microvascular anastomoses. Microsurgery 5:70, 1984

12. Rees TD, Liverett DM, Guy CL: The effect of cigarette smoking on skin-flap survival in the face lift patient. Plast Reconstr Surg 73:911, 1984

13. Ritchie JM: Central nervous system stimulants: the xanthines. p. 367. In Goodman LS, Gilman A (eds): The Pharmacological Basis of Therapeutics. 5th Ed. MacMillan, New York, 1975

14. MacDonald DJF: Anaesthesia for microvascular surgery. A physiological approach. Br J Anaesth 57:904, 1985

15. Phelps DB, Rutherford RB, Boswick JA: Control of vasospasm following trauma and microvascular surgery. J Hand Surg 4:109, 1979

16. Jakubowski M, Lamont A, Murray WB, De Wit SL: Anaesthesia for microsurgery. S Afr Med J 67:581, 1985

17. Puri VK, Howard M, Paidipaty BB, Singh S: Resuscitation in hypovolemia and shock: a prospective study of hydroxyethyl starch and albumin. Crit Care Med 11:418, 1983

18. Shatney CH, Deepika K, Militello PR et al: Efficacy of hetastarch in the resuscitation of patients with multisystem trauma and shock. Arch Surg 118:804, 1983

19. Haupt MT, Rackow EC: Colloid osmotic pressure and fluid resuscitation with hetastarch, albumin, and saline solutions. Crit Care Med 10:159, 1982

20. Physicians' Desk Reference. 45th Ed. Medical Economics Company, Montvale, NJ, 1991

21. Stump DC, Strauss RG, Henriksen RA et al: Effects of hydroxyethyl starch on blood coagulation, particularly factor VIII. Transfusion 25:349, 1985

22. Strauss RG, Stump DC, Henriksen RA, Saunders R: Effects of hydroxyethyl starch on fibrinogen, fibrin clot formation, and fibrinolysis. Transfusion 25:230, 1985

23. Symington BE: Hetastarch and bleeding complications. Ann Intern Med 105:628, 1986

24. Lineaweaver WC, Valauri FA: Pharmacology. p. 696. In Buncke HJ (ed): Microsurgery: Transplantation-Replantation. Lea & Febiger, Philadelphia, 1991

25. Robins DW: The anaesthetic management of patients undergoing free flap transfer. Br J Plast Surg 36:231, 1983

26. Sanders NR, Anderson KR: Anesthesia for microsurgery. p. 729. In Buncke HJ (ed): Microsurgery: Transplantation-Replantation. Lea & Febiger, Philadelphia, 1991

27. Flacke JW, Flacke WE: Inadvertent hypothermia: frequent, insidious, and often serious. Semin Anaesth 2:183, 1983

28. Bird TM, Strunin L: Anesthetic considerations for microsurgical repair of limbs. Can Anaesth Soc J 31:51, 1984

29. Goudsouzian NG, Morris RH, Ryan JF: The effects of a warming blanket on the maintenance of body temperatures in anesthetized infants and children. Anesthesiology 39:351, 1973

30. Stone DR, Downs JB, Paul WL, Perkins

HM: Adult body temperature and heated humidification of anesthetic gases during general anesthesia. Anesth Analg 60:736, 1981

31. Hynson JM, Sessler DI: Intraoperative warming therapies: a comparison of three devices. J Clin Anesth 4:194, 1992

32. Lennon RL, Hosking MP, Conover MA, Perkins WJ: Evaluation of a forced-air warming device. Anesth Analg 70:424, 1990

33. Neimkin RJ, May JW, Roberts J: Continuous axillary block through an indwelling Teflon catheter. J Hand Surg 9A:830, 1984

34. Raggi RP: Balanced regional anesthesia for hand surgery. Orthop Clin North Am 17:473, 1986

35. Geter RK, Winters RRW, Puckett CL: Resolution of experimental microvascular spasm and improvement in anastomotic patency by direct topical agent application. Plast Reconstr Surg 77:105, 1986

36. Aarts HF: Regional intravascular sympathetic blockade for better results in flap surgery: an experimental study of free flaps, island flaps, and pedicle flaps in the rabbit ear. Plast Reconstr Surg 66:690, 1980

37. Hickey RF, Eger EI II: Circulatory pharmacology of inhaled anesthetics. p. 649. In Miller RD (ed): Anesthesia. 2nd Ed. Churchill Livingstone, New York, 1986

38. Aps C, Cox RG, Mayou BJ, Sengupta P: The role of anaesthetic management of enhancing peripheral blood flow in patients undergoing free flap transfer. Ann R Coll Surg Engl 67:177, 1985

39. Finseth F: Clinical salvage of three failing skin flaps by treatment with a vasodilator drug. Plast Reconstr Surg 63:304, 1979

40. Pang CY, Neligan PC, Nakatsuka T, Sasaki GH: Pharmacologic manipulation of the microcirculation in cutaneous and my-ocutaneous flaps in pigs. Clin Plast Surg 12:173, 1985

41. Kerrigan CL, Daniel RK: Pharmacologic treatment of the failing skin flap. Plast Reconstr Surg 70:541, 1982

42. Harris GD, Finseth F, Buncke HJ: The hazard of cigarette smoking following digital replantation. J Microsurg 1:403, 1980

43. Rapoport S, Glickman MG, Salomon JC,. Cuono CB: Aggressive postoperative pharmacotherapy for vascular compromise of replanted digits. AJR 144:1065, 1985

44. Moore PL, Cockings E: Use of transarterial axillary sheath distension as an aid to catheter placement. Anesthesiology 65:131, 1986

45. Gaumann DM, Lennon RL, Wedel DJ: Continuous axillary block for postoperative pain management. Reg Anesth 13:77, 1988

46. Strecker WB, Wood MB, Wedel DJ: Epidural anesthesia during lower extremity free tissue transfer. J Reconstr Microsurg 4:327, 1988

47. Matsuda M, Kato N, Hosoi M: Continuous brachial plexus block for replantation in the upper extremity. Hand 14:129, 1982

48. van Twisk R, Gielen MJM, Pavlov PW, Robinson PH: Is additional epidural sympathetic block in microvascular surgery contraindicated? A preliminary report. Br J Plast Surg 41:37, 1988

49. Davis WJ, Lennon RL, Wedel DJ: Brachial plexus anesthesia for outpatient surgery procedures on an upper extremity. Mayo Clin Proc 66:470, 1991

50. Hagenouw RRPM, Bridenbaugh PO, van Egmond J, Stuebing R: Tourniquet pain: a volunteer study. Anesth Analg 65:1175, 1986

51. Kaufman RD, Walts LF: Tourniquet induced hypertension. Br J Anaesth 54:333, 1982

11

Outpatient Surgery

William J. Davis
Robert L. Lennon

There has been a significant increase in the number of surgical procedures performed in the outpatient setting since James Nicholl[1] published the results of 8,988 outpatient procedures on children in 1909 and Ralph Waters opened the first outpatient anesthesia clinic in Sioux City, Iowa, in 1916. Inpatient surgical procedures in the United States declined from 16.05 to 13.07 million between 1983 and 1986, while outpatient procedures increased from 5.03 to 8.82 million. In 1988, there were 984 Medicare-participating freestanding outpatient surgery centers, at which 1,702,397 operations were performed. This is a dramatic increase since the first totally self-sufficient, freestanding surgical center was opened in 1970 by anesthesiologists Wallace Reed and John Ford in Phoenix, Arizona.[2]

In 1984 the Society of Ambulatory Anesthesia was organized as a subspecialty in anesthesia and is now represented in the American Society of Anesthesiologists.

RATIONALE FOR OUTPATIENT SURGERY

The impetus behind the growth of outpatient surgery has been primarily economic. Insurance companies, government agencies, and other third-party payers are attracted by the purported decrease in hospital costs for surgical procedures performed on an outpatient basis. They have, therefore, applied financial incentives to encourage both physicians and consumers to accept outpatient rather than inpatient surgery.

Many patients, as well as their families, find outpatient surgery more convenient and less disruptive than inpatient treatment. Other factors in favor of outpatient surgery include the possibility that respiratory complications such as pneumonia and pulmonary embolus may be decreased.[3] It is also claimed that pediatric and immunocompromised patients have a decreased exposure to nosocomial contamination and cross-infection in an ambulatory facility.

Cost–benefit analysis is a complex issue requiring analysis of both direct costs (e.g., personnel, equipment, supplies) and indirect costs (e.g., facility maintenance, rent, utilities). Costs to the patients and their families (e.g., postoperative home care, lost income) must also be included.[4] A study examining clinical outcome and costs for cataract removal performed in both inpatient and outpatient settings showed lower Medicare costs among the outpatients.[5] Similarly, cost savings from a change in physician pattern of practice was documented when comparable groups of patients having either knee arthroscopy or laparoscopy were studied. There were more preoperative tests performed for inpatients (four times greater cost) than for outpatients, and shorter operating room and postanesthetic recovery times in the outpatient group.[6]

However, other studies have questioned the benefits of ambulatory surgery. A Canadian study examined patient satisfaction, clinical outcome, and costs associated with herniorrhaphy, tubal ligation, and menisectomy in outpatients and inpatients. Similar clinical outcomes were found in all the groups, but a significantly higher proportion of the outpatients than their hospitalized counterparts would have preferred hospitalization. While there were decreased costs among the outpatient herniorrhaphy and tubal ligation groups, there was no cost saving in the menisectomy group. This was mainly due to higher costs for outpatient physiotherapy.[7] It is clear that a cost–benefit analysis should be made by each facility that intends to change its practice.

PATIENT SELECTION

The American Society of Anesthesiologists (ASA) Physical Status Classification has been used as a general guide in patient selection for ambulatory surgery but is not intended to indicate an estimate of patient risk (see also Ch. 2):

Class 1. A normal healthy patient
Class 2. A patient with a mild systemic disease (e.g., essential hypertension, diet-controlled diabetes mellitus, moderate obesity) with no functional impairment
Class 3. A patient with a severe systemic disease that limits activity, but is not incapacitating (e.g., moderate pulmonary insufficiency, stable angina pectoris, morbid obesity)
Class 4. A patient with an incapacitating systemic disease that is a constant threat to life (e.g., unstable angina pectoris, severe pulmonary insufficiency, congestive heart failure)
Class 5. A moribund patient not expected to survive 24 hours with or without operation (e.g., ruptured abdominal aortic aneurysm, severe cerebral trauma)

In the event of emergency operation, the class number is preceded by an E.

While patients in ASA classes 1 and 2 are the usual types of patients accepted for outpatient surgery, occasionally patients in class 3 are also approved. Generally, class 3 patients can be accepted if (1) their illness is stable and well controlled, (2) appropriate intra- and postoperative monitoring and treatment are readily available, and (3) there is a suitable home situation after discharge.

A variety of approaches can be taken to ensure proper preoperative patient evaluation. An outpatient preanesthetic clinic can be established. All patients referred there by the surgeon would be evaluated by an anesthesia care provider and would undergo appropriate laboratory tests before the planned day of surgery. Kaplan[8] found that routine preoperative or protocol testing did not add to the information obtained by even a partial history. It was noted that 60 percent of routinely ordered tests would not have been performed if testing had been for recognizable indications. Only 0.22 percent of these tests revealed abnormalities that might have influenced perioperative management. In view of the low return from routine testing, a useful approach for minimal effective preoperative testing is outlined in Table 11-1.[9] These recommendations would also result in significant cost savings.

Table 11-1. Minimal Effective Preoperative Testing

Selected Disease/ Disorder	HGB M	HGB F	WBC	PT/PTT	PLT, BT	Elect	Creat/BUN	Glucose	SGOT/ALK PTASE	X-Ray	ECG	Pregnancy	T/S
Surgical procedure With blood loss	X	X											X
Without blood loss													
Neonates	X	X											
Age <40 yr		X											
40–59		X									±		
≥60 yr	X	X								X	X		
Cardiovascular disease							X			X	X		
Pulmonary disease										X	X		
Malignancy	X	X	*	*						X			
Radiation therapy			X	X						X	X		
Hepatic disease				X					X				
Exposure to hepatitis									X				
Renal disease	X	X				X	X						
Bleeding disorder				X	X								
Diabetes						X	X	X			X		
Smoking ≥20 pk-yr history	X	X								X			
Possible pregnancy												X	
Diuretic use						X	X						
Digoxin use						X	X				X		
Steroid use						X		X					
Anticoagulant use	X	X		X									

±, maybe; *, leukemias only; X, obtain; HGB, hemoglobin; WBC, white blood (cell) count; PT/PTT, prothrombin time/partial thromboplastin time; PLT, platelet count; BT, bleeding time; Elect, sodium, potassium, chloride, carbon dioxide, proteins; Creat/BUN, creatinine or blood urea nitrogen; SGOT/ALK PTASE, serum glutamic oxaloacetic transaminase/alkaline phosphatase; T/S, blood typing and screen for unexpected antibodies.

(From Roizen & Rupani,[57] with permission.)

Wilson et al[10] developed the following simple questions whose negative answers correlated well with a consensus of fitness for anesthesia among a group of anesthesiologists:

1. Do you feel unwell?
2. Have you had any serious illness in the past?
3. Do you get more short of breath on exertion than other people of your age?
4. Do you have any cough?
5. Do you have any wheeze?
6. Do you have any chest pain on exertion (angina type)?
7. Do you have ankle swelling?
8. Have you taken any medications in the past 3 months?
9. Have you any allergies?
10. Have you had an anesthetic in the past 2 months?
11. Have you or your relatives had any problems with anesthesia?

As the authors noted, "Patients who are thought to be perfectly fit on the basis of simple questions usually prove to be so after the traditional preoperative history and investigations. This suggests that a questionnaire might be developed for use in surgical outpatients to select patients for day surgery."

Whichever method is selected for preoperative evaluation of patients for planned outpatient anesthesia, the process not only allows for appropriate screening of patients, but also allows an opportunity for the anesthesia care provider to answer any questions the patient or family may have. At the same time, policies regarding eating or drinking prior to surgery and continuing essential medications can be explained clearly to the patient and reinforced with written instructions.

Pediatric patients gain special benefit from the advantages of outpatient surgery, in particular the reduced period of separation from their families and the de-creased exposure to nosocomial infections. There are, however, some children who may not be suitable candidates for outpatient surgery:

1. Infants born prematurely are more likely than mature infants to have postanesthetic apneic episodes. Welborn et al[11] noted that infants less than 44 weeks' conceptual age are at high risk for developing postoperative ventilatory dysfunction and bradycardia.
2. Children with a history of respiratory distress syndrome often have residual lung disease with decreased lung compliance and increased airway resistance. These children usually have hyperreactive airways and may also have subglottic stenosis from previous intubation. Infants who had respiratory distress syndrome complicated by bronchopulmonary dysplasia also have impaired lung function with hyperreactive airways and have an increased risk of sudden infant death syndrome, possibly associated with apneic episodes and decreased responsiveness to hypoxia.
3. Children with unstable asthma.
4. Children with an active respiratory infection associated with fever (greater than 38°C) and cough often have hyperreactive airways, which can persist for 4 weeks after the acute illness.
5. Children who are susceptible to malignant hyperthermia and who would benefit from overnight observation.
6. Children who are morbidly obese.
7. Children with uncontrolled seizures.

PREOPERATIVE FASTING

Pediatric Patients

Fasting instructions must be clearly explained to the patient and family to avoid having the child present for outpatient surgery with a full stomach. Because traditional fasting instructions could lead to significant dehydration, they have been modified on the basis of recent studies. Maltby et al[12] found that prolonged fasting did not provide a safe gastric pH, and that the ingestion of 150 ml of water actually reduced residual gastric volume. Preoperative pediatric feeding instructions used at the Mayo Clinic are shown in Figure 11-1.

Adult Patients

Anesthesia care providers also instruct adults to refrain from oral intake for at least 8 hours prior to induction of anesthesia to prevent possible pulmonary aspiration of vomited or regurgitated stomach contents. The risk of aspiration and the severity of pulmonary injury are thought to be increased when the pH of the gastric aspirate is less than 2.5 and the volume of aspirate exceeds 0.4 ml/kg. It is still appropriate to caution adult patients to avoid solids, foods such as milk, which can form solids in the stomach, and liquids with suspensions (e.g., juice with pulp). However, a recent study by Shevde and Trivedi[13] found that a 2-hour period was all that was necessary for the volume of stomach content to return to less than 25 ml after ingestion of moderate amounts (240 ml) of clear liquids. They concluded that if healthy patients have ingested a moderate amount of clear liquids it is safe to conduct general anesthesia after a 2-hour fast. Patients at higher risk for aspiration, such as diabetic, pregnant, and obese patients, should avoid any oral intake for the customary 8 hours before the induction of anesthesia.

PROCEDURES

A wide variety of orthopedic surgical procedures has been performed in outpatient facilities (Table 11-2). The deci-

---

For your child's safety, it is important that you follow these instructions. If these feeding instructions are not followed, your child's operation may be delayed.

At midnight the evening before surgery, **Stop all food,** including the following:

Solid food, candy and chewing gum
Milk, milk products, and formulas
Orange juice and any juice with pulp
Soda (pop, soft drinks, carbonated beverages)

Breastfeeding
    May continue until 3 hours before the time you are told to be at the hospital.

Clear fluids
    May be continued until 1 1/2 hours before the time you are told
    to be at the hospital.

Clear fluids include
    Water   Clear broth
    Apple juice   Pedialyte
    Clear juice drinks   Ice Popsicles
    Plain gelatin

Fig. 11-1. Preoperative feeding instructions for children 14 years of age or younger.

Table 11-2.   Orthopedic Outpatient Surgical Procedures

Arthroscopic debridement	Flexor tendon sheath release
Arthroscopic lateral release	Hammer-toe correction
Arthroscopic meniscectomy	Hardware removal
Arthroscopic shelf release	Median nerve decompression
Bone biopsy	Muscle biopsy
Bone-spur excision	Olecranon bursectomy
Bunionectomy	Olecranon spur excision
Carpal tunnel release	Open reduction/internal fixation of fingers
Cast change, with or without manipulation	Prepatelar bursectomy
Closed reduction	Release of Dequervain's hand
Cyst removal (e.g., Baker cyst)	Release of Dupuytren's contracture
Debridement	Release of trigger thumb
Diagnostic arthroscopy	Removal of foreign body
Epidural steroid injection	Removal of nails, pins, plates, screws, wires
Excision and removal of foreign body	Simple tendon repair
Excision of exostosis	Syndactylization of toes
Excision of ganglion	Synovectomy
Excision of lesion	Tendon exploration
Fasiectomy (finger, palm)	Ulnar nerve transfer
Finger-joint replacement	Z-plasty
Finger amputation and revision	

sion whether to perform any particular procedure on an outpatient basis depends on several factors. The importance of proper preoperative evaluation has been discussed already. Other significant considerations include the availability of (1) all necessary surgical facilities and equipment, and (2) blood and blood products for the planned procedure. Honest appraisal of the capabilities of the surgical facility and personnel must be made, including thoughtful provision to deal with any unexpected complications before undertaking any procedure.

It is also obvious that despite one of the primary motivations in establishing an outpatient facility being cost savings, no compromises must be made in ensuring all necessary anesthetic equipment is available for safe patient care. Established standards approved by bodies such as the American Society of Anesthesiologists should be followed at a minimum. Basic professional considerations, apart from medicolegal realities, mandate the provision of modern anesthesia machines

and patient monitors. These must include pulse oximetry, gas oximetry, capnography, neuromuscular blockade monitors, and equipment needed to deal with a difficult airway. A fiberoptic bronchoscope or laryngoscope is also recommended by some practitioners.

CHOICE OF ANESTHETIC TECHNIQUE

Premedication

A variety of approaches may be taken regarding the issue of premedication for outpatients. At the Mayo Clinic hospitals, routine premedication is not prescribed for ambulatory patients. Anesthesia care providers prefer to order anxiolytics or other drugs on an individual basis after individual evaluation. This has the advantage of producing predictable responses in a short period of time if medications are given intravenously. A prolonged recovery can be avoided by using centrally acting drugs judiciously. Another advantage of preoperative assessment by the anesthesia care provider is the beneficial effect of reducing patient anxiety. Egbert[14] noted that the anesthesia care provider's preoperative visit was more successful in reducing anxiety than intramuscular barbiturate.

Anxiolytics

Many practitioners find benzodiazepines beneficial in decreasing anxiety as well as producing amnesia, sedation, and muscle relaxation. Numerous studies have demonstrated the effectiveness of anxiolytics (e.g., diazepam) in decreasing preoperative apprehension without prolonging recovery time after surgery.[15] There are, however, reports indicating that recovery after diazepam is prolonged and incomplete 3 to 5 hours after intravenous administration as assessed by a variety of motor and cognitive tests.[16] Midazolam, a water-soluble benzodiazide, is a widely used anxiolytic having a number of advantages over diazepam. These include absence of pain when given parenterally, increased potency, quicker onset of action, shorter duration of action, and amnesia.[17] Midazolam is more potent than diazepam and it is recommended that the depressant effects of the drug be carefully monitored. This may include the use of pulse oximetry as well as the usual clinical measurements. Prudence dictates that midazolam should be titrated in small increments (0.5 to 1 mg IV), particularly in elderly patients.

Droperidol, a butyrophenone, is a potent neuroleptic drug. It is often used for its sedative and powerful antiemetic action (the latter effect via the chemoreceptor trigger zone). Droperidol produces a state of suppressed spontaneous movement with intact spinal and central reflexes. There is dissociation from the environment, and while the patient usually appears tranquil, an unpleasant mental agitation may occur in some instances. This can be relieved, if recognized, by opioid or benzodiazepine administration.

Onset of action of droperidol is usually within 5 to 10 minutes of an intravenous injection and duration of action may exceed 10 to 12 hours. Usual doses for premedication are 0.625 to 1.25 mg in adults (0.005 to 0.015 mg/kg). This dose of droperidol has been shown to be effective in reducing the incidence of postoperative vomiting in children[18] and adults without significant side effects, such as excessive sedation or extrapyramidal symptoms.

H$_2$ Receptor Antagonists, Antacids, and Dopamine Antagonists

The risk of aspiration, and recommendations regarding fasting to decrease this risk, are discussed above. Some anesthesia care providers regard all outpatients as having potential full stomachs and take all precautions, including intubation, to protect the airway. This degree of caution has not been shown in the scientific literature to be warranted for all patients. However, certain groups of patients, such as those with hiatal hernia, obesity, diabetes, and pregnancy, may be at particular risk of aspiration. Pharmacologic approaches to decrease gastric volume and increase gastric pH are appropriate for these patients, and include (1) histamine (H$_2$) receptor antagonists (cimetidine, ranitidine, and famotidine), (2) antacids, and (3) dopamine antagonists. These approaches may be used separately or in combination.

H$_2$ receptor antagonists decrease the volume and acidity of gastric fluid. Drug interactions due to impairment of drug metabolism and decreased liver blood flow have to be considered when using cimetidine, while such interactions are not thought to be significant with the newer H_2 receptor antagonists (ranitidine and famotidine).

Soluble or nonparticulate antacids such as sodium citrate are widely used in obstetric anesthesia and can also be used in ambulatory anesthesia. Doses of 15 to 30 ml sodium citrate solution have been shown to increase gastric pH to greater than 2.5 in more than 90 percent of patients when given up to 60 minutes before surgery[19]; however, this approach has the drawback of potentially increasing gastric volume.

Metoclopramide, a dopamine antagonist, has the effect of increasing lower esophageal sphincter tone, increasing gastric motility, and acting as a central antiemetic. It has been found more effective, in combination with cimetidine, in reducing gastric volume and increasing gastric pH than either drug alone.[20]

While all these pharmacologic maneuvers can be of value in decreasing the risk of gastric acid aspiration, they do not eliminate the need for careful anesthetic care to protect the airway throughout the anesthetic period.

General Anesthesia

The challenges of outpatient general anesthesia are (1) to provide a pleasant, rapid induction of surgical anesthesia; (2) to maintain stable conditions intraoperatively, including analgesia and amnesia; and (3) to allow prompt, smooth recovery to allow safe discharge home as soon as possible. General anesthesia typically provides a large percentage of all outpatient anesthetics. A commonly used technique is "balanced anesthesia." This involves the use of intravenous drugs, opioids, and/or hypnotics to supplement inhalational agents. Muscle relaxants are often used to provide suitable conditions for endotracheal intubation. They may also be used to provide skeletal muscle relaxation to reduce the doses of other anesthetic drugs in the hope of providing more rapid postoperative recovery.

Intravenous Induction Agents

All intravenous agents currently available may be used in outpatient anesthesia. Table 11-3 summarizes the pharmacokinetic variables of these drugs.

Sodium Thiopental Sodium thiopental remains the standard against which agents are compared. Recovery is rapid after a single dose because of redistribution to tissues other than the brain. However, after large or repeated doses, recovery may be slow because of a redistribution, represented by a long terminal elimination half-life (10 to 12 hours) and large volume of distribution.

Methohexital Methohexital is a methylated oxybarbiturate having a higher clearance and shorter elimination half-life than thiopental. Cumulation is less likely after repeated doses and recovery is generally more rapid in comparison to thiopental. However, complete recovery of fine motor skills may be as delayed with methohexital as it is with thiopental.[21] Disadvantages of methohexital include the occasional occurrence of dyskinetic muscle movements, coughing, and hiccupping. These effects can be reduced by slow injection of a dilute (0.5 percent) solution or by prior administration of an opioid (fentanyl 1 to 2 μg/kg). Cardiovascular and respiratory depression also occur, but are less than that usually associated with thiopental. Methohexital is therefore commonly used for induction of anesthesia when rapid recovery is desirable.

Etomidate Etomidate is a carboxylated imidazole compound with a high clearance and large volume of distribution. The main advantage of etomidate in healthy patients is that it produces less

Table 11-3.   Doses and Pharmacokinetic Variables of Intravenous Agents Used for Induction of General Anesthesia in Outpatients

Drug	Induction Dose (mg/kg)[a]	Distribution Half-Life (min)	Elimination Half-Life (hr)	Clearance (ml/min)	$V_{d,ss}$ (L)
Thiopental	3.0–6.0	2–4 (rapid) 30–60 (slow)	10–12	180–200	100–200
Methohexital	1.0–20	5–6	1.5–4	700–900	60–08
Etomidate	0.2–0.4	2–4	1.5–5	800–1,400	200–400
Ketamine	0.75–1.5	11–17	2–3	1,250–1,400	200–250
Midazolam	0.1–0.2	7–15	2–2.5	300–550	70–130
Propofol	1.25–2.5	2–4	1–3	1,400–2,800	200–500

$V_{d,ss}$, volume of distribution, steady state.

[a] Lower dosages recommended when used in combination with narcotic analgesics benzodiazepines or when administered to geriatric outpatients.

(From Apfelbaum et al,[58] with permission.)

cardiovascular depression than other intravenous induction agents. Disadvantages include pain on injection and myoclonic movements. The myoclonic movements can be prevented by prior administration of a benzodiazepine (midazolam 0.07 mg/kg) or an opioid (fentanyl 1 to 2 μg/kg). Suppression of cortisol synthesis by the adrenal glands has been reported after prolonged infusions. The pain on injection can be prevented by prior intravenous injection of 10 mg lidocaine. There may be postoperative nausea and vomiting, which can be alleviated by prophylactic antiemetics (which may, however, delay discharge). While etomidate can be used for outpatient anesthesia, these disadvantages make it unsuitable in most instances.

Ketamine   Ketamine is a phencyclidine derivative that produces a state of sedation, immobility, amnesia, and marked analgesia. This state is known as *dissociative anesthesia*, which is different from the generalized central nervous system depression produced by the other induction agents.[22] Ketamine is extremely lipid soluble, and an intravenous injec-

tion induces anesthesia within 30 to 50 seconds and produces unconsciousness for 10 to 15 minutes. It can also be given intramuscularly. Hallucinations and emergence delirium may occur with a prolonged recovery. It is, therefore, rarely useful in an ambulatory setting.

Midazolam   Midazolam[23] is a water-soluble benzodiazepine with a rapid onset (distribution half-life 7 to 15 minutes) and short duration of action (elimination half-life about 2.5 hours). Midazolam used for induction of anesthesia in outpatients is associated with a slower onset of action, a more prolonged recovery period, and a higher incidence of postoperative amnesia than thiopental[24] and methohexital. Midazolam is most useful when used as an anxiolytic and amnesic agent. Amnesia may persist for a variable time after administration, especially after the larger doses required for induction of anesthesia. This can be a problem as patients, especially the elderly, may not be able to recall postoperative instructions.

Flumazenil is a specific benzodiazepine antagonist. It has been shown to reverse midazolam sedation and may prove to be useful in modifying the effects of midazolam.[25]

Propofol Propofol is an extremely lipid-soluble phenol derivative, virtually insoluble in water, and formulated in a white, aqueous emulsion. It is supplied in ampules containing 200 mg propofol in 20 ml (10 mg/ml). Propofol has a large volume of distribution and is rapidly eliminated via hepatic metabolism. Renal and possibly lung elimination may be involved. This rapid onset and short duration of action has made propofol useful in outpatient anesthesia. There appear to be fewer postoperative adverse effects compared to thiopental and methohexital. Recovery from propofol-induced anesthesia has been found to be significantly faster in comparison in thiopental. In one study, the propofol group was more responsive and able to sit and stand more rapidly than the thiopental patients.[26]

Adverse effects of propofol may include a cardiovascular depression greater than that associated with barbiturate use, especially in hypovolemic patients and in the elderly. Apnea is also more common and lasts longer than with the barbiturates. Pain on injection is common and can be reduced by prior administration of 10 mg lidocaine into a large vein or a fast-running intravenous infusion.

Controlled intravenous infusion of propofol (0.1 to 0.2 mg/kg/min) has been used for maintenance of anesthesia. Best results are obtained by titrating the rate of infusion of propofol to the desired clinical effect rather than using a fixed infusion rate. Reports have shown that propofol infusion for outpatient surgery results in a significantly shorter recovery room stay in comparison to a standard thiopental–isoflurane technique.[27]

Opioid Analgesics

Opioids (Table 11-4) are powerful analgesic drugs that bind to receptors distributed throughout the central nervous system. The use of opioids in general anesthesia has been advocated to reduce the dosage of sedative and inhalational agents perioperatively, and to decrease the need for postoperative pain medication.[28] Opioids appear to allow faster patient recovery after outpatient anesthesia.

Morphine is sometimes used for outpatients, but its 3- to 6-hour half-life can result in prolonged sedation and possible delay in recovery and discharge. Only the potent shorter-acting opioid analgesics fentanyl, alfentanil, and sufentanil are discussed here in relation to their use for outpatient anesthesia.

Fentanyl Fentanyl is a phenylpiperidine approximately 100 times more potent than morphine. It is very lipid soluble and has a rapid onset of action (1 to 2 minutes). After a single dose its duration of action is limited to approximately 20 to 30 minutes by redistribution. Dosages of 1 to 3 μg/kg IV are appropriate for outpatients. Larger bolus doses or infusions may prolong its effects for 2 to 5 hours (in the elderly as long as 9 hours).

A group of outpatients who received intravenous fentanyl and droperidol were compared to a group receiving isoflurane. The fentanyl–droperidol group experienced faster awakening and orientation and decreased need for postoperative analgesics.[28]

Adverse effects of fentanyl include acute respiratory depression with decreased responsiveness to increases in arterial carbon dioxide tension. Delayed respiratory depression may occur, possibly due to sequestration of fentanyl in gastric juice with subsequent reabsorption from the small intestine. Chest wall rigidity may occur after high doses, but is rare after the low doses usually used for outpatient surgery.

Fentanyl Derivatives *Sufentanil* is a potent fentanyl derivative with an analgesic potency 5 to 10 times that of fen-

Table 11-4. Pharmacokinetic Variables of Opioids Often Used in Outpatient Anesthesia

Drug	Relative Potency	Distribution Half-Life (min)	Elimination Half-Life (hr)	Clearance (ml/min)	$V_{d,ss}$ (L)
Fentanyl	100	1–2 (rapid) 10–15 (slow)	3–4	700–900	200–300
Sufentanil	700	1–3 (rapid) 10–15	2–4	600–900	140–200
Alfentanil	15	1–3	1–2	200–500	30–70

$V_{d,ss}$, volume of distribution steady state.
(From Apfelbaum et al,[58] with permission.)

tanyl but with a shorter elimination half-life. This is associated with a more rapid recovery and shorter postanesthesia care unit (PACU) stay when compared to isoflurane, and a decreased postoperative analgesic requirement.[29] Sufentanil has adverse effects similar to fentanyl. The commercially available ampules of sufentanil are produced in the same concentration as fentanyl (50 μg/ml). A useful safety maneuver is, therefore, to dilute each milliliter of sufentanil with saline to 10 ml (= 5 μg sufentanil/ml). The optimal preinduction dose of sufentanil for short outpatient procedures is 10 μg IV with supplemental doses of 5 μg IV given as needed during the operation.[30]

Alfentanil, another synthetic derivative of fentanyl, is 6 to 8 times *less* potent than fentanyl. It has a rapid onset and brief duration of action because of its relatively small volume of distribution and short elimination half-life via rapid redistribution and hepatic metabolism. Alfentanil is used in high doses to induce anesthesia (30 to 50 μg/kg) and in small doses to provide analgesia as part of a "balanced" anesthetic (10 to 20 μg/kg with bolus increments of 5 μg/kg if required). It can also be used by continuous intravenous infusion alone or with nitrous oxide for maintenance of anesthesia. In this case a loading dose of 10 to 30 μg/kg

is followed by 0.5 to 3.0 μg/kg/min titrated to patient response. Coe et al[31] demonstrated that alfentanil administered by infusion rather than intermittent bolus resulted in a 38 percent lower total dose. There was also a decrease in time to ambulation, and no difference in adverse effects between the two techniques.[31] Patients receiving alfentanil have also been noted to recover faster than patients treated with the volatile inhaled anesthetics.[32] Disadvantages associated with the use of alfentanil are similar to those of the other opioids and include ventilatory depression, nausea, vomiting, and chest wall rigidity.

Antagonist Naloxone, an opioid antagonist, will effectively reverse all the effects of all opioids. In low doses (25- to 30-μg increments) naloxone reverses opioid-induced ventilatory depression without clinically affecting pain relief. Adverse effects of naloxone include termination of analgesia, precipitation of withdrawal symptoms in opioid-dependent subjects, dysrhythmias, hypertension, and pulmonary edema.

Muscle Relaxants

Some degree of mild muscle relaxation is obtained from modern inhalational agents and may be adequate for most orthopedic procedures. Neuromuscular blockade may have to be employed to facilitate tracheal intubation. Another advantage of using muscle relaxants is to obtain optimal surgical conditions while reducing the doses of other anesthetic agents. This results in more rapid patient recovery and earlier discharge.

Succinylcholine Succinylcholine, a depolarizing muscle relaxant, has remained in wide use because of its rapid onset of action (±30 seconds when given intravenously, usual dose 0.5 to 1.0 mg/kg) and short duration of action (3 to 5 minutes). It is rapidly hydrolyzed by plasma cholinesterase. Its main use is to facilitate endotracheal intubation, particularly for those at risk of pulmonary aspiration (e.g., patients with a hiatal hernia, pregnancy, or obesity). As with all muscle relaxants, a nerve stimulator should be available to monitor the effects of the drug. This will detect the uncommon patient with plasma cholinesterase deficiency or abnormality that impairs succinylcholine hydrolysis and prolongs the neuromuscular blockade. It will also detect the development of phase II block after repeated boluses or by prolonged infusion.

Succinylcholine is the most potent triggering agent of malignant hyperthermia in susceptible patients. The incidence of this condition is higher in children than adults; therefore many anesthesia care providers prefer not to use succinylcholine in children unless no other option is available. A treatment protocol for malignant hyperthermia, cooling equipment, and dantrolene should be available for immediate use in all areas where general anesthesia is administered. The address of the Malignant Hyperthermia Association of the United States (MHAUS) is MHAUS, P.O. Box 3231, Darien, CT 06820. A hotline is available at (209) 634-4917 for emergency consultations at any time.

Postfasciculation muscle pains can be significant after succinylcholine, especially in muscular patients, females, and in outpatients who are encouraged to ambulate soon after their surgery. The incidence of these myalgias is reduced if a small-dose "pretreatment" of a nondepolarizing muscle relaxant (e.g., *d*-tubocurarine 0.05 mg/kg) is given 5 minutes before the succinylcholine.

Succinylcholine may cause potassium release in paraplegic or spastic patients and those who have certain peripheral neuropathies, burns, or extensive muscle trauma. This hyperkalemia may cause cardiac dysrhythmias or arrest. Succinylcholine itself can cause bradycardia and even asystolic cardiac arrest via a vagal mechanism in children given repeated doses. This response can be prevented by pretreatment with atropine or glycopyrrolate. Increases in intragastric, intracranial, and intraocular pressure related to striated muscle fasciculation can occur after succinylcholine administration and may be prevented by pretreatment with a nondepolarizing relaxant, as above.

Nondepolarizing Muscle Relaxants *Mivicurium* is a short-acting, nondepolarizing neuromuscular blocking agent, whose action is terminated by rapid plasma cholinesterase hydrolysis. Ideal conditions for intubation after a dose of 0.2 to 0.25 mg/kg IV are usually reached 2.5 minutes after injection, with spontaneous recovery occurring in about 30 minutes. The short duration of action of mivacurium may be useful for outpatient anesthesia, but it is not superior to succinylcholine for rapid intubation in emergency situations. Mivacurium's mild histamine-releasing effects can result in a decrease in blood pressure, but this effect can be minimized by giving the drug slowly over 1 minute. Mivacurium infusion produces a similar degree of neuromuscular blockade as vecuronium; however, recovery time is significantly faster.

Atracurium is an intermediate-acting nondepolarizing neuromuscular blocking agent. The ED_{95} (dose required to produce 95 percent twitch height suppression) is 0.2 mg/kg, which lasts 30 to 45 minutes. Intubation requires doses of 0.5 mg/kg. Recovery of 95 percent twitch height occurs in 50 to 70 minutes. Atracurium is spontaneously inactivated by Hofmann elimination and ester hydrolysis, with an elimination half-life of about 20 minutes. It is, therefore, useful in outpatient procedures lasting longer than 20 minutes. As atracurium lacks cumulative effects, it can be given by continuous infusion.[33] Histamine release can occur, but atracurium rarely causes hypotension if doses less than 0.5 mg/kg are used. Volatile anesthetics augment the neuromuscular blockade produced by atracurium.

Vecuronium, another intermediate-acting nondepolarizing neuromuscular blocking drug, is an analog of the longer-acting steroid relaxant pancuronium. ED_{95} is 0.05 mg/kg, and the duration of action is approximately 30 minutes. A dose of 0.1 mg/kg produces good conditions for intubation within 3 minutes with approximately 45 minutes duration of action.

Inhalational Anesthetics

Three volatile inhalational agents (halothane, enflurane, and isoflurane) and one gas (nitrous oxide) are in general use as inhalational anesthetics. Standard anesthetic texts provide full information on these agents, but some comments on the use of inhalational anesthetics for outpatients follow.

Nitrous oxide is a gas with a low solubility (blood-gas partition coefficient 0.47) resulting in a rapid uptake and elimination from the body via the lungs. However, it has been associated with an increased incidence of postoperative nausea and vomiting. This might delay discharge after outpatient surgery. However, a recent randomized prospective study found no decrease in postoperative emesis when nitrous oxide was omitted from an isoflurane anesthetic technique.[34]

Isoflurane has the lowest blood-gas partition coefficient (1.4) of the three volatile anesthetics. This allows for rapid induction and recovery from anesthesia. Isoflurane's pungency limits its use as an inhalational induction agent for children. Despite this, isoflurane is widely used because of its advantages, which include cardiovascular stability, minimal biotransformation, and rapid recovery from anesthesia.

Desflurane, an isoflurane analog, is a product of recent research into inhalational agents with improved properties. Desflurane has a very low blood-gas partition coefficient (0.42), which should allow for rapid induction of and recovery from anesthesia. While it has a boiling point of 23.5°C and cannot be used in conventional vaporizers, desflurane is chemically stable, undergoes little biometabolism, and has an etheral but not pungent odor. Desflurane may prove to be a useful inhalational agent for outpatient anesthesia.

Regional Anesthesia

Regional anesthetic techniques offer a number of potential advantages when contrasted with general anesthesia for outpatients, but careful patient selection is essential for success (see also Chs. 4, 12, and 13).

Advantages claimed for regional anesthesia for outpatients include the following[35]:

1. Postoperative analgesia–regional anesthetic techniques can block postoperative pain for some hours after

surgery, decreasing the need for analgesics.

2. Recovery time after regional and local anesthesia can be significantly shorter than after general anesthesia and decreased hospital admission after regional anesthesia has also been reported.

3. The incidence of complications sometimes seen after general anesthesia such as nausea and vomiting, "hangover," or impaired coordination and dizziness, as well as sore throat from intubation and muscle pain due to succinylcholine administration, is reduced.

4. The risk of pulmonary aspiration in patients with full stomachs is reduced.

5. General anesthesia can be avoided by those patients who would prefer not to be unconscious during surgery.

6. Immunosuppression is less when compared to general anesthesia and therefore the incidence of postoperative infections may be decreased.[36]

The patient must be adequately informed in advance regarding the technique involved in performing the regional anesthetic block. Possible complications, such as headache after spinal anesthesia, and what to expect in the operating room while the surgery is proceeding must be discussed. It is useful to have a supportive surgeon who will suggest and explain the option of regional anesthesia at the preoperative visit. Significant factors that might limit the use of regional blocks include morbid obesity and rheumatoid arthritis, which may obscure landmarks, making regional anesthesia difficult to perform. Some patients may be unable to maintain a particular position for prolonged periods without added sedation or even general anesthesia. Regional anesthesia may be contraindicated in patients with pre-existing neurologic disease, particularly if unstable. Central neuraxial blocks should be avoided in anticoagulated patients because of the possible risk of subarachnoid or epidural hematoma.

Preoperative medication for adult outpatient regional anesthesia may be indicated to relieve anxiety. As noted above,[14] an anesthesia care provider's preoperative visit may be more effective than sedative administration in reassuring the patient. Intravenous sedatives such as midazolam may be given with a regional block to allay patient anxiety and to decrease discomfort when the block is only partially effective. The resulting increased sedation and amnesia may prolong recovery and delay discharge after the surgery is completed.

Premedication is commonly used for pediatric outpatient surgery, as the ability of children to cooperate during regional anesthesia may be poor. Intramuscular injections should be avoided for administration of premedication to children. Oral sedatives (e.g., diazepam suspension 0.2 to 0.4 mg/kg) have been found useful, and an anticholinergic (e.g., atropine or glycopyrrolate 0.02 mg/kg) can be given by mouth if indicated. Adequate time (1 to 2 hours) must be allowed for these drugs to reach their full effect. Alternatives include giving sedatives rectally (e.g., methohexitol 25 mg/kg of a 10 percent solution) or transmucosal administration of short-acting narcotics (e.g., oral fentanyl "lollipop" 15 to 20 μg/kg, nasal sufentanil 1.5 to 3.0 μg/kg,[37] or nasal or sublingual midazolam 0.2 mg/kg in Hershey's strawberry syrup 5 ml),[38] although published experience with the transmucosal routes of administration is still limited.

Local Infiltration

Local infiltration is often used by surgeons and occasionally by anesthesia care providers for anesthesia prior to removal of superficial lesions or scars and also for

Table 11-5. Doses of Local Anesthetic for Infiltration

Drug	Concentration (%)	Plain Solutions		Solutions With Epinephrine	
		Maximum Adult Dose (mg)	Maximum Dose (mg/kg)	Maximum Adult Dose (mg)	Maximum Dose (mg/kg)
Lidocaine	0.5–1	300	4	500	7
Bupivacaine	0.25–0.5	175	2.5	225	3

hardware removal (e.g., pins). This is a safe technique and intermediate-acting agents such as lidocaine or longer-acting bupivacaine are effective for this purpose.

Table 11-5 gives appropriate doses of local anesthetics used for infiltration.

Toxic reactions to local anesthetics can be avoided by keeping below the maximum recommended dosages for the drug and by carefully avoiding intravascular injection.

Central Neuraxial Blockade

Spinal Anesthesia   Spinal anesthesia offers a number of advantages when used for surgical procedures on the lower extremities. Spinal blocks are quick to perform and result in excellent analgesia and good surgical operating conditions. Onset is rapid and there is high reliability. Postoperative complications such as nausea and vomiting are less common after spinal anesthesia compared to general anesthesia.[39] This is a significant advantage as postoperative nausea and vomiting is an important cause of hospital admission after outpatient anesthesia.[40] Decreased postoperative pain and analgesic requirement is also a useful benefit of spinal anesthesia.

The main drawback to spinal anesthesia for outpatients is post-dural puncture headache (PDPH). The incidence of PDPH has been reported as 18 percent in all outpatients after dural puncture, and 39 percent in patients under 40 years of age despite use of a 26-gauge needle.[41] Variables include patient age, needle size, needle bevel (the conical point's spreading of dural fibers might be less traumatic than the cutting edge of a pointed needle). PDPH can be a significant cause of postoperative disability. Patients need to have a clear explanation of this potential complication during preoperative evaluation. However, a recent study by Dahl et al[39] of patients undergoing arthroscopy of the knee reported a similar incidence of PDPH when comparing a group of patients aged 18 to 49 years who received spinal anesthesia using a 29-gauge spinal needle (11 percent) to a similar group who had the surgery performed under general anesthesia (15 percent). Of note, 96 percent of the patients receiving spinal anesthesia indicated that they would prefer the same anesthetic for a similar procedure in the future. A prudent approach suggested by Charlton[42] is a combination of careful technique, small needles, and restriction of use of spinal anesthesia to older patients (over 50 years). However, should PDPH occur, epidural blood patch is an effective treatment for most patients.

Other potential effects of spinal anesthesia include hypotension and bradycardia due to sympathetic blockade and related to the extent of the spinal block. Patient fear of paralysis or nerve injury should be overcome by an honest discussion of all available options. Prolonged block can occur when long-acting agents such as bupivacaine or tetracaine are used. Urinary retention is common after prolonged spinal anesthesia. Postoperative backache may be minimized by using sufficient local anesthetic infiltration in preparation for the spinal anesthetic, avoiding the periosteum, and using the smallest needle possible.

Agents used for spinal anesthesia for outpatients are listed in Table 11-6.

Lumbar Epidural Anesthesia   Lumbar epidural anesthesia is a useful alternative to spinal or general anesthesia for lower extremity procedures, particularly for knee arthroscopy, in outpatients. It has been reported to provide more rapid ambulation and discharge compared to spinal or general anesthesia, and significantly less postoperative nausea or vomiting compared to general anesthesia.[43] The caudal approach to the epidural space can be considered for surgical procedures on the foot.

Advantages of epidural anesthesia include a gradual onset of action allowing for careful titration of the extent of anesthesia, which will limit the extent of sympathetic blockade hypotension. Catheter techniques, while somewhat more complex, offer the advantage of allowing maintenance of the anesthetic should the surgery last longer than anticipated. The incidence of headache is also significantly lower after epidural anesthesia than after spinal anesthesia.

While PDPH is less frequently encountered after epidural anesthesia, this complication may be seen if inadvertent dural puncture occurs. The well-known complication of inadvertent intravascular or subdural injection of local anesthetic while performing an epidural block can be minimized by careful attention to technique and incremental injection (see Ch. 15).

Recently Levy et al[44] have reported back pain after chloroprocaine was used for epidural anesthesia in outpatients undergoing knee arthroscopy. This may be a contraindication to the use of chloroprocaine.

Local anesthetics used for outpatient epidural anesthesia are listed in Table 11-7.

Peripheral Nerve Block

Brachial plexus blockade is frequently suitable for orthopedic procedures on the upper extremity. Axillary block is safe and effective for procedures on the hand and forearm. A low incidence of complications and high success rate using a variety of techniques was found in a recent Mayo Clinic survey.[45] Surgery on the elbow or shoulder is best managed by subclavian brachial plexus block. How-

Table 11-6.   Local Anesthetics Used for Spinal Anesthesia

Agent	Concentration	Usual Adult Dose	Baricity	Usual Duration (min)
Lidocaine	5% in 7.5% glucose	50–100 mg (1–2 ml)	Hyperbaric	45–80
	2%	40–60 mg (2–3 ml)	Isobaric	60–100
Bupivacaine	0.75% in 8.25% glucose	9–15 mg (1.2–2 ml)	Hyperbaric	90–240
	0.5%	15 mg (3 ml)	Isobaric	90–240
Tetracaine	0.5% in 5% glucose	10–20 mg (2–4 ml)	Hyperbaric	150–300
	0.5%	10–20 mg (2–4 ml)	Isobaric	
	0.1%	10 mg (10 ml)	Hypobaric	

Table 11-7. Local Anesthetics Used for Epidural Anesthesia

| Agent | Concentration (%) | Maximum Adult Dose | | Duration (min) |
		Plain Solution	With Epinephrine	
Chloroprocaine	2–3	≤800 mg (40 ml 2%)	≤900 mg (30 ml 3%)	30–75
Lidocaine	1–2	≤300 mg (30 ml 1%)	≤500 mg (50 ml 1%)	50–120
Mepivacaine	1–2	≤300 mg (30 ml 1%)	≤500 mg (50 ml 1%)	60–150
Bupivacaine	0.25–0.75	≤175 mg (35 ml 0.5%)	≤225 mg (45 ml 0.5%)	120–240

ever, the potential complication of pneumothorax (which can be delayed for some hours) may make this an inappropriate block for outpatients. Interscalene block is effective for shoulder or upper arm surgery and is useful for reduction of a dislocated shoulder. However, the ulnar nerve distribution to the elbow and hand may be missed with this block. Complications of interscalene block include central neuraxial blockade via the epidural or subarachnoid space, pneumothorax, recurrent laryngeal block (resulting in hoarseness), cervical sympathetic nerve block (leading to Horner syndrome), and convulsions after vertebral artery injection.

Patients must be warned to protect the anesthetized limb until full sensation has returned, and may need to be supplied with a padded sling until sensation and motor control have returned.

Bier block (intravenous regional block) is useful for procedures lasting 1 hour or less on the forearm or hand. It is a reliable technique that results in rapid onset of anesthesia with rapid recovery after tourniquet deflation. The main complication is related to inadvertent premature release of the tourniquet with resultant loss of the anesthetic and potential systemic toxicity.

Lower extremity blocks can be used for outpatients and to avoid the complications noted for central neuraxial blockade; however, nerve blocks of the leg wear off unpredictably and may delay the patient's ability to ambulate for 24 to 72 hours.

Ankle block is a useful technique for operations on the foot,[46] especially procedures on the sole of the foot, which is a very sensitive area but difficult and painful to infiltrate with local anesthetic.

Table 11-8 lists local anesthetics used for outpatient peripheral nerve blocks (epinephrine-containing solutions should not be used in the hand, foot, or penis because of the risk of ischemia).

Regional anesthetic techniques are finding increasing application in children. They may be conveniently administered after induction of general anesthesia. This combination will allow a lighter plane of general anesthesia to be used, with the advantages for outpatients of quicker recovery from general anesthesia and excellent pain relief postoperatively. The regional anesthetic techniques commonly used for orthopedic procedures in children are axillary blocks and intravenous regional (Bier) block for upper limb surgery, and femoral, sciatic, and peripheral nerve blocks at the knee or ankle for lower limb surgery. Caudal and epidural central neuraxial blocks may be used for orthopedic procedures on the pelvic girdle and lower extremities. Peripheral nerve blocks are safely used in children presenting for muscle biopsy to determine susceptibility to malignant hyperthermia. Wedel[47] found that femoral and lateral femoral cutaneous nerve block was well accepted by parents, surgeons,

Table 11-8. Local Anesthetics Used for Peripheral Nerve Blocks

Agent	Concentration (%)	Plain Solution (Adult Doses)	With Epinephrine	Duration (min)
Chloroprocaine	2–3	≤800 mg (40 ml 2%)	≤1000 mg (50 ml 1%)	30–75
Lidocaine	1–2	≤300 mg (30 ml 1%)	≤500 mg (50 ml 1%)	50–120
Mepivacaine	1–2	≤300 mg (30 ml 1%)	≤500 mg (50 ml 1%)	120–300
Bupivacaine	0.25–0.5	≤175 mg (35 ml 0.5%)	≤225 mg (45 ml 0.5%)	300–720

and the children undergoing muscle biopsy as outpatients, with moderate sedation facilitating the placement of the block. There have been a number of recent reviews on the subject of regional anesthesia for pediatric patients,[48,49] confirming our view that it is a safe and effective technique.

RECOVERY AND DISCHARGE

Unexpected hospital admission after outpatient surgery is usually related to the surgery itself (e.g., prolonged surgery, need for overnight observation) or after complications such as excessive bleeding. Admission can also be needed for anesthesia-related complications such as severe postoperative pain, persistent nausea or vomiting, and excessive sedation. Exacerbation of pre-existing medical problems such as asthma, diabetes, or angina pectoris may also require admission.

Postoperative Pain Management

As mentioned above, regional anesthetic techniques have the advantage of extending anesthesia into the postoperative period and decreasing the need for recovery room narcotic administration (see also Ch. 15). Local or regional nerve blocks are an option for controlling postoperative pain. Administration of fentanyl or other opioids during the perioperative period can decrease the need for inhalational agents for surgery. This may result in decreased sedation, quicker recovery, and decreased analgesic requirement in the PACU. The use of short-acting opioids such as fentanyl is also effective in treating pain in the PACU. By the time of discharge, pain should be controlled by the use of oral analgesics such as acetaminophen and/or codeine, and/or nonsteroidal anti-inflammatory analgesics. Hospital admission may be needed for further pain management.

Ketorolac[50] is a recently released potent nonsteroidal anti-inflammatory analgesic that acts by inhibiting prostaglandin synthesis. It is given parenterally and does not have any of the disadvantages of opioids (e.g., respiratory depression). Doses of 30 and 60 mg ketorolac have analgesic efficacy equal or superior to 12 mg morphine and last longer than the morphine. Adverse effect of ketorolac include gastrointestinal disturbance (pain, nausea, and gastritis in 3 to 9 percent of patients), edema, somnolence, and dizziness. Inhibition of platelet aggregation occurs. However, ketorolac is also considerably more expensive than morphine or fentanyl at present.

Excessive postoperative sedation is usually related to the drugs used for anesthesia. As noted earlier, a disadvantage of anxiolytics prior to surgery is prolonged drowsiness, which may delay discharge. Impaired psychomotor and cognitive function has been found after the use of long-acting drugs such as diazepam and meperidine in patients discharged from the hospital.[16] Newer intravenous induction agents such as propofol, which can be given by infusion, are useful for outpatient anesthesia. Recovery to readiness for discharge is faster than propofol than after inhalational agents.[27]

Nausea and vomiting can delay discharge after surgery. They do not often result in hospital admission after outpatient surgery.[51] Nausea is often related to postoperative pain and is often relieved when the pain is controlled. Droperidol in low doses (0.25 to 0.5 mg IV) is an effective antiemetic that does not delay recovery or discharge home. Droperidol 20 μg/kg has been recommended as the optimal antiemetic dose that did not prolong recovery time due to excessive sedation.[52]

Discharge Criteria

Minimal criteria for safe discharge have been recommended by Korttila[59]:

1. Vital signs must have been stable for at least 1 hour.
2. Patients must have no evidence of respiratory depression.
3. Patients must be
   Oriented to person, place and time
   Able to ingest oral fluids without nausea or vomiting
   Able to void
   Able to dress unassisted
   Able to walk without assistance
4. Patients must not have
   More than minimal nausea or vomiting
   Excessive pain
   Bleeding
5. Patients must be discharged both by the person who gave anesthesia and performed surgery or by their designees. Written instructions for the postoperative period at home, including a contact place and person, need to be reinforced.
6. Patients must have a responsible "vested" adult to escort them home and to stay with them at home.

The same discharge criteria required for patients recovering from general anesthesia must be met by patients recovering from regional anesthesia. Pflug et al[53] developed criteria for safe ambulation after subarachnoid block that could be also applied after epidural block:

1. Return of pinprick sensation in the perianal area (S4-S5)
2. Plantar flexion of the foot (while supine) at preanesthetic levels of strength
3. Return of big toe proprioception
4. The patient is not hypovolemic or sedated
5. The patient is able to void

High doses of local anesthetics can impair psychomotor skills for a number of hours. Lidocaine (200 mg) impaired the psychomotor skills of volunteers, while 500 mg with epinephrine did not result in similar impairment.[54] While such effects would usually not delay discharge, it is essential for the practitioner to be aware of these subtle effects of local anesthetics.

Psychomotor impairment after general anesthesia and regional anesthesia with sedation led to the recommendation that patients should refrain from activities requiring mental alertness such as driving a car or operating machinery. If the duration of anesthesia was less than 30 minutes, a 24-hour recovery period is recommended, and for anesthesia lasting 2 hours or more, patients should be advised not to drive for 48 hours.[55] Documentation that the patient was carefully assessed prior to discharge is essential. Litigation occurred when, after falling and sustaining a fracture while unaccompanied, a patient was judged to have been prematurely discharged.[56]

Anesthesia care providers have responded to the challenge presented by the increased demand for outpatient surgery with flexibility and imagination. Ongoing research and refinement of technique promise continuing improvement in professional anesthetic care that will be offered to the outpatient in the future.

REFERENCES

1. Nicholl JH: The surgery of infancy. Br Med J 2:753, 1909
2. Henderson J: Ambulatory surgery: past, present and future. p. 11. In Wetchler BV (ed): Anesthesia for Ambulatory Surgery. JB Lippincott, Philadelphia, 1985
3. White PF: Outpatient anesthesia—an overview. p. 1. In White PF (ed): Outpatient Anesthesia. Churchill Livingstone, New York, 1990
4. Orkin T: Economic and regulatory issues. p. 87. In White P (ed): Outpatient Anesthesia. Churchill Livingstone, New York, 1990
5. Bloom BS, Krueger N: Cost and quality effects of outpatient cataract removal. Inquiry 25:383, 1988
6. Kitz DS, Slusarz-Ladden C, Lecky JH: Hospital resources used for inpatient and ambulatory surgery. Anesthesiology 69:383, 1988
7. Pineault R, Contandriopoulos AP, Valois M et al: Randomized clinical trial of one-day surgery: patient satisfaction, clinical outcome, and costs. Med Care 23:171, 1985
8. Kaplan EB, Sheiner LB, Boeckmann AJ et al: The usefulness of preoperative laboratory screening. JAMA 253:3576, 1985
9. Roizen MF, Kaplan EB, Schreider BD et al: The relative roles of the history and physical examination, and laboratory testing in preoperative evaluation for outpa-

tient surgery: the "Starling Curve" of preoperative laboratory testing. Anesthesiol Clin North Am 5:15, 1987
10. Wilson ME, Williams NB, Baskett PJF et al: Assessment of fitness for surgical procedures and the variability of anaesthetists' judgments. Br Med J 280:509, 1980
11. Welborn LG, Ramirez N, Oh TH et al: Postanesthetic apnea and periodic breathing in infants. Anesthesiology 65:658, 1986
12. Maltby JR, Sutherland AD, Sale JP, Shaffer EA: Preoperative oral fluids: is a five-hour fast justified prior to elective surgery? Anesth Analg 65:1112, 1986
13. Shevde K, Trivedi N: Effects of clear liquids on gastric volume and pH in healthy volunteers. Anesth Analg 72:528, 1991
14. Egbert LD, Battit GE, Turndorf H, Beecher HK: The value of the preoperative visit by an anesthetist. JAMA 185:553, 1963
15. Jakobsen H, Hertz JB, Johansen JR et al: Premedication before day surgery: a double-blind comparison of diazepam and placebo. Br J Anaesth 57:300, 1985
16. Korttila K, Linnoila M: Psychomotor skills related to driving after intramuscular administration of diazepam and meperidine. Anesthesiology 42:685, 1975
17. Reinhart K, Dallinger-Stiller G, Dennhardt R et al: Comparison of midazolam, diazepam and placebo IM as premedication for regional anesthesia: a randomized double-blind study. Br J Anaesth 57:294, 1985
18. Rita L, Goodarzi M, Seleny F: Effect of low dose droperidol on postoperative vomiting in children. Can Anaesth Soc J 28:259, 1981
19. Dewan DM, Floyd HM, Thistlewood JM et al: Sodium citrate pretreatment in elective cesarean section patients. Anesth Analg 64:34, 1985
20. Rao TLK, Suseela M, El-Etr AA: Metoclopramide and cimetidine to reduce gastric juice pH volume. Anesth Analg 63:264, 1984
21. Korttila K, Linnoila M, Ertama P, Hakkinen S: Recovery and stimulated driving after intravenous anesthesia with thiopental, methohexital, propanidid or alphadione. Anesthesiology 43:291, 1975

22. Reich DL, Silvay G: Ketamine: an update on the first twenty-five years of clinical experience. Can J Anaesth 36:186, 1989

23. Richter JJ: Current theories about the mechanisms of benzodiazepines and neuroleptic drugs. Anesthesiology 54:66, 1981

24. Fragen RJ: The uses of midazolam. Anesthesiol Rev 12:29, 1986

25. Alon E, Baitella L, Hossil G: Double-blind study of the reversal of midazolam-supplemented general anesthesia with RO15-1788. Br J Anaesth 59:455, 1987

26. MacKensie N, Grant IS: Propofol for intravenous sedation. Anaesthesia 42:3, 1987

27. Korttila K, Faure E, Apfelbaum J et al: Recovery from propofol versus thiopental/isoflurane in patients undergoing outpatient anesthesia. Anesthesiology 69:A564, 1988

28. Pollard J: Clinical evaluation of intravenous vs inhalational anesthesia in the ambulatory surgical unit: a multicenter study. Curr Therap Res 36:617, 1984

29. Zuurmond WWA, van Leeuwen L: Recovery from sufentanil anaesthesia for outpatient arthroscopy: a comparison with isoflurane. Acta Anaesthesiol Scand 31:154, 1987

30. White PF, Sung ML, Doze VA: Use of sufentanil in outpatient anesthesia—determining an optimal preinduction dose. Anesthesiology 63:A202, 1985

31. Coe V, Shafer A, White PF: Techniques for administering alfentanil during outpatient anesthesia: a comparison with fentanyl. Anesthesiology 59:A347, 1983

32. Zuurmond WWA, van Leeuwen L: Alfentanil vs. isoflurane for outpatient arthroscopy. Acta Anaesthesiol Scand 30:329, 1986

33. Shanks CA: Pharmacokinetics of the nondepolarizing neuromuscular relaxants applied to calculation of bolus and infusion dosage regimens. Anesthesiology 64:72, 1986

34. Korttila K, Hovorka J, Erkola O: Omission of nitrous oxide does not decrease the incidence or severity of emetic symptoms after isoflurane anesthesia. Anesth Analg 66:S98, 1987

35. Bridenbaugh LD: Regional anaesthesia for outpatient surgery. A summary of 12 years experience. Can Anaesth Soc J 30:548, 1983

36. Edwards AE, Gemmell LW, Mankin PP et al: The effects of three differing anaesthetics on the immune response. Anaesthesia 39:1071, 1984

37. Henderson JM, Brodsky DA, Fisher DM et al: Pre-induction of anesthesia in pediatric patients with nasally administered sufentanil. Anesthesiology 68:671, 1988

38. Wilton NCT, Leigh J, Rosen DR, Pandit UA: Preanesthetic sedation of preschool children using intranasal midazolam. Anesthesiology 69:972, 1988

39. Dahl JB, Schultz P, Anker-Moller E et al: Spinal anaesthesia in young patients using a 29-gauge needle: technical considerations and an evaluation of postoperative complaints compared with general anaesthesia. Br J Anaesth 64:178, 1990

40. Gold BS, Kitz DS, Lecky JH, Neuhaus JM: Unanticipated admission to the hospital following ambulatory surgery. JAMA 262:3008, 1989

41. Clarke GA, Power KJ: Spinal anaesthesia for day case surgery. Ann R Coll Surg Engl 70:144, 1988

42. Charlton JE: Local anaesthesia for day stay surgery. p. 697. In Healy TEJ (ed): Anaesthesia for Day Case Surgery. Vol. 4. No. 3. Bailliere Tindall, London, 1990

43. Randel GI, Levy L, Kothary SP et al: Epidural anesthesia is superior to spinal or general for outpatient knee arthroscopy. Anesthesiology 71:A769, 1989

44. Levy L, Randel GI, Pandit SK: Does chloroprocaine (Nesacaine MPF) for epidural anesthesia increase the incidence of blockade? Anesthesiology 71:476, 1989

45. Davis WJ, Lennon RL, Wedel DJ: Brachial plexus anesthesia for outpatient surgical procedures on an upper extremity. Mayo Clin Proc 66:470, 1991

46. Schurman DJ: Ankle-block anesthesia for foot surgery. Anesthesiology 44:348, 1976

47. Wedel DJ: Femoral and lateral femoral cutaneous nerve block for muscle biopsies in children. Reg Anesth 14:63, 1989

48. Dalens B: Regional anesthesia in children. Anesth Analg 68:654, 1989

49. Yaster M, Maxwell LG: Pediatric regional anesthesia. Anesthesiology 70:324, 1989

50. Litvak K, McEvoy GK: Ketorolac, an injectable nonnarcotic analgesic. Clin Pharm 9:921, 1990

51. Kortilla K: Practical discharge criteria. Prob Anesth 2:144, 1988

52. Pandit SK, Kothary SP, Pandit UA et al: Dose-response study of droperidol and metoclopramide as antiemetics for outpatient anesthesia. Anesth Analg 68:798, 1989

53. Pflug AE, Aasheim GM, Foster C: Sequence of return of neurological function and criteria for safe ambulation following subarachnoid block (spinal anaesthetic). Can Anaesth Soc J 25:133, 1978

54. Korttila K: Psychomotor skills related to driving after intramuscular lidocaine. Acta Anaesthesiol Scand 18:290, 1974

55. Korttila K: How to assess recovery from outpatient anesthesia. p. 16. In Barash PG (ed): ASA Refresher Courses in Anesthesiology. Vol. 16. JB Lippincott, Philadelphia, 1988

56. Montedonico J, Tazzara PM: Legal considerations of outpatient anesthesia. Anesthesiol Clin North Am 5:227, 1987

57. Roisen M, Rupani G: Preoperative assessment of adult outpatients. p. 181. In White P (ed): Outpatient Anesthesia. Churchill Livingstone, New York, 1990

58. Apfelbaum JL, Kallar SK, Wetchler BV: Adult and geriatric patients. p. 214. In Wetchler BV (ed): Anesthesia for Ambulatory Surgery. JB Lippincott, Philadelphia, 1991

59. Korttila K: Recovery from day case anaesthesia. p. 715. In Healy TEJ (ed): Anaesthesia for Day Case Surgery. Vol. 4. No. 3. Balliere Tindall, London, 1990

12

Peripheral Nerve Blocks*

Denise J. Wedel

Orthopedic surgical procedures are especially well-suited to regional anesthetic techniques. Peripheral nerve blocks are often considered to be the best anesthetic choice for procedures limited to the extremities. Contraindications are few, complications are relatively rare when good technique and reasonable precautions are employed, and excellent surgical anesthesia and postoperative analgesia without major organ system involvement are provided.

Techniques for peripheral nerve blockade can be traced to the earliest history of regional anesthesia. Halstead and Hall, American surgeons in the late 1800s, described injection of cocaine for the purpose of surgical anesthesia into a variety of peripheral sites, including the ulnar, musculocutaneous, supratrochlear, and infraorbital nerves.[1,2] Use of a tourniquet to arrest blood flow, thus prolonging the anesthetic blockade, was described by Corning in 1885[3]; in 1903 Braun[4] reported the use of epinephrine as a "chemical tourniquet" to accomplish a similar purpose. Braun also introduced the term *conduction anesthesia* in his 1905 textbook on local anesthesia that describes a wide variety of regional anesthetic techniques.[5]

Though the initial history of regional anesthesia primarily involved surgeons, the organization of anesthesiology as a specialty resulted in major new developments in the pharmacology of local anesthetics as well as their practical application. These advances were aided by the introduction of the anesthesia record, credited to Sydney Ormand Goldan,[6] who designed an intraoperative chart for recording the effects of "intraspinal cocainization." The French anesthetist, Gaston Labat, author of the famous text on regional anesthesia bearing his name, was another early pioneer in this field. His influence extended to North America following his acceptance of William Mayo's invitation to lecture at the Mayo Clinic in the 1920s.

Peripheral nerve block techniques are a well-accepted part of the anesthetic management of orthopedic procedures. These techniques can be applied to all age groups, and are particularly useful in patients with multisystem disease processes, who may be at increased risk of complications from general anesthesia. Orthopedic surgeons are generally cognizant of the benefits of nerve blocks in their patient population, and are often enthusiastic in their preparation of the pa-

* Modified from Wedel and Brown,[47] with permission.

tient prior to the anesthetic preoperative evaluation. Patients, too, are more sophisticated in their approach to anesthetic care, and are usually open to discussions concerning the relative advantages of this form of anesthetic management. The additional benefits of postoperative analgesia, particularly in the continuously expanding outpatient population, provide an added incentive for offering these techniques as part of the anesthesia care provider's armamentarium. Familiarity with the available pharmacologic agents, new techniques and alternatives, and attendant side effects or complications is an important aspect of providing appropriate anesthetic care to the orthopedic patient population.

UPPER EXTREMITY BLOCKS

Peripheral nerve blocks of the upper extremities are a mainstay of the orthopedic anesthesia care provider's technical armamentarium. Successful neural blockade of the upper extremity requires extensive anatomic knowledge of the brachial plexus, from its origin as the roots emerge from the intervertebral foramina to its eventual termination in the distal peripheral nerves of the hand. Detailed anatomic knowledge enables the anesthesia care provider to choose the appropriate technique for the intended surgical procedure, and salvage "inadequate" blocks with appropriate supplementation. Without a mastery of the anatomy, luck rather than skill will be the primary determinant of successful neural blockade. Also important is a knowledge of the side effects and complications of peripheral nerve blocks in the upper extremity as well as the clinical application of available local anesthetics for these blocks. Fi-

nally, one must not underestimate the role of appropriate sedation during placement of the block as well as during the surgical procedure. Many a "perfect" regional anesthetic technique has been undone by inadequate management of sedation.

Anatomy

The brachial plexus derives from the anterior primary rami of the fifth, sixth, seventh, and eighth cervical and the first thoracic nerves, with variable contributions from the fourth cervical and second thoracic nerves.

On leaving the intervertebral foramina, these nerves course anterolaterally and inferiorly to lie between the anterior and middle scalene muscles. The phrenic nerve lies in close approximation to the plexus in its position over the anterior scalene muscle, thus explaining its vulnerability to blockade during interscalene techniques. The anterior scalene muscle arises from the anterior tubercles of the cervical vertebrae and passes caudad and laterally to insert onto the scalene tubercle of the first rib. The middle scalene muscle, arising from the posterior tubercles of the cervical vertebrae, inserts onto the first rib posterior to the subclavian artery, which passes between these two scalene muscles within the subclavian groove. Both the anterior and middle scalene muscles are invested with prevertebral fascia, which fuses laterally to enclose the brachial plexus within a fascial sheath at the level of the neck.

The nerve *roots* making up the brachial plexus form three *trunks* as they course between the scalene muscles, the superior (C5-C6), middle (C7), and inferior (C8-T1). These trunks leave the interscalene groove to lie cephaloposterior to the subclavian artery as it courses along the first rib. This cephaloposterior orientation is in contrast to the inaccurate, but common, depiction of the trunks of the brachial plexus lying in a horizontal formation along the first rib. At the lateral edge of the rib, each trunk forms anterior and posterior *divisions*, which pass below the midportion of the clavicle to enter the axilla. Once in the axilla, the divisions form the medial, lateral, and posterior *cords*, named according to their positional relationship to the second part of the axillary artery. The medial cord is a continuation of the anterior division of the inferior trunk, the lateral cord derives from the superior divisions of the superior and middle trunks, and the inferior divisions from all three trunks form the posterior cord.

The three cords divide into the peripheral *nerves* of the upper extremity at the lateral border of the pectoralis minor muscle. The medial cord gives rise to the medial head of the median nerve, as well as the ulnar, medial antebrachial, and medial brachial cutaneous nerves; the lateral cord gives rise to the lateral head of the median nerve and the musculocutaneous nerve; and the posterior cord divides into the axillary and radial nerves (Fig. 12-1).

Several other nerves arise as branches from the roots of the brachial plexus and provide innervation to nearby anatomic structures. These include the branches providing motor innervation to the rhomboid muscles (C5), the subclavian muscles (C5-C6), and the serratus anterior muscle (C5–C7). The suprascapular nerve (C5-C6) innervates the dorsal aspect of the scapula as well as provides a significant contribution to the sensory supply of the shoulder joint. These

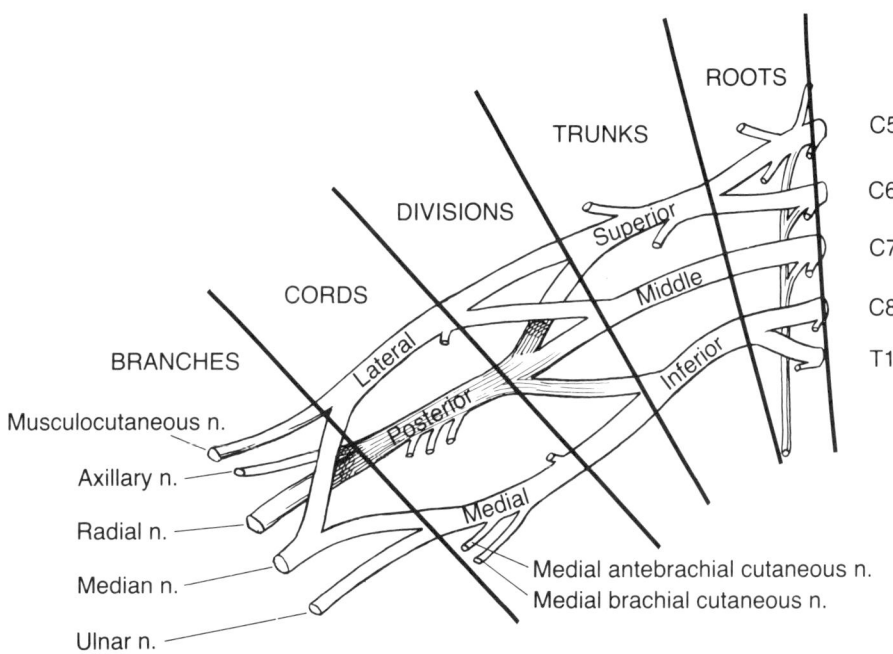

Fig. 12-1. Roots, trunks, divisions, cords, and branches of the brachial plexus. (From Wedel & Brown,[47] with permission.)

branches may be blocked with the inter-scalene approach to the brachial plexus, but are not reliably anesthetized with more caudal approaches. Sensory distributions of the cervical roots and peripheral nerves of the upper extremity are shown in Figure 12-2.

Knowledge of the neuroanatomy must be supplemented by familiarity with adjacent soft tissue structures in order to safely and reliably perform regional anesthesia. The brachial plexus courses between the anterior and middle scalene muscles, lying superior and posterior to the second and third parts of the subclavian artery. The dome of the pleura lies anteromedial to the inferior trunk. Other structures will be discussed in relation to the specific approaches to the brachial plexus.

Brachial Plexus Blocks

Interscalene Block

Clinical Applications The interscalene approach to the brachial plexus is best suited to surgery on the shoulder in which a block of the cervical plexus is also desirable. While this approach can be used for forearm and hand surgery, blockade of the inferior trunk (C8-T1) is often incomplete, requiring supplementation at the ulnar nerve for adequate surgical anesthesia in that distribution. This block is technically easy because necessary landmarks can be readily palpated and can be performed with the arm in any position, which is an advantage in cases involving upper extremity trauma or other painful conditions.[7] Use of a nerve

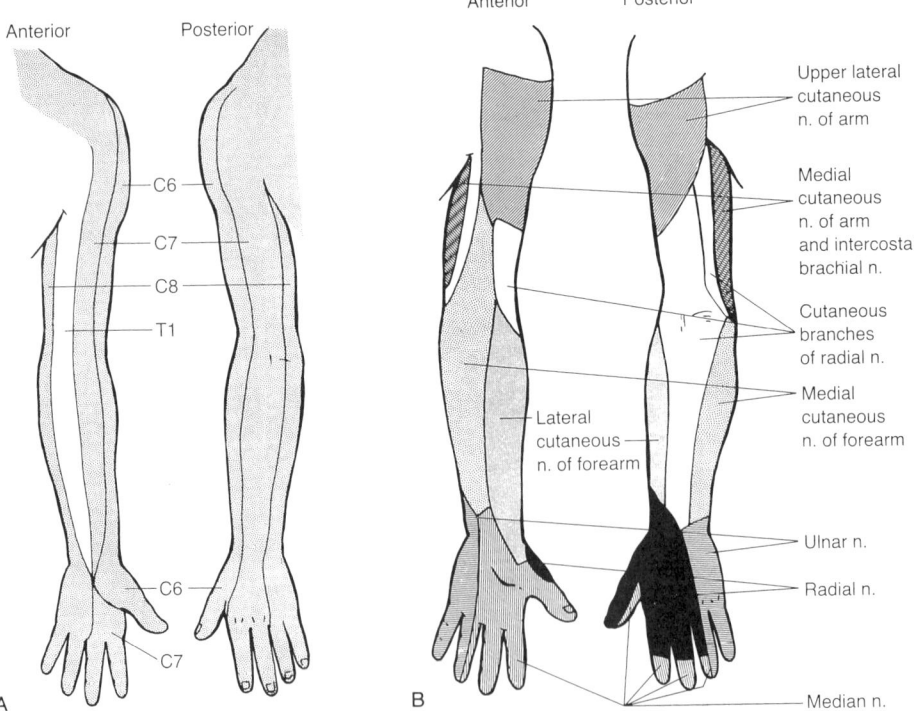

Fig. 12-2. (A) Cutaneous distribution of the cervical roots. (B) Cutaneous distribution of the peripheral nerves. (From Wedel & Brown,[47] with permission.)

stimulator or elicitation of paresthesias is recommended with this technique in order to place the local anesthetic solution accurately. The risk of pneumothorax is low when the needle is correctly placed at the C5 or C6 level because of the distance from the dome of the pleura.

This approach is ideally suited for management of postoperative pain after shoulder surgery. The block can be performed prior to surgery, thus providing surgical anesthesia as well, or may be placed in the recovery room after the patient has awakened from general anesthesia. The latter approach may be desirable in cases in which the surgical approach involves neurologic risk to the brachial plexus (e.g., total shoulder replacements). In such cases, the surgical service should ascertain and document that no neurologic damage has occurred before the block is performed.

Side Effects/Complications   Nerve damage or neuritis can occur secondary to needle trauma or pharmacologic toxicity, but is uncommon and usually self-limited. Local anesthetic toxicity as a result of intravascular injection should be guarded against by careful aspiration and incremental injection. Seizure activity secondary to this complication is particularly undesirable in a patient with a newly repaired rotator cuff, which can theoretically be undone by the associated muscular activity.

The phrenic nerve is blocked in up to 100 percent of interscalene blocks, probably because of its anatomic proximity on the anterior surface of the anterior scalene muscle.[8] While this is usually not associated with significant symptoms, the patient may complain of subjective shortness of breath. Pneumothorax, while rare with this approach, should be considered whenever dyspnea is observed following a block performed in the neck or thorax region. Patients with compromised re-

spiratory function may have more severe symptoms and should be observed carefully for respiratory failure. Most patients will feel subjectively improved in the sitting position. Bilateral blocks at the interscalene level are contraindicated.

Involvement of the vagus, recurrent laryngeal, and cervical sympathetic nerves is rarely significant, but the patient experiencing symptoms related to these side effects may require reassurance. Epidural and intrathecal injections have been reported during interscalene block; maintaining a caudad needle angle is an important preventive measure.

Technique   With the patient in the supine position, the head is turned away from the side to be blocked. The lateral border of the sternocleidomastoid muscle is palpated and marked; identification is facilitated by having the patient lift the head briefly. The interscalene groove may be palpated by rolling the fingers posterolaterally from the muscle border, over the belly of the anterior scalene muscle. In a slender patient, the scalene muscles can sometimes be visualized during a deep breath, which recruits the accessory muscles of respiration. A line is then extended laterally from the cricoid cartilage to intersect the vertical line of the interscalene groove; this represents the level of the C6 transverse process. The external jugular vein often crosses at this level, but is not a reliable anatomic landmark.

Using sterile precautions, a skin wheal is injected at the described site and a 22-gauge, 4-cm, short-beveled needle is inserted perpendicular to skin at a 45-degree caudad and slightly posterior angle (Fig. 12-3). The needle is advanced until a paresthesia is obtained or, if a nerve stimulator is being used, a motor response is observed in the forearm or hand. The brachial plexus is usually quite superficial in the interscalene area (1 to

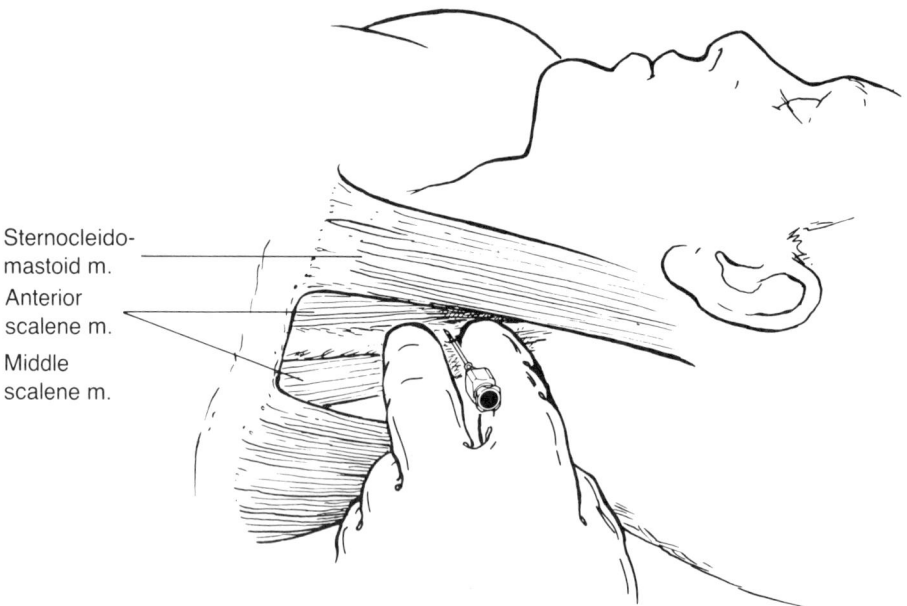

Sternocleido-
mastoid m.

Anterior
scalene m.

Middle
scalene m.

Fig. 12-3. Interscalene block. The fingers palpate the interscalene groove, and the needle is inserted with a caudad and slightly posterior angle. (From Wedel & Brown,[47] with permission.)

2 cm deep). A "click" may be felt as the blunt needle penetrates the prevertebral fascia, giving another confirmation of accurate needle location. If the needle encounters bone within 2 cm of the skin surface, this is likely the transverse process, and the needle should be gently "walked off" anteriorly. The needle is immobilized when its correct location is confirmed by the methods described above, and following negative aspiration a test dose of the local anesthetic is injected. A length of flexible intravenous tubing between the needle and syringe is helpful in minimizing needle movement during injection. The remainder of the local anesthetic (10 to 40 ml) should be injected incrementally with frequent aspiration. While studies with radiographic dye suggest that injection of 40 ml of solution in this area should be associated with complete anesthesia of the brachial and cervical plexus,[9] clinical reports indicate variable block of the inferior trunk even

with larger volumes.[10] Caudad spread of the local anesthetic may be facilitated by maintaining digital pressure proximal to the injection site and placing the patient in a head-up position during or following blockade. A variety of local anesthetics are suitable for interscalene blockade; the specific choice should take into consideration the duration and intensity of block needed for a given clinical situation.

Supraclavicular Block

Clinical Applications Because of the compact arrangement of the trunks of the brachial plexus at the level of the first rib, the supraclavicular approach is extremely efficient; relatively small volumes of local anesthetic result in rapid and profound neural blockade when injected accurately. This block is performed with the arm at the patient's side, although it should be maximally extended for best results. Technically, this is considered the most difficult approach to the brachial plexus to learn and teach. Observation of an experienced regional anesthetist is perhaps the most effective way of learning the technique. The supraclavicular approach provides excellent surgical anesthesia for the elbow, forearm, and hand.

Side Effects/Complications The major complication associated with supraclavicular blockade is pneumothorax, which usually presents in the postoperative period. Routine chest radiography is not justified because of the delayed presentation. The incidence ranges from 0.5 to 6 percent, decreasing with the experience of the practitioner. Patients who are uncooperative or cannot tolerate any degree of respiratory compromise would be poor candidates for this procedure.

Block of the phrenic (50 to 60 percent), recurrent laryngeal, and cervical sympathetic nerves is a minor inconvenience requiring only reassurance. Nerve damage is uncommon and usually transient. Intravascular injection is largely preventable by careful technique, including use of test doses, aspiration, and incremental injection.

Technique As previously described, at the level of the first rib, the three trunks are compactly arranged cephaloposterior to the subclavian artery, which can often be palpated in the slender patient. With the arm extended at the patient's side, the brachial plexus lies inferior to the clavicle approximately at its midpoint. The first rib has an anteroposterior orientation and is short, flat, and broad; it acts as a medial barrier to the needle reaching the dome of the pleura.

The patient is positioned supine with the head turned away from the side to be blocked and the arm adducted and stretched as far as possible toward the ipsilateral knee. In the classic descrip-

tion, the midpoint of the clavicle is marked. The lateral border of the sternocleidomastoid muscle is identified (aided by the patient lifting the head) and the interscalene groove palpated by rolling the fingers back from the muscle border over the anterior scalene muscle. A mark is then made 1.5 to 2.0 cm posterior to the clavicle at its midpoint within the interscalene groove. Palpation of the subclavian artery, if possible, provides further verification of the correct needle placement.

After sterile precautions, the anesthesia care provider stands on the side to be blocked, facing the patient's head. A 22-gauge, 4-cm, short-beveled needle is directed in a caudad, slightly medial and posterior direction until a paresthesia or the first rib is encountered. This needle orientation lies in a plane parallel to a line joining the skin entry site and the patient's ear. If the first rib is encountered prior to elicitation of a paresthesia the needle can be walked anteriorly and posteriorly along the rib until a paresthesia or the subclavian artery is encountered (Fig. 12-4). If the artery is located, the needle should be redirected in a more posterolateral direction, a maneuver that usually results in elicitation of a paresthesia. A nerve stimulator can also be used to aid in needle placement.

The first rib is usually encountered at a needle depth of 3 to 4 cm; however, this depth may be exceeded in an obese patient or in the case of distortion caused by hematoma or local anesthetic injection.

The "plumb-bob" approach has been recommended as a modification of the classic supraclavicular block technique.[11] The reported advantages are the ease of this method as well as a theoretical decrease in the risk of pneumothorax. The needle entry site is at the point of intersection between the clavicle and the lateral border of the sternocleidomastoid muscle. The needle is inserted in a

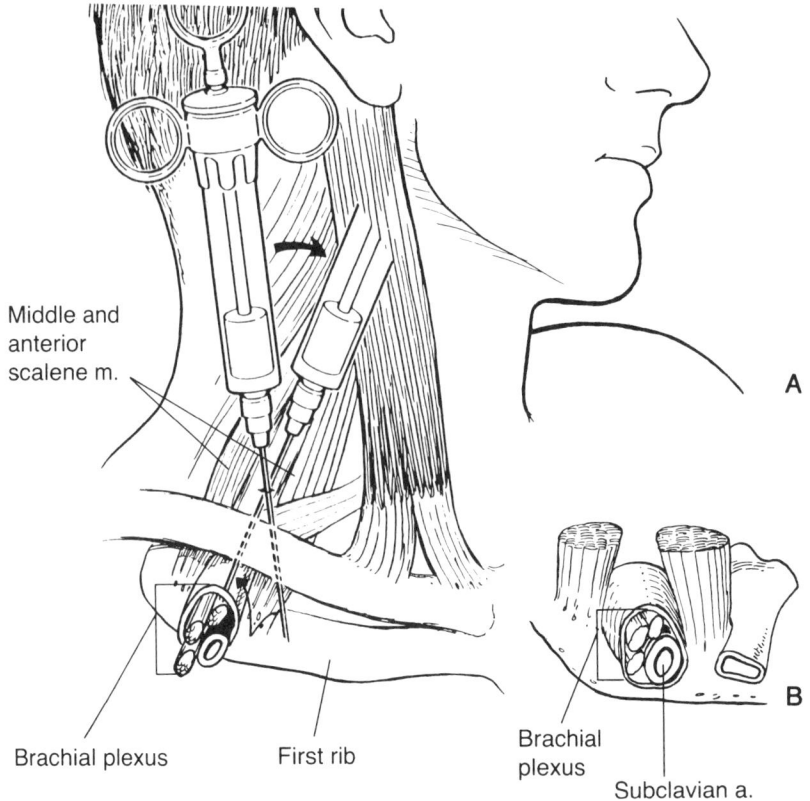

Fig. 12-4. (**A**) Supraclavicular block. The needle is systematically walked anteriorly and posteriorly along the rib until the plexus is located. (**B**) The three trunks are compactly arranged at the level of the first rib. (From Wedel & Brown,[47] with permission.)

"plumb-bob" orientation (Fig. 12-5); a paresthesia is often elicited on the first needle pass. If not, the needle is reinserted at a slightly cephalad angle. If a paresthesia does not result, the needle is walked caudad in small steps until the first rib is contacted.

Axillary Block

Clinical Applications Of all the approaches to the brachial plexus, the axillary block is most often employed because of its ease of performance, safety, and reliability, particularly for hand and forearm surgery.[10] It is well-suited to both outpatient and pediatric popula-

tions.[12,13] A variety of approaches to the axillary block have been described, including elicitation of paresthesias, transarterial injection, sheath blocks, and use of a nerve stimulator, and in experienced hands all seem to be reasonably successful. Use of this technique is confined to patients who are able to abduct their arms sufficiently to allow access to the neurovascular bundle within the axilla. While providing excellent anesthesia below the elbow, the axillary block is not reliable for surgery at the elbow and is not suitable for shoulder procedures. The musculocutaneous nerve may not always be blocked with this approach, but can be supplemented either at the level of the

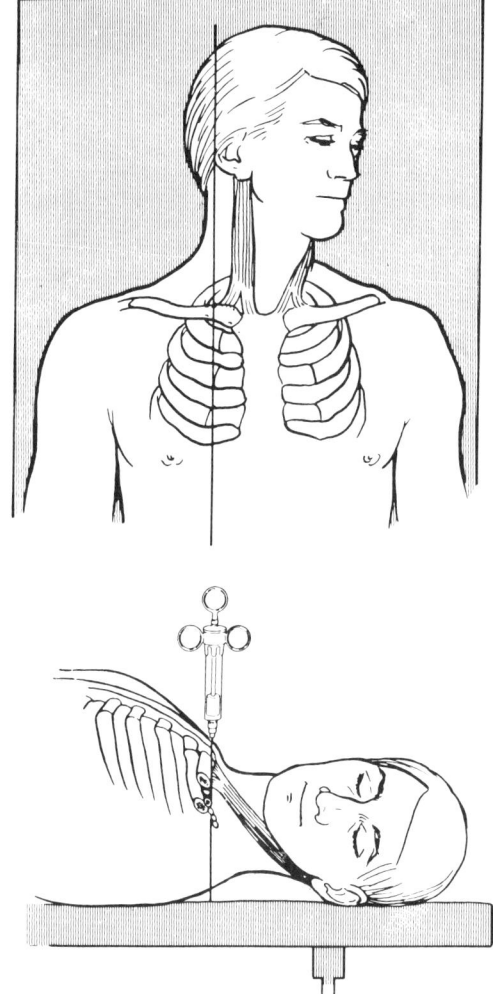

Fig. 12-5. Supraclavicular block. Plumb-bob approach. (From Wedel & Brown,[47] with permission.)

coracobrachialis muscle or as it courses superficially above the interepicondylar line at the elbow.

The axillary approach can be used in patients with disturbances of coagulation when indicated, as direct pressure can be applied to the area should a hematoma occur.

Side Effects/Complications Because of the large volumes of local anesthetic

often recommended for axillary blocks, the proximity of large blood vessels, and the popularity of "immobile" needle techniques, local anesthetic toxicity due to rapid uptake or intravascular injection may be a higher risk with this technique compared with other approaches to the brachial plexus. Frequent aspiration combined with incremental injection is an important feature of any method used in this block. Hematoma, sometimes with associated vascular compromise of the upper extremity, and infection are rare but reported complications. The assertion that paresthesia techniques are associated with a higher risk of neural complications has not been substantiated by available data.[14]

Technique It is helpful to review relevant anatomic points prior to discussing the technical methods described for axillary block.

1. The axillary neurovascular bundle is multicompartmental[15] (Fig. 12-6).
2. The peripheral nerves in the axilla lie in predictable orientation to the axillary artery, which is usually easily palpable. When the arm is abducted, the *radial nerve* is posterior and somewhat lateral (behind), the *median nerve* superior, and the *ulnar nerve* posterior to the axillary artery (Fig. 12-7).
3. The ulnar and median nerves are very superficial (0.25 to 1 cm deep) in most patients.
4. At the level of the axilla, the musculocutaneous nerve lies in the substance of the coracobrachialis muscle.
5. Adequate sensory block for tourniquet pain requires blockade of the intercostobrachialis nerve, a branch of the T2 intercostal nerve. This can be most easily accomplished by extending the skin wheal over the axillary artery 1 to 2 cm in the superior and inferior directions.

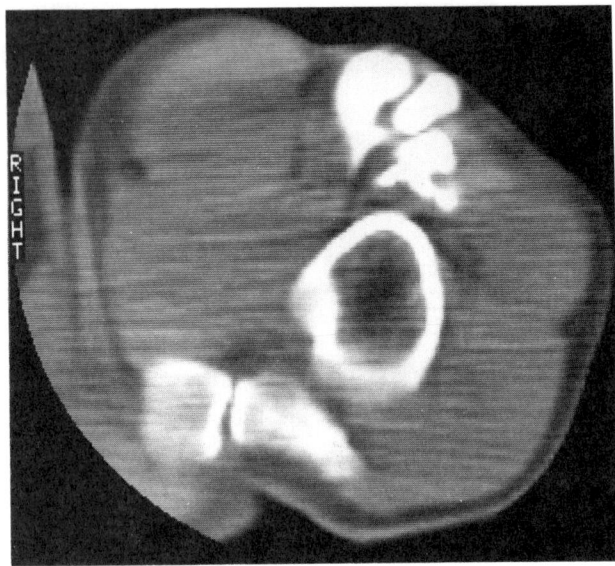

Fig. 12-6. Axillary block. Computed tomogram after axillary block with 0.5 percent bupivacaine and iodothalamate. Separate injections of 10-ml solution were made after obtaining median and radial nerve paresthesias and transarterially. Contrast medium appears to remain in three separate compartments. (From Wedel & Brown,[47] with permission.)

For all approaches to the axillary block, the patient is positioned supine with the arm to be blocked abducted at right angles with the body and the elbow flexed to 90 degrees. The dorsum of the hand may rest on the bed or a pillow; the tendency to place the hand under the patient's head, thus hyperabducting the arm, should be avoided as this position will frequently obliterate the pulse.

The axillary artery is palpated as close to the axillary crease as possible and a line is drawn tracing its course distally. Using sterile technique, the artery is fixed against the humerus at the level of the axillary crease by the index and middle fingers of the nondominant hand and a skin wheal raised. Placement of the needle proximal to the fingers along with maintenance of distal pressure encourages proximal spread of the local anesthetic solution, increasing the likelihood of blocking the musculocutaneous nerve.

At this point several different tech-

niques of axillary blockade may be employed singly or in combination.

Paresthesia techniques involve elicitation of single or multiple paresthesias with a small-gauge (22- to 25-gauge), 2-cm needle. Longer needles are not recommended or required as the peripheral nerves are quite superficial. A minimum volume of 10 ml of local anesthetic is carefully injected at each paresthesia. Following elicitation of paresthesias, initial injection of local anesthetic should be done cautiously to ascertain that there is no pain in the distribution of the nerve, which would suggest an intraneural injection. There is some evidence that smaller needles have a lower associated risk of nerve injury.[14]

The assertion by some practitioners that paresthesia techniques are associated with a higher risk of postblock nerve injury has not been substantiated.[13,16] Unintentional paresthesias are often elicted during nonparesthesia tech-

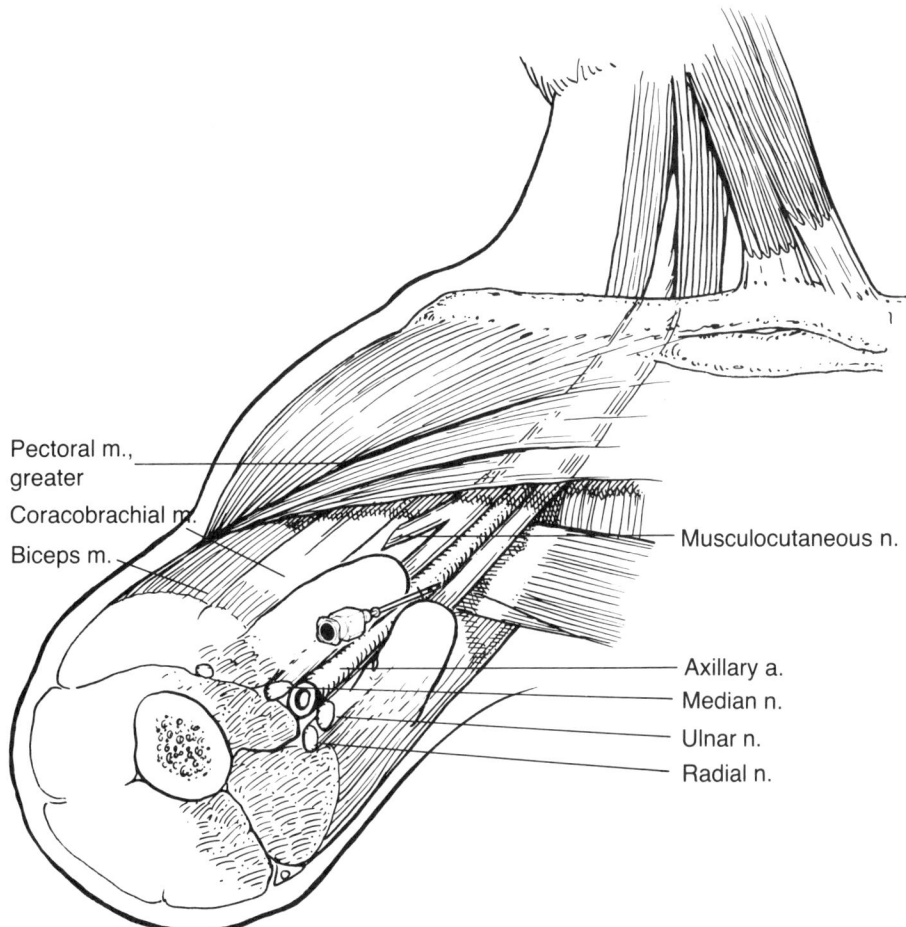

Pectoral m.,
greater

Coracobrachial m.

Biceps m.

Musculocutaneous n.

Axillary a.

Median n.

Ulnar n.

Radial n.

Fig. 12-7. Axillary block. The arm is abducted at right angles to the body. Distal digital pressure is maintained during needle placement and injection of local anesthetic. (From Wedel & Brown,[47] with permission.)

niques; repositioning of the needle without injection when this occurs would disregard the best locator of the brachial plexus. Furthermore, reported success rates with single-injection "sheath" techniques may not be clinically acceptable.[17,18] Demonstration of multicompartments in the axillary sheath would be consistent with poor diffusion of local anesthetic solutions injected in a single site.[15]

At the completion of the axillary block, the arm should be immediately adducted to prevent obstruction of proximal flow of the local anesthetic solution by the humeral head. The musculocutaneous nerve is not reliably blocked, even with large volumes,[19] and may require supplementation in the axilla or at the elbow.

Nerve stimulator techniques can be employed using a Teflon-coated (insulated) needle and commercially available nerve stimulators. This technique avoids sensory paresthesias, but requires additional equipment.[20]

Sheath techniques are advocated by

those experts who downplay the anatomic relevance of the multicompartmental nature of the axillary sheath. In this technique a short-beveled needle is slowly advanced in proximity to the axillary artery until the "axillary sheath" is entered, as evidenced by a "fascial click." At this point the total volume of local anesthetic is injected after negative aspiration.[10,21] This method theoretically lowers the risk of nerve damage by avoiding paresthesias; however, paresthesias are often obtained with needle placement.[14] This technique is associated with a slow and often incomplete onset of surgical anesthesia, but is quite effective in pediatric axillary blocks, in which patient cooperation may be absent and heavy sedation is often required.

Transarterial techniques have been described involving placement of a sharp needle through the axillary artery and injecting local anesthetic (40 to 50 ml) behind the artery or, in some descriptions, dividing the total volume behind and in front of the artery. Obviously, great care must be taken to avoid intravascular injection with this technique, particularly since the pressure of injection within the compartments of the axillary sheath may move anatomic structures in relation to the "immobile" needle. Unintentional arterial puncture can occur with all the described techniques, and since the radial nerve is reliably located behind the artery, it is reasonable to place local anesthetic in this location if the artery is punctured. Some practitioners avoid intentional arterial puncture in the belief that it is unnecessarily traumatic.

Field block of the brachial plexus with a fanwise injection of 10 to 15 ml of local anesthetic solution on each side of the artery is a variation of the sheath technique. While paresthesias are not specifically sought, they may be encountered with this technique and provide evidence of correct needle placement.

Infraclavicular Block

Clinical Applications This approach to the brachial plexus was described by Raj et al,[22] and can be used for surgery of the elbow, forearm and hand. The technique is particularly well-suited to placement of an indwelling catheter because of the minimal tissue movement around the catheter insertion site over the lateral thorax during patient activity. There is a theoretical lowered risk of pneumothorax when the block is done correctly and a reportedly high rate of blockade of the axillary and musculocutaneous nerves. No special arm position is required. A nerve stimulator is required as there are no palpable landmarks to aid in directing the needle placement.

Side Effects/Complications If the needle is directed too medially, pneumothorax may result. As in other approaches to the brachial plexus, intravascular injection is a risk, requiring standard precautions as described earlier.

Technique The midpoint of the clavicle is identified, and using standard sterile technique, an insulated needle is inserted at a point 2 cm below this point and advanced in a lateral direction. A nerve stimulator is used to identify the brachial plexus. A line drawn between the axillary artery (with the arm abducted) and the C6 tubercle is helpful in visualizing the course of the brachial plexus. Once the plexus is identified, an injection of 20 to 30 ml of local anesthetic solution should provide surgical anesthesia. Modifications of this technique involving more lateral placement of the needle may decrease the rate of success of musculocutaneous nerve block.

Brachial Plexus Catheters

The concept of providing prolonged pain relief along with upper extremity sympathectomy with brachial plexus catheterization has applicability in both post-surgical and pain patient populations. A variety of methods for providing continuous brachial plexus anesthesia has been described for many years,[23] including needles secured in place with corks, various-length catheters, and over and through the needle methods. Commercial kits providing the needle, catheter, and stimulating electrode for use with a nerve stimulator are now available. The longer catheter has theoretical advantages of being easier to secure as well as providing a more reliable block due to the proximal position of the catheter in the brachial plexus.[24]

Theoretical complications include infection, hematoma, kinking or curling of the catheter, migration of the catheter intravascularly, and nerve injury during placement. Technical problems include difficulty in securing the catheter and keeping it in place because of arm motion and the presence of sweat glands at the site of insertion. Postoperative pain control with this technique is excellent; however, application to surgical anesthesia is somewhat less satisfactory because of the slow onset of anesthesia and partial blockade requiring supplementation.

Peripheral Blocks at the Elbow and Wrist

Clinical Applications Brachial plexus block at one of the sites described above is superior to peripheral nerve block at the elbow or wrist for surgical anesthesia of the upper extremity because there is usually adequate tourniquet anesthesia with a brachial plexus block and the block is easier to perform at the brachial plexus, where the upper extremity nerves are clustered anatomically. However, peripheral nerve blocks at the elbow or wrist can be very useful when a very limited surgical approach is anticipated, when approaches to the brachial plexus are contraindicated (because of infection, coagulation abnormalities, bilateral surgery, difficult anatomy, etc.), or for supplementation of an inadequate brachial plexus block.

Side Effects/Complications In general, distal peripheral blocks are associated with a lower risk of complications. However, intravascular injection can occur, and the usual precaution of incremental injection after aspiration is recommended. The risk of nerve damage is hypothesized to be higher when nerves are blocked more distally, perhaps because of their smaller size and anatomic placement between bony and ligamentous structures that tend to limit the movement of the nerve away from the probing needle tip.

Elbow versus Wrist The forearm cutaneous nerves arise in the upper arm, and will not be anesthetized by block of the peripheral nerves at the elbow. Hence, there is no advantage to either elbow or wrist techniques; both will provide sensory anesthesia of the hand.

Median Nerve Block
The sensory distribution of the median nerve supplies the palmar aspects of the thumb and index fingers, middle finger, radial half of the ring finger, and the nailbeds of all digits except the little finger. The motor distribution of this nerve involves the muscles of the thenar eminence and lumbrical muscles of the first and second digits; in addition, when the block is performed at the elbow, the median-innervated wrist flexor muscles of the forearm are blocked.

Elbow Technique With the arm placed in the anatomic position (palm up), a line is drawn connecting the medial and lateral epicondyles of the humerus. The bra-

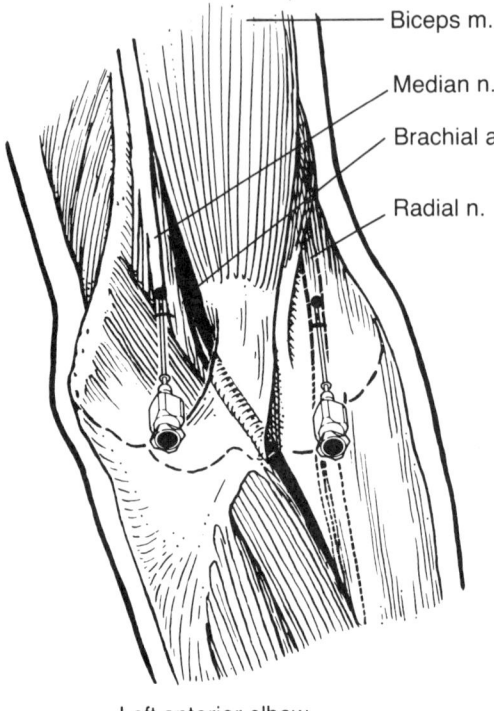

Biceps m.

Median n.

Brachial a.

Radial n.

Left anterior elbow

Fig. 12-8. Anatomic landmarks for median and radial nerve block at the elbow. (From Wedel & Brown,[47] with permission.)

chial artery is located and marked medial to the biceps tendon along the interepicondylar line. The median nerve lies medial to the artery and can be blocked with 3 to 5 ml of local anesthetic solution after a paresthesia is elicted, or with 5 to 10 ml of solution injected fanwise medial to the artery (Fig. 12-8).

Wrist Technique The median nerve lies between the flexor carpi radialis and palmaris longus tendons and can be blocked at a point 2 to 3 cm proximal to the wrist crease (Fig. 12-9). (The palmaris longus is not an invariable anatomic structure; it may be congentially or postsurgically absent in some patients.) As the needle passes through the flexor retinaculum a loss of resistance will be felt, at which point 2 to 4 ml of solution are in-

jected. An additional 1 ml of solution should be injected superior to the retinaculum as the needle is withdrawn to anesthetize the superficial palmar branch of the median nerve, which supplies sensation to the skin of the thenar eminence. Elicitation of paresthesias is contraindicated in this area because of the physical confinement of the nerve in the carpal tunnel, increasing the risk of nerve injury.

Radial Nerve Block

The radial nerve supplies sensation to the lateral aspect of the dorsum of the hand (thumb side) and the proximal portion of the thumb, index, middle, and lateral half of the ring fingers.

Elbow Technique The radial nerve courses over the anterior aspect of the lateral epicondyle at the elbow and can be blocked by a fanwise injection of 3 to 5 ml of solution at this site. The interepicondylar line and the lateral edge of the biceps tendon are palpated and marked. A 3- to 4-cm needle is advanced through a point 2 cm lateral to the line marking the border of the biceps tendon and advanced until bone is encountered (Fig. 12-8). The local anesthetic is injected fanwise along this needle course.

Wrist Technique Multiple peripheral branches of the radial nerve descend along the dorsum and radial side of the wrist; therefore block of this nerve requires a fanwise field block injection. The patient is asked to extend the thumb to allow identification of the extensor pollicus longus tendon. The needle is inserted over the tendon at the base of the first metacarpal. All injections of local anesthetic are made superficial to the tendon; 2 ml are injected proximally along the tendon and an additional 1 ml is injected as the needle passes at right angles across the "anatomic snuffbox" (Fig. 12-10).

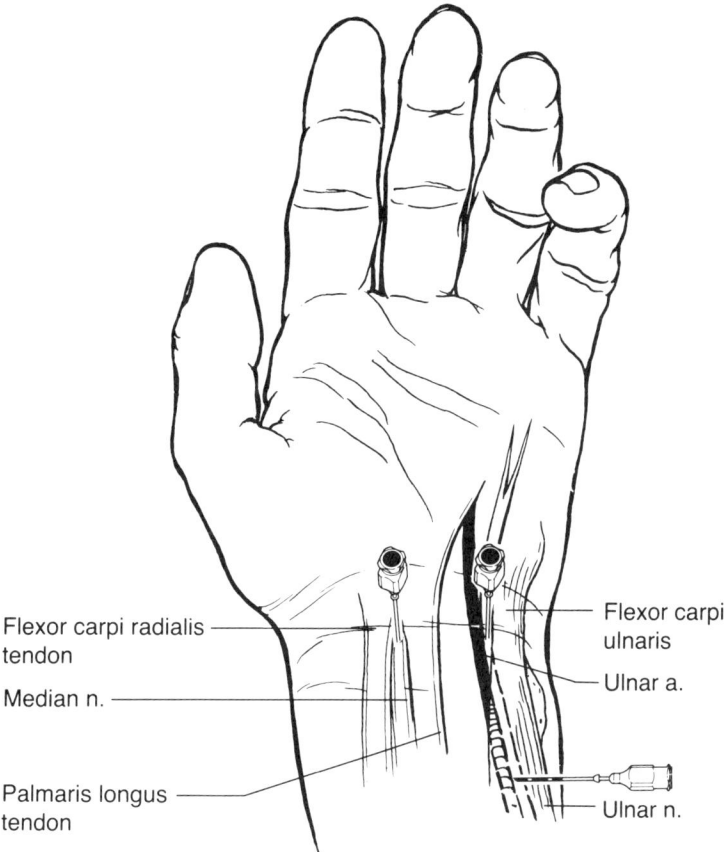

Flexor carpi radialis tendon

Median n.

Palmaris longus tendon

Flexor carpi ulnaris

Ulnar a.

Ulnar n.

Fig. 12-9. Anatomic landmarks for median and ulnar nerve block at the wrist. An alternative method for ulnar nerve block, from the ulnar side of the wrist, is shown. (From Wedel & Brown,[47] with permission.)

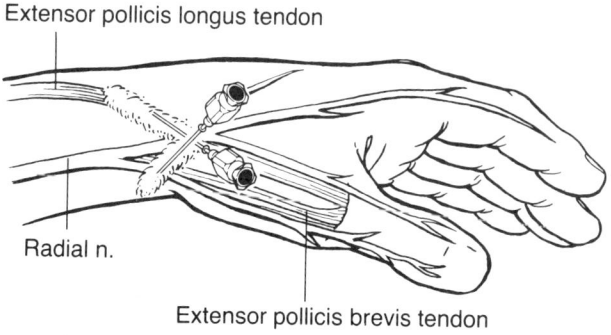

Extensor pollicis longus tendon

Radial n.

Extensor pollicis brevis tendon

Fig. 12-10. Anatomic landmarks and method of needle insertion for radial nerve block at the wrist. (From Wedel & Brown,[47] with permission.)

Ulnar Nerve Block

The ulnar nerve provides sensory innervation to the ulnar side of the hand and the little and the ulnar side of the ring fingers, and motor innervation to all of the small muscles of the hand except the thenar eminence and the first and second lumbrical muscles.

Elbow Technique   The ulnar nerve is easily accessible in its subcutaneous position posterior to the medial epicondyle; however, blockade at this site is associated with a high risk of neuritis. This is probably due to the anatomic position of the nerve, which is surrounded by fibrous tissue at this site, encouraging injection of local anesthetic intraneurally because of the lack of distensible soft tissues. If the nerve is blocked at this location, very small volumes of solution are required (1 ml); however, it is preferable to block the nerve 3 to 5 cm proximal to the elbow with a larger volume. An injection of 5 to 10 ml of local anesthetic injected in a fanwise fashion without elicitation of a paresthesia is recommended.

Wrist Technique   The ulnar nerve lies beneath the flexor carpi ulnaris tendon between the ulnar artery and the pisiform bone. At this site it has already given off palmar cutaneous and dorsal branches. The nerve is blocked by injection of 3 to 5 ml of local anesthetic in a fanwise fashion medially from the radial side of the tendon (Fig. 12-9). Elicitation of a paresthesia is not necessary, but confirms correct needle placement.

Musculocutaneous Nerve Block

The musculocutaneous nerve is often missed in block techniques performed at the level of the axilla. Supplementation of this nerve at the elbow, where it becomes the lateral cutaneous nerve of the forearm and provides sensation to the skin on the radial side of the forearm up to the radiocarpal joint, may be necessary for surgery involving this area.

Elbow Technique   The lateral cutaneous nerve of the forearm is the sensory termination of the musculocutaneous nerve, which lies in a superficial position at the level of the elbow. It can be blocked with 3 to 5 ml of local anesthetic by a fanwise subcutaneous injection 1 cm proximal to the interepicondylar line just lateral to the biceps tendon.

Intravenous Regional (Bier) Block

The injection of local anesthetic into a vein distal to a tourniquet as a means of inducing regional anesthesia was first described by the German surgeon, August Bier,[25] in 1908. Early techniques involved a proximal and distal tourniquet with injection of the local anesthetic, procaine. Reliable brachial plexus block techniques largely replaced the "Bier block" because of time limitations for surgical anesthesia associated with the latter method.

Clinical Applications   The advantages of the intravenous regional technique include ease of administration, low cost, control over the extent of anesthesia, applicability to all age groups, and rapidity of onset and offset of surgical anesthesia.

Side Effects/Complications   Accidental or early deflation of the tourniquet or use of excessive doses of local anesthetics can result in toxic reactions. Injection of the drug as distally as possible at a slow rate has been shown to decrease blood levels and theoretically increase safety.[26,27] The use of bupivacaine for intravenous regional anesthesia has been associated with local anesthetic toxicity and death[28,29] and is not recommended. Cyclic deflation of the tourniquet at 10-

second intervals has been shown to increase the time to peak arterial lidocaine levels, which may decrease potential toxicity.[30] Other problems associated with this technique include development of compartment syndrome,[31] loss of limb,[32] tourniquet pain, lack of postoperative pain relief, difficulty in providing a bloodless surgical field, and the need to exsanguinate the affected limb prior to onset of anesthesia.

Technique Two intravenous cannulas are inserted, one in the contralateral extremity for injection of sedative and resuscitative drugs, and the second in the affected extremity as distally as possible. A double tourniquet fitted with a reliable pressure gauge and secure closures is placed on the operative extremity. The extremity is then exsanguinated. This can be done by wrapping the extremity tightly with an Esmarch bandage, which will be most effective but may cause excessive pain to the patient with a broken bone or open laceration. Alternatively, the arm can be exsanguinated by elevation of the limb for several minutes or by application of an air splint, which is available in most emergency rooms, to above systolic pressure. These techniques will usually provide adequate exsanguination for closed procedures or bone pinning, but may result in unsatisfactory surgical conditions for open procedures. Some authors recommend re-exsanguination of the arm with an Esmarch bandage following institution of the intravenous regional anesthetic with a brief deflation and reinflation of the tourniquet, a technique that reportedly results in minimal leakage of local anesthetic.[33]

Following exsanguination of the arm, and while compression is still applied to the limb, the proximal tourniquet cuff is inflated to approximately 150 mmHg higher than the patient's systolic pressure. Absence of the radial pulse confirms adequate tourniquet pressure. Obese patients may require higher pressures. The calculated dose of local anesthetic, usually 0.5 percent lidocaine or prilocaine, is injected slowly. When or if the patient complains of tourniquet pain (usually after 10 to 30 minutes), the distal tourniquet overlying anesthetized skin is inflated and checked prior to deflating the proximal cuff. This procedure can be reversed later in the procedure if the patient complains of tourniquet pain again, although the usual duration of the block is 60 to 150 minutes. Wider single-cuffed tourniquets may have an advantage over double cuffs in that the inflation pressures will be lower, decreasing the risk of neurologic injury.[34] In small children, because a double tourniquet is usually too large for the arm, a single child-sized cuff may be used. The tourniquet may be safely released 20 to 25 minutes after injection of the local anesthetic. As previously discussed, cyclic deflations may afford a greater margin of safety during deflation.[30]

LOWER EXTREMITY BLOCKS

Blocks of the lower extremity have not achieved the popularity and widespread clinical application of upper extremity block techniques. One explanation for this difference lies in the well-accepted safety and efficacy of central neuraxial blocks for lower extremity surgery. The introduction of smaller needles for intrathecal blockade designed to decrease the incidence of dural puncture headache, the flexibility achieved with continuous spinal and epidural techniques, the ease with which central neuraxial techniques are learned and performed, the increased utilization of continuous techniques to provide analgesia into the postoperative period, and the proven safety of a variety of local anesthetic agents delivered to the central neuraxis have all contributed to the popularity of these techniques for lower extremity surgery. Furthermore, unlike the brachial plexus, the nerves supplying the lower extremity are not anatomically clustered where they can be easily blocked with a relatively superficial injection of local anesthetic. Because of the anatomic considerations, these blocks are technically more difficult and require more training and practice before expertise is acquired. Finally, persistent block of any of the major nerves of the lower extremity results in the patient being unable to ambulate, an unacceptable side effect in the outpatient population.

However, there are advantages associated with nerve blocks of the lower extremity. Surgical anesthesia can be provided in one limb without complete sympathectomy, in contrast to central neuraxial block. Peripheral nerve blocks of the lower extremity usually result in a prolonged duration of anesthesia, especially if long-acting agents are used, and thus provide excellent postoperative pain relief for selected patients. Knowledge of the anatomy and application of nerve blockade techniques to the lower extremity is an important component of comprehensive anesthesia care, providing the anesthesia care provider with an array of options when faced with lower extremity surgical cases.

Anatomy

The lower extremity nervous supply arises from the lumbar and sacral plexuses. The lumbar plexus is formed from the anterior rami of the first four lumbar nerves, often including a branch from T12 and occasionally from L5 (Fig. 12-11). The plexus courses through the psoas compartment, which is the potential space between the psoas major and quadratus lumborum muscles.

The anterior and medial hip are supplied by the lower components of the lumbar plexus (L2–L4). The *obturator nerve* is formed by the anterior divisions of L2–L4, the *femoral nerve* by the posterior divisions of the same roots, and the *lateral femoral cutaneous nerve* from the posterior divisions of L2-L3.

The remainder of the leg is supplied by the lower lumbar and sacral roots. The *sciatic nerve* and *posterior cutaneous nerve of the thigh* are derived from the S1–S3 roots plus branches from the anterior rami of L4 and L5, respectively. These two nerves course through the pelvis and greater sciatic foramen together and are blocked by the same technique. The sciatic nerve is made up of two large nerves, the *tibial nerve* (ventral branches of the anterior rami of L4-L5 and S1–S3) and the *common peroneal nerve* (dorsal branches of the anterior rami of L4-L5 and S1–S3), which separate at or above the popliteal fossa, where the tibial nerve passes medially and the peroneal nerve laterally.

The cutaneous distributions of the lumbosacral roots and peripheral nerves of the lower extremities are illustrated in Figure 12-12.

Hip, Thigh, and Knee Block

Psoas Compartment Block

Clinical Applications This technique provides anesthesia of the hip and lateral thigh without the disadvantage of sympathectomy associated with blocks of the central neuraxis, and with a single needle insertion.[35] If entire lower extremity anesthesia is desired, a block of the sciatic nerve must also be performed.

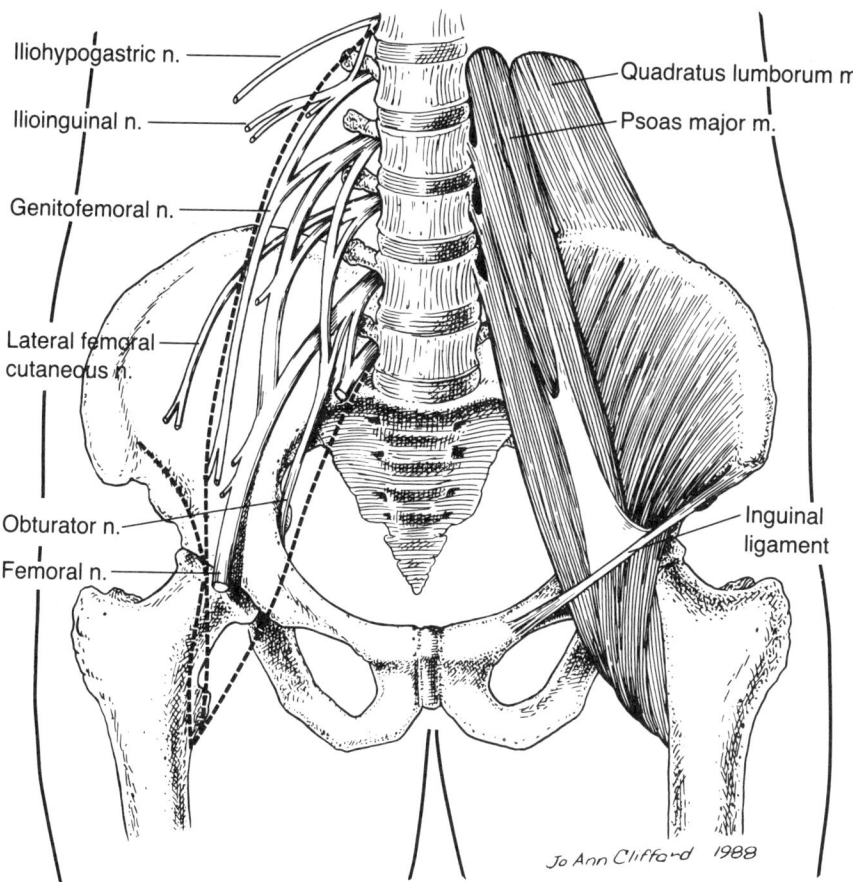

Iliohypogastric n.

Ilioinguinal n.

Genitofemoral n.

Lateral femoral cutaneous n.

Obturator n.

Femoral n.

Quadratus lumborum m.

Psoas major m.

Inguinal ligament

Jo Ann Clifford 1988

Fig. 12-11. The lumbar plexus lies in the psoas compartment between the psoas major and quadratus lumborum muscles. (From Wedel & Brown,[47] with permission.)

Side Effects/Complications The combination of large volumes of local anesthetic required and the deep needle insertion increases the risk of intravascular, epidural, or intrathecal injection and its potentially adverse effects. Spread of the local anesthetic can also result in significant sympathetic blockade. Peripheral nerve injury is a potential risk of this technique.

Technique The lumbar nerves course between the quadratus lumborum and psoas major muscles, where they can be blocked by a paravertebral approach posteriorly. The nerve roots continue into the femoral canal, where they are surrounded by a fascial sheath. At this point they can be blocked by a cephalad spread of local anesthetic injected distal to the femoral canal using the so-called perivascular approach. These two techniques are described below.

Posterior Approach to the Psoas Block The patient is positioned laterally with the hips flexed and the operative leg uppermost. A line is drawn connecting the iliac crests (intercristal line), which will usually cross the L4 spine or the L4-L5 interspace. Using sterile technique, a skin wheal is raised at a point 3 cm caudad and

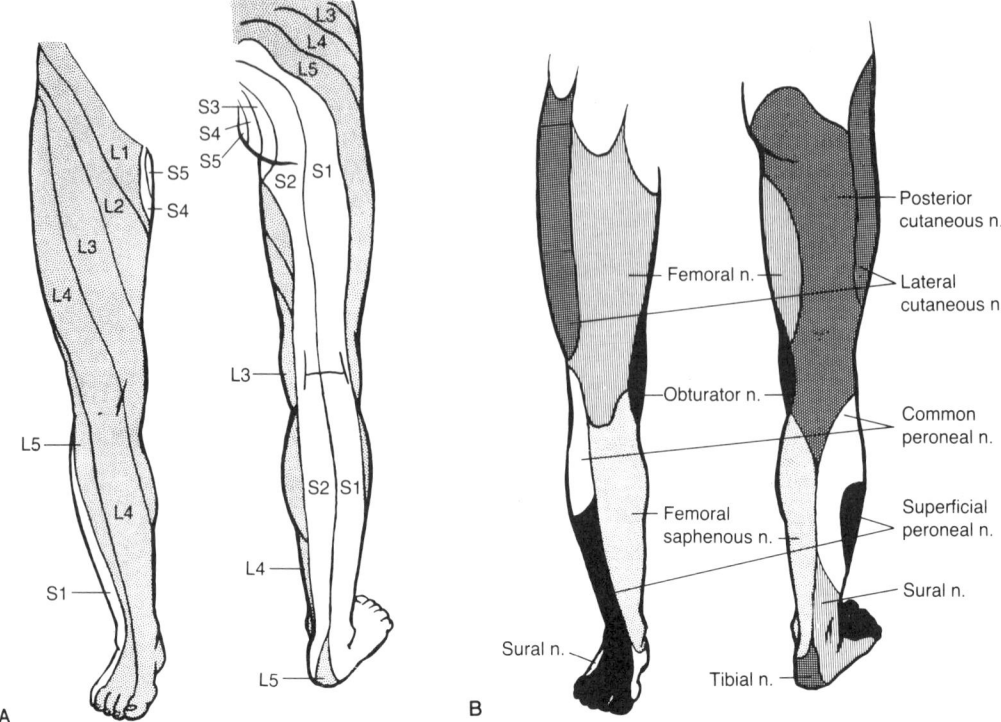

Fig. 12-12. (**A**) The cutaneous distribution of the lumbosacral nerves. (**B**) The cutaneous distribution of the peripheral nerves of the lower extremity. (From Wedel & Brown,[47] with permission.)

5 cm lateral to the spinal midline on the side to be blocked (uppermost). A long (15-cm) 22-gauge needle is advanced perpendicular to the skin until bone is contacted, representing the L5 transverse process. The needle is redirected cephalad in small steps until it slides off the transverse process. It is advanced until a paresthesia is elicted. A nerve stimulator can also be used with this technique. The needle depth is usually about 5 to 6 cm. Dilation of the compartment with 20 ml of air may facilitate spread of local anesthetic solution (30 to 40 ml).

Perivascular Technique The perivascular technique ("3-in-1 block") is based on the premise that injection of a large volume of local anesthetic within the femoral canal while maintaining distal pressure will cause proximal spread of the solution into the psoas compartment, resulting in a lumbar plexus block.[36] The key anatomic assumption is that the fascial sheath surrounding the lumbar roots extends into the femoral canal and acts as an enclosed conduit for the spread of local anesthetic solutions.

With the patient in the supine position, a line representing the inguinal ligament is drawn between the palpated anterior superior iliac crest and the pubic tubercle. A second line is drawn at right angles to the inguinal ligament, representing the femoral artery. Using sterile precautions, a skin wheal is made 1 cm lateral to the femoral artery and 2 cm distal to the inguinal ligament. A 22-gauge, 5-cm short-beveled needle is advanced in the cephalad direction at a 30- to 45-degree angle to skin until a paresthesia is obtained. Alternatively a nerve stimulator can be used to locate the femoral nerve. Once the needle is correctly located, firm pressure is applied just distal to the skin entry with the fingers of the other hand while the needle is held immobile. A total of 20 to 40 ml of local anesthetic is injected incrementally following negative aspiration. Reportedly reliable anesthesia of the femoral and lateral femoral cutaneous nerves is achieved with 20 ml of solution, while obturator nerve block requires volumes greater than 30 ml.[36]

Femoral Nerve Block

Clinical Applications   The femoral nerve is formed within the psoas major muscle by the posterior divisions of L2–L4, emerges from the lateral border of that muscle, and descends in the groove between the psoas and iliacus muscles. It enters the thigh lateral to the femoral artery and divides into anterior and posterior branches distal to the inguinal ligament. The femoral nerve supplies the anterior compartment muscles of the thigh (quadriceps, sartorius) and skin of the anterior thigh from the inguinal ligament to the knee. Below the knee it supplies sensation to the medial side of the leg, extending to the big toe in the distribution of the saphenous nerve.

Because of its limited sensory distribution, the femoral nerve block is usually combined with other peripheral blocks in clinical practice. However, it can be used alone for muscle biopsies of the quadriceps muscle or other surgical procedures limited to the anterior thigh, and its use has been described for anesthetic management of knee arthroscopy and surgical repair of fractures of the midfemoral shaft.[37,38]

Side Effects/Complications   The proximity of the femoral artery to this nerve may increase the risk of hematoma and intravascular injection. However, anatomically the nerve and artery are located in separate sheaths approximately 1 cm apart. In most patients with normal anatomy the femoral artery can be easily palpated, allowing correct, safe needle positioning lateral to the pulsation. Blockade of the femoral nerve should probably be avoided in patients who have undergone femoral vascular grafts, as the anatomy is distorted, and needle injection may cause excessive bleeding or infection. Nerve damage from needle trauma or drug toxicity is an unlikely complication from this block.

Technique   With the patient positioned supine, a line is drawn between the anterior superior iliac crest and the pubic tubercle, indicating the inguinal ligament. A second line is drawn at right angles to the inguinal ligament at the site of palpation of the femoral artery. Using a sterile approach, a skin wheal is raised 1 cm lateral to the artery and 2 cm distal to the inguinal ligament. A 22-gauge, 3- to 5-cm short-beveled needle is advanced until a paresthesia is obtained (Fig. 12-13A). A nerve stimulator may also be used to correctly place the needle. Arterial pulsations transmitted to the hub of the needle from the femoral artery can often be observed when the needle is in position. Local anesthetic solution (10 to 20 ml) is injected incrementally through the needle after negative aspiration, including 5 to 10 ml of solution injected fanwise laterally to block branches of the femoral nerve, which can divide high at the level of the inguinal ligament.

Lateral Femoral Cutaneous Nerve Block

Clinical Applications   The lateral femoral cutaneous nerve arises from L2-L3, emerging at the lateral border of the psoas

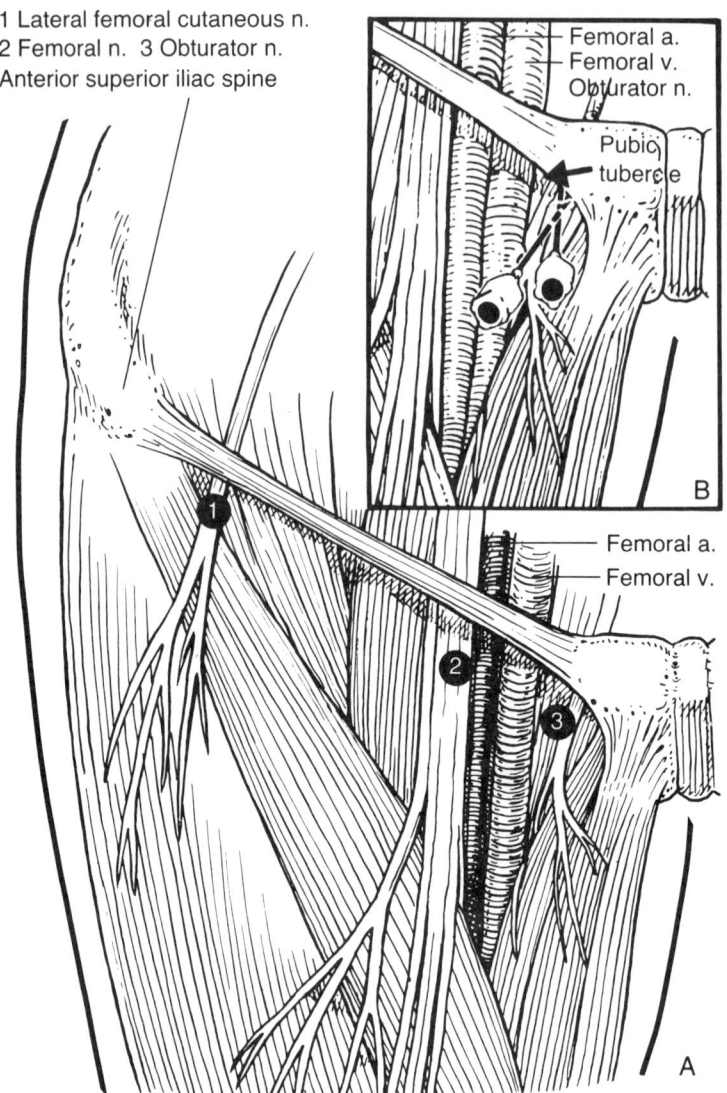

1 Lateral femoral cutaneous n.
2 Femoral n. 3 Obturator n.
Anterior superior iliac spine

Femoral a.
Femoral v.
Obturator n.

Pubic
tubercle

B

Femoral a.
Femoral v.

A

Fig. 12-13. (A) Anatomic landmarks for lateral femoral cutaneous, femoral, and obturator nerve blocks. (B) Obturator nerve block. The needle is walked off the inferior pubic ramus in a lateral and caudad direction until it passes into the obturator canal. (From Wedel & Brown,[47] with permission.)

muscle inferior to the ilioinguinal nerve. It courses beneath the iliac fascia, entering the thigh deep to the inguinal ligament 1 to 2 cm medial to the anterior superior iliac spine. The nerve emerges from the fascia lata 7 to 10 cm caudad to the spine and divides into anterior and

posterior branches. The anterior branches supply the skin of the anterolateral thigh to the knee, while the posterior branch supplies the skin of the lateral thigh from the hip to the midthigh.

This block is usually combined with other lower extremity blocks; however, it can provide adequate anesthesia for superficial procedures involving the skin of the anterolateral thigh such as skin graft harvests. It is an important part of lower extremity blockade when a thigh tourniquet will be used.

Side Effects/Complications Neuritis of this nerve secondary to needle trauma or drug toxicity is a potential but unlikely complication. There are no large blood vessels in the vicinity of this nerve; therefore the likelihood of rapid uptake or intravascular injection is very small.

Technique The anterior superior iliac spine is palpated and a mark made at a point 2 cm medial and 2 cm caudad to this landmark. Using sterile technique, a 4-cm, 22-gauge short-beveled needle is advanced through a skin wheal in an orientation perpendicular to the skin. As the needle is advanced the fascia lata will be encountered at a depth of 1 to 3 cm, with a sudden release indicating passage through this structure. Local anesthetic (10 to 20 ml) is injected above and below the fascia at several points as the needle is slowly moved fanwise laterally and medially (Fig. 12-13A).

The success rate of this block can be increased by depositing an additional 10 ml of solution just medial and posterior to the anterior superior iliac crest. The needle is advanced to the medial edge of the spine and then redirected to walk underneath the spine. The lateral femoral cutaneous nerve is a pure sensory nerve, so a nerve stimulator is not helpful in performing this block. Paresthesias elicted during needle placement confirm that the needle depth is correct.

Obturator Nerve Block

Clinical Applications The obturator nerve is primarily derived from L3-L4, with variable minor contributions from L2. It lies deep in the obturator canal after descending from the medial psoas muscle border. Anterior and posterior branches form as it leaves the obturator canal. The anterior branch supplies an articular branch to the hip, the anterior adductor muscles, and a variable cutaneous branch to the lower medial thigh. The posterior branch supplies the deep adductor muscles, with a variable articular branch to the knee.

Usually the obturator nerve is blocked as part of regional anesthesia for knee surgery. Because it is primarily a motor nerve, it is rarely blocked on its own; however, obturator nerve block can be useful in treating or diagnosing the extent of adductor spasm in patients with cerebral palsy and other muscle or neurologic diseases affecting the lower extremities prior to surgical intervention (adductor tenotomy).

Side Effects/Complications Because of the deep location of the nerve in the obturator canal, it is a difficult block to learn and perform. An inadequate blockade of this nerve can mar an otherwise elegant regional anesthetic for knee surgery. The obturator canal contains vascular and neural structures, increasing the potential risk of intravascular injection or nerve damage.

Technique With the patient in the supine position a mark is made 1 to 2 cm lateral and 1 to 2 cm caudad to the palpated pubic tubercle. Using sterile technique a skin wheal is raised and a 22-gauge, 8- to 10-cm short-beveled needle is advanced slightly medially toward the pubic tubercle. Usually the inferior pubic ramus will be encountered at a depth of 2 to 4 cm. At that point the needle is walked laterally and caudad in small steps until it drops into the obturator canal. The obturator nerve is located 2 to 3 cm past the point of contact with the pubic ramus (Fig. 12-13). Local anesthetic solution (10 to 15 ml) is injected after negative aspiration.

A nerve stimulator is very useful for accurate location of this motor nerve; a twitch will be observed in the medial thigh adductor muscles as the needle approaches the obturator nerve.

Sciatic Nerve Block

Clinical Applications   The sciatic nerve derives from L4-L5 and S1–S3. It is a large peripheral nerve with a width of 2 cm. It exits the pelvis with the posterior cutaneous nerve of the thigh, passes through the sacrosciatic foramen beneath the piriformis muscle, and courses between the greater trochanter of the femur and the ischial tuberosity. At the lower border of the gluteus maximus muscle, the sciatic nerve becomes superficial as it begins its descent down the posterior thigh toward the popliteal fossa. The sciatic nerve supplies sensation to the largest area of the lower extremity, including the posterior thigh and everything below the knee with the exception of a thin medial strip supplied by the saphenous nerve (terminal branch of the femoral nerve).

Because of its wide sensory distribution, the sciatic nerve block can be used alone for any surgery below the knee that does not require a thigh tourniquet. It can also be combined with other peripheral nerve blocks to provide anesthesia for surgical procedures involving the thigh and knee. This form of anesthesia avoids the sympathectomy associated with central neuraxial blocks, and therefore its use may be advantageous in patients in whom any shift in hemodynamics might be deleterious, such as those with significant aortic stenosis.

Side Effects/Complications   Block of the sciatic nerve is technically difficult to perform and can be quite painful. Adequate sedation is an important component if this procedure is to meet with patient and surgeon satisfaction; however, in the classic approach the patient is in a lateral position, which may complicate airway management during sedation. Hematoma formation and nerve damage are potential risks. Because of the large area of blockade with sciatic nerve block, vasodilation with venous pooling will occur in the affected extremity. This may be associated with hemodynamic changes in patients with decreased intravascular volume or low cardiac outputs.

Technique

Classic Approach of Labat[39] (*Posterior*) The patient is positioned laterally, with the leg to be blocked fully flexed and rolled forward so that the heel of the upper (operative) leg rests on the knee of the dependent (nonoperative) leg, which is stretched out in a straight line with the torso (Fig. 12-14). A line is drawn between the palpated posterior superior iliac spine and the greater trochanter of the femur. This line is bisected with a perpendicular line extending approximately 5 cm caudad. Next a line is drawn between the greater trochanter of the femur and the sacral hiatus, which will cross the perpendicular at a point 3 to 5 cm along the line. This represents the point of needle insertion. Using sterile technique, a 22-gauge, 10- to 12-cm short-beveled needle is advanced perpendicular to skin until a paresthesia is elicited or bone is encountered (Fig. 12-15). If bone is contacted the needle is redirected to systematically sweep in a lateral-medial direction until the nerve is located. A nerve stimulator is helpful in ascertaining the correct needle position. When the sciatic nerve has been located, a total of 25 to 30 ml of local anesthetic solution is injected.

Anterior Approach[40]   This technique is

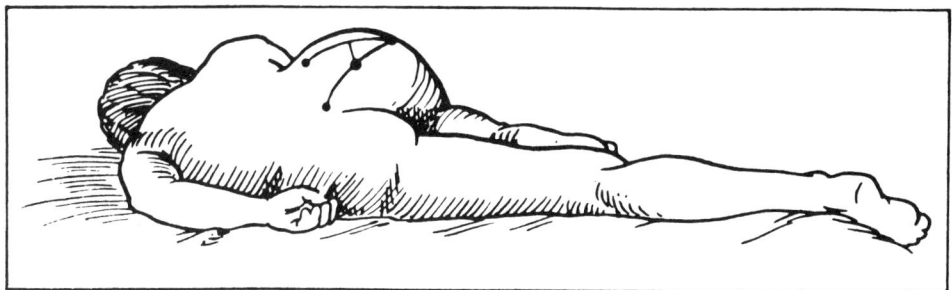

Fig. 12-14. Posterior approach to the sciatic nerve: patient positioning. (From Wedel & Brown,[47] with permission.)

useful for patients who cannot be positioned for the classic posterior approach because of pain or lack of cooperation. If the femoral nerve is blocked first, this approach will be more comfortable for the patient.

The patient is placed in the supine position and a line drawn between the anterior superior iliac spine and the pubic tubercle, representing the inguinal ligament. This line is trisected, and a second parallel line drawn from the point of the tuberosity of the greater trochanter of the hip. The intersection of this second line

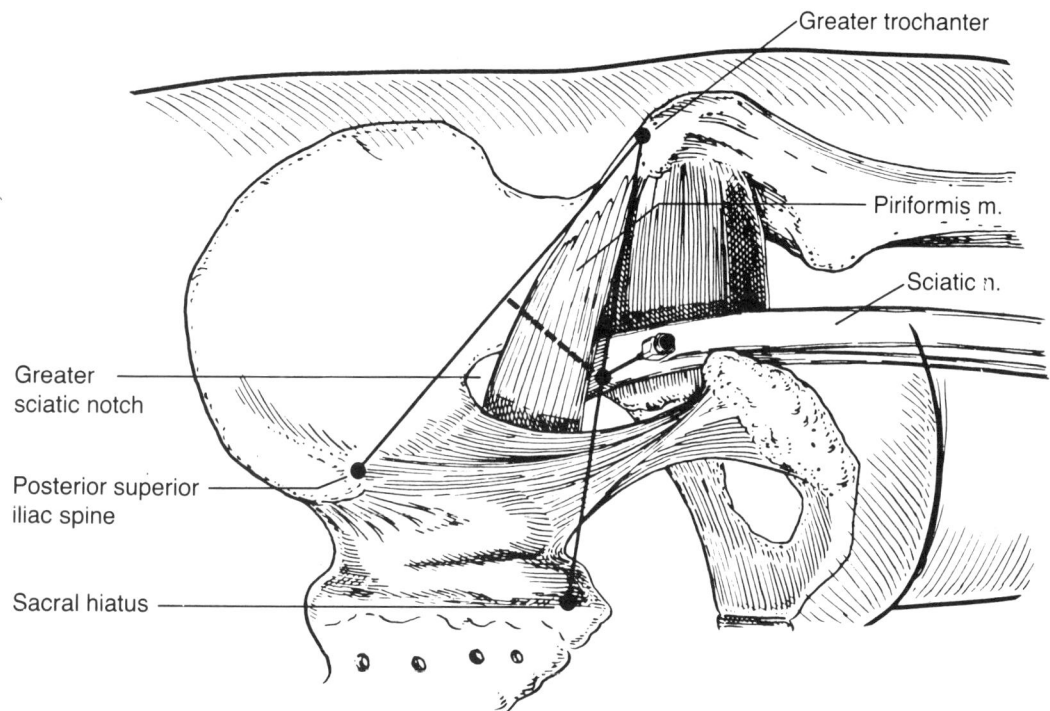

Fig. 12-15. Anatomic landmarks for the posterior approach to sciatic nerve block. (From Wedel & Brown,[47] with permission.)

with the more medial of the perpendicular lines represents the point of needle entry (Fig. 12-16). Using sterile technique, a 22-gauge, 10- to 12-cm short-beveled needle is advanced with a slight lateral angulation until the lesser trochanter of the hip is encountered. At this point the needle is redirected slightly medially, walked off the femur, and advanced until a paresthesia is elicited (approximately 5 cm past bone). A total of 20 to 25 ml of local anesthetic solution is injected incrementally after careful aspiration. A nerve stimulator is useful in locating the sciatic nerve in this technique.

Other Techniques   Blockade of the sciatic nerve in the lateral (patient supine)[41] and lithotomy[42] positions has been described but is rarely applied clinically.

Peripheral Nerve Blocks at the Ankle

Clinical Applications   Peripheral nerve blocks at the ankle are low-risk, simple forms of regional anesthesia that are effective for surgical procedures of the foot in which a leg tourniquet is not required.

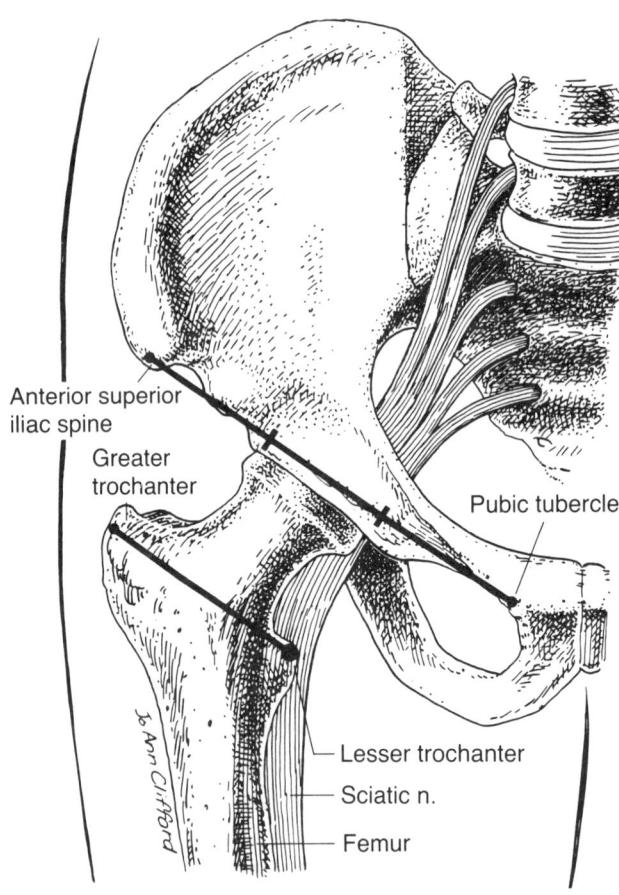

Anterior superior iliac spine

Greater trochanter

Pubic tubercle

Lesser trochanter

Sciatic n.

Femur

Fig. 12-16. Anatomic landmarks for the anterior approach to sciatic nerve block. (From Wedel & Brown,[47] with permission.)

The saphenous nerve is the distal termination of the femoral nerve. All of the other four nerves innervating the foot are branches of the sciatic nerve: the posterior tibial and sural nerves and the superficial and deep peroneal nerves. The sciatic nerve divides into the common peroneal and tibial nerves at the apex of the popliteal fossa or higher. The common peroneal nerve winds around the head of the fibula, where it is susceptible to trauma (surgical, pressure, etc.) because of its superficial position, and divides into the superficial and deep peroneal nerves. The tibial nerve divides into the posterior tibial and sural nerves in the lower leg. The sural nerve emerges lateral to the Achilles tendon, while the posterior tibial nerve can be blocked at the medial border of the Achilles tendon, where it lies near the artery of the same name. It is not always necessary to block all five nerves at the ankle. Knowledge of the anatomy of the foot will allow the anesthesia care provider to choose the appropriate combination of blocks required for a given surgical procedure.

Side Effects/Complications   Multiple needle-stick techniques can be quite uncomfortable for the patient if sedation is inadequate. Persistent paresthesias can occur, but are usually self-limiting. The presence of edema or induration in the area of the ankle block can make palpation of landmarks impossible. Intravascular injection is possible but unlikely if aspiration for blood is negative. The volume of local anesthetic used is small, decreasing the risk of local anesthetic toxicity.

Posterior Tibial Nerve Block

Technique   The patient can be positioned prone or supine for this block. The posterior tibial nerve supplies sensation to the heel, plantar portion of the toes,

and the sole of the foot as well as muscular branches. It can be blocked by palpating the tibial artery and inserting a 22-gauge, 1- to 3-cm short-beveled needle posterolateral to the artery at the level of the medial malleolus (Fig. 12-17A & B). Elicitation of a paresthesia is confirmation of correct needle placement, although it is not necessary for satisfactory blockade. If a paresthesia is obtained, 3 to 5 ml of local anesthetic should be injected; otherwise 7 to 10 ml of solution should be injected as the needle is slowly withdrawn back from the posterior aspect of the tibia.

Sural Nerve Block

Technique   The sural nerve innervates the lateral side of the foot, including the lateral aspect of the little toe. It is located superficially between the lateral malleolus and the Achilles tendon. A 25-gauge, 3-cm needle is inserted lateral to the malleolus and local anesthetic injected as the needle is advanced slowly toward the Achilles tendon. A total of 7 to 10 ml of local anesthetic is deposited in a fanwise fashion in the same direction as the initial needle pass (Fig. 12-17A & C).

Deep Peroneal, Superficial Peroneal, and Saphenous Nerve Block

Technique   All three of these nerves can be blocked through a single needle entry site with the patient in the supine position. A line connecting the malleoli is drawn across the dorsum of the foot. The patient is asked to dorsiflex the big toe to allow easy identification of the tendon of the anterior tibial muscle. The anterior tibial artery, accompanied by the deep peroneal nerve, lies between this tendon and the tendon of extensor hallucis longus (Fig. 12-18A). Using sterile technique, a skin wheal is raised between the

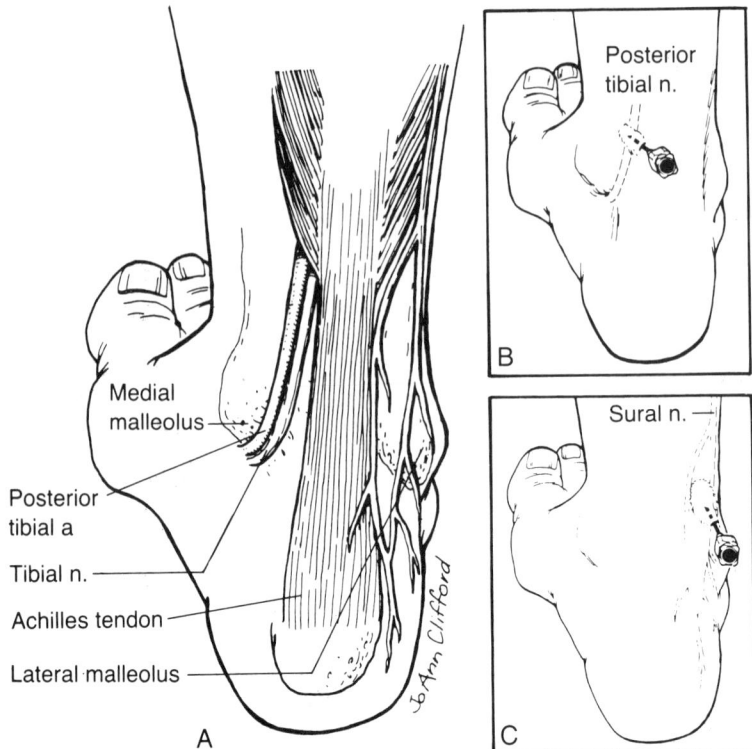

Fig. 12-17. (**A**) Anatomic landmarks for block of the posterior tibial and sural nerves at the ankle. (**B**) Posterior tibial nerve. Method of needle placement for block at the ankle. (**C**) Sural nerve. Method of needle placement for block at the ankle. (From Wedel & Brown,[47] with permission.)

two tendons at the level of the intermalleolar line and lateral to the arterial pulsation if it can be palpated. A 25-gauge, 3-cm needle is advanced perpendicular to skin, through the extensor retinaculum, which will be perceived as a definite resistance. A total of 3 to 5 ml of local anesthetic solution is injected deep into this structure after careful aspiration to block the deep peroneal nerve, which innervates the skin between the first and second toes and the short extensors of the toes.

The needle is then withdrawn, directed laterally though the same skin wheal, and 3 to 5 ml of solution is injected subcutaneously. This will result in a block of the superficial peroneal nerve, which supplies the dorsum of the foot and toes with the exception of the first interdigital cleft.

The needle is now reinserted in the medial direction, and a further 3 to 5 ml of solution injected subcutaneously to anesthetize the saphenous nerve, which innervates a strip of skin along the medial aspect of the foot (Fig. 12-18B).

MISCELLANEOUS BLOCKS

Accessory Nerve Block

Clinical Applications/Technique The accessory nerve (cranial nerve 11) supplies motor innervation to the trapezius

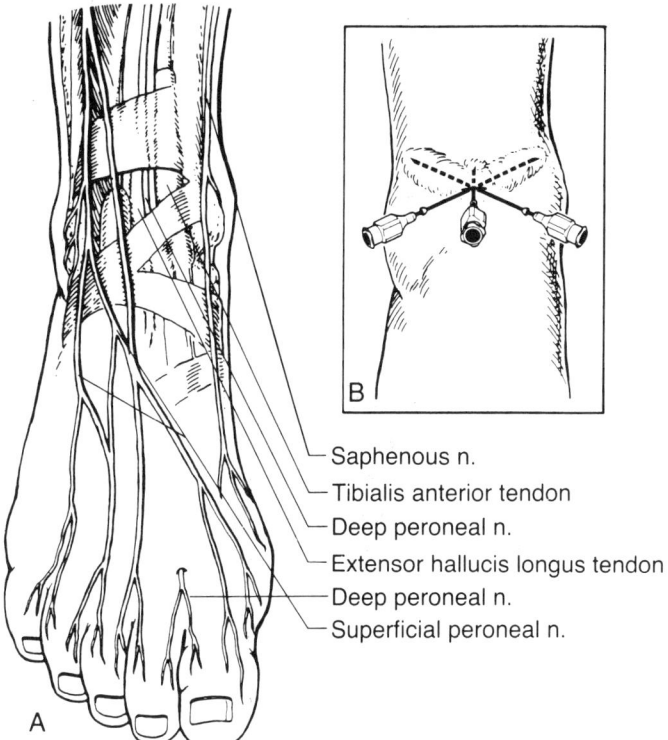

Saphenous n.
Tibialis anterior tendon
Deep peroneal n.
Extensor hallucis longus tendon
Deep peroneal n.
Superficial peroneal n.

Fig. 12-18. (**A**) Anatomic landmarks for block of the deep peroneal, superficial peroneal, and saphenous nerves at the ankle. (**B**) Method of needle placement for block of the deep peroneal, superficial peroneal, and saphenous nerves through a single needle entry site. (From Wedel & Brown,[47] with permission.)

muscle. Block of this nerve is sometimes used in concert with the interscalene block of the brachial plexus to ensure relaxation of this muscle during shoulder surgery. The accessory nerve crosses the posterior triangle of the neck (an anatomic area defined by the posterior border of the. sternocleidomastoid muscle, middle third of the clavicle, and anterior border of the trapezius muscle) as it emerges from the body of the sternocleidomastoid muscle at the junction of the superior and middle thirds of that muscle's posterior border. At this point the accessory nerve is very superficial and can be readily blocked with 5 to 10 ml of local anesthesia solution.

Side Effects/Complications Because of

the small amount of local anesthetic solution used for this block, risks are minimal. Intravascular injection is theoretically possible.

Stellate Ganglion Block

Clinical Applications While sympathetic block of the upper extremity is not a part of orthopedic anesthesia for surgery, it does play an important part in management of common postsurgical and pain conditions such as reflex sympathetic dystrophy and the desirability of increased blood flow following replantation.

Side Effects/Complications The stellate ganglion is located in an anatomic area where there is a high density of neurovascular structures. As a result, extravasation of local anesthetic solution can result in anesthesia of the brachial plexus, recurrent laryngeal nerve, and (infrequently) phrenic nerve. Epidural and subarachnoid blockade,[43] as well as intravascular injection and hematoma formation, are also possible. The vertebral artery is very accessible to the needle with this technique, and small volumes of local anesthetic (less than 1 ml) can cause immediate seizure activity because of the direct route to the brain. Because this complication is not always preventable, stellate ganglion blocks require full monitoring and the capability for complete resuscitation.

Technique   The patient lies supine with the neck slightly extended. The tubercle of C6 (Chassaignac's tubercle), which is the most easily palpated tubercle in the neck, is identified between the sternocleidomastoid muscle and the trachea. The tubercle is firmly palpated between the index and middle fingers while the carotid artery is pushed laterally. Using sterile technique, a skin wheal is raised over the C6 tubercle and a 22- or 25-gauge, 2- to 3-cm short-beveled needle is directed onto the tubercle. Once bone is contacted, the needle is withdrawn 3 mm and fixed in place. After careful aspiration, 8 to 12 ml of local anesthetic is injected incrementally (Fig. 12-19).

Physical signs associated with correct placement of local anesthetic include ipsilateral Horner syndrome, anhydrosis, vascular congestion of the conjunctiva,

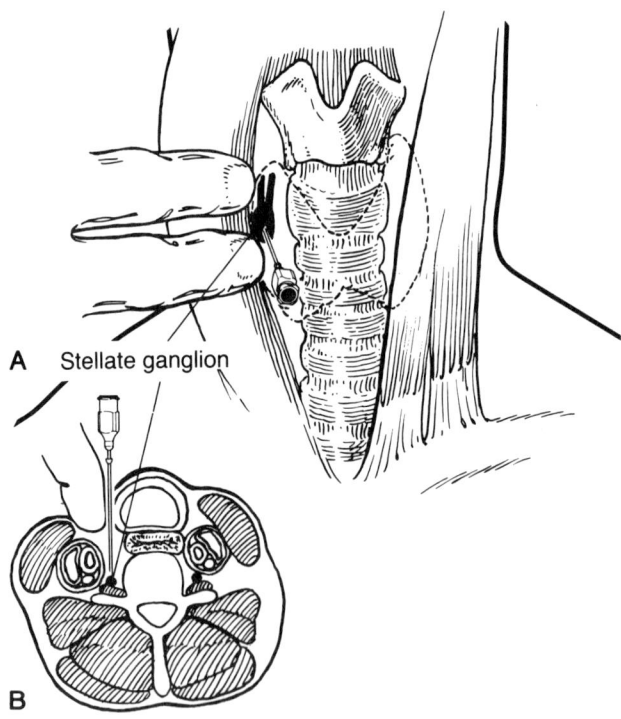

A Stellate ganglion

B

Fig. 12-19. (A) Anatomic landmarks and method of needle placement for stellate ganglion block. (B) Stellate ganglion block: cross-sectional view. (From Wedel & Brown,[47] with permission.)

nasal stuffiness, vasodilation of the facial and upper extremity skin, and increased temperature of the blocked limb.

Paravertebral Block

Clinical Applications   The paravertebral block has limited application to orthopedic practice. However, it can be used as supplementation to other block techniques to provide isolated areas of surgical anesthesia, for example, to provide anesthesia for bone graft harvesting from the iliac crest in a patient undergoing upper extremity surgery under brachial plexus blockade.

Side Effects/Complications   Because of the close proximity of the central neuraxis, epidural or subarachnoid injection of local anesthetic is a risk of this procedure. Intravascular injection into the lumbar vessels, aorta, or vena cava can also occur if the needles are inaccurately placed.

Technique   Lumbar nerves exit the ver-

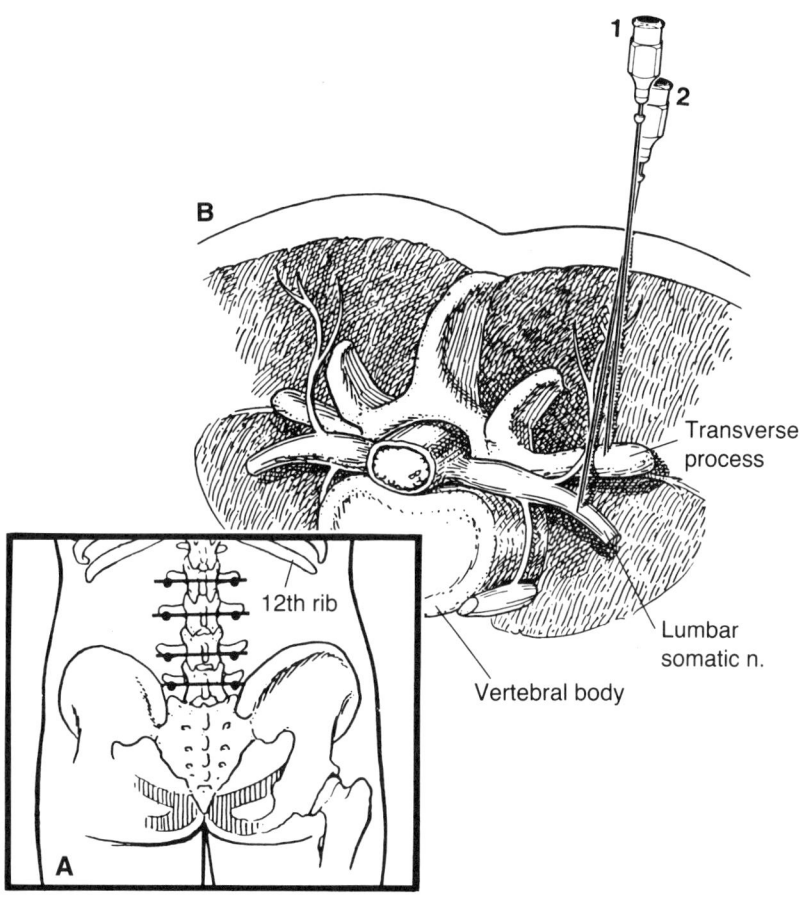

Fig. 12-20. (A) Paravertebral nerve block: patient position and surface landmarks. (B) Paravertebral nerve block: the needle is advanced perpendicularly until it contacts the transverse process. It is redirected to walk off the caudad edge of the transverse process and advanced 1 to 2 cm. (From Wedel & Brown,[47] with permission.)

tebral foramina inferior to the caudad edge of the transverse process before dividing into anterior and posterior branches. The anterior branches of L1–L4 (with a contribution from T12) form the lumbar plexus.

The patient is placed in the prone position with a pillow under the hips to straighten out the lumbar curve. Lines are drawn across the cephalad edge of the lumbar vertebral spinous processes. These will lie opposite the caudad edges of the homologous transverse processes (Fig. 12-20A). Using sterile technique a skin wheal is raised 3 cm lateral to midline on the line corresponding to the chosen lumbar nerve. A 20- or 22-gauge, 6- to 8-cm short-beveled needle is advanced perpendicular to skin until bone (the transverse process) is contacted at a depth of approximately 3 to 5 cm. The needle is then withdrawn and redirected caudad in small steps until the tip walks off the edge of the transverse process. At a depth of 1 to 2 cm beyond this caudad edge, 6 to 10 ml of local anesthetic is injected (Fig. 12-20B). Elicitation of a paresthesia or use of a nerve stimulator is helpful in confirming accurate needle placement.

CHOICE OF LOCAL ANESTHETIC

The choice of local anesthetic for a nerve block requires evaluation of a number of factors: anticipated length of surgery, need for postoperative pain relief, admission status, and patient medical conditions. The use of catheter techniques allows a greater flexibility in choice since the block can be reinjected as desired. Whatever agent is chosen, careful attention must be paid to the total dosage so that toxic blood levels are avoided (Table 12-1). Outpatient procedures can usually be performed under

short- to medium-duration local anesthetics; however, in certain peripheral blocks, long-duration agents may be used to provide extended pain relief. If this is done, patients must be instructed verbally and in writing in care of the anesthetized limb in order to avoid unintentional injury that is not recognized.

Peripheral nerves are quite susceptible to the blocking effects of local anesthetics. High concentrations are not necessary to achieve surgical anesthesia, and may be deleterious. Therefore, 0.75 percent bupivacaine, 2 percent lidocaine and mepivacaine, and 3 percent 2-chloroprocaine are not recommended for peripheral nerve blocks. The lowest commercially available concentrations of common agents (0.25 percent bupivacaine, 1 percent lidocaine and mepivacaine) will usually provide good sensory block, but variable motor blockade. Again the choice will depend on the extent of surgery, need for muscle relaxation to accomplish the procedure, and to some degree, surgeon preference. Mixing of short- and long-duration agents to provide a "perfect" intermediate drug with rapid onset and long duration has given contradictory results.[44,45]

Vasoconstrictors, usually epinephrine, can be added to local anesthetics to improve onset, increase sensory and motor blockade, prolong duration, and decrease vascular uptake. They should not be used for blocks involving end arteries (penis, digits, ears) because of the risk of ischemia. If epinephrine is used it may be more advantageous to add it to the solution at the time the block will be performed rather than using commercially prepared solutions.[46] The proposed mechanism for the observed decrease in onset time seen with freshly added epinephrine compared with the commercial preparations is related to the lower pH in the commercial solutions. This causes an increase in the percentage of ionized mol-

Table 12-1. Local Anesthetics for Peripheral Nerve Block

Drug	Maximum Dose (with epinephrine) (mg)	Concentration (%)	Duration (hr)
2-Chloroprocaine	1,000	1–2	0.5–1
Lidocaine	500	0.5–1.5	1–3
Mepivacaine	500	0.5–1.5	2–3
Bupivacaine	250	0.25–0.5	4–24
Etidocaine	400	0.5–0.75	3–12

(From Wedel & Brown,[47] with permission.)

ecules of the local anesthetic. Since these are the form of local anesthetic less likely to cross the neural membrane the onset is prolonged.

In conclusion, peripheral nerve blocks are ideally suited to the orthopedic surgical practice. They are applicable to all age groups and provide excellent intraoperative anesthesia with the added benefit of postoperative pain relief in many cases. However, clinical application requires a firm knowledge of the relevant anatomy and pharmacology so that these blocks can be used appropriately and confidently.

REFERENCES

1. Hall RJ: Hydrochlorate of cocaine. NY Med J 40:643, 1884
2. Halsted WS: Practical comments on the use and abuse of cocaine; suggested by its invariably successful employment in more than a thousand minor surgical operations. NY Med J 42:294, 1885
3. Corning JL: On the prolongation of the anaesthetic effect of the hydrochlorate of cocaine, when subcutaneously injected. An experimental study. NY Med J 42:317, 1885
4. Braun H: Über den Einfluss der Vitalität der Gewebe auf die örtlichen und allgemeinen Giftwirkungen local anästhesi- render Mittel und über die Bedeutung des Adrenalins für die local anästhesie. Arch Klin Chir 69:541, 1903
5. Braun H: Local Anesthesia: Its Scientific Basis and Practical Use. 3rd Ed. Lea & Febiger, Philadelphia, 1914
6. Goldan SO: Intraspinal cocainization for surgical anesthesia. Philadelphia Med J 6:850, 1900
7. Winnie AP: Interscalene brachial plexus block. Anesth Analg 49:455, 1970
8. Urmey WF, Talts KH, Sharrock NE: One hundred percent incidence of hemidiaphragmatic paresis associated with interscalene brachial plexus anesthesia as diagnosed by ultrasonography. Anesth Analg 72:498, 1991
9. Lanz E, Theiss D, Jankovic D: The extent of blockade following various techniques of brachial plexus block. Anesth Analg 62:55, 1983
10. de Jong RH: Axillary block of the brachial plexus. Anesthesiology 22:215, 1961
11. Brown DL, Bridenbaugh LD: Physics applied to regional anesthesia results in an improved supraclavicular nerve block: the "plumb-bob" technique. Anesthesiology 69:A376, 1988
12. Serlo W, Haapanemi L: Regional anesthesia in paediatric surgery. Acta Anaesthesiol Scand 29:283, 1985
13. Eriksson E: Axillary brachial plexus anaesthesia in children with Citanest. Acta Anaesthesiol Scand (Suppl) 16:291, 1965
14. Selander D, Edshage S, Wolff T: Paresthesiae or no paresthesiae: nerve lesions

after axillary blocks. Acta Anaesthesiol Scand 23:27, 1979

15. Thompson GE, Rorie DK: Functional anatomy of the brachial plexus sheaths. Anesthesiology 59:117, 1983

16. Selander D, Dhuner KG, Lungborg G: Peripheral nerve injury due to injection needles used for regional anesthesia: an experimental study of the acute effects of needle point trauma. Acta Anaesthesiol Scand 21:182, 1977

17. Vester-Andersen T, Christiansen C, Srensen M, Eriksen C: Perivascular axillary block. I. Blockade following 40 ml 1% mepivacaine with adrenaline. Acta Anaesthesiol Scand 26:519, 1982

18. Vester-Andersen T, Christiansen C, Srensen M et al: Perivascular axillary blocks. II. Influence of injected volume of local anaesthetic on neural blockade. Acta Anaesthesiol Scand 27:95, 1983

19. Vester-Andersen T, Husum B, Lindeburg T et al: Perivascular axillary block. IV. Blockade following 40, 50, or 60 ml of mepivacaine 1% with adrenaline. Acta Anaesthesiol Scand 28:99, 1984

20. Montgomery SJ, Raj PP, Nettles D, Jenkins MT: The use of the nerve stimulator with standard unsheathed needles in nerve blockade. Anesth Analg 52:827, 1973

21. Winnie AP, Collins VJ: The subclavian perivascular technique to brachial plexus anesthesia. Anesthesiology 25:353, 1964

22. Raj PP, Montgomery SJ, Nettles D, Jenkins MT: Infraclavicular brachial plexus block: a new approach. Anesth Analg 52:897, 1973

23. Ansbro PF: A method of continuous brachial plexus block. Am J Surg 71:716, 1946

24. Gaumann DM, Lennon RL, Wedel DJ: Continuous axillary block for postoperative pain management. Reg Anesth 13:77, 1988

25. Bier A: Über einen neuen Weg Lokalanasthesie an den gliedmassen zu Erzcugen. Verh Dtsch Ges Chir 27:204, 1908

26. Duggan J, McKeown DW, Scott DB: Venous pressures in intravenous regional anesthesia. Reg Anesth 9:70, 1984

27. El-Hassan KM, Hutton P, Black AMS: Venous pressure and arm volume changes during simulated Bier's block. Anaesthesia 39:229, 1984

28. Davies JAH, Wilkey AD, Hall ID: Bupivacaine leak past inflated tourniquets during intravenous regional analgesia. Anaesthesia 39:996, 1984

29. Palas TAR, Els M: Intravenous regional anesthesia (IVRA) with an additive-free 0.5% chloroprocaine solution. Reg Anesth 15:16, 1991

30. Sukhani R, Garcia CJ, Munhall RJ et al: Lidocaine disposition following intravenous regional anesthesia with different tourniquet deflation technics. Anesth Analg 68:633, 1989

31. Hastings H II, Misamore G: Compartment syndrome resulting from intravenous regional anesthesia. J Hand Surg 12A:559, 1987

32. Luce EA, Mangubat E: Loss of hand and forearm following Bier block: a case report. J Hand Surg 8:280, 1983

33. Rawal N, Hallén J, Amilon A, Hellstrand P: Comparison between IVRA and reexsanguination IVRA (Re-IVRA) using three different local anesthetics. Reg Anesth 15:18, 1991

34. Moore MA, Garfin SR, Hargens AR: Wide tourniquets eliminate blood flow at low inflation pressures. J Hand Surg 12A:1006, 1987

35. Chayden D, Nathan H, Chayden M: The psoas compartment block. Anesthesiology 45:95, 1976

36. Winnie AP, Ramamurthy S, Durrani Z: The inguinal paravascular technique of lumbar plexus anesthesia: the "3-in-1 block". Anesth Analg 52:989, 1973

37. Patel NJ, Flashburg MH, Paskin S, Grossman R: A regional anesthetic technique compared to general anesthesia for outpatient knee arthroscopy. Anesth Analg 65:185, 1986

38. Berry FR: Analgesia in patients with fractured shaft of femur. Anaesthesia 32:576, 1977

39. Labat G: Regional Anesthesia: Its Technique and Clinical Application. WB Saunders, Philadelphia, 1924

40. Beck GP: Anterior aproach to sciatic nerve. Anesthesiology 24:222, 1963
41. Ichiyanagi K: Sciatic nerve block: lateral approach with the patient supine. Anesthesiology 20:601, 1959
42. Raj PP, Parks RI, Watson TD, Jenkins MT: New single position supine approach to sciatic-femoral nerve block. Anesth Analg 54:489, 1975
43. Scott DL, Ghia JN, Teeple E: Aphasia and hemiparesis following stellate ganglion block. Anesth Analg 62:1038, 1983
44. Raj PP, Rosenblatt R, Miller J et al: Dynamics of local-anesthetic compounds in regional anesthesia. Anesth Analg 56:110, 1977
45. Cohen SE, Thurlow A: Comparison of a chloroprocaine-bupivacaine mixture with chloroprocaine and bupivacaine used individually for obstetric epidural analgesia. Anesthesiology 51:288, 1979
46. DiFazio CA, Carron H, Grosslight KR et al: Comparison of pH-adjusted lidocaine solutions for epidural anesthesia. Anesth Analg 65:760, 1986
47. Wedel DJ, Brown DL: Nerve Blocks. p. 1407. In Miller RD (ed): Anesthesia. 3rd Ed. Churchill Livingstone, NY, 1990

13

Spinal and Epidural Blocks*

David L. Brown
Lance A. Proctor

Often, central neuraxial blocks (spinal, epidural, and caudal) are believed to be "one and the same" block. This misperception seems to occur because they all result in sensory and motor block following insertion of a needle in the plane of the central neuraxis. In spite of this misperception by many physicians and patients, there are significant physiologic and pharmacologic differences between spinal, epidural, and caudal anesthetics. For example, spinal anesthesia requires only a small mass of drug that is almost devoid of systemic pharmacologic effect. Epidural anesthesia demands the use of a mass of local anesthetic that often produces pharmacologically active systemic blood levels. These plasma concentrations of local anesthetic may be associated with side effects and complications unknown with spinal anesthesia. In spite of the differences between epidural and spinal anesthesia, orthopedic surgical patients provide many opportunities for anesthesia care providers to use these blocks comprehensively in their practice.

* Modified from Brown and Wedel,[111] with permission.)

INDICATIONS

Fundamentally, central neuraxial blocks are indicated whenever a surgical procedure can be carried out with a sensory level of anesthesia that is not associated with unfavorable outcomes. The prescription of a central neuraxial block must also include the amount and type of supplemental medications that will be needed to ensure effective sedation and anxiolysis during the surgical procedure. When choosing the central neuraxial block for a patient, the level of sensory analgesia that the surgical procedure demands is of central importance. It is clear that low spinal anesthesia (that is, a T10 or lower sensory level) has a different impact on a patient than does a block performed to produce high (above T5) spinal anesthesia.[1] The indications for central neuraxial blocks in orthopedic surgical patients include almost all patients undergoing lower extremity procedures. In this group of patients, in whom a central neuraxial block is virtually uniformly indicated, it is most often a patient's specific contraindication that will modify that anesthetic prescription. In addition

291

to the lower extremity procedures, central neuraxial block may also be used successfully in many patients undergoing procedures on the lumbar spine.

CONTRAINDICATIONS

There are a few absolute contraindications to the central neuraxial blockade. The most significant ones include patient refusal; patient inability to maintain stillness during the lumbar puncture, thus exposing the neural structures to unacceptable risk of injury; and raised intracranial pressure, which theoretically may predispose to brain stem herniation. Relative contraindications that must be balanced against the potential benefits include coagulopathy, both intrinsic and idiopathic, such as that occurring with the administration of warfarin or heparin; skin or soft tissue infection at the site of needle insertion; severe hypovolemia; and lack of anesthesia care provider experience. The commonly cited relative contraindication of pre-existing neurologic disease (e.g., neuropathies of the lower extremities) seems primarily based on legal considerations rather than sound medical criteria.

PHILOSOPHY OF CENTRAL NEURAXIAL BLOCKADE

Although most anesthetics in the United States are performed with general anesthesia, when anesthesia care providers are questioned about their preference for anesthetic technique they overwhelmingly prefer regional anesthesia for themselves.[2] It seems likely that this dichotomy can be explained by an incomplete appreciation of what physicians expect from regional anesthetics. There seems to be a misconception that a regional block is a failure if intravenous or inhaled supplementation has to be titrated following a regional anesthetic. This misconception is probably the single most important impediment to a more comprehensive and appropriate use of regional anesthesia. During the early years of regional anesthesia at the turn of the century, this concept was not in vogue; rather, physicians at that time believed combining regional anesthetics with other amnestic and sedative agents was the desired goal. Crile believed his concept of *anociassociation* prevented morbidity.[3] *Balanced anesthesia* at that time implied a combination of regional and general anesthesia.[4] Since that time, the fundamental flaw in our understanding of comprehensive anesthetic care has entered anesthetic practice. For far too many of our colleagues, regional anesthetics are prescribed to "stand alone," without the useful adjunct of appropriate intravenous or inhalational sedation.

Perhaps this has occurred because all anesthetic techniques have become safer since those early years, and thereby one of the principal advantages of regional techniques became less important. In spite of these observations, there is a renewed interest in regional techniques, seemingly driven by increased concerns over ineffective postoperative analgesia. Investigators are documenting that the use of regional analgesic techniques may provide for both decreased morbidity and mortality, as well as lower postoperative costs.[5,6]

An anesthesia care provider can become frustrated during attempts to prescribe regional anesthesia, since it appears many patients simply will not accept a block technique. Our own observations are this "lack of acceptance" is based on a lack of experience and lack of confidence that anesthesia care providers unavoidably communicate to patients during their preoperative discussions. The lack of confidence that anesthesia care providers often express is not often directly their responsibility. One of the problems in establishing a more comprehensive anesthetic practice is that many anesthesia care providers receive limited training and experience in regional anesthesia during their residencies.[7]

One of the solutions to performing more comprehensive regional anesthesia is to appropriately use intravenous sedatives prior to performing the block. Since central neuraxial blocks do not require the elicitation of a paresthesia, sedation can be administered so that most patients do not have a recollection of the needle insertion. Often the titration of an intravenous benzodiazepine (e.g., midazolam) and narcotic (e.g., fentanyl) will adequately prepare the patient for the block technique.

Another necessity for comprehensive use of central neuraxial blocks is the development of a method of checking the block prior to surgical incision and ascertaining appropriate supplementation needs. The sensory level of these blocks should initially be checked within 3 to 5 minutes of administration to determine whether the level is developing as expected. This can often be effectively accomplished by using an alcohol wipe to determine at what level temperature discrimination changes. The determination of sensory levels should not stop following surgical incision; rather it should be part of the anesthetic monitoring throughout the case. Nevertheless, emphasis should be placed on carrying out this determination in a reassuring manner, rather than an inquisitive or tentative one, which may lead the patient to wonder whether the anesthesia care provider questions if the block will work. Again for this reason, the surgeon should refrain from "checking" the block prior to incision in an inquisitive manner but should instead be reassured by the anesthesia care provider that adequate surgical anesthesia will be provided in all cases.

ANATOMY OF CENTRAL NEURAXIAL BLOCKS

Subarachnoid local anesthetics produce their sensory block at the spinal cord, which is continuous cephalad with the brain stem via the foramen magnum and terminates distally in the conus medullaris. The caudad termination, because of differential growth rates between the bony vertebral canal and the central nervous system, varies from L3 in the infant to the lower border of L1 in adults. In the bony vertebral column, the spinal cord is surrounded by three membranes, which from within to the periphery are the pia mater, arachnoid mater, and dura mater. The pia mater is a vascularized membrane that closely invests the spinal cord (and brain). The arachnoid mater is a nonvascular delicate membrane closely attached to the outermost layer, the dura. Between the two innermost membranes is the area of interest in spinal anesthesia, the subarachnoid space. Contained in this space are the cerebrospinal fluid (CSF), spinal nerves, a trabecular network between the two membranes, blood vessels that supply the spinal cord, and the lateral extensions of the pia mater, the dentate ligaments. These ligaments supply lateral support from the spinal cord to the dura mater throughout the length of the vertebral column. Although the spinal cord ends at the lower border of L1 in adults, the subarachnoid space continues to the level of S2. The outermost membrane in the spinal canal is the longitudinally organized fibroelastic membrane, the dura mater (or theca). This layer is the direct extension of the cranial dura mater

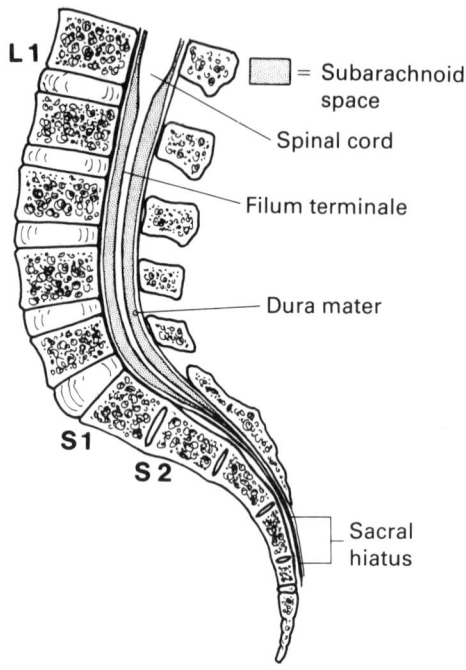

L1

☐ = Subarachnoid
space

Spinal cord

Filum terminale

Dura mater

S1

S2

Sacral
hiatus

Fig. 13-1. Distal central neuraxial anatomy. In adults the spinal cord ends at lower border of L1, with the subarachnoid space continuing to S2. (From Brown & Wedel,[111] with permission.)

and extends as spinal dura mater from the foramen magnum to S2, where the filum terminalae (an extension of the pia mater beginning at the conus medullaris) blends with the periosteum of the coccyx (Fig. 13-1). There is a potential space between the dura mater and the arachnoid, the subdural space, which contains only small amounts of serous fluid to allow the dura and arachnoid to move over each other. Anesthesia care providers do not intentionally use this space, although injection into it during spinal anesthesia may explain the occasional failed spinal anesthetic and the rare slow-to-develop total spinal block following epidural anesthesia, when there is no indication of errant injection of local anesthetic into the CSF.

Surrounding the dura mater is another space that is important to anesthesia care providers, the epidural space. This space extends from the foramen magnum to the sacral hiatus and surrounds the dura mater anteriorly, laterally, and more usefully, posteriorly. Contents of the epidural space include the nerve roots that traverse it from the foramina to peripheral locations, as well as fat, areolar tissue, lymphatics, and blood vessels, which include the well-organized venous plexus of Batson. Posterior to the epidural space is the yellow ligament or ligamentum flavum. This ligament also extends from the foramen magnum to the sacral hiatus. Classically, many have portrayed the ligamentum flavum as a single ligament. In reality, it is composed of two ligamenta flava, the right and the left, which join in the middle forming an acute angle with a ventral opening[8] (Fig. 13-2). The ligamenta flavum is not uniform from skull to sacrum, nor even within an intervertebral space. The ligament thickness, distance to dura, and skin to dura distance vary with the area of the vertebral canal (Table 13-1). Immediately posterior to the ligamenta flavum are either lamina and spinous processes of the vertebral bodies or the interspinous ligaments. Extending from the external occipital protuberance to the coccyx posterior to these structures is the supraspinous ligament, which joins the vertebral spines (Fig. 13-3). An anatomic clarification that has been made through epiduroscopy and epidurography confirms some of our prior clinical observations that occasionally unilateral anesthesia follows apparently adequate epidural technique.[9,10] Blomberg,[11] via epiduroscopy, identified the universal appearance of a dorsomedian connective tissue band in the midline of the epidural space. Anatomic dissection and computed tomography (CT)-epidurography have also documented epidural space septa (Fig. 13-4). Additionally, Blomberg[13] utilized fiberoptic tech-

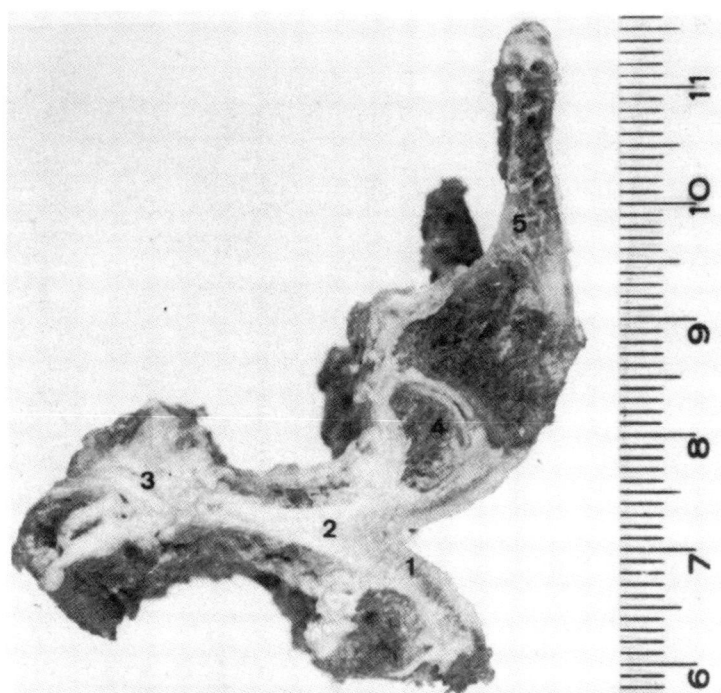

Fig. 13-2. Lumbar segment of the vertebral column in horizontal section. 1, Ligamentum flavum (the two leaves of the ligament make an approximately 90-degree angle as they join); 2, interspinous ligament; 3, supraspinous ligament; 4, articular process; and 5, transverse process. (From Zarzur,[8] with permission.)

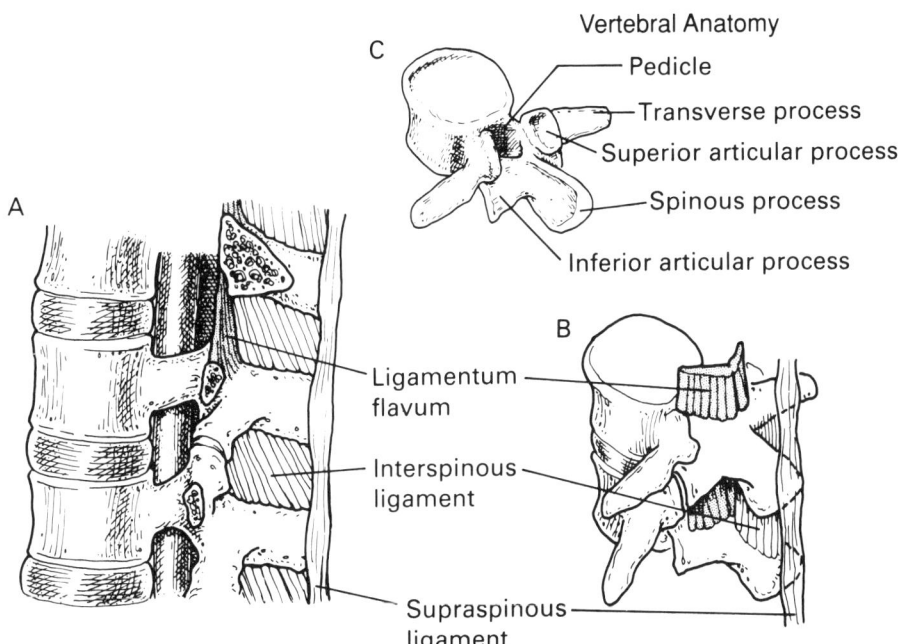

Vertebral Anatomy

Pedicle

Transverse process

Superior articular process

Spinous process

Inferior articular process

Ligamentum flavum

Interspinous ligament

Supraspinous ligament

Fig. 13-3. Vertebral anatomy. **(A)** Sagittal view; **(B)** oblique view of lumbar vertebra showing ligamentum flavum thickening in the caudad extent of intervertebral space and in the midline; **(C)** oblique view of single lumbar vertebra. (From Brown & Wedel,[111] with permission.)

Table 13-1. Characteristics of Ligamentum Flavum at Different Vertebral Levels

Site	Skin to Ligament (cm)	Thickness of Ligament (mm)
Cervical	—	1.5–3.0
Thoracic	—	3.0–5.0
Lumbar	3.0–8.0[a]	5.0–6.0[b]
Caudal	Variable	2.0–6.0

[a] Distance is 4 cm for 50% of patients and 4–6 cm for 80% of patients.
[b] Within each interlaminal space the ligamentum flavum varies in thickness from cephalad to caudad: near the rostral lamina 1.3–1.6 mm, near the caudad lamina 6.9–9.1 mm. (Data from Bromage,[72] Cousins and Bromage,[71] and Reynolds et al.[73])

niques to demonstrate that the subdural extra-arachnoid space is easily entered in two-thirds of autopsy attempts in humans. In spite of this high frequency, it seems to be an infrequent clinical problem with epidural anesthesia.

When caudal anesthesia is chosen, it calls for an expanded understanding of epidural anatomy and especially the frequent variations in sacral hiatus anatomy. The sacrum results from the fusion of the five sacral vertebrae. The sacral hiatus, which is the failure of the lamina of S5 and usually part of S4 to fuse in the midline, is the center of interest during caudal anesthesia (Fig. 13-5). The sacral hiatus results in a variably shaped and sized inverted V-shaped bony defect. This opening is covered by the posterior sacrococcygeal ligament, which is a functional counterpart to the ligamentum flavum. The bony defect of the sacral hiatus allows access to the sacral canal; the needle insertion through this opening may be made difficult by the frequent variations in anatomy of the hiatus (Fig. 13-6). For example, the shape of the space may vary from a slit-like opening to a wide-based inverted V, and in 5 percent of patients

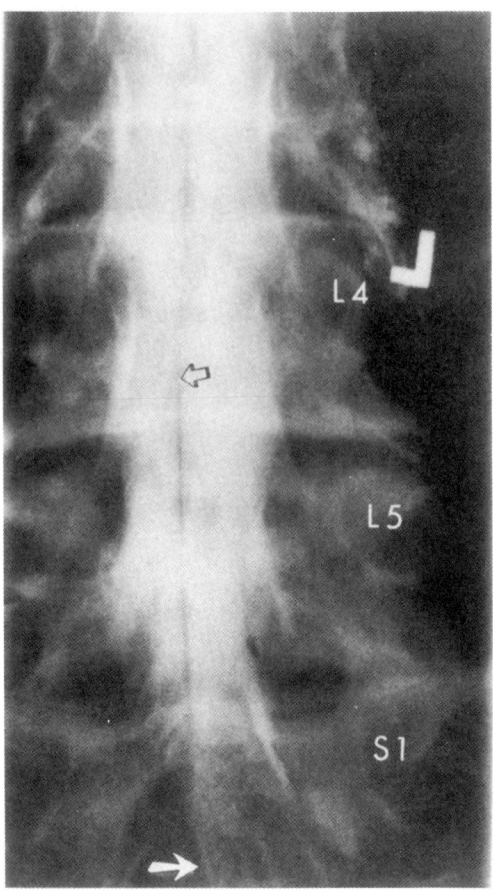

Fig. 13-4. Anteroposterior view of lumbosacral epidural space after contrast injection. Arrow indicates a median dorsal band in the epidural space. (From Savolaine et al,[12] with permission.)

the bony defect may be absent, precluding the usual caudal approach.[14,15] Within the sacral canal is the terminal portion of the dural sac, which usually ends cephalad to a line joining the posterior superior iliac spines or S2. Similar to most anatomic features of the central neuraxis, there is variation in the distal extent of the dural sac. Its termination may be lower in children, although the ease of palpating the sacral hiatus in these young patients may make pediatric caudal technique overall easier to learn. In addition

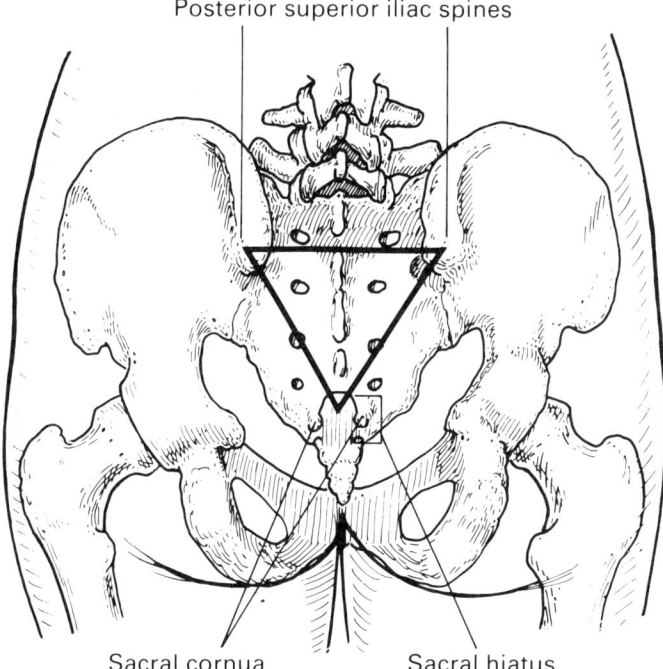

Fig. 13-5. Sacral surface anatomy. An equilateral triangle can be drawn to connect the posterior superior iliac spines and the sacral hiatus. This can be useful in confirming palpation of the sacral hiatus. (From Brown & Wedel,[111] with permission.)

to the dural sac, the sacral canal also contains a venous plexus that is part of the valveless internal vertebral venous plexus. Once one develops an understanding of central neuraxial anatomy, it is often tempting to immediately begin administering spinal or epidural anesthesia. Nevertheless, to administer these anesthetics safely, an appreciation for the physiologic changes accompanying these blocks is necessary.

PHYSIOLOGIC EFFECTS OF CENTRAL NEURAXIAL BLOCKS

Often physiologic effects of central neuraxial blocks are mislabeled as complications. An example of this is hypoten-sion, which is listed as a complication of the technique rather than a side effect.[16] It is important that anesthesia care providers understand this distinction, since accurate determination of the risk/benefit ratio for an individual patient requires it.

Cardiovascular Effects

Central neuraxial blocks produce many of the same effects that intravenous α_1- and β-adrenergic blockers do, including decreases in heart rate and arterial blood pressure. The sympathectomy associated with central neuraxial blocks is dependent on the height of the block, with the sympathectomy typically described as extending for two to six dermatomes above the sensory level with spinal anesthesia and nearly at the same level during epi-

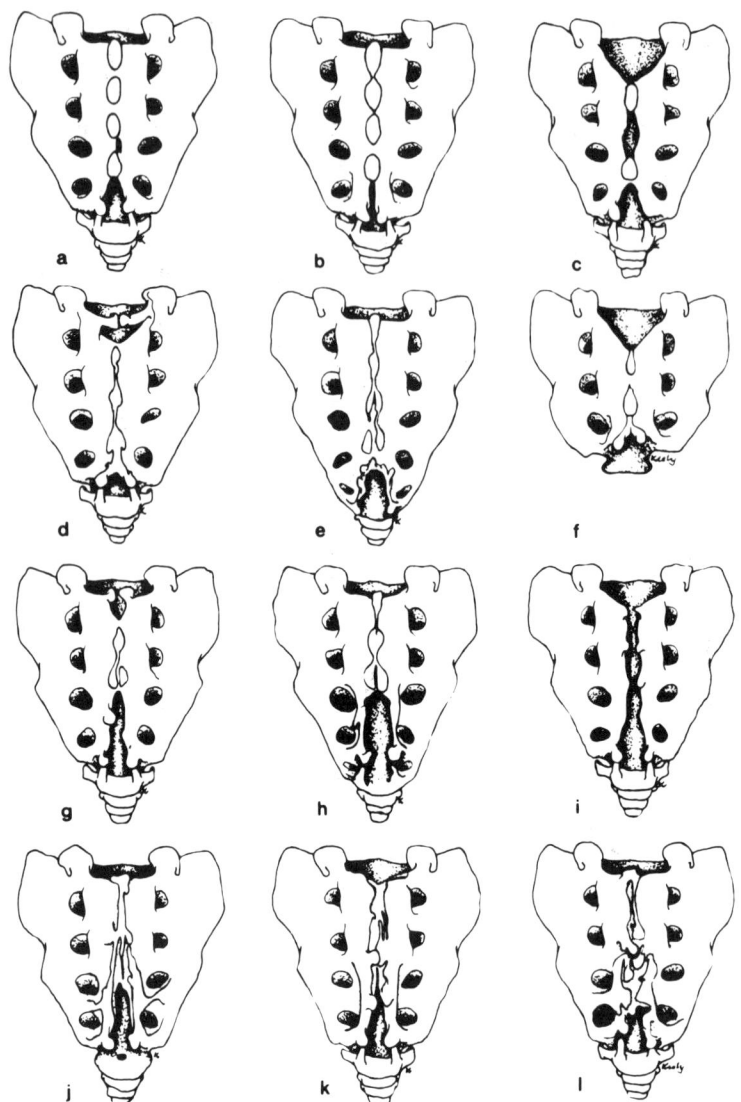

Fig. 13-6. Anatomic variants of sacrum and sacral hiatus. Sacral hiatus variants: **(A)** normal; **(B)** longitudinal slitlike hiatus; **(C)** second midline hiatus; **(D)** transverse hiatus; **(E)** large hiatus with absent cornua; **(F)** transverse hiatus with absent coccyx and two prominent cornua, and two proximal "decoy hiatuses lateral to the cornua"; **(G–I)** large midline defects contiguous with sacral hiatus; **(J–L)** enlarged longitudinal hiatuses, each with an overlying "decoy" hiatus. (From Willis,[110] with permission.)

dural anesthesia.[17] Although the sympathectomy results in both venous and arterial vasodilatation, the venodilatory effect predominates since approximately 75 percent of the total blood volume is contained in the venous system. Additionally, this is a result of the limited amount of smooth muscle in venules, whereas the vascular smooth muscle on the arterial side of the circulation retains a considerable degree of autonomous tone even in the face of sympathectomy. In normovolemic patients, even with near-total sympathectomies, if normal cardiac output is maintained, total peripheral resistance should decrease only 15 to 18 percent during central neuraxial techniques. During these techniques, heart rate typically decreases as a result of blockade of the cardioaccelerator fibers arising from T1–T4. Another reason that heart rate may decrease following central neuraxial block is a result of a decrease in right atrial filling. This decreased filling limits the outflow from intrinsic chronotropic stretch receptors located in the right atrium and great veins, thus further decreasing the heart rate.[17]

Is the blood pressure decrease accompanying central neuraxial blocks less worrisome than a similar fall in blood pressure accompanying general anesthetic techniques? At this time, this question is unanswerable. It does seem clear that blood loss during many lower extremity procedures can be decreased by utilizing a central neuraxial block and that the risk/benefit ratio of lower blood pressure and patient morbidity has yet to be definitively answered. Nevertheless, we believe that the key during decreases in blood pressure associated with central neuraxial block is the maintenance of normovolemia. In spite of our beliefs, there are some data available to help determine the extent to which arterial blood pressure should be allowed to decrease during central neuraxial block. Kety and colleagues[18] studied both normotensive and hypertensive patients during low and high spinal anesthesia. During their studies, coronary blood flow paralleled the decrease in mean arterial pressure in both groups of patients, although the percentage extraction of myocardial oxygen was unchanged during the hypotension. The reason the extraction of oxygen was unchanged is that myocardial work paral-

leled the decrease in mean arterial pressure and coronary flow.[19] Cerebral blood flow in these patients was unchanged in the normotensive group; however, an approximate 20 percent decrease in cerebral blood flow occurred in the untreated hypertensive patients.[18,20] Sivarajan and coworkers[21] performed organ blood flow studies via microsphere techniques in rhesus monkeys during both low and high spinal anesthesia. When spinal anesthesia was maintained at a T10 level, there was no significant change in the organ blood flow; during the T1 spinal anesthetics, with a 22 percent decrease in mean arterial pressure, cerebral and myocardial blood flows were insignificantly altered.[21] Overall, prevention of decreases in mean arterial pressure of more than 30 percent (the often-cited recommendation) has some basis, but the data supporting this recommendation were collected in severely hypertensive and presumably untreated patients. For normotensive and treated hypertensive patients, a wider, though undocumented margin of safety probably exists. Once arterial blood pressure falls to the level for which treatment is believed necessary, ephedrine (a mixed adrenergic agonist) provides more appropriate therapy for the noncardiac circulatory sequela of central neuraxial block than do either a pure α- or pure β-adrenergic agonist.[22] The fall in blood pressure following these blocks can be minimized by administration of crystalloids intravenously prior to administering the block. The amount of crystalloid indicated will depend on the hydration of the patient, concurrent cardiovascular disease, and type of central neuraxial block chosen.

Respiratory Effects

In healthy patients following central neuraxial block, the alteration in pulmonary variables is usually of little clinical consequence. It seems clear that tidal volume, respiratory rate, and minute ventilation are minimally changed during central neuraxial block.[23] Vital capacity does decrease a small amount and is likely a result of the decrease in expiratory reserve volume related to paralysis of abdominal muscles necessary for forced exhalation, rather than a decrease in phrenic or diaphragmatic function.[1] The rare respiratory arrest associated with spinal anesthesia is also unrelated to phrenic or inspiratory dysfunction, but rather to hypoperfusion of the respiratory centers in the brain stem. Supportive evidence for this concept is seen following resuscitation, when apnea almost always disappears as soon as pharmacologic and fluid therapies have restored cardiac output in blood pressure. This would not be the case if phrenic paralysis was the mechanism of respiratory arrest.[1] Central neuraxial block can be used in respiratory cripples in spite of some paralysis of respiratory muscles. Except for the severely compromised patient with respiratory failure, inspiratory muscle function during central neuraxial blocks should be adequate to maintain ventilatory function. The physiologic consideration most related to muscle paralysis with central neuraxial block is the expiratory muscle function in these severely compromised patients. This is important since these expiratory muscles are necessary for effective coughing and clearing of intrapulmonary secretions.[24,25]

Gastrointestinal Function

Other organ system physiology affected during central neuraxial block involves the gastrointestinal tract. Nausea and vomiting may occur in up to 20 percent of patients undergoing central neuraxial block, and seems primarily related to gastrointestinal hyperperistalsis due to un-opposed parasympathetic activity. This is given credence since atropine is effective in treating nausea associated with high spinal anesthesia in almost every case.[26] This gastrointestinal hyperperistalsis does produce a contracted gut, which may be an advantage during intra-abdominal surgery, but should be of limited importance during most orthopedic surgical procedures. Hepatic blood flow during central neuraxial blocks should parallel the decrease in mean arterial pressure accompanying the techniques.[27]

Renal Function

Renal function has a remarkably wide physiologic reserve. Although there are predictable decreases in renal blood flow during central neuraxial blockade, the decrease seems to be of little physiologic importance. One aspect of genitourinary function that is of clinical importance is the belief that central neuraxial blocks frequently cause urinary retention. This is important since urinary retention often delays the discharge of outpatients or necessitates bladder catheterization in inpatients. It is evident that lower concentrations of local anesthetic are necessary for paralysis of bladder function than for motor nerves to lower extremities. Nevertheless, the clinical applicability of this concept is in question. As an example, orthopedic patients undergoing hip replacement demonstrated that bladder catheterization was no more frequent after central neuraxial (spinal or epidural) block than after general anesthesia followed by narcotic analgesia.[28] Still, it is important to avoid excessive administration of crystalloid solutions intravenously to patients undergoing central neuraxial blocks.

Physiologic Effects Specific to Epidural and Caudal Anesthesia

The physiologic effects of epidural and caudal anesthesia are similar to those for spinal anesthesia, with the exception that local anesthetic blood levels reach concentrations sufficient to produce systemic effects on their own. For example, intravenously administered lidocaine resulting in blood levels similar to those following continuous epidural analgesia does decrease postoperative narcotic requirements.[29] When blood levels are excessive, adverse central nervous system and cardiovascular effects can occur. Clinically, a common concept promoted is that the decrease in arterial blood pressure following epidural or caudal anesthesia is more gradual and of less magnitude than that following spinal anesthesia to comparable levels. In spite of this belief, there is evidence that when tetracaine (10 mg) spinal anesthesia was compared to lidocaine (20 to 25 ml at 1.5 percent) epidural anesthesia, arterial blood pressure fell more, approximately 10 percent, with the epidural technique than with the spinal technique.[30] Proponents of a lesser fall of blood pressure with continuous epidural and caudal techniques suggest that anesthesia care providers are able to administer a decreased volume of local anesthetic with the initial epidural therapeutic dose, and then by titrating subsequent doses, minimize the fall in arterial blood pressure. In many instances there seems to be a "clinical logic fault" with this concept. We believe that often following the initial decreased epidural therapeutic dose, anesthesia care providers are prone to administer additional epidural local anesthetic when the block height does not rise as rapidly as clinical situations dictate. Anesthesia care providers then find themselves loading this epidural anesthetic with even more local anesthetic than would have been required if an appropriate initial dose had been administered. In spite of this caution in selected patients this concept may be indicated.

SPINAL ANESTHESIA

Equipment

Spinal anesthesia remains unparalleled in the way a small mass of drug, devoid of systemic pharmacologic effect, produces effective surgical anesthesia. Further, by altering the small mass of drug, very different spinal anesthetics can be produced. In order to place the small mass of spinal drug into the CSF, the proper equipment must be used. Most anesthesia care providers practice in a setting in which disposable regional block trays are used. It is our belief that the most effective use of regional block trays involves adding specialized needles and drugs to a basic tray. This is in contrast to supplier-prepared specific spinal trays, in which drug and needle are preselected, and thus often are unable to be individualized to specific patients or procedures.

Spinal needles fall into two principal categories: those that cut the dura and those designed to spread dural fibers. The former include the "traditional" disposable spinal needle, the Quincke-Babcock needle, while the latter contain the needles with a cone-shaped tip, including the Greene and the Whitacre needles (Fig. 13-7). If a continuous spinal technique is chosen, the use of a needle with a lateral facing tip (e.g., Tuohy) needle will facilitate passage of the catheter. The continuous spinal catheters range in size from those identical to our continuous epidural catheters (approximately 20-gauge) to those as small as a 32-gauge catheter

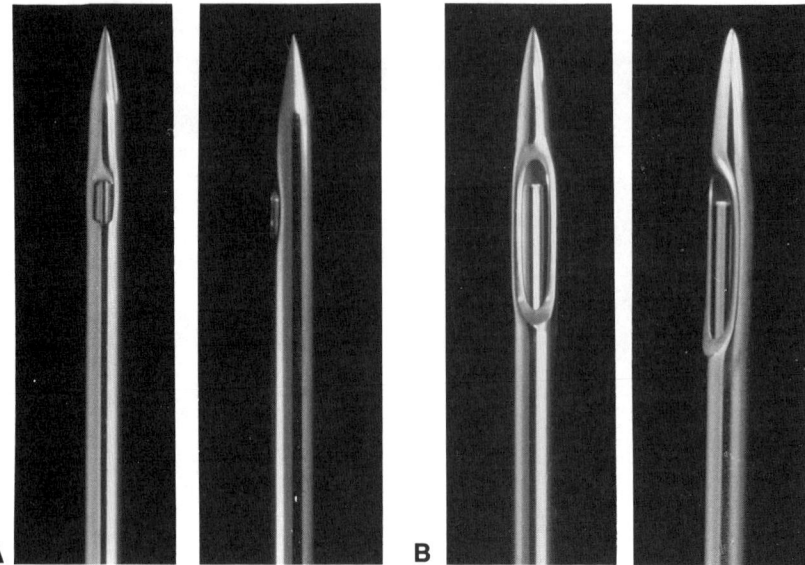

Fig. 13-7. Selected spinal needles in anteriorposterior and oblique views: (**A**) 22-gauge Whitacre, (**B**) 22-gauge Sprott. (*Figure continues.*)

(microcatheters).* The use of the microcatheters is promoted by some anesthesia care providers as significantly reducing the incidence of post-dural puncture headache (PDPH) during continuous spinal anesthesia. It should be emphasized that small needles reduce the incidence of PDPH, whereas larger needles improve the tactile "feel" of needle placement. If the use of a smaller needle increases the number of dural punctures necessary to appreciate correct needle position, the difference between small and large needles in producing PDPHs may be minimal. There may also be a difference in PDPH incidences among needle tip designs, even when needle sizes are comparable.[31] In spite of these observations, as the facility with spinal anesthesia increases, the use of a smaller,

similarly "tipped" needle will decrease PDPH incidence if the number of dural punctures does not increase. Often overlooked with spinal anesthesia is the advisability of using a spinal needle introducer. Many anesthesia care providers seem to have discarded the use of an introducer, presumably thinking it unnecessary. We believe that the use of a short, disposable 18- to 20-gauge introducer (appropriate for the size of the spinal needle chosen) allows a more systematic approach to reinsertion of a spinal needle if CSF placement is not achieved on the first needle pass.

Positioning

Positioning of patients for spinal anesthesia is often the most inadequately managed part of the spinal technique. This seems to be the case for at least two reasons: first, the assistant often does not understand the rationale for positioning

---

* The Food and Drug Administration withdrew permission for clinical use of small-bore catheters (smaller than 27 gauge) for continuous spinal anesthesia in May of 1992.

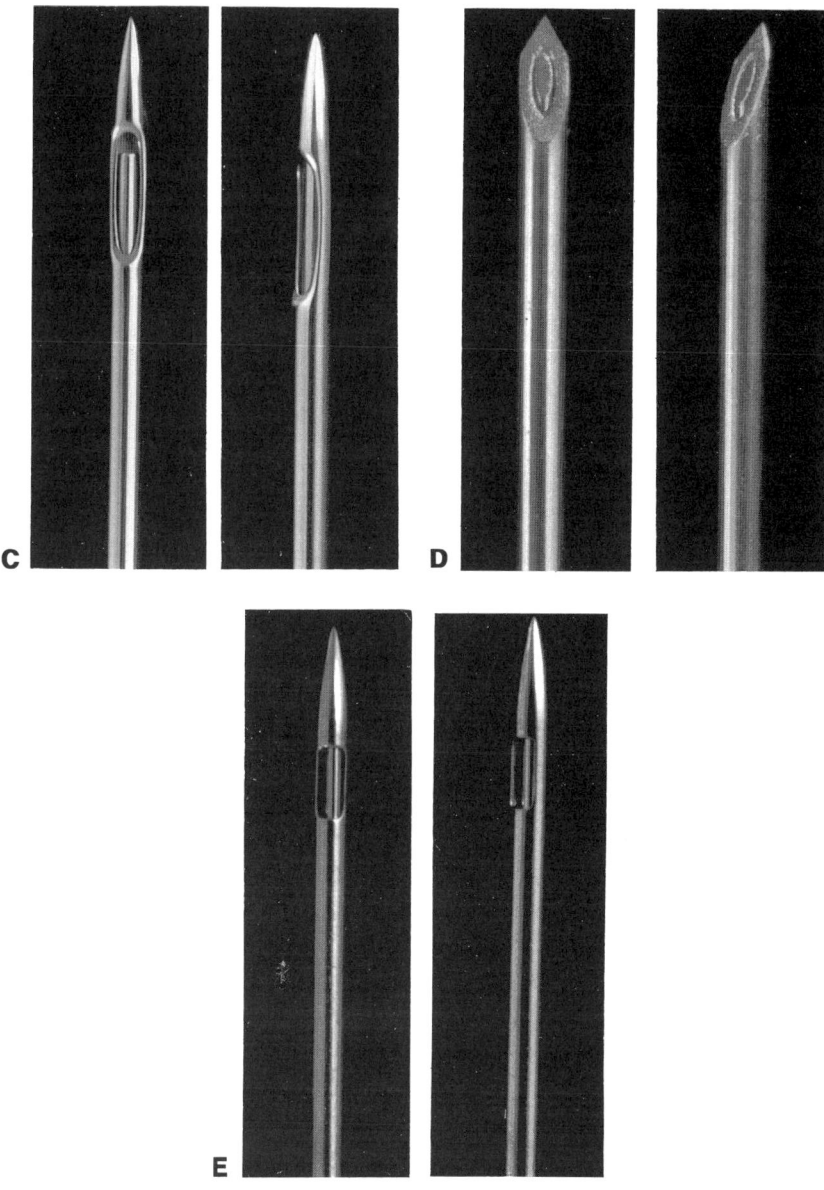

Fig. 13-7 (*Continued*). **(C)** 24-gauge Sprott, **(D)** 25-gauge Quincke, **(E)** 25-gauge Whitacre. All spinal needles photographed at same magnification.

the patient and second, patients are often inadequately or excessively sedated, making cooperation poor. The three methods of patient positioning for spinal anesthesia include the lateral decubitis, sitting, and prone positions. Each has advantages in specific surgical procedures or patients. The lateral decubitis position is probably the most commonly used since it allows administration of more sedation and is less dependent on a well-trained assistant than the sitting position.

The patient should be encouraged to assume the "fetal" position with the back parallel to the edge of the operating table nearest the anesthesia care provider. Often the assistant may be invaluable during this positioning by assisting the patient in assuming this ideal lateral decubitis position (Fig. 13-8). The sitting position is often appropriate when low lumbar and sacral levels of sensory anesthesia are desired. Another indication for the sitting position is obesity, which makes identification of the patient's midline anatomy difficult in the lateral position. Optimal positioning for the sitting approach is made practical if the patient's feet are placed on a footrest, and a pillow placed in the lap. The assistant then assists the patient in maintaining the vertebral midline in the vertical plane while flexing the patient's neck and arms over the pillow to reduce lumbar lordosis (Fig.

13-9). If a sitting position is chosen to keep the sensory level low, the patient should be maintained sitting for approximately 5 minutes; if this position is chosen because of difficulties with midline identification and a higher sensory level is needed, the patient may be placed supine immediately after subarachnoid injection by manipulating the table appropriately. If difficulties are encountered identifying the midline with the patient in the sitting position, it is most likely that the patient has been allowed to slump, causing the advantage of the improved midline identification to be lost.

The prone position is often indicated when the patient is to be maintained in that position (often with jackknife modification) during the surgical procedure. An additional advantage of using the hypobaric technique in this position is that patients can help in the initial positioning

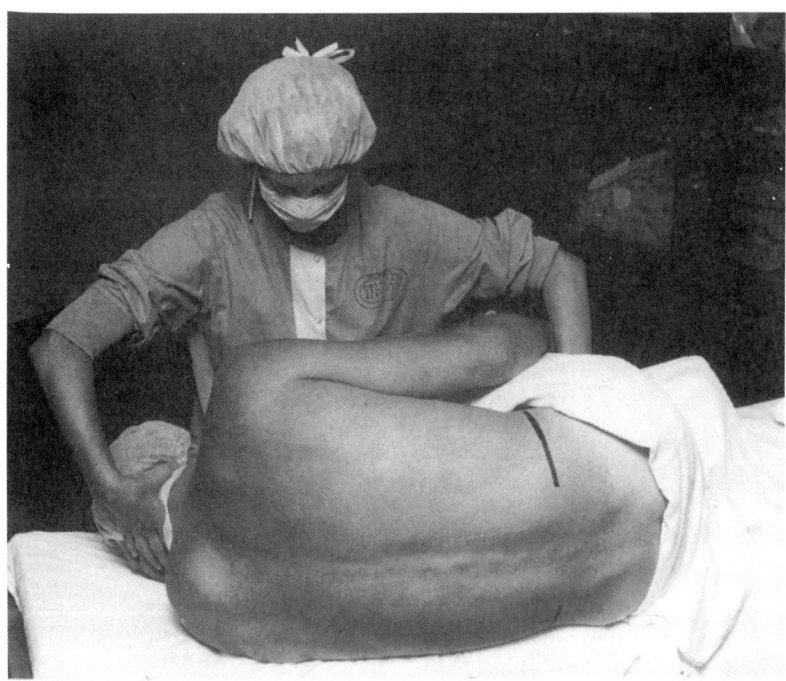

Fig. 13-8. Lateral decubitus positioning for centralneuraxial block. The assistant can help the patient assume the ideal position of "forehead-to-knees." (From Brown & Wedel,[111] with permission.)

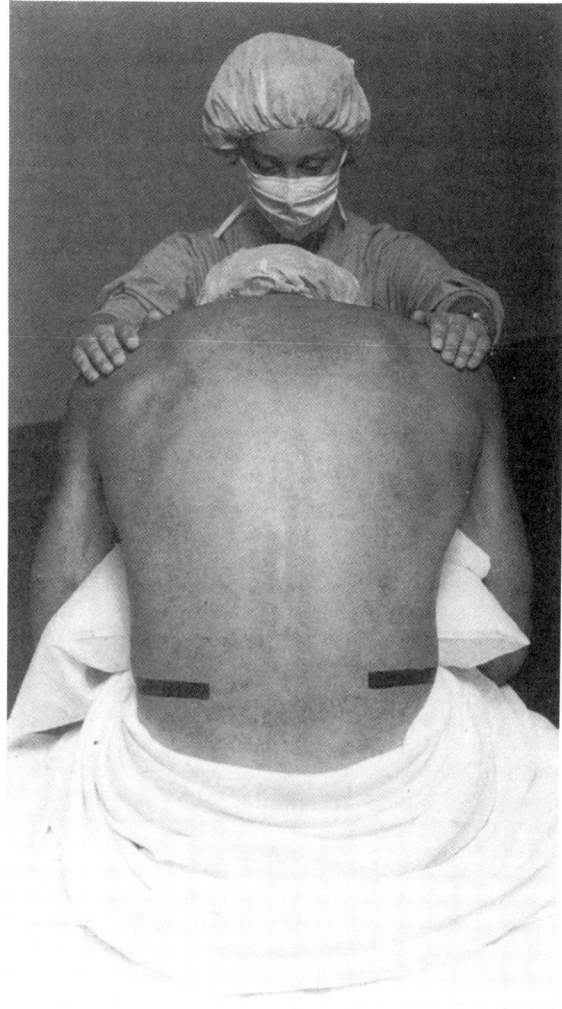

Fig. 13-9. Sitting position for central neuraxial block. The assistant proves the patient with a foot rest (stool) and pillow, and prevents the patient from slumping to either side. (From Brown & Wedel,[111] with permission.)

on the operating table, thus potentially minimizing the opportunity for positioning injuries. Using the prone position often means the paramedian approach to the subarachnoid space is the most efficient method of needle placement. Also, one may need to aspirate for CSF since CSF pressures are minimized when lumbar needle insertion is carried out in the prone position.

Spinal Technique

The most common approach to a spinal anesthesia uses a midline needle insertion (Fig. 13-10); perhaps because many find it easier to "work" in two planes rather than the addition of a third plane necessary for paramedian needle insertion. The midline approach is made eas-

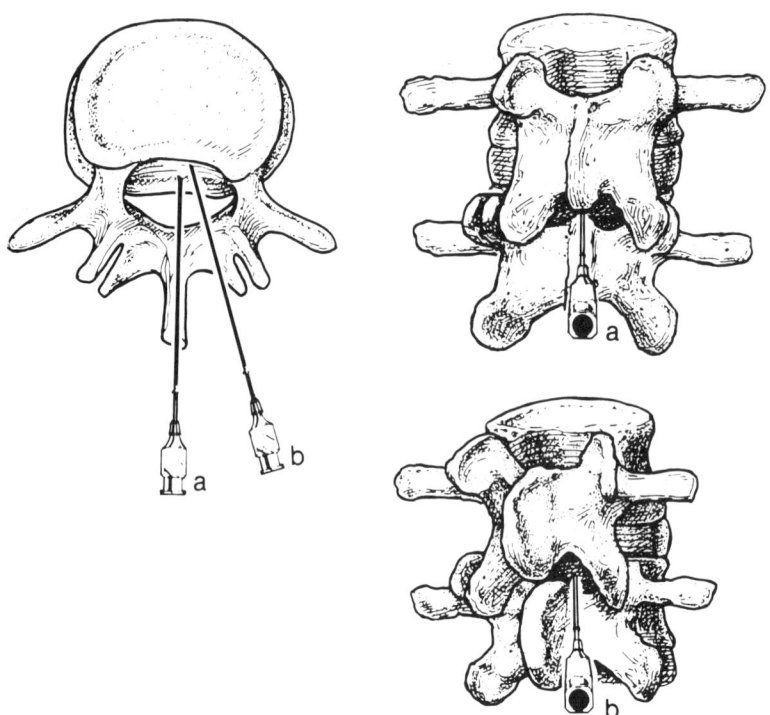

Fig. 13-10. Vertebral anatomy of midline and paramedian approaches to central neuraxial blocks. (**A**) The midline approach requires anatomic projection in only two planes, sagittal and horizontal. (**B**) The paramedian approach requires an additional oblique plane to be considered, although it has the benefit of a larger subarachnoid target. (From Brown & Wedel,[111] with permission.)

ier by patients and assistants who are able to minimize lumbar lordosis, which allows access to the subarachnoid space usually between adjacent spinous processes at the L2-L3, L3-L4, or sometimes the L4-L5 interspace. The anesthesia care provider's palpating fingers (usually the index and third fingers) should identify the interspinous area by the caudad extent of the more cephalad spine and the midline by rolling the fingers medial to lateral (Fig. 13-11). After the skin and subcutaneous tissues are anesthetized, an introducer is inserted into the substance of the interspinous ligament. The introducer is grasped with the palpating fingers and steadied, while the other hand is used to insert the spinal needle through the introducer and into the subarachnoid space. This is often most effectively accomplished by holding the spinal needle like a dart, while the fifth ("little") finger is used as a tripod against the patient's back to prevent patient movement from unintentionally altering needle direction or depth. If a needle with a bevel is used, the bevel is inserted parallel to the longitudinal dural fibers and is advanced slowly to increase the anesthesia care provider's sense of tissue planes traversed and to prevent injury to nerve roots until the characteristic change in resistance is noted as the needle passes through the ligamentum flavum and dura. Once a chance in resistance is noted, the stylet is removed and CSF should appear

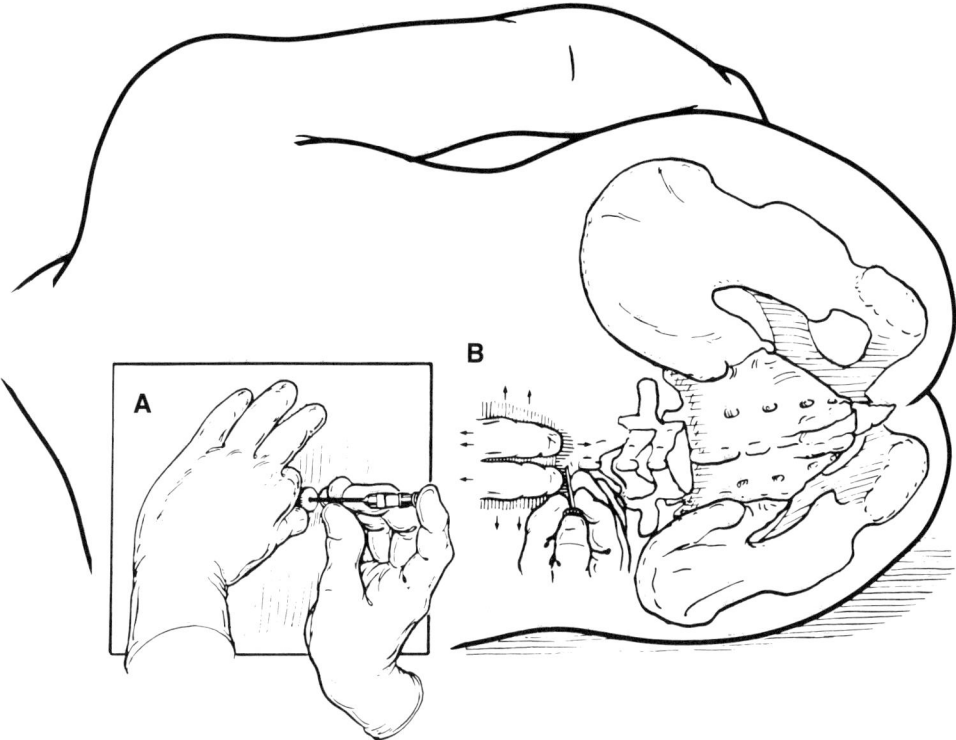

Fig. 13-11. Spinal needle insertion. (**A**) The palpating fingers are "rolled" in both a side-to-side and cephalad-to-caudad direction to identify interspinous space. (**B**) During needle insertion, the needle should be stabilized in a tripod fashion while placed in the hand, similar to a dart being thrown. (From Brown & Wedel,[111] with permission.)

at the needle hub. If it does not, the needle is rotated in 90-degree increments until CSF appears or it is clear that the needle should be advanced since the subarachnoid space has not been reached. If CSF does not appear, yet the needle is at a depth appropriate for the patient, the needle introducer should be withdrawn and insertion steps repeated. This is important since the most common reason for lack of CSF return is an off-midline insertion of the needle. Once the CSF is freely obtained, the anesthesia care provider's nondominant hand is steadied against the patient's back while gripping the needle hub. The syringe containing the therapeutic dose of spinal anesthetic is then attached to the needle

and a check for free CSF aspiration is made. Once CSF is freely aspirated, the spinal anesthetic dose is injected at a rate of approximately 0.2 ml/s. Once the entire dose has been injected, 0.2 ml of CSF is again aspirated into the syringe and reinjected subarachnoid, both to reconfirm location and to clear the needle of any remaining local anesthetic. At this point, the patient and operating table should be placed in positions appropriate for the surgical procedure and drugs chosen.

If difficulties are encountered with midline needle insertion, the paramedian approach is often indicated. An advantage of the paramedian route is that it does not require the same level of patient cooperation or reversal of lumbar lordosis that the midline requires. The paramedian approach is useful since if a needle is inserted slightly lateral to the midline it is possible to utilize the larger "subarachnoid target" that exists (Fig. 13-10). Nevertheless, a common error made with the paramedian technique is that the needle insertion is carried out too far off the midline, making the vertebral lamina barriers to needle insertion rather than guides to insertion. During the paramedian technique, a mark should be made approximately 1 cm lateral and 1 cm caudad to the caudad edge of the cephalad spinous process at the space chosen for needle insertion. A skin wheal should be raised at this point and then a longer needle (e.g., 1.5 in.) is then used to infiltrate the deeper tissues in a cephalomedial direction. The spinal introducer and needle are then inserted 10 to 15 degrees off the sagittal plane in a cephalomedial attitude. As with the midline technique, the single most frequent error is to angle the needle too far cephalad on initial needle insertion. To perform properly, the needle should contact bone (the vertebral lamina) and then be redirected slightly in a steplike fashion in a cephalad direction. With this technique, if bone is contacted but at a deeper level each time, the cephalad angulation is continued since it is likely the needle is being "walked up" the lamina. Similar to the midline approach, the ligaments and dura should have a characteristic "feel," although the angle of needle insertion will require more of the needle to be used. Once CSF is obtained, the block is carried out in a manner similar to that described for the midline approach. One variation on the paramedian technique is the lumbosacral approach described by Taylor[32] (Fig. 13-12). This technique is performed at the L5-S1 interspace, which is the largest interlaminal interspace of the vertebral column. A skin wheal should be raised approximately 1 cm me-

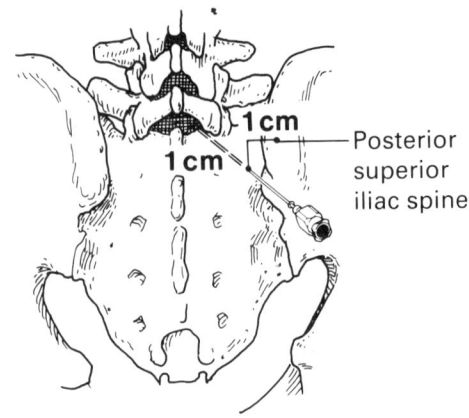

Fig. 13-12. Anatomy of the Taylor approach, which is really a paramedian approach at L5-S1 level. (From Brown & Wedel,[111] with permission.)

dial and 1 cm caudad to the lowermost prominence of the posterior-superior iliac spine. Infiltration with a longer needle is then carried out in a cephalomedial direction through this skin wheal. A 5-in., 22-gauge spinal needle is then inserted, again in a cephalomedial direction, until bone is encountered. If bone is encountered on this initial insertion, the needle is walked off the sacrum into the subarachnoid space similar to that "needle walking" used during lumbar paramedian spinal anesthesia. Once CSF is obtained with the Taylor approach, the steps of drug injection are similar to those previously outlined.

Pharmacology

Drugs
In the United States, three drugs comprise the most used spinal anesthetics: lidocaine (Xylocaine), tetracaine (Pontacaine), and bupivacaine (Marcaine or Sensorcaine). Lidocaine is a short- to intermediate-acting spinal drug; tetracaine and bupivacaine provide intermediate- to long-duration blockade.

Lidocaine is often appropriate for procedures, such as bunionectomy, that can be completed in 1 hour or less. This drug has a measurable effect in less than 5 minutes after injection and is frequently used as the 5 percent solution in 7.5 percent dextrose. In the past it was thought that epinephrine did not prolong the length of spinal anesthesia with lidocaine since duration was most often defined by two-segment regression* in thoracic dermatomes. In spite of lidocaine not prolonging the duration of spinal anesthesia as defined by thoracic dermatomal two-segment regression, addition of epinephrine (0.2 mg) has been found to prolong the length of lidocaine spinal anesthesia at the operative site.[33] Additionally, the use of epinephrine with spinal drugs may do more than simply prolong the duration of the block at the operative site. It is likely that the quality of blockade improves as well.[34,35] In dogs, subarachnoid lidocaine (plain) increases spinal cord blood flow, whereas when epinephrine is added to lidocaine no statistically significant change in spinal cord blood flow results.[36]

Tetracaine has been used during spinal anesthesia for years and is available as both niphanoid crystals (20 mg) and as a 1 percent solution (20 mg). This drug has an onset of 5 to 10 minutes after subarachnoid injection and is appropriate for procedures lasting up to 2 to 3 hours when epinephrine is added, and for up to 5 hours for lower extremity procedures when phenylephrine (5 mg) is utilized. If niphanoid crystals are chosen, a 1 percent solution is formulated by adding 2 ml of

sterile water (without preservatives) to the crystals. Then the prescribed milligram dose of 1 percent solution is mixed in equal volumes of 10 percent dextrose to produce a 0.5 percent tetracaine solution weighted with 5 percent dextrose. Subsequently, the vasoconstrictor may be added. Once again, epinephrine and phenylephrine both prolong spinal anesthesia with tetracaine[37] (Table 13-2). In dogs, subarachnoid tetracaine increases spinal cord blood flow, while addition of epinephrine to tetracaine leaves blood flow unaltered.[38]

Bupivacaine spinal anesthesia is performed using a number of distinct formulations. Hyperbaric bupivacaine is commonly carried out with a 0.75 percent solution in 8.25 percent dextrose. The 0.75 percent (plain) bupivacaine solution is also used as a near-isobaric formulation. Bupivacaine 0.5 percent, with or without dextrose weighting, has also been used, with a plain solution acting as a near-isobaric solution. Bupivacaine is appropriate for procedures lasting up to 2 to 2.5 hours.[39] Subarachnoid bupivacaine in dogs decreases lumbosacral spinal cord blood flow with or without added epinephrine.[40] In spite of this laboratory finding, the clinical significance of the spinal cord blood flow alteration seems minimal.

Additives

Some anesthesia care providers express concern that the use of additives, particularly vasoconstrictors, may add an unacceptable risk to spinal anesthesia. The concept is that epinephrine and phenylephrine have such potent vasoconstrictive action as to put the blood supply of the spinal cord in jeopardy. There are no human data supporting this theory. Kozody and co-workers[41] have shown that administering subarachnoid epinephrine

---

* Two-segment regression is a measure of the duration of central neuraxial blocks, or the time from injection of the local anesthetic mixture until the spinal or epidural anesthetics maximum level (usually thoracic) has decreased by two dermatome levels.

Table 13-2. Drug Selection for Hyperbaric Spinal Anesthesia

Local Anesthetic Mixture	Dose[a] (mg)		Duration (min)	
	to T10	to T4	Plain	0.2 mg Epinephrine
Lidocaine (5% in 7.5% dextrose)	50–60	75–100	60	75–100
Tetracaine (0.5% in 5% dextrose)	6–8	10–16	70–90	100–150
Bupivacaine (0.75% in 8.5% dextrose)	8–10	12–20	90–110	100–150

[a] Doses are for use in a 70-kg adult male of average height.
(From Brown & Wedel,[111] with permission.)

(0.2 mg) and phenylephrine (5 mg) does not decrease spinal cord blood flow in dogs. These traditional vasoconstrictors are not the only adrenergic agents being studied. Clonidine, an α_2 agonist, prolonged motor block associated with tetracaine spinal anesthesia in dogs as much as epinephrine, while prolonging sensory blockade for even a longer interval.[42] The mechanism for this effect may involve vasoconstriction, or antinociception from α_2 stimulation.

Traditionally, epinephrine was believed to prolong only tetracaine spinal anesthesia, but not bupivacaine or lidocaine spinal anesthesia.[43] This belief was held because of the differences in vasodilatory actions of the local anesthetic drugs: plain lidocaine and bupivacaine cause vasodilatation, whereas plain tetracaine does not. Additionally, the original investigations of spinal anesthetic duration used two-dermatome regression in the thoracic region to establish spinal anesthetic duration.[44,45] More recently, it has become clearer that two-dermatome regression in the mid-to-high thoracic dermatomes may be misleading when establishing spinal anesthetic duration in the lower thoracic and lumbar dermatomes. Data are available showing that spinal anesthesia with lidocaine is prolonged by epinephrine when measured by two-dermatome regression in the lower thoracic dermatomes and by occurrence of pain at the operative site for procedures carried out at the level of the lumbosacral dermatomes.[33,46]

When epinephrine is compared to phenylephrine as a means of prolonging spinal anesthesia, conflicting information appears to exist. Concepcion and co-workers[47] compared epinephrine (0.2 and 0.3 mg) and phenylephrine (1 and 2 mg) added to tetracine and did not find a difference in increased duration with the two vasoconstrictors. Nevertheless, Caldwell and colleagues[37] used a higher dose of each vasoconstrictor, epinephrine at 0.5 mg and phenylephrine at 5 mg, and showed that phenylephrine prolonged tetracaine spinal anesthesia significantly more than epinephrine (Table 13-3). It also seems clear that during lower extremity surgery that epinephrine will prolong bupivacaine spinal anesthesia.[48]

Another additive that can be added to spinal anesthetic mixtures is preservative-free sterile water. By adding sterile water to a spinal anesthetic mixture, a hypobaric solution can be created. In order to make a drug hypobaric to CSF, it must be less dense than the CSF. This means it must have a baricity appreciably less than 1.0000 or a specific gravity appreciably less than 1.0069 (the mean value of CSF specific gravity). To understand hypobaric formulation, one must understand some additional terminology. The *density* of any solution is the weight in grams of 1 ml of the solution at a standard temperature. *Specific gravity* is the den-

Table 13-3.   Effect of Adding Epinephrine or Phenylephrine to
Tetracaine Spinal Anesthesia

| | Duration of Blockade[a] | |
	T10 (min)	L1 (min)
Group 1		
Tetracaine (plain)	159 ± 41	230 ± 55
Group II		
Tetracaine (+ epinephrine 0.5 mg)	234 ± 59[b]	327 ± 72[b]
Group III		
Tetracaine (+ phenylephrine 5 mg)	273 ± 90[b]	406 ± 63[b,c]

[a] Duration of blockade is defined as that time between administration of
the spinal anesthesia and regression of the blockade to T10 or L1.
[b] Significant difference from group I (P < 0.01).
[c] Significant difference from group II (P < 0.025).
(Modified from Caldwell et al,[37] with permission.)

sity of a solution compared in a ratio to the density of water. By contrast, *baricity* is the ratio comparing the density of one solution to another. If the other solution happens to be water, the baricity will be the same as the specific gravity.

In the United States, the most common method of formulating a hypobaric solution is to mix tetracaine in a 0.1 to 0.33 percent solution with sterile water. This produces a solution with a baricity of less than 0.9977 and allows clinically useful anesthesia to be produced. During orthopedic procedures, the most common indication for hypobaric spinal anesthesia is a patient undergoing hip repair in the lateral position. In these patients, 6 to 8 mg of selected hypobaric dilution is often adequate. There are conflicting data regarding the rate of injection of hypobaric solution and the eventual block height. Atchison and colleagues[49] demonstrated that a slow injection of hypobaric tetracaine via a 22-gauge Whitacre needle produced lower levels of spinal anesthesia than those resulting from fast injection. There was a 25-fold difference in injection speed in their patients; slow injections required 250 seconds while fast injections were conducted over 10

seconds.[49] Stienstra and Van Poorten[50] showed that a 10-fold difference in speed of injection (fast approximately 0.54 ml/s, slow at 0.05 ml/s) does not significantly affect subarachnoid spread of isobaric 0.5 percent bupivacaine administered via a 25-gauge needle.

Whichever local anesthetic solution and additives are selected for subarachnoid injection, special care should be taken to ensure that one knows what substance is being injected and that all procedures have been carried out aseptically.

Complications

One of the most feared complications following spinal anesthesia is neurologic dysfunction. Neurologic injury after spinal anesthesia received considerable media attention in the 1940s and 1950s, when the widely publicized "Wooley and Roe" case in England and the "investigation" published by Kennedy in 1950 in the United States were made available.[51] Many of our current orthopedic patients were in their formative years when these "complications" were in the headlines.

Not making the headlines was information from Marinacci, whose investigation was performed after Kennedy's publication. Marinacci, a neurologist, evaluated 542 patients who were believed to have neurologic complications related to a previous spinal anesthetic.[52] After neurologic evaluation, in only 4 of the 542 patients was there any indication that the prior spinal anesthetic was the cause of the postoperative neurologic change. It should be emphasized that the total number of patients undergoing spinal anesthesia that resulted in the four cases of neurologic symptoms following spinal anesthesia is unknown.

In spite of Marinacci's study not having a denominator, there are reports that outline both the numerator and denominator of neurologic change following spinal anesthesia. Vandam and Dripps[53] documented 10,098 patients who underwent spinal anesthesia and reported no severe neurologic sequela related to the anesthetics. Similarly, Moore and Bridenbaugh[31] failed to find a single permanent neuropathy after spinal anesthesia in 11,574 patients undergoing spinal anesthesia. A review of neurologic complications associated with central neuraxial blocks, prompted by the chloroprocaine epidural controversy in the early 1980s, tabulated 65,304 patients following spinal anesthesia with only one permanent lesion potentially related to the anesthetic (a lumbar plexus injury).[54] Nevertheless, these large series documenting only one rare neurologic lesions after spinal anesthesia should not provide one with a false sense of security. For example, Rigler and colleagues[55] documented four cases of cauda equina syndrome occurring after continuous spinal anesthetics. They postulated that a maldistribution of local anesthetic combined with a relatively high dose of the spinal anesthetic drug resulted in a neurotoxic injury.[55]

It is clear that neurologic changes can occur following spinal anesthesia; the important point is that severe neurologic change can also occur after general anesthesia. The risk/benefit ratio of anesthesia and neurologic injury must include those cases of neurologic injury (e.g., hypoxic central nervous system lesions), that are possible during general anesthesia if a logical and well-informed decision based on neurologic outcome is to be made for our patients.

A more common complication of spinal anesthesia is postoperative headache. PDPHs are not exclusively related to spinal anesthetics, but occur after myelography and diagnostic lumbar puncture as well. Factors increasing the incidence of PDPHs, or unrelated to its development, are listed in Table 13-4.[56]

Mihic's investigation of bevel direction during insertion of a spinal needle clearly demonstrated that splitting, rather than cutting, the longitudinally directed dural fibers resulted in a lower incidence of PDPH[57] (Fig. 13-13). Mihic did not specify needle type in the report, but it is likely that a Quinke-type needle was used. PDPHs have also not been found to be lessened by patients assuming some arbitrary period of recumbency following the spinal anesthetic.[58] Some data indicate that early ambulation may actually decrease the incidence of PDPH.[59,60] Possibly more important than knowing all the variables resulting in an increased incidence of PDPH is an understanding of how and when to carry out the definitive therapy—epidural blood patch—for this complication.[61] It seems to us that far too many anesthesia care providers avoid a useful anesthetic technique, spinal anesthesia, because of a reluctance to use epidural blood patch therapy. The successful use of spinal anesthesia necessitates the early use of epidural blood patching when indicated. This therapy appears to have a greater than 90 percent efficacy in

Table 13-4.   The Relationship Among Variables and Post-Dural Puncture Headache

Factors *related* to increased incidence of post-dural puncture
    headache

Age:	Younger more frequent
Gender:	Females > males
Needle size:	Larger > smaller
Needle bevel:	More when dural fibers cut transversely
Pregnancy:	More when pregnant
No. dural punctures:	More with multiple punctures

Factors *not increasing* post-dural puncture headache incidence
    Continuous spinals
    Timing of ambulation

(From Brown & Wedel,[111] with permission.)

relieving headache with each epidural blood patch treatment.[62–64] One question that has not been fully answered since epidural blood patch therapy was introduced is the volume of blood most effective in balancing blood patch efficacy and risks. Szeinfeld and colleagues[65] have shown via radionucleotide-labeled red blood cells injected epidurally that approximately 15 ml of blood provides efficacy and allows spread over a mean distance of nine spinal segments, thus

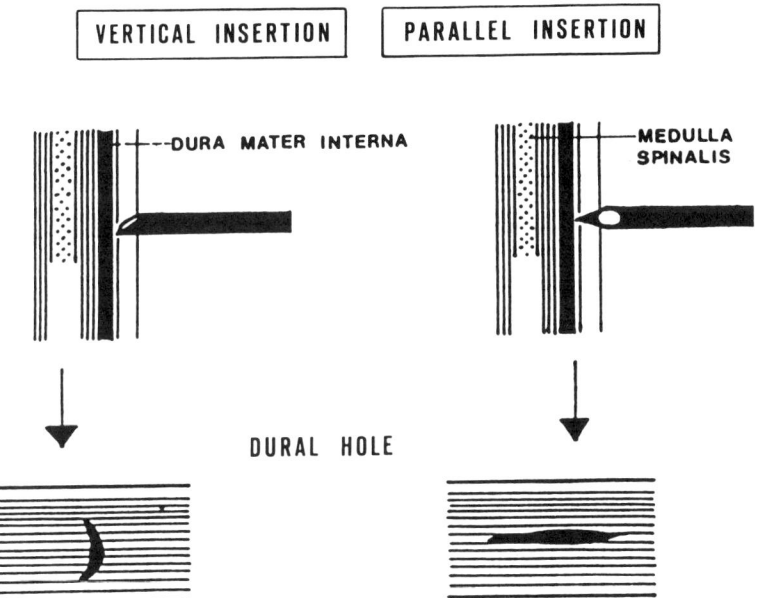

Fig. 13-13. Types of needle insertion in Mihic's report. In the vertical versus parallel insertion, the bevel of the spinal needle is inserted through the dura mater internal perpendicular to, instead of parallel to, the long axis of the vertebral column. (From Mihic,[57] with permission.)

providing some latitude for blood patch needle placement. They demonstrated that blood was spread over more segments in the cephalad direction than the caudad direction. As a result, they recommend inserting the blood patch needle in a more caudad site if it is impossible to insert the needle at the same level as that of the prior dural puncture.

Another fear that many of our patients articulate during preoperative discussion of anesthetic options is that a spinal anesthetic will provide lifelong backache. There are no data to suggest this happens. Brown and Elman[66] demonstrated that approximately 25 percent of all our surgical patients undergoing anesthesia, regardless of anesthetic technique, experience backache in the immediate postoperative period. There was no difference between those undergoing spinal anesthesia and those undergoing general anesthesia. Thus, backache after central neuraxial block should not immediately be attributed to needling of the back.

Caplan and colleagues[67] identified 14 cases of sudden cardiac arrest in healthy patients receiving spinal anesthesia through review of the American Society of Anesthesiologists' closed claims database. Because these cases seemed to appear suddenly after stable hemodynamic status existed intraoperatively, they concluded that a poorly understood potential exists for sudden cardiac arrest in healthy patients. It can be debated whether this represented a lack of vigilant monitoring in treatment as opposed to some mysterious physiologic explanation.[68] In either case, it should be emphasized that cardiovascular changes can occur rather suddenly during spinal anesthesia. These changes can occur near or remotely from the time of injection. It does seem clear that ventilatory inadequacy does not need to exist for these changes to occur.[69]

EPIDURAL ANESTHESIA

Equipment

When selecting a method of epidural anesthesia, the first decision that must be made is whether a continuous or single-shot technique will be used. This consideration is the principle determinant of needle selection. If a single-shot epidural technique is used, a Crawford needle is appropriate; if a continuous catheter technique is indicated, either a Tuohy or another needle with a lateral facing opening is chosen (Fig. 13-14). If a continuous technique is prescribed, another decision that must be made is what type of catheter to use. The major division of epidural catheters are into those with a single-endhole design or a closed-tip multiple-sidehole design. Either of these catheters can also be obtained with a removable stylet if so desired. If a loss-of-resistance is used for identifying the epidural space, an additional decision on type of syringe (glass versus plastic, Luer-lok versus friction hub) is required. We believe the theoretical ideal is the Luer-lok, finely ground glass syringe, since it minimizes the chance of misidentification of the epidural space.

Positioning

The patient positions indicated for epidural puncture are the same as those for spinal anesthesia, with the exception of the prone position for the caudal approach to the epidural space. Deserving emphasis again is that inadequate positioning of the patient will negate otherwise meticulous epidural technique and should be prevented. The limitation of block spread (height) is not as clinically predictable with position alterations during epidural anesthesia as with spinal anesthesia. Gravity and solution baricity

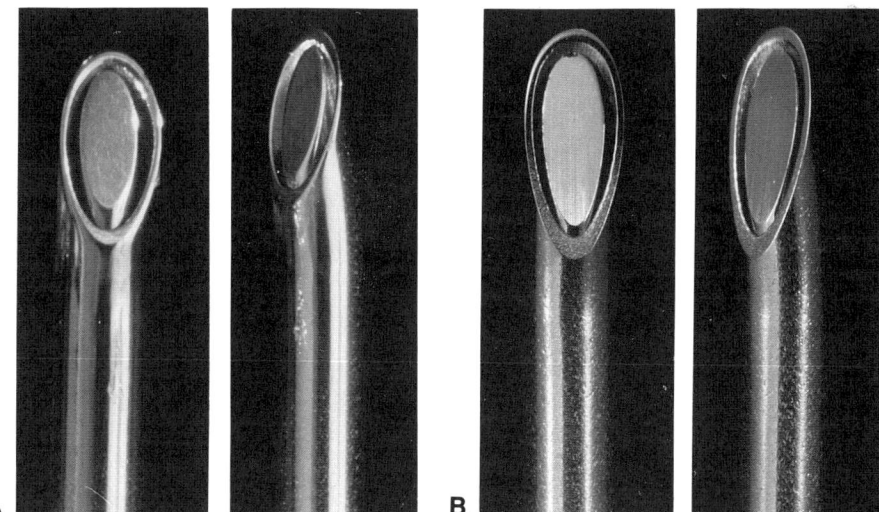

Fig. 13-14. Selected epidural needles in anteroposterior and oblique views; (**A**) 18-gauge Hustead; (**B**) 17-gauge Tuohy.

are not as intimately related to block spread, thus the mandate that the operative leg be dependent during the epidural cannulation is not absolute. In spite of these observations, Seow and co-workers[70] have demonstrated slightly faster onset times for epidural block in patients dependent by regions when the lateral decubitus position was used during the regional technique.

Three positions are available for caudal anesthesia, with the prone position most often chosen in adults, the lateral position in children, and the knee–chest position infrequently used today. The lateral decubitus position is often indicated in children since it is easier to maintain a patent airway in this position than in the prone position. This is pertinent to children since typically caudal anesthesia is administered following induction of general anesthesia, or conversely, during emergence from general anesthesia when maintenance of a patent airway is still important. By contrast, a caudal block is often administered during preoperative sedation in adults when the prone posi-

tion is applicable. When placing a patient in the prone position, a pillow should be inserted beneath the iliac crests to rotate the pelvis and make cannulation of the caudal canal easier. One additional positioning help is for patients to position their lower extremities about 20 degrees apart with heels rotated laterally. This minimizes gluteal muscle contraction and eases needle insertion (Fig. 13-15). Additionally, caudal cannulation can be uncomfortable for patients and the prone position allows liberal sedation to be used.

Epidural Technique

The use of epidural anesthesia requires placement of the needle tip into the ligamentum flavum for both loss-of-resistance and hanging-drop methods. Placing the needle (with stylet) into the ligamentum flavum prior to attaching the syringe or placing solution into the needle hub, allows an improved appreciation of epidural anatomy for the operator if performed systematically. If the needle is

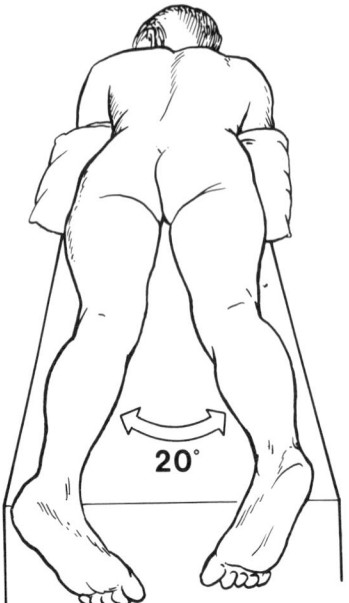

Fig. 13-15. Prone position for caudal technique. Pillow used under anterior iliac crests to rotate pelvis, legs spread 20 degrees to ease identification of sacral hiatus, and heels rotated laterally to relax gluteal musculature. (From Brown & Wedel,[111] with permission.)

merely inserted into the supraspinous ligament and then either loss-of-resistance or hanging-drop insertion begun, an increased chance of false identification of the epidural space seems more likely. During anesthesia for orthopedic surgical patients, a lumbar approach is most common. The depth from the skin to ligamentum flavum commonly approaches 4 cm, and ranges in most (80 percent) patients between 3.5 and 6 cm. In this region, the ligamentum flavum is 5 to 6 mm thick in the midline, thus requiring needle control if unintentional dural puncture is to be prevented[71–73] (Table 13-1). The preferred method of carrying out the loss-of-resistance technique involves inserting the needle to the ligamentum flavum and then attaching a 3- to 5-ml glass syringe filled with 2 ml saline

and a small (0.25-ml) air bubble. The needle hub is then grasped with the nondominant hand and pulled toward the epidural space, while the dominant hand (thumb) applies constant steady pressure on the syringe plunger, compressing the air bubble. If the needle tip is not abutting or within the ligamentum flavum, compression of the air bubble is not likely. If the technique outlined is used, when the epidural space is entered the pressure applied to the syringe plunger will allow the solution to flow without resistance into the epidural space (Fig. 13-16).

An alternative, although with a less precise endpoint in our opinion, is the technique of hanging-drop identification of entry into the epidural space. With this technique, once the needle is placed into the ligamentum flavum, a drop of solution is placed within the hub of a needle. When the needle is advanced into the epidural space the solution should be "sucked in." The theory behind this maneuver has been attributed to a subatmospheric pressure in the epidural space. This subatmospheric pressure has been related to the expansion of the epidural space as the needle pushed the dura away from ligamentum flavum during needle passage.

Whichever method is chosen for needle insertion, when one chooses to cannulate the epidural space with a catheter, success may be increased by advancing the needle 1 to 2 mm once the space has been identified. Additionally, the incidence of unintentional intravenous cannulation with an epidural catheter may be lessened by injecting air or solution prior to threading the catheter.[74,75] Unless radiographic guidance is utilized for some special reason, epidural catheters should be inserted only 2 to 3 cm into the epidural space, since threading more catheter may increase the likelihood of catheter malposition. In spite of an adequately posi-

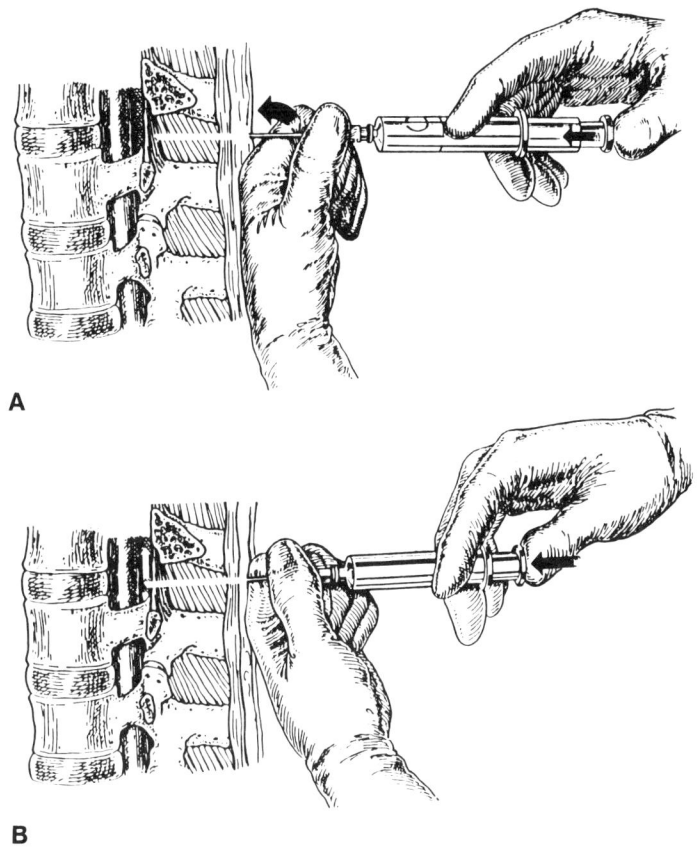

A

B

Fig. 13-16. Loss-of-resistance technique. (**A**) Needle "seated" in interspinous ligament and ligamentum flavum, with constant, steady pressure applied to syringe plunger; (**B**) entry of needle into epidural space is noted by loss of resistance to syringe plunger pressure, and solution entering the space easily. (From Brown & Wedel,[111] with permission.)

tioned catheter during the first use of local anesthetic, each subsequent injection should be preceded by aspiration and an epidural test dose, since catheter migration into vessels and subarachnoid or subdural spaces does occur.

Caudal Technique

Caudal anesthesia requires the identification of the sacral hiatus. The sacral hiatus lies cephalomedial to the sacral cornu and is covered by an extension of the ligamentum flavum, the sacrococcygeal ligament. To locate the cornu, the posterior superior iliac spines should be located, and, by using the line between them as one side of an equilateral triangle, the location of the sacral hiatus approximated (Fig. 13-17). Once the sacral hiatus is identified, the index and middle finger of the palpating hand are placed on the sacral cornu and the caudal needle is inserted at an angle of approximately 45 degrees to the sacrum. While advancing the needle, a decrease in resistance to needle insertion should be appreciated as

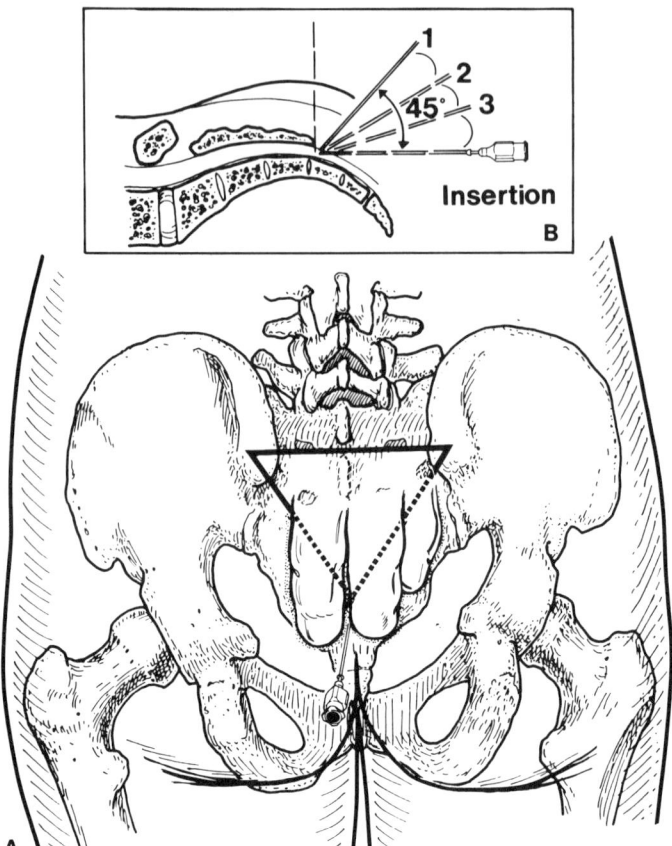

Fig. 13-17. Caudal technique. (**A**) Palpating fingers locate the sacral cornua by using equilateral triangle (shown in Fig. 13-5); (**B**) needle insertion is carried out by insertion and withdrawal in stepwise fashion ("1-2-3 insertion"), until needle can be advanced into the caudal canal and solution can be injected easily (without creation of a subcutaneous "lump" of fluid). (From Brown & Wedel,[111] with permission.)

the needle enters the caudal canal. The needle is advanced until bone (the dorsal aspect of the ventral plate of the sacrum) is contacted, and then slightly withdrawn, and the needle redirected so that the angle of insertion relative to the skin surface is decreased. In males this angle is almost parallel to the operative table (or coronal plane); in females a slightly steeper angle (15 degrees) is necessary because of the difference between male and female sacral anatomy. During redi-

rection of the needle and once loss of resistance is again encountered, the needle is advanced approximately 1 to 2 cm into the caudal canal. Further advance is not necessary, since dural puncture and unintentional intravascular cannulation become more likely with deeper needle insertion. Prior to the injection of the therapeutic dose of caudal anesthetic, a test of needle placement should be undertaken. Rapid injection of 5 ml of preservative-free saline should be administered through the caudal needle while the anesthesia care provider's other hand overlies the sacrum. It should not be possible to feel a midline "bulge" during saline injection if the needle is appropriately placed within the caudal canal. If a midline bulge is appreciated with this technique, the needle should be withdrawn and reinserted. This saline "test dose," we believe, will help in caudal canal identification, especially in those gaining experience in the technique. Additionally, prior to the injection of the therapeutic dose of anesthetic, aspiration and an epinephrine test dose should be administered since, as in lumbar epidural anesthesia, a vein or subarachnoid space can be entered unintentionally.

Pharmacology

Drugs

Appropriate prescription of drugs for epidural anesthesia requires an understanding of the local anesthetic potency and duration, as well as estimation of surgical requirements and duration and postoperative analgesia requirements. Similar to any choice of anesthetic, the surgeon, anesthesia care provider, procedure, and anesthetic technique must all be included in the drug choice equation.

Drugs available for epidural use can be categorized into short-, intermediate-, and long-acting agents, and with the addition of epinephrine to these agents, surgical anesthesia ranging from 45 to 240 minutes is possible (Table 13-5). Chloroprocaine, an ester local anesthetic, is a short-acting agent that was associated with neurotoxicity (adhesive arachnoiditis) when unintentionally injected in large volumes subarachnoid prior to a formulation change.[76,77] Since 1985, reduced bisulfite concentrations have been available, and since 1987 bisulfite-free 2-chloroprocaine has been available. Since these formulation changes, there have not been reports of neurotoxicity attributable to 2-chloroprocaine. In the era of ever-increasing numbers of surgical outpatients, combining 2-chloroprocaine and a catheter technique allows an efficient matching of surgical procedure and duration of epidural analgesia. This also enables patients to spend a minimal recovery time in the postanesthesia care unit. This drug is available in 2 and 3 percent concentrations, with the latter preferable for surgical anesthesia and the former for techniques not requiring muscle relaxation. Lidocaine is the prototypical amide local anesthetic and is used in 1.5 to 2 percent concentrations epidurally. Mepivacaine is similar to lidocaine in the concentrations necessary for epidural anesthesia and lasts 15 to 30 minutes longer than lidocaine when used as a single injection. Epinephrine significantly prolongs the duration of surgical anesthesia, approximately 50 percent, with both lidocaine and mepivacaine.[71] Both of these drugs are able to bridge the gap between the shorter-acting 2-chloroprocaine and the longer-acting bupivacaine.

Bupivacaine is the most widely used long-acting local anesthetic. It is often used in 0.5 and 0.75 percent concentrations for surgical anesthesia, with the latter used during the initial injection via the needle in patients in which muscle relaxation is important for the anesthetic. Analgesic techniques can be performed with concentrations from 0.125 to 0.25 percent bupivacaine. The duration of bupivacaine is less consistently prolonged by addition of epinephrine, although up to 240 minutes of surgical anesthesia can be obtained from a single injection when epinephrine is added. In 1983, the Food and Drug Administration stated that 0.75 percent bupivacaine was no longer rec-

Table 13-5. Comparative Onset Times and Analgesic Durations of Local Anesthetics Administered Epidurally in 20- to 30-ml Volumes

Drug	Concentration (%)	Onset (min)	Duration (min) Plain	Duration (min) 1:200,000 Epinephrine
2-Chloroprocaine	3	10–15	45–60	60–90
Lidocaine	2	15	80–120	120–180
Mepivacaine	2	15	90–140	140–200
Bupivacaine	0.5–0.75	20	165–225	180–240
Etidocaine	1	15	120–200	150–225

(Data from Cousins & Bromage[71] and other sources.)

ommended in obstetric anesthesia, as a result of a perception that systemic toxicity with that concentration resulted in more difficult resuscitations than occurred with lower concentrations. The evidence for this remains controversial, although it does appear that bupivacaine and etidocaine may be more likely to impair myocardial performance and conduction than the other local anesthetics when systemic toxicity occurs.[78,79] In spite of these observations, we believe that 0.75 percent bupivacaine remains a useful drug for orthopedic anesthesia when administered through an epidural needle. Once a catheter is in place, we do follow the Physicians' Drug Reference recommendations that 0.75 percent bupivacaine not be administered via a catheter.

Etidocaine, another long-acting local anesthetic, is infrequently used by most anesthesia care providers. It appears that this is principally because of the perception, and some data, that motor blockade is more profound than sensory block with the drug.[80] The reason for this may be that etidocaine is less effective than bupivacaine in producing small fiber blockade.[81] Nevertheless, when muscle relaxation needs to be accentuated during epidural block, 1 to 1.5 percent etidocaine may be injected in 8- to 12-ml volumes to improve the muscle relaxation.

Additives

Similar to spinal anesthetic drug mixtures, some advocate combining agents with local anesthetics to make epidural anesthesia last longer, improve quality of blockade, or to accelerate onset of the block. Epinephrine will increase the duration of epidural anesthesia with all the agents, although the proportional effect is greatest with lidocaine, mepivacaine, and 2-chloroprocaine, while a lesser effect is shown with bupivacaine and etidocaine (Table 13-5). Phenylephrine has been used in epidural anesthesia less frequently than during spinal anesthesia, perhaps because it does not reduce peak blood levels of local anesthetic as effectively as epinephrine during epidural use.[82]

Carbonation of the local anesthetic solution during epidural anesthesia has been suggested as a means of increasing both speed of onset and quality of block by producing more rapid intraneural diffusion and more rapid penetration of connective tissue surrounding the nerve trunk.[83,84] There are data suggesting that there are no clinical advantages of the carbonated solutions,[85] and some disadvantages since peak blood levels of the drug are higher after carbonation of the local anesthetic and blood pressures decreases may occur more rapidly.[86,87]

The addition of bicarbonate has also been suggested as a means of raising the pH of local anesthetic solution, thus increasing the concentration of nonionized free base, which will theoretically increase the rate of diffusion of the drug and speed the onset of block. Clinically, the addition of 1 mEq of sodium bicarbonate to each 10 ml of commercially prepared 1.5 percent lidocaine solution produces a significantly faster onset of anesthesia and more rapid spread of sensory block.[88] The clinical necessity for this modification remains to be justified. One other alteration of local anesthetic mixture for epidural use involves combining long- and short-acting drugs. Theoretically, this is to gain the benefit of both quick onset and long duration. This practice does not seem necessary or prudent, since familiarity with the local anesthetics and additives available allows a spectrum of block lengths to be produced. Further, the purported advantages of faster onset with the combinations of local anesthetics seems clinically inconsequential. Additionally, the dilution of otherwise useful concentrations of local anesthetic during the mixing procedure we believe makes the predictability of the epidural anesthetic less exact.

Complications

Epidural anesthesia, in contrast to spinal anesthesia, has the potential to produce local anesthetic systemic toxicity, principally through the unintentional injection of local anesthetic into an epidural vein. The toxic effects of local anesthetics primarily impact the central nervous and cardiovascular systems, with the central nervous system (CNS) affected at a lower blood level. As an example, four to seven times the dose of local anesthetic necessary to produce convulsions in dogs is required to produce cardiovascular collapse.[89] The CNS stimulation is a result of local anesthetic-induced inhibition of the CNS. The initial excitatory phase of a systemic toxic reaction is due to selective inhibition of inhibitory neurons in the cerebral cortex, thus allowing facilitory neurons to discharge in an unopposed fashion.[90] Once blood levels increase high enough, both inhibitory and facilitory pathways are inhibited, leading to CNS depression. For many years, the potential for local anesthetic-induced toxicity, both CNS and cardiovascular, was believed to parallel anesthetic potency.[91,92] However, current information suggests that bupivacaine and etidocaine may be proportionally more cardiotoxic than their anesthetic potency predicts.[93,94] This proportional increase in cardiotoxicity appears to result from more potent electrophysiologic effects of the long-acting amides.

If CNS toxicity or frank convulsions occur following an epidural local anesthetic injection, a number of steps must be followed efficiently if adverse outcomes are to be prevented. Early in local anesthetic-induced seizures hypoxemia, hypercarbia, and acidosis are present and therefore symptomatic treatment of the toxicity must involve treatment of these factors. Oxygen should be given via bag and mask, but tracheal intubation is not mandated unless ventilation is ineffective.[95] The next step in treatment of local anesthetic toxicity remains controversial, with either succinylcholine or anticonvulsant administered. Succinylcholine is often recommended since the local anesthetic-induced seizures are usually short-lived, and the muscle relaxation obtained facilitates ventilation and decreases the magnitude of metabolic acidosis from skeletal muscle contraction.[95] Nevertheless, it does not decrease cerebral metabolism; thus, CNS oxygen requirements remain increased. Others suggest that diazepam is effective in con-

trolling local anesthetic-induced seizures, although 2 to 3 minutes is required
to control seizures once administered.[96,97] The most effective method of
treating toxic reactions is prevention.
One of the methods that has been effective in limiting the number of local anesthetic-induced seizures is appropriate
use of test doses. Considerable research
has been undertaken to find the ideal test
dose for continuous epidural catheter
use. Currently, in patients not receiving
β blockers it appears that 15 μg of epinephrine is a clinically useful marker of
intravascular placement.[98] In addition to
the use of a test dose, incremental injection of the therapeutic local anesthetic
dose (in 5-ml increments) also appears to
provide a margin of safety, without adversely affecting block height.[99]

Another adverse effect of unintentionally administering an epidural local anesthetic errantly is an injection into the
spinal fluid. The most dramatic example
of such an injection is the neurologic
changes (cauda equina syndromes) that
followed the subarachnoid injection of 2-
chloroprocaine in the late 1970s and early
1980s.[54] Most subarachnoid injections of
epidural local anesthetics are less dramatic: rather, the issue is how one should
treat the cardiopulmonary effects resulting from such an injection. Similar to any
central neuraxial block that reaches high
levels, arterial blood pressure and heart
rate should be supported pharmacologically. The Trendelenburg position
should be instituted to maximize venous
return and intravenous atropine and
ephedrine are often effective in tempo-
rizing until there is time to administer a
more potent catecholamine, if needed. If
the entire dose (20 to 25 ml) of local anesthetic has been administered into the
CSF, tracheal intubation and mechanical
ventilation are indicated since these patients may require approximately 1 to 2
hours of mechanical ventilation before

adequate spontaneous ventilation is
maintained consistently. One caution is
that after a large dose of local anesthetic
into the CSF, patients will also develop
dilated pupils. To the less experienced,
this may seem to indicate CNS injury if
this phenomenon is not recognized for
what it is. The pupils will return to baseline state as the high block recedes. For-
tuitously, the necessity for sedation during the period of tracheal intubation and
mechanical ventilation is minimal, since
these patients generally do not recall
such events.[100]

If an epidural anesthetic is performed
and higher-than-expected sensory levels
develop only after a delay of 15 to 30 minutes, subdural placement of the local anesthetic must be considered. Treatment
is once again symptomatic; the most difficult aspect is recognizing the possibility
of a subdural injection.

With the exception of the publicity surrounding the 2-chloroprocaine-induced
adhesive arachnoiditis, epidural anesthesia has not been linked with neurologic injury more frequently than other
anesthetics, regional or general.[54] No
specific local anesthetic, needle versus
catheter technique, addition or omission
of epinephrine, or location of epidural
puncture seems to be associated with an
increased incidence of neurologic injury.
Nevertheless, neurologic injury is often
feared and epidural anesthesia avoided in
patients in whom antiplatelet drugs or
other anticoagulant drugs have been used
preoperatively. Is this justified? There
are no data in patients taking antiplatelet
drugs such as aspirin or nonsteroidal anti-
inflammatory drugs, as do many of our orthopedic patients, that there is an increased incidence of neurologic injuries
secondary to epidural bleeding (hematoma) when epidural anesthesia is used.
It seems doubtful that the lack of data indicates that the problem has been overlooked, since epidural anesthesia is fre-

quently used in patients undergoing orthopedic procedures. However, there are isolated case reports of neurologic injury after both epidural and spinal anesthesia in patients in whom antiplatelet drugs were used. It may be significant that in these case reports the initial central neuraxial technique was abandoned after technical difficulties with needle placement.[101,102]

In patients receiving anticoagulants preceding orthopedic anesthesia (e.g., the patient receiving subcutaneous heparin therapy) the risk/benefit ratio remains undetermined at this time. There are data from Odoom and Sih[103] who used continuous epidural anesthesia in a thousand vascular operations without problems, in patients receiving preoperative oral anticoagulants. Nevertheless, in orthopedic patients receiving anticoagulants preoperatively the risk/benefit ratio must be determined on an individual basis. Some speculate that proof of minimal systemic effect from the subcutaneous heparin (normal partial thromboplastin time) is necessary prior to central neuraxial block.[104]

CLINICAL APPLICATIONS

Patients undergoing orthopedic surgical procedures typically fall into three principal groups. One group consists of pediatric patients with significant orthopedic disease, including those with cerebral palsy, juvenile rheumatoid arthritis, the varied forms of scoliosis, or long bone or spine deformities. A second group consists of primarily healthy patients, both pediatric or adult, undergoing surgical procedures for orthopedic trauma related to day-to-day life or sporting injuries. A final broad category of orthopedic surgical patients are those older patients undergoing joint replacement procedures for joint diseases such as degenerative arthritis or rheumatoid arthritis. Each of these subgroups of patients brings unique problems or concerns to the anesthesia care provider. Pediatric patients with significant orthopedic abnormalities often require an anesthesia care provider's patience and reassurance that everything possible will be done to minimize the perioperative pain and discomfort. "Healthy" patients undergoing repair of a traumatic orthopedic injury often will arrive in the operating room with a full stomach and significant pain. Efforts in these patients must be directed toward perioperative pain management, as well as getting them back to their preinjury state as soon as possible. In the final, broad subgroup of patients, those requiring total joint replacement, the anesthesia care provider must focus on their pre-existing medical problems, such as cardiovascular and/or pulmonary disease, obesity, hypertension, diabetes, or other chronic conditions.

In this latter group of patients, in addition to concern over their medical conditions, attention must be focused on their ongoing drug therapy. These patients are often receiving antiplatelet drugs for their significant arthritis, therefore, as outlined earlier, a risk/benefit decision must be made regarding the appropriateness of a central neuraxial block. It may be appropriate to administer a spinal anesthetic via a midline approach with a small-gauge needle in a patient with significant cardiopulmonary disease undergoing a hip replacement procedure, whereas, in a patient receiving chronic warfarin therapy for a prior history of deep venous thrombosis who requires a knee arthroscopy, a central neuraxial technique should be avoided.

This same subgroup of patients, those receiving total joint replacements, have a significant incidence of hypertension. They may be receiving adrenergic blockers, calcium channel blockers, or other antihypertensives, which needs to be taken into consideration prior to the prescription of an anesthetic. The classic report on anesthesia and hypertension by Goldman and Caldera[105] needs to be understood before it is interpreted for orthopedic patients undergoing regional anesthesia. Their study involved only general anesthetics. This report did identify that as long as patients' diastolic blood pressures remained consistently below 110 mmHg, their risk of perioperative cardiovascular events was not excessive. Nevertheless, it must be emphasized that these data were acquired in a group of patients above the age of 40 years undergoing only general anesthesia. The applicability to patients undergoing regional anesthesia is yet to be established.

One final, yet often overlooked, pharmacologic implication in orthopedic patients is the prior use of steroids. Many of the patients, especially those with significant rheumatoid arthritis, have received steroids over a long period of time. Generally, it is still advised to prescribe a "stress-dose" of hydrocortisone for this group of patients when undergoing major surgical procedures. A "stress-dose" for lesser procedures, such as outpatient procedures, does not appear indicated; however, this decision must be individualized to each patient.

Rheumatoid Arthritis

Patients with rheumatoid arthritis present a number of challenges to anesthesia care providers.[106] Many of these challenges involve seemingly routine aspects of care, such as tracheal intubation, epidural and subarachnoid cannulation, intravenous catheter placement, and positioning on the operating table. The disease is seemingly of immunologic, au-

toimmune origin, and tracheal intubation is often a concern in these patients since atlantoaxial subluxation may develop from ligamentous erosion by rheumatoid involvement of the bursa surrounding the odontoid process of C2. Subluxation of this joint occurs with flexion of the neck and anesthetic management should be directed toward preventing flexion of the cervical spine. This may be accomplished by using an "awake"–sedated–spontaneously ventilating intubation or the help of an assistant to hold the head in a neutral position during gentle, direct visualization of the trachea by an experienced laryngoscopist.

Arthritides

Another form of arthritis that does impact the use of central neuraxial blocks is ankylosing spondylitis. This disease involves ossification of ligaments at their attachment to bone. This progressive arthritis involves the joint cartilage and disc space of the axial skeleton with eventual ankylosis. The arthritis may progress to develop in the hips, shoulders, and costovertebral joints.[107] Once again, there is a risk of cervical spine instability in these patients, so attention to positioning and tracheal intubation must again be central in anesthetic decision-making. This is one patient population in which caudal anesthesia may be more easily obtained than either lumbar epidural or spinal anesthesia. Nevertheless, in a subgroup of these patients spinal anesthesia can be accomplished by the use of Taylor's approach to the subarachnoid space. In spite of this observation, it is difficult to predict in an individual patient whether this approach will be successful.

In patients with diffuse osteoarthritis, the principle anesthetic consideration is often positioning. These patients are frequently more difficult to position for central neuraxial blockade, and it is almost mandatory that a well-trained assistant be present to assist the anesthesiologist during block placement. Additional positioning concerns are primarily directed to the length of the surgical procedure. If a central neuraxial block is chosen in this subgroup of patients, it is often necessary and advantageous to plan significant intravenous and/or inhalational sedation to allow patient comfort through the length of what is often a 2- to 4-hour procedure.

Obesity

Obese patients have many of the same considerations that patients with significant arthritis present anesthesia care providers. In a sense, our arthritic patients have a disease of their endoskeleton, whereas our obese patients have a limitation of skeletal movement via a adipose-filled "exoskeleton." These obese patients often come for hip or knee total joint replacement and present many of the same positioning problems that arthritic patients experience. In addition, airway management concerns are also frequent in this subgroup of orthopedic patients. Additionally, obese patients present to anesthesia care providers technical difficulties that demand increased skills in central neuraxial midline identification. It is in these patients that the sitting position for spinal or lumbar epidural cannulation can be used to advantage.

Miscellaneous Orthopedic Concerns

Patients undergoing surgical procedures to correct orthopedic trauma emergently are often those involved in motor vehicle accidents. In this subgroup of patients, one must be vigilant for signs of closed-head trauma accompanying their other orthopedic injuries. It is often advisable to forego a central neuraxial technique if there is any concern over closed-head injury, since increased intracranial pressure may be present and would contraindicate subarachnoid puncture. In this group of trauma patients, it is also advisable to pay particular attention to the patient's intravascular volume. Long bone fractures can easily be responsible for 1 to 2 L of concealed blood loss, and this may not become evident until a sympathectomy is produced by the use of a central neuraxial block. It should not be construed that trauma contradicts central neuraxial blockade. These blocks can often be useful in the trauma setting as long as careful attention to volume status is maintained.

Another group of patients that often can benefit from central neuraxial blockade are those undergoing some form of lower extremity amputation. There is evidence that phantom-limb pain may be reduced if a central neuraxial block is maintained perioperatively.[108] It often seems that anesthesia care providers avoid the use of central neuraxial blocks during procedures in which an amputation is to be performed; however, we believe adequate sedation coupled with the central neuraxial block provides excellent operating conditions and, managed comprehensively, may have the additional advantage of reducing the incidence of phantom-limb pain. Another subgroup of patients in whom general anesthesia often seems to be reflexive choice are those patients undergoing orthopedic cancer surgery. Once again, if appropriate intravenous or inhalational sedation is chosen to complement a central neuraxial block, there seems little reason why these techniques cannot be used for lower extremity cancer surgery.

Hospitalization Status

Often it seems outpatient orthopedic surgical patients are steered away from central neuraxial blocks because of the fear of PDPH. In spite of this observation, central neuraxial blocks are often useful anesthetic techniques in this group of patients if the occasional headache is efficiently treated with an epidural blood patch.[109] In a busy outpatient orthopedic surgical practice in which many patients are undergoing arthroscopic knee evaluation, spinal anesthesia is often one of the most time-efficient ways to anesthetize patients. It has an advantage over epidural anesthesia in that the block develops rapidly, and if lidocaine is used as the spinal anesthetic, it has a relatively short duration of action. Nevertheless, comprehensive use of spinal anesthesia in outpatients demands that epidural blood patch therapy be able to be administered in a time-efficient fashion. In a patient living at a distance from such facilities, perhaps it is more useful to choose epidural anesthesia, and under special circumstances, general anesthesia. If a central neuraxial block is chosen in an outpatient orthopedic patient, the patient should be able to ambulate without orthostatic changes and void prior to discharge from the outpatient unit.

Finally, probably the most important factor for the successful use of central neuraxial blocks in orthopedic anesthesia is that they be time-efficient. These blocks cannot measurably add to the surgical day if nurses and surgeons are to be coadvocates of the technique. To achieve this goal, one should plan ahead to maximize anesthetic efficiency. Often overlooked in this planning is that the patient preparation for surgery can begin almost as soon as the block is administered if patient sedation is at an appropriate level.

Inpatients are often ideal candidates for central neuraxial blocks, particularly continuous epidural techniques. They are excellent candidates for these techniques since perioperative analgesic techniques can be administered via the epidural catheter. Many patients undergoing lower extremity orthopedic surgical procedures can take advantage of advances in epidural opioid or opioid/local anesthetic mixtures. It is our belief that the advances in perioperative analgesia are one of the principal advantages of central neuraxial blocks in the orthopedic surgical patient. More on this aspect of orthopedic care can be found in Chapter 16.

To have central neuraxial blocks accepted in a specific institution, a plan must be in place to prevent prolongation of the patient's recovery room stay. This is important because if recovery of central neuraxial block patients is not understood, unnecessary introduction of institutional inefficiency can result. Inpatients should not be forced to completely "wear off" their central neuraxial block prior to discharge to the floor. Inpatients should be allowed to leave the recovery room after central neuraxial blockade once it can be demonstrated that their block is receding appropriately (at least four dermatomes regression or less than T10 level), they are hemodynamically stable, and they are comfortable.[110] In this way, postanesthesia care unit nurses will also become coadvocates of the technique rather than central neuraxial block detractors.

REFERENCES

1. Greene NM: Perspectives in spinal anesthesia. Reg Anesth 7:55, 1982
2. Broadman LM, Mesrobian R, Ruttimann U et al: Do anesthesiologists prefer a regional or general anesthetic for themselves? Reg Anesth 11:A57, 1986

3. Crile GW: Nitrous oxide anaesthesia and a note on anociassociation, a new principle in operative surgery. Surg Gynecol Obstet 13:170, 1911

4. Lundy JS: Balanced anesthesia. Minn Med 9:399, 1926

5. Yeager MP, Glass DD, Neff RK et al: Epidural anesthesia and analgesia in high risk surgical patients. Anesthesiology 66:729, 1987

6. Pflug AE, Murphy TM, Butler SH et al: The effects of postoperative peridural analgesia on pulmonary therapy and pulmonary complications. Anesthesiology 41:8, 1974

7. Bridenbaugh LD: Are anesthesia resident programs failing regional anesthesia? Reg Anesth 7:26, 1982

8. Zarzur E: Anatomic studies of the human lumbar ligamentum flavum. Anesth Analg 63:499, 1984

9. Santos DJ, Bridenbaugh PO, Heins S, Pai U: Unilateral epidural analgesia for labor. Reg Anesth 10:41, 1985

10. Nunn G, Mackinnon RPG: Two unilateral epidural blocks (letter). Anesthesia 41:439, 1986

11. Blomberg RG: The dorsomedian connective tissue band in the lumbar epidural space of humans: an anatomic study using epiduroscopy in autopsy cases. Anesth Analg 65:747, 1986

12. Savolaine ER, Pandya JB, Greenblatt SH, Conover SR: Anatomy of the human lumbar epidural space: new insights using CT-epiduroscopy. Anesthesiology 68:217, 1988

13. Blomberg RG: The lumbar subdural extraarachnoid space of humans: an anatomical study using spinaloscopy in autopsy cases. Anesth Analg 66:177, 1987

14. Thompson JE: An anatomical and experimental study of sacral anesthesia. Ann Surg 66:718, 1917

15. Trotter M: Variations of the sacral canal: their significance in the administration of caudal anesthesia. Anesth Analg 26:192, 1947

16. Murphy TM: Spinal, epidural and caudal anesthesia. p. 1061. In Miller RD (ed): Anesthesia. 2nd Ed. Churchill Livingstone, New York, 1986

17. Greene NM: Physiology of Spinal Anesthesia. 3rd Ed. Williams & Wilkins, Baltimore, 1981

18. Kety SS, King BD, Horvath SM et al: The effects of an acute reduction in blood pressure by means of differential spinal sympathetic block on the cerebral circulation of hypertensive patients. J Clin Invest 29:403, 1950

19. Hackel DB, Sancetta S, Kleinerman J: Effect of hypotension due to spinal anesthesia on coronary blood flow and myocardial metabolism in man. Circulation 13:92, 1956

20. Kleinerman J, Sancetta SM, Hackel DB: Effects of high spinal anesthesia on cerebral circulation and metabolism in man. J Clin Invest 37:285, 1958

21. Sivarajan M, Amory DW, Lindbloom LE et al: Systemic and regional blood-flow changes during spinal anesthesia in the rhesus monkey. Anesthesiology 43:78, 1975

22. Butterworth JF, Piccione W Jr, Berrizbeitia LD et al: Augmentation of venous return by adrenergic agonists during spinal anesthesia. Anesth Analg 65:612, 1986

23. Steinbrook RA, Concepcion M: Respiratory effects of spinal anesthesia: resting ventilation and single-breath CO_2 response. Anesth Analg 72:182, 1991

24. Harrop-Griffiths AW, Ravalia A, Browne DA, Robinson PN: Regional anaesthesia and cough effectiveness. Anaesthesia 46:11, 1991

25. Egbert LD, Tamersoy K, Deas TC: Pulmonary function during spinal anesthesia: the mechanism of cough depression. Anesthesiology 22:882, 1961

26. Ward RJ, Kennedy WF, Bonica JJ et al: Experimental evaluation of atropine and vasopressors for the treatment of hypotension of high subarachnoid anesthesia. Anesth Analg 45:621, 1966

27. Greene NM, Bunker JP, Kerr WS et al: Hypotensive spinal anesthesia: respiratory, metabolic, hepatic, renal and cerebral effects. Ann Surg 140:641, 1954

28. Walts LF, Kaufman RD, Moreland JR et al: Total hip arthroplasty: an investigation of factors related to postoperative

urinary retention. Clin Orthop 194:280, 1985

29. Cassuto J, Wallin G, Hogstrom S et al: Inhibition of postoperative pain by continuous low-dose intravenous infusion of lidocaine. Anesth Analg 64:971, 1985

30. Defalque RJ: Compared effects of spinal and extradural anesthesia upon the blood pressure. Anesthesiology 23:627, 1962

31. Moore DC, Bridenbaugh LD: Spinal (subarachnoid) block: a review of 11,574 cases. JAMA 195:907, 1966

32. Taylor JA: Lumbrosacral subarachnoid tap. J Urol 43:561, 1940

33. Moore DC, Chadwick HS, Ready LB: Epinephrine prolongs lidocaine spinal: pain in the operative site the most accurate method of determining local anesthetic duration. Anesthesiology 67:416, 1987

34. Smith HS, Carpenter RL, Bridenbaugh LD: Failure rate of tetracaine spinal anesthesia with and without epinephrine. Anesthesiology 65:A193, 1986

35. Abouleish EI: Epinephrine improves the quality of spinal anesthesia of bupivacaine. Anesthesiology 65:A375, 1986

36. Kozody R, Swartz J, Palahniuk RJ et al: Spinal cord blood flow following subarachnoid lidocaine. Can Anaesth Soc J 32:472, 1985

37. Caldwell C, Nielsen C, Baltz T et al: Comparison of high-dose epinephrine and phenylephrine in spinal anesthesia with tetracaine. Anesthesiology 62:804, 1985

38. Kozody R, Palahniuk RJ, Cumming MO: Spinal cord blood flow following subarachnoid tetracaine. Can Anaesth Soc J 32:23, 1985

39. Moore DC, Spinal anesthesia: bupivacaine compared with tetracaine. Anesth Analg 59:743, 1980

40. Kozody R, Ong B, Palahniuk RJ et al: Subarachnoid bupivacaine decreases spinal cord blood flow in dogs. Can Anaesth Soc J 32:216, 1985

41. Kozody R, Palahnuik RJ, Wade JG et al: The effect of subarachnoid epinephrine and phenylephrine on spinal cord blood flow. Can Anaesth Soc J 31:503, 1984

42. Bedder MD, Kozody R, Palahniuk RJ et al: Clonidine prolongs tetracaine spinal anesthesia. Can Anaesth Soc J 33:591, 1986

43. Greene NM: Uptake and elimination of local anesthetics during spinal anesthesia. Anesth Analg 62:1013, 1983

44. Chambers WA, Littlewood DG, Logan MR et al: Effect of added epinephrine on spinal anesthesia with lidocaine. Anesth Analg 60:417, 1981

45. Chambers WA, Littlewood DG, Scott DB: Spinal anesthesia with hyperbaric bupivacaine: effect of added vasoconstrictors. Anesth Analg 61:49, 1982

46. Leicht CH, Carlson SA: Prolongation of lidocaine spinal anesthesia with epinephrine and phenylephrine. Anesth Analg 65:365, 1986

47. Concepcion M, Maddi R, Fancis D et al: Vasoconstrictors in spinal anesthesia with tetracaine—a comparison of epinephrine and phenylephrine. Anesth Analg 63:134, 1984

48. Racle JP, Benkhadra A, Poy JY, Gleizal B: Effect of increasing amounts of epinephrine during isobaric bupivacaine spinal anesthesia in elderly patients. Anesth Analg 66:882, 1987

49. Atchison SR, Wedel DJ, Wilson PR: Effect of injection rate on level and duration of hypobaric spinal anesthesia. Anesth Analg 69:496, 1989

50. Stienstra R, Van Poorten F: Speed of injection does not affect subarachnoid distribution of plain bupivacaine 0.5%. Reg Anesth 15:208, 1990

51. Kennedy F, Effron AS, Perry G: The grave spinal cord paralyses caused by spinal anesthesia. Surg Gynecol Obstet 91:385, 1950

52. Marinacci AA: Neurologic aspects of complications of spinal anesthesia. Los Ang Neurol Soc Bull 25:170, 1960

53. Vandam LD, Dripps RD: A long-term follow-up of patients who received 10,098 spinal anesthetics. II. Incidence and analyses of minor sensory neurologic defects. Surgery 38:463, 1955

54. Kane RE: Neurologic deficits following epidural or spinal anesthesia. Anesth Analg 60:150, 1981

55. Rigler ML, Drasner K, Krejcie TC et al: Cauda equina syndrome after continuous spinal anesthesia. Anesth Analg 72:275, 1991

56. Denny N, Masters R, Pearson D et al: Postdural puncture headache after continuous spinal anesthesia. Anesth Analg 66:791, 1987

57. Mihic DN: Postspinal headache and relationship of the needle bevel to longitudinal dural fibers. Reg Anesth 10:76, 1985

58. Jones RJ: The role of recumbency in the prevention and treatment of postspinal headache. Anesth Analg 53:788, 1974

59. Thornberry EA, Thomas TA: Posture and post-spinal headache: a controlled trial in 80 obstetric patients. Br J Anaesth 60:195, 1988

60. Baumgarten RK: Should caffeine become the firstline treatment for postdural puncture headache (letter)? Anesth Analg 66:913, 1987

61. Gormley JB: Treatment of postspinal headache. Anesthesiology 21:565, 1960

62. DiGiovanni AJ, Dunbar BS: Epidural injections of autologous blood for post-lumbar puncture headache. Anesth Analg 49:268, 1970

63. DiGiovanni AJ, Galbert MW, Wahle WM: Epidural injection of autologous blood for post-lumbar puncture headache. II. Additional clinical experiences and laboratory investigation. Anesth Analg 51:226, 1972

64. Ostheimer GW, Palahniuk RJ, Shnider SM: Epidural blood patch for post-lumbar-puncture headache (letter). Anesthesiology 41:307, 1974

65. Szeinfeld M, Ihmeidan IH, Moser MM et al: Epidural blood patch: evaluation of the volume of spread of blood injected into the epidural space. Anesthesiology 64:820, 1986

66. Brown EM, Elman DS: Postoperative backache. Anesth Analg 40:683, 1961

67. Caplan RA, Ward RJ, Posner K, Cheney FW et al: Unexpected cardiac arrest during spinal anesthesia: a closed claims analysis of predisposing factors. Anesthesiology 68:5, 1988

68. Zornow MH, Scheller MS: Cardiac arrest during spinal anesthesia. II. Anesthesiology 68:970, 1988

69. Mackcy DC, Carpcntcr RL, Thompson GE et al: Bradycardia and asystole during spinal anesthesia: a report of three cases without morbidity. Anesthesiology 70:866, 1989

70. Seow LT, Lips FJ, Cousins MJ: Effect of lateral posture on epidural blockade for surgery. Anaesth Intensive Care 11:97, 1983

71. Cousins MJ, Bromage PR: Epidural neural blockade. p. 255. In Cousins MJ, Bridenbaugh PO (eds): Neural Blockade in Clinical Anesthesia and Management of Pain. JB Lippincott, Philadelphia, 1988

72. Bromage PR: Epidural Anesthesia. WB Saunders, Philadelphia, 1978

73. Reynolds AF, Roberts PA, Pollay M, Stratemeier PH: Quantitative anatomy of the thorocolumbar epidural space. Neurosurgery 17:905, 1985

74. Philip BK: Effect of epidural air injection on catheter complications: experience in obstetric patients. Reg Anesth 10:21, 1985

75. Verniquet AJW: Vessel puncture with epidural catheters. Anaesthesia 35:660, 1980

76. Ravindran RS, Bond VK, Tasch MD et al: Prolonged neural blockade following regional anesthesia with 2-chloroprocaine. Anesth Analg 59:447, 1980

77. Moore DC, Spierdijk J, vanKleef JD et al: Chloroprocaine neurotoxicity: four additional cases. Anesth Analg 61:155, 1982

78. Lynch C: Depression of myocardial contractility in vitro by bupivacaine, etidocaine, and lidocaine. Anesth Analg 65:551, 1986

79. Kasten GW: Amide local anesthetic alterations of effective refractory period temporal dispersion: relationship to ventricular arrhythmias. Anesthesiology 65:61, 1986

80. Moore DC, Bridenbaugh PO, Bridenbaugh LD et al: A double-blind study of bupivacaine and etidocaine for epidural (peridural) block. Anesth Analg 53:690, 1974

81. Stanton-Hicks M, Murphy TM, Bonica JJ et al: Effects of extradural block: comparison of the properties, circulatory effects and pharmacokinetics of etidocaine and bupivacaine. Br J Anaesth 48:575, 1976

82. Stanton-Hicks M, Berges PU, Bonica JJ: Circulatory effects of peridural block. IV. Comparison of the effects of epinephrine and phenylephrine. Anesthesiology 39:308, 1973

83. Park WY, Hagins FM: Comparison of lidocaine hydrocarbonate with lidocaine hydrochloride for epidural anesthesia. Reg Anesth 11:128, 1986

84. Bokesch PM, Raymond SA, Strichartz GR: Dependence of lidocaine potency on pH and PCO_2. Anesth Analg 66:9, 1987

85. Brown DT, Morison DH, Covino BG, Scott DB: Comparison of carbonated bupivacaine and bupivacaine hydrochloride for extradural anaesthesia. Br J Anaesth 52:419, 1980

86. Martin R, Lamarche Y, Tetreault L: Effects of carbon dioxide and epinephrine on serum levels of lidocaine after epidural anaesthesia. Can Anaesth Soc J 28:224, 1981

87. Parnass SM, Curran MA, Becker GL: Comparison of hypotensive responses of the carbonated and hydrochloride salts of lidocaine in epidural blocks. Anesth Analg 66:S134, 1987

88. Di Fazio CA, Carron HO, Grosslight KR et al: Comparison of pH adjusted lidocaine solutions for epidural anesthesia. Anesth Analg 65:760, 1986

89. Liu PL, Feldman HS, Giasi R et al: Comparative CNS toxicity of lidocaine, etidocaine, bupivacaine, and tetracaine in awake dogs following rapid intravenous administration. Anesth Analg 62:375, 1983

90. Tanaka K, Yamasaki M: Blocking of cortical inhibitory synapses by intravenous lidocaine. Nature 209:207, 1966

91. Munson ES, Tucker WK, Ausinsch B, Malagodi MH: Etidocaine, bupivacaine, and lidocaine seizure thresholds in monkeys. Anesthesiology 42:471, 1975

92. Block A, Covino B: Effect and local anesthetic agents on cardiac conduction and contractility. Reg Anesth 6:55, 1981

93. de Jong RH, Ronfeld RA, DeRosa RA: Cardiovascular effects of convulsant and supraconvulsant doses of amide local anesthetics. Anesth Analg 61:3, 1982

94. Kotelko DM, Shnider SM, Dailey PA et al: Bupivacaine-induced cardiac arrhythmias in sheep. Anesthesiology 60:10, 1984

95. Moore DC, Bridenbaugh LD: Oxygen: the antidote for systemic toxic reactions from local anesthetic drugs. JAMA 174:842, 1960

96. Munson ES, Wagman IH: Diazepam treatment for local anesthetic-induced seizures. Anesthesiology 37:523, 1972

97. Moore DC, Balfour RI, Fitzgibbons D: Convulsive arterial plasma levels of bupivacaine and the response to diazepam therapy. Anesthesiology 50:454, 1979

98. Moore DC, Batra MS: The components of an effective test dose prior to epidural block. Anesthesiology 55:693, 1981

99. Batra MS, Bridenbaugh LD, Levy S: Epidural anesthesia for cesarean section: Comparison of bolus and fractionated injection. Reg Anesth 10:32, 1985

100. Evans TI: Total spinal anesthesia. Anaesth Intensive Care 2:158, 1974

101. Mayumi T, Dohi S: Spinal subarachnoid hematoma after lumbar puncture in a patient receiving antiplatelet therapy. Anesth Analg 62:777, 1983

102. Greensite FS, Katz J: Spinal subdural hematoma associated with attempted epidural anesthesia and subsequent continuous spinal anesthesia. Anesth Analg 59:72, 1980

103. Odoom JA, Sih IL: Epidural analgesia and anticoagulant therapy: experience with one thousand cases of continuous epidurals. Anaesthesia 38:254, 1983

104. Owens EL, Kasten GW, Hessel EA: Spinal subarachnoid hematoma after lumbar puncture and heparinization: a case report, review of the literature, and discussion of anesthetic implications. Anesth Analg 65:1201, 1986

105. Goldman L, Caldera DL: Risks of gen-

eral anesthesia and elective operation in the hypertensive patient. Anesthesiology 50:285, 1979

106. Sullivan M, Edelist G: Anesthesia and the inflammatory arthropathies: rheumatoid arthritis and ankylosing spondylitis. Probl Anesth 5:25, 1991

107. McCarthy DJ: Ankylosing spondylitis. p. 934. In McCarthy DJ (ed): Arthritis and Allied Conditions. 11th Ed. Lea & Febiger, Philadelphia, 1989

108. Bach S, Noreng MF, Tjelídeu NU: Phantom limb pain in amputees during the first 12 months following limb amputation, after preoperative lumbar epidural blockade. Pain 33:297, 1988

109. Ravindran RS: Epidural autologous blood patch on an outpatient basis (letter). Anesth Analg 63:962, 1984

110. Willis RJ: Caudal epidural block. p. 361. In Cousins MJ, Bridenbaugh PO (eds): Neural Blockade in Clinical Anesthesia and Management of Pain. JB Lippincott, Philadelphia, 1988

111. Brown DL, Wedel DJ: Spinal, epidural, and caudal anesthesia. p. 1377. In Miller RD (ed): Anesthesia. 3rd Ed. Churchill Livingstone, NY, 1990

14

Complications

Denise J. Wedel

Complications associated with orthopedic surgical procedures include an extensive array of surgical problems such as infection, bleeding, reactions to pharmacologic agents, embolic phenomena (fat, air, and thrombus), and surgical trauma, as well as those specifically related to the anesthetic management. A complete discussion of all possible complications would fill the pages of a dedicated text. Many of these problems are common to all surgical specialties and anesthetics and are described in general texts concerning these specialities. This chapter limits itself to specifically addressing the complications associated with regional anesthesia and the risk of embolic phenomena associated with orthopedic procedures. Surgical and medical problems that can mimic anesthetic complications are also discussed, and a plan for evaluation and treatment is offered.

COMPLICATIONS OF REGIONAL ANESTHESIA

Risk Management

Complications associated with regional anesthesia can be due to effects of the injected agent (e.g., local anesthetic toxicity or allergy) or to incorrect placement of a needle or catheter causing direct tissue damage (e.g., pneumothorax).

It is important to differentiate complications from side effects, which are the normal physiologic effects of a drug or procedure. For example, hypotension associated with a thoracic spinal level is a side effect. However, hypotension due to the accidental injection of an epidural dose of local anesthetic into the subarachnoid space causing a total spinal block is a complication.

Adverse events related to the surgical procedure, positioning, or a patient's underlying medical condition can also present as possible complications of regional anesthesia. The importance of the postoperative anesthetic visit and careful evaluation of all reported postsurgical "complications" can not be overemphasized. The anesthesia care provider is in a unique position to participate as a knowledgeable consultant in all phases of the evaluation and treatment of adverse perioperative events. Finally, at all stages of the anesthetic care (preoperative, intraoperative, and postoperative), prevention is an important aspect of risk management (Table 14-1).

The often-overemphasized risk of serious complications associated with regional anesthesia along with their reported

333

Table 14-1. Complications of Regional Anesthesia and Their Prevention

---

Preoperative factors
  Patient selection
  Choice of technique and agent
  Familiarity with patient medical history
  Awareness of potential side effects/complications
Intraoperative factors
  Appropriate monitoring
  Availability of resuscitation equipment
Postoperative factors
  Appropriately timed postoperative evaluations
  Early intervention of multispecialty team for diagnosis and treatment

---

high frequency of medicolegal problems has often been used as a reason to avoid regional blockade in preference to general anesthesia. Anesthesia care providers who are wary of litigation or unskilled in regional anesthetic techniques can easily persuade a patient to choose to "just go to sleep" by weighting the preoperative presentation of anesthetic choices toward rare and devastating problems with regional anesthesia while downplaying the risks of general anesthesia. Many patients believe pre-existing societal myths concerning risks of spinal anesthesia and may be more than willing to be "protected" from neural blockade. However, the well-documented benefits to be gained by employing regional anesthetic techniques in the orthopedic surgical population, such as decreased blood loss,[1] decreased risk of thromboembolism,[2] and improved postoperative pain relief, are cogent arguments in favor of these techniques. Chapter 4 outlines these arguments in detail.

Furthermore, the serious risks of regional techniques are often overstated. When compared to general anesthesia, there is no evidence that regional anesthesia is associated with a higher incidence of complications. For example,

several studies have examined the safety of central neuraxial blockade (spinal, caudal, and epidural) in large groups of patients, all confirming the rarity of permanent neurologic injury associated with this type of anesthesia.[3–7] However, the common perception by the anesthesia care provider that injuries associated with regional anesthesia techniques are more likely to be associated with litigation than those due to general anesthesia is borne out by investigations of closed insurance claims.[8] This phenomenon is not clearly understood but may be due to a number of factors, including the lack of acceptance of regional anesthesia in the general population, unrealistic expectations concerning outcome by the surgical patient, the readiness of other medical and surgical specialists to ascribe all perioperative complications to the anesthetic if the etiology is unclear, and the devastating nature of a major neurologic complication in an otherwise healthy patient. As the popularity of regional anesthesia techniques increases, patients and medical care providers will gain in knowledge and understanding of the advantages and limitations of these techniques, which should ultimately result in decreased anxiety and more appropriate expectations concerning the application of this form of anesthesia.

What is the appropriate approach to informing the patient of anesthetic risks? Certainly, cataloging every known complication of general or regional anesthesia is excessive, and results in an increase in patient anxiety while only minimally protecting the anesthesia care provider in the event of medicolegal complications. A recommended approach is to inform the patient of those risks that are reasonably common (a suggested frequency of greater than 1 per 10,000 is considered acceptable by most authors). An equally important purpose of the preanesthetic consultation is to provide information about the advantages of various techniques in order to help the patient in arriving at a truly informed decision about the anesthetic management. However, the practice of anesthesia is far too complicated and the amount of information required to make "informed" decisions too vast to expect any patient other than a practicing anesthesia care provider to independently choose which anesthetic is "best." It is the responsibility of the anesthesia care provider to evaluate the individual patient and make an appropriate recommendation based on all the available information regarding anesthesia management. Finally, the level of familiarity, comfort, and expertise of the anesthesia care provider with the techniques should also be considered. The safest anesthetic technique for a given procedure is often the one with which the practitioner is most comfortable.

Anticipation and prevention of complications, along with their early diagnosis and treatment, are the most important factors in dealing with regional anesthetic risks. During the preoperative period, assessment of the patient, review of all medical conditions, and careful preparation for the chosen anesthetic procedure, including ensuring the availability of appropriate monitoring, are necessary factors in risk management. During the intraoperative phase, fastidious neural blockade techniques, vigilance in monitoring and observation, and early and appropriate interventions when problems occur will help decrease the incidence of complications and diminish the impact of those which do occur despite these precautions. Finally, appropriately timed follow-up visits during the postoperative period allow early diagnosis of delayed complications and facilitate intervention in those problems that may be reversible. The postoperative visit also permits the anesthesia care provider to reassure the patient about "minor" postsurgical prob-

lems, such as backache or urinary retention, which are frequently and often inappropriately ascribed to the anesthetic. These "minor" problems can be the focus of anxiety or even hostility in the individual patient suffering through a variety of postsurgical discomforts, and can set the stage for further misunderstandings and negative feelings about the anesthetic care.

Preoperative Assessment

Careful assessment of the patient in the preoperative period allows the anesthesia care provider to select the appropriate anesthetic technique and prepare the patient prior to surgery. Such preparation is important whether regional or general anesthesia is planned. However, it is especially critical in ensuring patient and surgeon satisfaction with regional block techniques, which may be viewed as "different" or a deviation from the "usual anesthetic." Preoperative preparation is also an important aspect of risk management.

The preoperative visit is a valuable opportunity for the clinician to evaluate the patient for organic, pharmacologic, and psychological/emotional disorders that may have an effect on the risk of complications of neural blockade. In rare cases, contraindications to regional anesthesia will be identified. This visit will also set the stage for a good patient–physician relationship. The importance of the development of confidence in the anesthesia care provider during this visit cannot be overemphasized. Such a relationship can be a major factor in risk management.

Contraindications to Regional Anesthesia
Some individuals may be poorly suited for regional anesthetic techniques because of physical, psychological, or emo-

Table 14-2.   Preoperative Assessment
for Regional Anesthesia

Absolute contraindications
  Patient refusal
  Infection at the site of needle insertion
Relative contraindications
  Progressive neurologic disease (e.g., mul-
    tiple sclerosis)
  Aortic or mitral valve stenosis (central
    neuraxial blockade)
  Severe or unstable psychiatric disease
  Severe emotional instability
  Clotting disorders (uncompensated)
  Hypovolemia
  Sepsis
Medical conditions that may affect anesthetic
    choice
  Stable pre-existing neurologic disease
    (i.e., documented peripheral neuropa-
    thy, cerebral vascular accident)
  Diabetes mellitus
  Medications (e.g., antihypertensives, an-
    tiplatelet drugs)
  Cardiovascular disease
  Stable psychiatric and/or emotional dis-
    orders

---

tional conditions (Table 14-2). A number
of "absolute" and "relative" contraindications to regional anesthesia have been
cited. This list varies in length and con-
servatism according to the enthusiasm
and experience of the practitioner.

Absolute Contraindications

Two conditions that must be considered
absolute contraindications to neural
blockade in my opinion are (1) patient refusal and (2) infection at the site of the
needle injection. The wisdom of avoiding
bacterial contamination is obvious. However, proceeding with a block technique
in the face of steadfast patient refusal is
legally considered battery in most states.
If the best attempts at convincing the patient of the advantages and safety of regional anesthesia fail, it would be prudent to proceed with an appropriate
general or local anesthetic. There are no

data that unassailably prove that regional
techniques are superior or safer than a
carefully administered general anesthetic.

Relative   Contraindications   Other
relative contraindications may take on
"absolute" characteristics when applied
to specific patients. For example, the patient with severe aortic stenosis is a poor
candidate for single-shot spinal anesthesia because of the risk of cardiac ischemia and death resulting from the sudden onset of sympathetic blockade.
However, there may be situations in
which a cautiously administered continuous spinal technique may be preferable
to a general anesthetic in such a patient.
The risk/benefit ratio must be carefully
weighed and applied to the individual
case. The patient with underlying clotting disorders presents a similar dilemma.
If general anesthesia techniques are
equally safe, the risk of hematoma from
needle placement may well dissuade the
conservative practitioner from choosing a
central neuraxial blockade technique.
However, in the face of other medical
problems where the benefits of a regional
technique may be more impressive, the
risk of intraspinal hematoma may become
the lesser concern.

Medical Conditions Affecting
Regional Anesthesia

All medical illnesses or drug therapies
that may affect the risks of regional anesthesia should be discussed with the patient preoperatively. Some specific conditions merit special attention with
regard to regional anesthetic techniques.
In this section a number of other medical
conditions and pharmacologic therapies
that may affect the choice of regional
anesthesia in the preoperative period are
discussed.

Neurologic Disease   Patients with progressive neurologic disease such as mul-

tiple sclerosis or amyotrophic lateral sclerosis may develop new neurologic lesions coincidentally during or following a regional anesthetic or surgery. Subsequent symptoms may be difficult to differentiate from nerve injuries resulting from the surgical procedure, positioning, or anesthetic. In general, the safest and most conservative approach would be to avoid nerve blocks in such patients. However, if regional anesthesia is indicated because of other medical reasons or patient request, an exhaustive discussion concerning neurologic complications associated with the anesthetic and surgical procedures, as well as the risks of progression of the underlying disease process that can occur coincidentally, should be fully documented in the patient's chart. The preoperative neurologic status should be fully documented also.

Pre-existing stable neurologic lesions (e.g., a hemiparetic motor deficit following a cerebrovascular accident, or peripheral neuropathy associated with diabetes mellitus) that are appropriately evaluated and documented are not contraindications to neural blockade. However, the underlying etiology of such lesions deserves careful evaluation. While hemiparesis, for example, is not a contraindication to a spinal anesthetic, the underlying cerebrovascular pathology would indicate the need for careful monitoring of the cerebral perfusion pressure and management of the potential hypotensive side effects of the expected sympathectomy associated with central neuraxial blockade. Hence, the choice of regional technique will also be affected; a continuous spinal or epidural technique may be favored over a single-shot method in order to control the height and onset of blockade, thus attenuating or avoiding the sympathetic block. While such technicalities of management may seem challenging at first glance, in this example the advantage of being able to monitor the ad-equacy of cerebrovascular perfusion pressure in the awake patient may well be a deciding factor in choosing a block technique.

Diabetes Mellitus   Diabetes mellitus has known pathologic effects on neural tissue due to the effects of high serum glucose as well as the associated microvascular disease. Neurologic symptoms may occur coincidentally at the time of anesthesia or in the postoperative period, and neural tissue is more susceptible to injury in the perioperative period and is slower to recover. Because of these factors, management of the diabetic patient requires special attention to decreasing the risk of neural injury in the operating room. Careful positioning on the operating table with padding at all neurologically vulnerable sites (see Ch. 5) is especially important. The addition of epinephrine to the local anesthetic solution for peripheral or spinal blockade should be evaluated in relation to the advantages and possible complications. The vasoconstrictive properties of this additive are theoretically undesirable in the presence of diabetic microvascular disease. However, there are no data specifically linking neurologic complications with the use of epinephrine, and the advantages of predicting intravascular injections as well as improvement of block quality may outweigh the unknown risk of complications. Another theoretical concern in the diabetic patient is the use of paresthesias in performing peripheral nerve blocks. Some experts caution that paresthesia techniques are associated with a higher risk of peripheral nerve injury.[9] This concern may be highlighted in the diabetic patient, in whom nerve injury is frequently evident clinically, often making the elicitation of paresthesias difficult if not impossible. Again there is little evidence to influence the practitioner in either direction. It is safe to say that caution should be employed in all nerve blocks to avoid direct needle trauma and intraneural injection of local anesthetic solutions. Because the diabetic patient is at inherent increased risk for neurologic damage, such precautions are especially important. The preoperative physical examination and history will aid the anesthesia care provider in choosing the appropriate technique and agents. A candid discussion of the possible risks with the patient is also important. Once again, as with the example of the patient with cerebrovascular disease, the advantages of a regional technique, allowing awake monitoring of the diabetic patient for signs of hypoglycemia, is a potent argument in the favor of neural blockade, in spite of theoretical risks.

Drug Therapy   Antiplatelet drugs are often self-administered for pain relief or prescribed for the treatment of rheumatoid arthritis or other bone and joint conditions in the orthopedic and aged population. Low-dose aspirin therapy is, recommended as prophylaxis for a variety of common medical conditions, resulting in almost universal use of this agent. While the effects of nonsteroidal anti-inflammatory agents are relatively short-lived and measured in days, the antiplatelet effects of aspirin may last for a week or longer after ingestion. The effect of antiplatelet therapy on hemorrhagic complications of neural blockade is unknown. However, some authors consider a history of such therapy a contraindication to central neuraxial blockade because of the theoretically greater risk of hematoma formation due to the prolongation in bleeding time.[10] These issues are addressed in depth in Chapter 3, and include the effects of other anticoagulant drugs as well as diseases that affect coagulation.

In summary, the controversy concerning management of the patient on preoperative antiplatelet medications has not yet been resolved and requires further prospective study. Because of the rarity of these complications and the known spontaneous occurrences of epidural hematoma in nonsurgical populations, a large series would be required to answer this question. The only large retrospective study published suggests that central neuraxial blockade is safe in patients taking these medications.[11] Appropriate preoperative evaluation of such patients should include determination of a history of abnormal bleeding or bruising, which would indicate further evaluation with a preoperative bleeding time.

A variety of other frequently prescribed medications can also influence the anesthetic management of the orthopedic surgical patient. Antihypertensive medications, especially diuretics and β-blocking agents, have physiologic effects that may influence the anesthetic approach. Diuretic therapy results in a decreased total blood volume, which, in the presence of sympathetic blockade induced by central neuraxial blockade, can result in significant hypotension. This effect can be modified by appropriate fluid and pharmacologic management in the perianesthetic period. β-blockers will interfere with interpretation of an epinephrine-containing local anesthetic test dose, which is used to determine whether intravascular injection has occurred. While β-blockade will prevent an increase in heart rate following intravascular injection of epinephrine, it will not block the increase in blood pressure observed. These examples illustrate the importance of a careful preoperative evaluation in the choice and management of a regional anesthetic.

Infection   Neurologic complications of central neuraxial blockade due to infection are extremely rare. Patients with bacteremia are theoretically at higher risk for this problem and should be identified in the preoperative period. The importance of a localized infection at a site distant from the site of needle insertion in the etiology of epidural or intrathecal infectious complications is unknown, but at best such an association is highly theoretical.

Cardiovascular Disease   Cardiovascular disease can affect the choice of anesthetic technique and management in a variety of ways. The presence of valvular disease, especially anatomic lesions that limit cardiac output, is usually considered a contraindication for central neuraxial blockade for the reasons outlined above. Ischemic cardiac disease is quite common in the elderly orthopedic population, and because of the patient's inability to exercise secondary to lower extremity joint disease and pain, it can be difficult to evaluate the extent of the ischemic disease based on history. In addition to problems associated with evaluation of this medical condition, these patients are often treated with a variety of pharmacologic agents that can interact with the anesthetic. Appropriate evaluation may include noninvasive and invasive modalities to assess ventricular function and the risk of ischemia as described in Chapter 1, which discusses general concepts of preoperative evaluation.

Psychiatric Disorders   Psychiatric illness may interfere with a patient's ability to give informed consent, particularly if distortions of reality (psychoses) are present. In such cases, a regional anesthetic may still be appropriate based on other medical factors; however, the patient's ability to tolerate an awake procedure should be considered. Heavy sedation or a concomitant light general anesthetic may be indicated. Similarly, patients who are emotionally unstable or have a high level of anxiety should also be identified in the preoperative period. Such individuals may be unsuitable candidates for neural blockade because of their underlying fear of loss of control or because of uncontrollable anxiety about the surgical procedure. While heavy sedation or light general anesthesia may provide a suitable background for neural blockade as the primary anesthetic technique, each situation must be handled individually. Psychogenic reactions during a regional anesthetic may mimic a serious complication. The possibility of a conversion reaction should be considered in the differential diagnosis, but this conclusion can only be safely determined by ruling out organic, treatable etiologies.

Intraoperative Complications

Anesthesia care providers tend to concentrate primarily on the intraoperative period when considering problems related to regional anesthesia. However, this is the stage of management over which the practitioner can exert the most control. Intraoperative anesthetic problems can be related to block technique, pharmacologic interventions, or patient management factors (Table 14-3). It is important to recall that coincidental events related to underlying medical conditions or the surgical procedure can also present intraoperatively. Patient positioning, surgical trauma, pharmacologic agents given at the request of the surgical team, and other surgically dictated treatments such as dressing or cast applications can also result in complications that may be attributed to neural blockade in the postoperative period.

Block Techniques

Inappropriate or mismanaged block techniques can result in acute vascular, cardiovascular, neurologic, and respiratory system changes that are deleterious to the patient. There can also be technical dif-

Table 14-3. Intraoperative Problems Associated with Neural Blockade

---

Block technique
    Intravascular injection
    Hematoma formation
    Block-induced sympathectomy
    Peripheral nerve injury
    Pneumothorax (early)
    Sheared/knotted/coiled catheter
    Needle breakage
    "Total" spinal or epidural
    Spinal cord trauma

Pharmacologic
    Oversedation
    Local anesthetic toxicity
    Drug allergy
    Injection of incorrect agent

Patient management
    Undersedation
    Patient decompensation
    Lack of appropriate monitoring

---

ficulties involving the needle or continuous catheter technique.

Vascular and Cardiac Complications

Local Anesthetic Toxicity While both intravenous and intra-arterial injection can cause acute local anesthetic toxicity, there are important differences. Intra-arterial injection into the carotid and vertebral arteries can occur during the performance of stellate block, interscalene block of the brachial plexus, and cervical plexus block. This results in central nervous system (CNS) toxicity and seizure activity with minimal volumes (0.5 to 2 ml) of local anesthetic caused by the immediate delivery of the drug to the brain. Other reported signs of direct CNS toxicity with small volumes of local anesthetic include aphasia, hemiparesis, and sudden unconsciousness.[12] While direct injection into the vertebral or carotid arteries is the mechanism in some cases, retrograde flow into the central cerebral circulation has been demonstrated in the head and neck region as well as in the brachial and femoral arteries. Careful re-

peated aspiration with slow incremental injections of small volumes should be employed to prevent this complication. However, because of the small volumes of local anesthetic required to produce toxicity, preventive measures may not always be successful. The anesthesia care provider must be prepared to diagnose and treat this complication whenever a block of the head and neck is being performed.

Intravenous injections of local anesthetics are more common than intra-arterial injections, and the margin of safety is greater in regard to the volume of drug required to cause CNS toxicity. This complication can occur during the performance of peripheral nerve blocks, through an epidural needle or catheter, and following the release of the tourniquet in an intravenous (Bier) block. Accidental intravenous injection through a needle or catheter can be avoided by frequent, gentle aspiration, slow injection of incremental doses of the local anesthetic, and the use of epinephrine in the solution as an intravascular marker. The observant practitioner will often detect prodromal signs of local anesthetic toxicity such as slurred speech due to numbness of the tongue, or receive from the patient complaints of dizziness, facial twitching, and perioral tingling prior to seizure activity. The injection can be interrupted at an early stage. Severe hypoxia and acidosis can be demonstrated early in the course of seizure activity following intravascular injection.[13] Early intervention is a critical factor in determining outcome.

The basic tenets of resuscitation from local anesthetic toxicity are similar to those recommended for any emergency situation, with emphasis on establishing an airway, ventilation with 100 percent oxygen, maintaining adequate perfusion pressures, and treating the seizure activity. If the patient does not have a full stomach and can be adequately ventilated with a mask and bag, intubation is not mandatory. Seizure activity is usually self-limited; however, a small dose of short-acting barbiturate or benzodiazepine can be given intravenously. Longer-acting antiepileptic agents are usually not necessary and will interfere with evaluation of the patient in the postictal period. The use of succinylcholine should be reserved for facilitating intubation. If a muscle relaxant is administered, it is important to remember that the apparent cessation of seizure activity is limited to the abolition of muscle movement; this treatment will not stop the central effects of seizure activity, including the attendant increase in cerebral oxygen consumption. Cardiovascular depression secondary to local anesthetic toxicity is related both to myocardial depression and peripheral vasodilatation. Elevating the patient's lower extremities will increase cardiac filling pressures and may improve cardiac output. However, if this maneuver does not promptly reverse the hypotension, a vasopressor should be given. Very large doses of local anesthetics injected intravascularly can cause depression of all physiologic functions and require active, prolonged intervention if a good outcome is to be achieved.

Bupivacaine toxicity can be associated with significant cardiovascular depression and dysrhythmias, which can be difficult to manage.[14–16] Electrophysiologic studies of the heart show marked depression of the rapid phase of depolarization of the cardiac action potential and prolongation of the recovery phase.[17] Guinea pig papillary muscle studies demonstrate inhibition of slow calcium channels by both bupivacaine and lidocaine.[18] These data suggest a possible unidirectional blockade of conducting pathways that ultimately results in a re-entrant type of ventricular dysrhythmia. Whatever the etiology, treatment of bupivacaine toxicity should be aggressive and sustained.

Closed chest massage and repeated cardioversion may be necessary; bretylium is probably more effective than lidocaine in treatment of dysrhythmias.

Complications from local anesthetic toxicity due to early, accidental tourniquet deflation during intravenous regional blockade can be avoided by scrupulous management of the tourniquet, informed choice of agent, and use of an appropriate dosage. The technique should only be performed by medical practitioners who are fully trained in resuscitation techniques, including airway management and treatment of local anesthetic toxicity (i.e., anesthesia care providers).

Cardiac Effects of High-Level Blockade   The cardiovascular system is directly and indirectly affected by local anesthetic agents as described above, as well as by the physiologic effects of neural blockade during the intraoperative period. Central neuraxial blockade can result in profound cardiac effects depending on the level of sympathetic blockade and the underlying medical condition of the patient. A sensory level at T4 or above results in a nearly complete block of the sympathetic nervous system, which can result in significant hypotension and compensatory tachycardia. Levels of blockade at and above T2 can interrupt all outflow to the cardioaccelerator fibers as well, resulting in bradycardia and the inability of the patient to respond normally to changes in blood volume, vascular tone, or cardiac filling pressures. Levels of blockade above T8 are rarely indicated for orthopedic surgical procedures on the lower extremities. High levels can often be avoided by careful titration of the total dose of anesthetic, use of continuous catheter techniques, and choice of isobaric or hypobaric spinal solutions to control the height of blockade. However, even the most carefully managed central neuraxial block will sometimes ascend to spinal levels that are associated with hemodynamic changes. Such blocks require close monitoring by the anesthesia care provider as well as a readiness to promptly intervene with pharmacologic agents, appropriate positioning, and intravascular volume expansion in order to counteract the physiologic effects of the sympathetic blockade. Reports of unexpected cardiac arrest during spinal anesthesia gathered from closed insurance claims suggest that life-threatening cardiac decompensation can occur suddenly and without clear warning.[19] While the etiology of such disastrous events is unclear, possible contributing factors include respiratory depression with resultant hypoxia and the effects of sedative agents on the cardiovascular system. Aggressive resuscitation, including the early administration of epinephrine, along with other appropriate steps is recommended. Appropriate intraoperative monitoring serves as an important preventive tool as well as an aid in early diagnosis and treatment of these potentially devastating complications.

Hematoma   Hematoma formation is usually not a cause of morbidity in peripheral blocks commonly used for orthopedic patients, as it is usually associated with anatomic locations having loose, highly vascular tissue such as the neck or scrotum. The use of small-gauge, sharp-beveled needles may diminish the risk of superficial hematoma formation secondary to direct needle trauma.[20] However, hematoma formation in the wall or lumen of peripheral vascular structures during nerve block can result from accidental, undetected intramural injection. This rare complication is described in a report of obliteration of the axillary artery[21] as well as in a reported aneurysmal obstruction of the axillary vein[22] following otherwise unremarkable brachial plexus block. In both reports, the lesion was undetected intraoperatively, the brachial plexus block provided adequate surgical anesthesia, and the vascular lesion presented in the postoperative period as vascular insufficiency.

The risk of epidural, intrathecal, or intracranial hematoma following regional anesthesia is small, but it is devastating if it does occur. The signs of these also usually present in the postoperative period. This rare complication is addressed in the major delayed neurologic complications section of this chapter.

Neurologic Complications   Neurologic complications are relatively rare in the practice of regional anesthesia, but when they occur, they are a major source of litigation. Most of these problems will present in the postoperative period. However, preventive measures and initial management are best instituted intraoperatively.

Careful technique is important in avoiding peripheral nerve injury. Claims that paresthesia techniques for nerve location are inherently dangerous remain unproven. However, direct nerve trauma with a large-gauge, sharp-beveled needle; injection of local anesthetic solutions intraneurally; or injection of an inappropriate drug are avoidable causes of nerve injury. Careful intraoperative positioning of the blocked limb is also important. Large studies have documented the risk of peripheral nerve injury associated with surgery under general anesthesia.[8,23,24] Coincidental nerve injuries have been reported in patients undergoing regional anesthesia as well. Marinacci reported that careful neurologic evaluation of 542 postoperative nerve injuries in patients who had undergone spinal anesthetics revealed only four lesions directly related to the block technique.[25]

Scrupulous documentation of paresthesias elicited during the block as well as the presence or absence of pain during injection of local anesthetic can be helpful in determining the etiology of postoperative neurologic complaints. Tourniquet duration and pressure; a description of the patient's position on the operating table, including documentation of efforts to pad vulnerable anatomic sites; and a record of local anesthetic injections by the surgeon should also be part of the permanent anesthesia record.

Respiratory Complications   Respiratory complications that occur intraoperatively can be due to effects of the sedation, side effects of the nerve block (e.g., phrenic nerve block following interscalene block), trauma to the lung (e.g., pneumothorax associated with supraclavicular block), or effects related to high central neuraxial blockade.

Respiratory Depression   Excessive sedation during regional anesthesia can cause respiratory depression if the airway is uncontrolled. The resulting hypercarbia and hypoxia can cause cardiac irritability, increased blood pressure, and increased intracranial pressure, and stress a variety of other organ systems. Hypercarbia may also increase the risk of local anesthetic toxicity by decreasing the threshold for seizure activity. The definition of "adequate" sedation will vary from patient to patient according to the level of anxiety expressed by the patient and surgeon, the experience and philosophy of the anesthesia care provider, and the drug tolerance of the patient. Sedation only causes respiratory complications if the level and effects are unmonitored and the airway is uncontrolled. For this reason, appropriate intraoperative monitoring of the patient is crucial, both for early intervention and prevention of critical events.

Pneumothorax   Pneumothorax is a well-documented complication of nerve blocks performed in close anatomic relationship to the pleura. In the orthopedic population these include stellate, cervical plexus, supraclavicular, and interscalene blocks. The incidence varies with the expertise of the practitioner as well as the block technique. A "routine" post-block chest x-ray has limited value in the asymptomatic patient as the pneumothorax is usually not detectable until 6 to 12 hours after the block. Treatment varies with the size of the pneumothorax and symptoms. Moore recommends aspirating any pneumothorax greater than 20 percent; larger volumes may require chest tube placement and suction.[26]

Disruption of Respiratory Mechanics   Regional blockade can also cause changes in respiratory status by interfering with the mechanics of respiration. Motor blockade of the intercostal muscles of respiration achieved with high central neuraxial blocks in patients with chronic lung disease may increase the risk of respiratory-related complications and should be used with caution. Since high sensory levels are rarely indicated for orthopedic surgical procedures on the lower extremities, steps should be taken to control the height of blockade. Phrenic nerve blockade is a common side effect following blocks of the brachial plexus, cervical plexus, or cervical sympathetic chain and may also cause respiratory distress in some patients. The interscalene approach to the brachial plexus has a reported incidence of complete ipsilateral phrenic nerve block ranging from 36 to 100 percent, with the higher incidence documented by ultrasonography.[27] While this is usually a benign, self-limited condition, persistence of phrenic nerve paresis for several years following interscalene block has been reported.[28] Performance bilaterally of blocks that have a risk of phrenic nerve block could result in paralysis of both diaphragms, and should be avoided in patients who are at risk for respiratory problems. Careful attention to technique, decreased volumes and concentrations of local anesthetic, and anticipation of potential problems should diminish the impact of this complication.

The effects of high spinal or total epidural block on the respiratory system are complex. High thoracic blockade does not affect arterial blood gas tensions, tidal volumes, or maximum inspiratory volume. However, it may cause decreases in maximum breathing capacity, expiratory volumes, and pressures during forced expiration, and these changes diminish the patient's ability to cough. Even midcervical levels of motor and sensory anesthesia do not appear to affect the function of the phrenic nerves. Respiratory depression seen in total spinal anesthesia is not due to the effect of the local anesthetic on the respiratory center or respiratory motor nerves. It appears to be secondary to medullary ischemia due to hypotension resulting from the decreased cardiac output. Total spinal anesthesia due to injection of an epidural dose of local anesthetic intrathecally can be avoided by careful aspiration and use of an appropriate test dose. The total sympathetic block achieved with high spinal and epidural levels may result in bronchospasm in the susceptible patient due to the unopposed parasympathetic tone of the airway muscles.

Faulty Equipment and Technique
Faulty equipment and technique can cause complications during the performance of a block. Attempted withdrawal of an epidural or intrathecal catheter through the needle can result in shearing of the catheter, leaving a portion of it in the epidural or intrathecal space. Currently marketed catheters are made of inert materials and can theoretically be left within the epidural space without causing damage. Surgical exploration is not recommended for pieces of catheter that are left in the epidural space, although the patient should be informed of the presence of the catheter remnant. Occasionally a catheter may break off at or just beneath the surface of the skin during removal. When this occurs, the catheter remnant acts as a theoretical conduit for bacteria from the surface of the skin into the epidural space. Because of the risk of infection extending into the epidural space, efforts to retrieve this catheter should be instituted. Early involvement of orthopedic and neurosurgical services will aid in the management of such patients. Inserting the catheter beyond the recommended 4 cm may result in coiling and subsequent knotting of the catheter in the epidural space. This problem will usually present as difficulty in removing the catheter, which will gradually attenuate as traction is applied. Epidural catheters are made of materials with high tensile strength, so that it is sometimes possible to apply gentle, continuous traction on the catheter until the knot becomes stretched enough to allow it to be pulled intact through the structures overlying the epidural space. While the risk of this maneuver is that the catheter will break, other options are limited. One case report described knotting of the catheter around the L2-L3 nerve root, resulting in radicular pain when removal was attempted.[29] It is best to avoid this complication altogether by limiting the length of catheter introduced into the epidural space to 4 cm.

Breakage of needles was more common in the past when the manufacturing process resulted in structural weakness at the junction of the needle hub and shaft. Modern needles are more resistant to breakage. However, recommendations concerning surgical exploration and removal in the event of a broken needle remain valid because of the propensity for needle points to migrate and cause potentially serious tissue damage.

A discussion of technical problems would not be complete without reference to the problem of the "failed" or "patchy" block. This outcome is often blamed on abnormalities of the patient's anatomy or ineffective drug batches, but is primarily due to the block technique used or the inexperience of the practitioner performing the block. When faced with an inadequate block, the clinician has several options, including repeating the block, manipulating the catheter in continuous techniques, supplementing with local anesthetic injection, deepening the level of sedation, and general anesthesia.

Pharmacologic Complications

The injection of local anesthetics intravascularly and the risks of oversedation have been addressed above. Rapid, early intervention and aggressive resuscitation are critical to a good outcome in these cases.

Inappropriate Choice of Anesthetic Drug Other pharmacologic-related problems involve clinical judgment concerning the choice of agent and additives. Inappropriate choice of a short-acting agent may result in an inadequate duration of blockade for a given procedure or surgeon. On the other hand, a prolonged peripheral nerve block in an outpatient may be equally undesirable because of the risk of nerve injury in the blocked but unprotected limb. The anesthesia care provider must have a working knowledge of the pharmacokinetic and pharmacodynamic features of local anesthetics. There must be familiarity with the usual duration of surgical procedures, and experience with the actual range of surgical time for individual surgeons is also valuable. A solid foundation in the pharmacology of local anesthetics will facilitate early diagnosis and treatment of problems related specifically to these agents. For example, knowledge of the as-

sociation of methemoglobinemia with prilocaine aids in recognition of this problem should it occur. Inappropriately large volumes of local anesthetics, particularly if highly concentrated, may cause toxicity due to high blood levels as well as increasing the risk of peripheral neurotoxicity. Knowledge of common additives to local anesthetics is also important. For example, addition of epinephrine is not recommended in anatomic areas such as the digits and penis, where vasoconstriction of terminal arteries may cause local tissue ischemia.

Allergic Reactions to Local Anesthetics
Allergic reactions to local anesthetics are exceedingly rare and are almost exclusively associated with the ester-type agents. However, methylparaben, a preservative commonly added to multiple-use vials of amide anesthetics, can cause a reaction in patients who are allergic to ester-type agents. The mechanics of this appear to be a common metabolic breakdown product with cross-reactivity. A common problem with which the anesthesia care provider is faced is managing the patient who is "allergic to novocaine." In most cases the "allergic" episode occurred in a dental office; a careful history will usually indicate that the likely pharmacologic culprit was epinephrine. Most dentists routinely use medium-duration amide local anesthetics (lidocaine, mepivacaine, prilocaine) with relatively high concentrations of epinephrine (1:60,000). While patients and medical practitioners alike use the term "novocaine" generically to indicate all local anesthetics, it is most unlikely that this agent was the cause of the reaction. A history of transient palpitations, dizziness, and anxiety in the absence of true signs of allergy such as angioedema, wheal and flare skin lesions, or bronchospasm will usually confirm the etiology of the reaction. Skin patch testing has

not been useful in determining allergic responses to local anesthetics. Some authors suggest intradermal injection of a dilute concentration (1:1,000) of a local anesthetic followed by progressively more concentrated solutions.[30] If this method is employed it is important to remember that sensitized patients may react to very small doses of allergen, so the practitioner should be prepared to treat anaphylaxis if it occurs. Multidose vials may contain preservatives other than methylparaben such as bisulfite, which can also cause allergic reactions in susceptible individuals. For this reason, solutions containing no preservative are recommended for any patient with an atopic history.

Accidental Injection of Nonanesthetic Agents Finally, the accidental injection of pharmacologic agents other than local anesthetics must be scrupulously avoided. Descriptions of mistakenly injected solutions, including potassium chloride,[31] and thiopentone,[32] among others, reinforce the importance of vigilance on the part of the practitioner.

Patient Management Factors
In spite of careful preoperative selection, a patient may emotionally decompensate when faced with surgery while awake under regional anesthesia. This anxiety reaction can take almost any form, including vasovagal syncope, hyperventilation, incoherent agitation, and frank hostility. The vital signs may remain stable in the face of apparent loss of consciousness, or may reflect a highly agitated or vagal state. Loss of control can occur at any time in the procedure, but is usually associated with the first sight of any needle, often the intravenous catheter. Most patients respond to calm reassurance and appropriate sedation such as intravenous midazolam and fentanyl. In rare cases, substitution of general anes-

thesia may be necessary. As previously mentioned, preoperative preparation is invaluable in forming a trusting relationship between the patient and the physician and is the best method to prevent this problem.

Postoperative Complications

Complications of regional anesthesia, such as nerve damage, frequently present in the postoperative period after the effects of the local anesthetic have worn off. In addition, in cases in which a continuous infusion of local anesthetic and/or narcotic is continued into the postoperative period, problems may be related to the infusion technique. Such problems can occur in the immediate recovery period or several hours to days after surgery. Careful follow-up and early intervention are critical components of risk management and good outcome (Table 14-4).

Complications in the Immediate Postoperative Period
The patient who has undergone regional anesthesia requires special care and monitoring in the immediate postoperative period. The residual effects of sedative and general anesthetic agents can be significant, and may result in respiratory and cardiovascular depression. Persisting sensory blockade renders affected anatomic sites vulnerable to inadvertent injury. The anesthetized limb requires careful positioning and padding, particularly if the local anesthetic is long-acting. A block of the somatic nerves interferes with the patient's ability to feel painful responses to surgically induced problems such as ischemia or compression of tissues (due to a tight cast, compartment syndrome, surgical dressing, etc.).

Following central neuraxial blockade,

Table 14-4. Postoperative Complications

Immediate (Recovery Room/Outpatient)	Delayed (12 Hours → Permanent)

Pharmacologic
    Sedation → respiratory depression
	Pharmacologic (continuous local anesthetic/
	    narcotic infusions)
	        Toxicity/respiratory depression
	        Catheter migration
	        Intravascular/intrathecal injection

Neurologic
    Delayed recovery
    Nerve ischemia
    Cast/dressing
    Positioning
	Neurologic
	    Minor
	        Postspinal headache
	        Persistent paresthesia (days–weeks)

Cardiovascular
    Sympathectomy → orthostatism
	Major
	        Permanent peripheral nerve injury
	        Anterior spinal artery syndrome
	        Intracranial hematoma
	        Epidural abscess/hematoma
	        Meningitis (septic vs. aseptic)
	        Chronic adhesive arachnoiditis

Respiratory
    Pneumothorax (early)
	Respiratory
	    Pneumothorax (late)

such as spinal or epidural anesthesia, variable degrees of sympathetic block also affect the postoperative management. Appropriate nursing care requires a complete understanding of these physiologic effects in order to avoid iatrogenic problems related to orthostatic changes following alterations in patient position. Management of hypotension in the recovery room requires a careful assessment of the patient's circulating blood volume status as well as the residual effects of the block. Careful evaluation of the patient's blood pressure responses with gradual sitting and standing is essential.

Neurologic complications of central neuraxial blockade are rare but devastating, and may be detected early in the postoperative period. Persistent motor blockade in the presence of recovery from sensory anesthesia may indicate anterior spinal artery occlusion or spasm. While lack of recovery from spinal or epidural blockade in the expected time interval has been reported as a side effect of the long-acting local anesthetic bupivacaine,[33,34] it can also be an early sign of epidural or subarachnoid hematoma. Since early intervention is the key to success in managing these potentially devastating complications, prompt neurologic evaluation may include magnetic resonance imaging, computed tomography, or myelography. It is essential to diagnose the etiology because early surgical intervention is indicated if a compressive lesion is present.

Most problems encountered in the recovery room period are residual effects of the local anesthetic, sedatives, or neural blockade associated with the regional anesthetic. An appropriately timed postoperative visit within 24 hours of the administration of a regional anesthetic is important in identifying complications that will appear when the effects of the local anesthetic and sedatives are completely worn off. A neurologic examination will reveal any major neurologic deficit, and the patient should be asked about somatic symptoms, such as persistent paresthesias. Appropriate notes should be made in the medical record of both the presence and absence of symptoms and signs.

Outpatient Management

The use of regional anesthesia in the outpatient population is associated with several theoretical benefits for the patient. Studies have demonstrated decreased nausea and vomiting, less drowsiness, improved pain control, and shorter stays in the outpatient unit. However, management of the outpatient regional anesthetic presents a number of unique problems as well. In many cases, residual blockade at the time of discharge is not desirable. This is particularly true when central neuraxial blockade is employed. In such cases, a local anesthetic should be chosen to provide a short duration of blockade, and the patient should be fully recovered by the time of discharge. *Full recovery* implies return of all motor and sensory function along with evidence that the sympathetic blockade has also dissipated. This can best be evaluated by performing orthostatic blood pressure checks, as well as assessing the patient's ability to stand upright and ambulate without assistance. It is also prudent to require that the patient be able to urinate prior to discharge to prevent overdistention of the bladder, and to demonstrate return of autonomic and somatic nerve function.

Return of full neurologic function may be less important immediately following peripheral nerve blocks. Persisting neural blockade provides excellent pain relief and increased blood flow to the surgical site, both of which may be desirable side effects. However, the risk of accidental nerve trauma in a blocked extremity is theoretically higher outside of the hospital environment. The patient should be informed of the risks and instructed in appropriate care of the extremity. Patients who are unable or unwilling to comply with recommended medical care may not be good candidates for regional anesthesia techniques, and should be fully recovered prior to discharge.

In all cases, a follow-up telephone call on the first postoperative day should include questions concerning residual areas of neural blockade or altered neural function such as paresthesias. Any patient concerns regarding the anesthetic or surgery should also be discussed. In the case of outpatient spinal anesthesia or accidental dural puncture during epidural anesthesia, the patient should be informed of the risk of postspinal headache and given a contact person in the anesthesia department to call if problems arise. Post-dural puncture headache should be managed conservatively for 24 to 72 hours with bed rest and rehydration. If it persists, epidural blood patch may be considered.

Complications Involving Pain Control in the Postoperative Period

An excellent method of postoperative pain control involves the use of continuous infusions of dilute local anesthetics and/or narcotics via catheters placed centrally (epidural or spinal) or peripherally. Such methods are often employed on the postsurgical wards and carry special risks that should be anticipated by nursing services and the pain management team.

Catheter migration is of particular concern when the epidural route of drug administration is used. An epidural catheter may migrate intrathecally, intravascularly, subdurally,[35] or, most commonly, subcutaneously. Intrathecal migration can result in a high spinal block with attendant cardiovascular instability, and respiratory depression due to intrathecal narcotic administration. Intravenous migration can result in local anesthetic toxicity and ineffective analgesia. Subcutaneous migration will result in poor pain control. This may require either replacement of the catheter or pain management by other methods. Catheters placed in more peripheral sites, such as the brachial plexus, may also migrate intravascularly or subcutaneously, with loss of analgesic effect, and potential for toxic reactions if the infusion rate is increased or the catheter is bolused in an attempt to obtain adequate analgesia.

Rarely, more serious neurologic problems have been reported with continuous epidural techniques. These include fistula formation,[36] epidural abscess,[37] lumbar root compression secondary to epidural air,[38] transient unilateral anterior spinal cord syndrome secondary to catheter irritation and spasm,[39] and masking of a compartment syndrome following free fibular transfer.[40]

These continuous analgesic techniques provide potentially superb benefits to the patient, but require a vigilant and efficient pain service for safe management. Any evidence of neurologic deficit requires a prompt evaluation. In some cases, removal or replacement of the catheter may resolve the problem. Radiographic procedures are often helpful in making the diagnosis of migration or mass effect, and choosing an appropriate intervention. Informed nursing care will help in early identification of problems associated with catheter infusions as well as those postsurgical problems, such as compartment syndrome, which may be masked by this form of analgesia.

Delayed Neurologic Complications

Neurologic complications of regional anesthetics are usually discovered after the patient has left the recovery room. They can be classified as "minor," such as postspinal headache or mild persistent paresthesias, or "major," often devastating, problems, as in the case of intraspinal hematoma, epidural abscess, or anterior

spinal artery syndromes, all of which can lead to paraplegia.

Diagnosis is often difficult, and outcome is frequently determined by the time between diagnosis and intervention. The most severe of these complications have attached a notoriety to complications of regional anesthesia that exceeds the lay response to death due to general anesthesia. Fortunately, several large series point to the rarity of significant neurologic problems after regional anesthesia[41] (Table 14-5).

"Minor" Neurologic Complications

Post-dural Puncture Headache   Post-dural puncture headache (PDPH) is a minor but relatively common complication of subarachnoid puncture. Reports of methods to prevent this problem at the time of recognized dural puncture include the injection of blood prophylactically within the epidural space (epidural blood patch)[42] or the institution of epidural saline infusions.[43,44] However, prophylaxis has not been consistently successful. The most reliable preventive factors are the use of small pencil-point needles (Table 14-6) and selection of older patients for this technique. Interestingly, intrathecal catheters placed through large-gauge epidural needles (18 gauge) do not have the anticipated high incidence of headache associated with this size needle.[45] The reasons for this discrepancy are not known, although a theoretical mechanism involving a fibroblastic reaction at the catheter site has been suggested. Early detection and aggressive management of PDPII is recommended, particularly in the outpatient. Conservative treatment with hydration and bed rest can be attempted. If this is unsuccessful, it should be followed by early epidural autologous blood patch after 1 to 3 days if the headache does not resolve. Treatment should not be delayed inordinately; case reports of intracerebral hematoma,[46] subdural

Table 14-5. Survey Reports of Neurologic Sequelae Following Central Neuraxial Blockade

Reference	No. of Patients	Anesthetics	Procedures	Neurologic Sequelae
Epidural/caudal				
Bleyaert et al[57]	3,000	Bupivacaine 0.125%, 1:800,000 epinephrine	Obstetric	None
Moore et al[58]	11,080	Bupivacaine 0.25%, 0.5%, or 0.75% with or without epinephrine	Surgical, obstetric, diagnostic	None
Holdcroft & Morgan[59]	1,000	Bupivacaine 0.5% or lidocaine 1.5% (32 pts)	Obstetric	1 foot drop; 1 paresthesia of thigh
Moore et al[60]	7,286	Lidocaine + tetracaine with epinephrine in 6,270 patients, various agents in remaining cases	Surgical, obstetric	1 bilateral paralysis of quadriceps muscles
Lund[3]	10,000	Lidocaine 2% (8,000 pts), chloroprocaine 3% (700 pts), hexylcaine 2% (200 pts)	Surgical, obstetric, diagnostic	1 paresis of 1 leg (subarachnoid hexylcaine); 4 paresthesias of thigh; 1 persistent numbness; 3 bladder or rectal incontinence
Eisen et al[61]	9,532	Lidocaine	Obstetric	16 paresthesias; 9 numbness of thigh; 1 paraplegia (1 of 5,091 surgical cases)
Bonica et al[62]	3,885	Various, mostly lidocaine	Surgical, obstetric, diagnostic	1 hypalgesia of trunk, weakness of leg (subarachnoid lidocaine); 1 paresthesia, numbness weakness of leg
Dawkins[4]	32,718	Unspecified	Obstetric, surgical	Epidural: 0.1% transient, 0.02% permament Caudal: 0.2% transient, 0.05% permament
Usubiaga[5]	780,000	Unspecified	Various	1:1100
Spinal Anesthesia				
Kortum et al[63]	2,592	Bupivacaine 0.5%	Surgical	1 lumbar plexus injury
Bergman[64]	10,000	Lidocaine, mepivacaine, bupivacaine	Various	None
Phillips et al[7]	10,440	Lidocaine	Obstetric, surgical	8 persistent peripheral neuropathy
Moore[65]	11,574	Tetracaine, dibucaine; with epinephrine or phenylephrine in 8,852	Surgical, obstetric	1 persistent muscular weakness of legs, impotence
Sadov et al[66]	20,000	Tetracaine, procaine, dibucaine	Various	1 paraplegia due to spinal tumor; 3 meningitis
Dripps[67] & Vandam[68-70]	10,098	Tetracaine, procaine, dibucaine; with epinephrine in 2,000		No major neurologic sequelae; 2 foot drop; 1 leg weakness (trauma); 12 exacerbation of previous neurologic disease
Brown[71]	600	Tetracaine	Surgical	2 peroneal paresis, unilateral
Noble & Murray[6]	78,746			3 transient

(Modified from Kane,[41] with permission.)

Table 14-6. Relationship of Gauge of Needle Used for Lumbar Puncture to Incidence of Spinal Headache

Needle Gauge	No. of Spinal Anesthetics	No. of Spinal Headaches	%
16	839	151	18
19	154	16	10
20	2,698	377	14
22	4,954	430	9
24	634	337	6

(From Vandam & Dripps,[99] with permission.)

hematoma,[47–50] and cranial nerve palsy[51] after PDPH suggest that significant loss of cerebrospinal fluid (CSF) may result in major morbidity in rare cases.

The use of caffeine in both oral and intravenous forms has also been recommended for treatment of PDPH.[52,53] While the initial positive therapeutic benefit is reportedly high for both methods, the rate of recurrence of symptoms exceeds 50 percent. While this therapeutic regimen has minimal side effects, it may delay the definitive epidural blood patch therapy. More recently, the use of theophylline has also been suggested. However, long-term benefits are likely to be similar to caffeine therapy.

Transient Persisting Paresthesias Transient persisting paresthesias following peripheral nerve blocks can result in symptoms varying from mild dysesthesias

Table 14-7. Causes of Neurologic Sequelae Unrelated to Anesthesia

Patient positioning
Surgical retractors
Surgical trauma
Tourniquet pressure
Cast or dressing application
Undiagnosed neurologic disease

lasting a few days to severe aching pain and permanent paresis. The mechanism is presumably direct nerve trauma from needle insertion or intraneural injection of local anesthetic. Selander et al[20] have shown axonal degeneration and damage to the blood–nerve barrier with intrafascicular injections of local anesthetic and saline solutions. In the same study, conventional sharp-beveled needles also appear to be associated with increased nerve damage when compared to blunt-beveled needles. However, the recommendation that paresthesia techniques should be avoided in all patients (because of this low risk of nerve injury[9]) may not be justified. There is a reported low incidence of postblock neuropathy following brachial plexus block in several large studies[54–56] in which no attempts were made to avoid paresthesias.

Measures that can be taken to help prevent peripheral nerve injury include (1) gentle needle techniques when paresthesias are being sought; (2) avoidance of intraneural injection by repositioning the needle if the patient experiences any pain or paresthesia with initial injection of 0.5 ml or less; and (3) appropriate choice of needle, local anesthetic agent, and patient. Persistent paresthesias often do not become evident until the second or third postoperative day. Other etiologies, such as improper positioning, ischemia due to prolonged tourniquet inflation or a tight cast or dressing, and surgical trauma, as well as underlying coincident medical problems such as undiagnosed peripheral neuropathies should be considered (Table 14-7). Fortunately, the outcome of this type of lesion is usually good, with full recovery within a few days to weeks being the norm.

"Major" Neurologic Complications
The most common postoperative complications of subarachnoid and epidural blocks are relatively minor and include

PDPH, backache, and urinary retention. Failure to recover from a central neuraxial blockade, or apparent return of blockade following recovery, may indicate a more serious problem such as compression of the spinal cord due to epidural or subdural abscess or hematoma or anterior spinal artery ischemia. However, large surveys specifically addressing neurologic complications attributed to central neuraxial blockade indicate that these devastating problems are exceedingly rare (Table 14-5). Other uncommon complications of blocks of the central neuraxis include meningitis, abscess, arachnoiditis, intracranial hemorrhage or thrombosis, and nerve root trauma. Peripheral nerve blocks are rarely associated with permanent nerve injury or other major neurologic complications.

Infectious Complications   Bacterial infection in the vicinity of the spinal cord can present as meningitis or cord compression secondary to abscess formation. The source can be exogenous (contaminated equipment or drugs) or endogenous (a bacterial source present in the patient with direct or hematogenous seeding to the site of needle or catheter placement). Indwelling catheters may also be contaminated from a superficial bacterial site in the skin or subcutaneous tissues, or from a nosocomial source in the hospitalized patient. Continuous catheters can serve as wicks for the spread of infection from the surface of the skin to the epidural space, particularly in patients who are immunocompromised.

Aseptic meningitis will present a similar course to infectious or septic meningitis. Analysis of CSF will determine the presence or absence of a bacterial organism. The most common organisms in bacterial meningitis are *Staphylococcus aureus*, coliforms, and *Pseudomonas*. Partial treatment with antibiotics prior to CSF examination may confuse the diagnosis by reducing the number of bacteria present. Aseptic meningitis is usually due to nonbacterial contamination of the CSF with an exogenous irritant (e.g., contamination of block equipment with detergent[72,73] or accidental injection of a chemical irritant such as phenol). However, a variety of apparently innocuous substances, such as starch powder from surgical gloves, have also been shown to induce an irritative response when introduced into the CSF. Analysis of the CSF in aseptic meningitis reveals mononuclear cells, normal protein and glucose levels, and absence of organisms.[73,74] Both bacterial and aseptic meningitis may present 24 to 48 hours after needle placement with fever, stiff neck, and signs of meningeal irritability. Analysis of CSF should be performed early so that appropriate antibiotic treatment can be instituted if bacteria are present.

Abscess formation following epidural or spinal anesthesia can be superficial, requiring limited surgical drainage and intravenous antibiotics. However, it can also occur deep in the epidural space with associated cord compression. The latter is fortunately a rare complication, but it requires aggressive, early surgical management (laminectomy and drainage) in order to achieve a satisfactory outcome. Superficial infections present with local tissue swelling, erythema, and drainage of purulent fluid, often associated with fever. They rarely cause neurologic problems unless left untreated with spread to neural structures. Epidural abscess formation usually presents several days after neural blockade with clinical signs of severe back pain, local tenderness, and fever associated with leukocytosis and white blood cells and bacteria in the CSF. Radiologic evidence of an epidural mass in the presence of variable neurologic deficit are diagnostic. Surgical intervention within 12 hours is associated with the best chance of neurologic recovery. Injection of epidural steroids may cause local immunosuppression, theoretically increasing the risk of epidural infection.[75,76] Patients who have underlying disease processes associated with immunocompromise may also be assumed to be at increased risk and should be observed carefully for signs of infection when a continuous epidural catheter is left in place for prolonged periods. Injection of local anesthetic or insertion of a catheter in an area at high risk for bacterial contamination, such as the sacral hiatus, may also increase the risk for abscess formation,[77] emphasizing the importance of meticulous aseptic technique.

Chronic adhesive arachnoiditis resulting in the devastating complication of cauda equina syndrome can be caused by a variety of factors, including bacteria, direct spinal cord trauma, ischemia of the cord, contaminants in injected fluids, direct local anesthetic toxicity, additives to local anesthetics such as bisulfite, accidental injection of nerve irritants such as distilled water, or blood. Clinical signs include bowel and bladder dysfunction, sensory loss in the perineum, and variable lower extremity paresis with constant pain. These symptoms can present slowly over days to weeks. The variable nature of the complaints and onset can result in a delay in diagnosis. Laboratory examination of the CSF and radiographic studies may not be helpful in determining the etiology or presence of this problem, but should be performed to rule out reversible anatomic or infectious causes. A cystometrogram will often show increased bladder volume and reduced sensation of urgency (neurogenic bladder). Electromyography may also be helpful in determining the extent of involvement and confirming the clinical findings. A recent report of four cases of postoperative cauda equina syndrome linked this rare complication with the use of spinal microcatheters.[78] The authors noted that

greater than normal doses of local anesthetic were administered through the catheter because of initial inadequate blockade. They concluded that although the etiology was unclear, the neural damage might have been caused by a combination of maldistribution of relatively high doses of local anesthetic to the sacral nerve roots.

Repeated applications of local anesthetics via an indwelling intrathecal catheter or by multiple single-shot spinal injections to improve on a patchy or failed block may be a potentially unsafe practice. In such cases, the pain usually caused by needle trauma or intraneural injection may not be elicited, and nerve damage may result. Precautions that may decrease the risk include (1) always confirming that CSF is obtained before injecting local anesthetic into the subarachnoid space; (2) evaluating the extent of blockade in the sacral dermatomes to determine whether the local anesthetic action might be preferentially distributed to that site; (3) limiting the local anesthetic dosage to a maximum precalculated "safe" dosage; (4) if an injection is repeated, modifying the technique to avoid reinforcement of the same drug distribution (change patient position, drug baricity, etc.); and (5) if CSF cannot be aspirated after injection, not repeating a "full' dose unless no sign of neural blockade (including the sacral area) is present on physical examination.[79] Because of the rarity of this complication, these recommendations are based on principles of prudent practice, rather than prospective epidemiologic studies.

Intraspinal Hemorrhage and Thrombosis
Epidural and subarachnoid hematomas may also present as neurologic deficits in the postoperative period if the hematoma itself causes cord compression. Epidural needles and catheters frequently (2.8 to 11.5 percent) cause vascular trauma as-

sociated with minimal bleeding that usually resolves without sequelae.[80,81] Patients with abnormal clotting abilities are theoretically at increased risk for development of epidural hematomas following even minor trauma. Reports of spontaneous epidural hematoma formation in anticoagulated as well as in normal patients illustrate the risk of coincidental hematoma development as well.[82] The safety of inserting epidural catheters prior to heparinization in patients undergoing major vascular surgery has been reported.[83,84] Allowing the local anesthetic epidural blockade to wear off prior to instituting continuous postoperative infusions, and consideration of the use of narcotic infusions when appropriate, permit ongoing evaluation of the patient's neurologic status during the postoperative period. Patient complaints of back pain or an increase in intensity of motor or sensory blockade, particularly the development of new paresis, require immediate and aggressive evaluation to rule out epidural hematoma formation.

Anterior spinal artery thrombosis or spasm causes a syndrome consisting primarily of lower extremity paresis with a variable sensory deficit. This is usually diagnosed in the immediate postoperative period as the neural blockade resolves. The etiology of this problem is uncertain, although direct trauma to the anterior artery and ischemia secondary to hypotension or vasoconstrictor agents may be causative factors. The clinical presentation can be difficult to differentiate from other hemorrhagic or infectious causes of cord compression (Table 14-8). Patient factors such as advanced age and a history of peripheral vascular disease may also be important etiologic factors. While the addition of vasoconstrictors to intrathecal local anesthetics has been implicated as a theoretical cause, it is unlikely to be the primary mechanism of this problem. Spinal cord perfusion studies do not show any deleterious effect of epinephrine.[85]

Nerve Root Trauma   Direct needle trauma to the spinal cord can be avoided by performing the dural puncture below L2 in adults and L4 in children. If the spinal cord or nerve root is traumatized during the course of a spinal or epidural needle or catheter placement, an awake patient will complain of severe lancinating pain in the dermatomes at or below the insertion site. Should this occur, the anesthesia care provider should abandon the nerve block and observe the patient closely for evidence of damage to neurologic structures. If signs develop, neurologic imaging is indicated.

Needle entry lateral to midline may result in paresthesias due to stimulation of the spinal nerve root in the dural cuff region. Complaints of unilateral paresthesias during needle or catheter placement should be treated by withdrawing the needle and repositioning it. If trauma to the nerve has occurred, the paresthesia may persist into the postoperative period. The patient should be followed carefully for evidence of neurologic damage. Usually these are transient problems, but appropriate documentation of the lesion and its progression are necessary components of risk management. Concerned follow-up will also help maintain a positive relationship with the patient.

Summary

Major complications of regional anesthesia are rare, but can be devastating to the patient and anesthesia care provider. Prevention and management begin in the preoperative period with a careful evaluation of the patient's medical history and appropriate preoperative patient education. This must include a frank discussion of risks, advantages, and disadvantages of

Table 14-8.   Differential Diagnosis of Epidural Abscess, Epidural Hemorrhage, and Anterior Spinal Artery Syndrome

	Epidural Abscess	*Epidural Hemorrhage*	*Anterior Spinal Artery Syndrome*
Age of patient	Any age	50% over 50 years	Any age
Previous history	Infection[a]	Efforts, anticoagulants	Arteriosclerosis
Onset	1–3 days	Sudden	Sudden
Generalized symptoms		None during epidural block; sharp, transient pain otherwise	None
Sensory involvement	None or paresthesias		
Motor involvement	Flaccid paralysis, later spastic	Flaccid paralysis	Flaccid paralysis
Segmental reflexes	Exacerbated[a]: later obtunded	Abolished	Abolished
Queckenstedt's sign and myelogram	Signs of extradural compression	Signs of extradural compression	Normal
Cerebrospinal fluid	Increased cell count	Normal	Normal
Blood data	Rise in red blood cell sedimentation rate	Prolonged coagulation time[a]	Normal

[a] Infrequent findings.
(From Usubiaga,[100] with permission.)

available anesthetic techniques. Preparation for the intraoperative period requires appropriate monitoring and resuscitation equipment as well as careful management of the technical and pharmacologic aspects of the nerve block.

Complications of neural blockade can occur hours to days after the completion of the surgical procedure. Anticipation of these problems when the risk is increased and timely postoperative evaluations are critical to early diagnosis and management. Most major neurologic complaints benefit from a multispeciality approach involving neurology, radiology, internal medicine, and surgery to assist in appropriate and timely evaluation and treatment.

COMPLICATIONS RELATED TO ORTHOPEDIC SURGERY

Embolic Phenomena

Orthopedic surgical procedures are associated with a variety of complications due to embolic phenomena. Reported emboli occurring intra- and postoperatively include fat, cement, air, and thrombus. These may be caused by multiple factors such as positioning, fracture of long bones, injection of cement under pressure, and predisposing medical conditions. Venous air embolus is a potentially life-threatening condition caused by entrainment of air into the venous system when the surgical site is elevated above the level of the right atrium. This complication can occur in orthopedic surgical patients undergoing spine surgery in the prone position and shoulder surgery in the sitting position. Serious morbidity and mortality may occur if the amount of entrained air is large, thus blocking the right ventricular outflow tract, or the patient has a patent foramen ovale, permitting air to cross over to the left side of the heart and enter the systemic arterial circulation. This complication is extensively reviewed in Chapter 8, which discusses management of orthopedic spinal surgery.

Pulmonary Thromboembolus

Pulmonary thromboembolus (PTE) resulting from deep venous thrombosis (DVT) is a serious complication associated with orthopedic surgery involving the lower extremities. The risk of DVT associated with total hip arthroplasty (THA) has been reported to range from 20 to 80 percent.[86-89] There is an estimated risk of 50 percent associated with total knee replacement.[90] The cited risk of fatal PTE associated with hip fracture is estimated at 4 to 7 percent, and with THA at 0.3 to 2.4 percent.[91] Autopsy studies indicate that PTE is the major cause of death in patients undergoing THA, and major thrombi in the thigh and iliofemoral region are considered the most important cause of PTE. Recommended prophylactic measures such as oral anticoagulants, intravenous dextran, external pneumatic compression devices, and adjusted-dose heparin have decreased but not abolished this life-threatening complication. Medical conditions that significantly increase the risk for DVT include advanced age, obesity, presence of malignancy, congestive heart failure, acute myocardial infarction, a history of prior DVT or PTE, estrogen therapy, presence of varicose veins, and immobilization.

Operative factors such as blood and fluid replacement, intraoperative positioning of the patient, and surgical technique may also play a role.

Several studies show a decrease in the incidence of both DVT and PTE in patients undergoing hip surgery under epidural[2,86] and spinal[87-89] anesthesia. Similar findings have been reported for knee surgery performed under epidural anesthesia.[90,92] Proposed mechanisms for this effect include (1) rheologic changes resulting in hyperkinetic lower extremity blood flow, reducing venous stasis and preventing thrombus formation; (2) beneficial circulatory effects from epinephrine added to the local anesthetic solutions; (3) altered coagulation and fibrinolytic responses to surgery under central neuraxial blockade, resulting in a decreased tendency for blood to clot and better fibrinolytic function[93]; (4) the absence of positive pressure ventilation and its concomitant effects on circulation; and (5) direct local anesthetic effects such as decreased platelet aggregation. While the improved lower extremity rheology associated with spinal and epidural anesthesia seems self-evident, other cited mechanisms are difficult to prove. Interpretation of studies that examine these factors must take into consideration variations in surgical techniques, fluid management, patient positioning, and other parameters. For example, the reported enhancement of fibrinolysis with epidural anesthesia[93] has not been consistently observed in all studies involving orthopedic surgical patients. Coagulation changes may be subtle, possibly involving single variables such as the more rapid postoperative return to normal of antithrombin III demonstrated in another study of similar patients.[88] Finally, most of the studies examining the value of epidural and spinal anesthesia in preventing DVT and PTE involved patients who were not receiving presently recommended pharmacologic prophylaxis. The role of regional anesthesia needs to be re-evaluated in this population to determine the extent of protection as well as the risk of performing neural blockade in partially anticoagulated patients so that a reasonable risk/benefit ratio can be determined.

Fat Embolism

Fat embolism syndrome (FES) is associated with multiple traumatic injuries and surgery involving long-bone fractures.[94] Risk factors include gender and age (males, age 20 to 30), hypovolemic shock, intramedullary instrumentation, rheumatoid arthritis,[95] THA utilizing the technique of cementing femoral stems designed for press-fit application,[96] and bilateral total knee surgery.[97] The incidence of FES in isolated long bone fractures is 3 to 4 percent, and mortality associated with this condition is significant, ranging from 10 to 20 percent.

Clinical and laboratory signs of FES have been classified by Gurd[98] as major or minor (Table 14-9), with a diagnosis requiring at least one major and four minor criteria as well as the exclusion of other post-traumatic causes of hypoxemia. Major signs of the syndrome include the presence of axillary or subconjunctival petechiae, significant hypoxemia, central nervous system depression in excess of that expected because of the level of hypoxemia, and pulmonary edema. Classified as minor signs are tachycardia, hyperthermia, retinal fat emboli on fundoscopic examination, urinary fat globules, an unexplained decrease in hematocrit or platelets, an increased erythrocyte sedimentation rate, and fat globules in the sputum. Symptoms usually occur 12 to 40 hours after the injury and can range from mild dyspnea to frank coma. Decreased arterial oxygen tension is the most consistent abnormal laboratory value.[94] Fulminant episodes can occur within hours of the traumatic

Table 14-9. Criteria for Diagnosis of Fat Emboli Syndrome[a]

Major
 Axillary/subconjunctival petechiae
 Hypoxemia ($PaO_2 < 60$ mmHg;
  $FiO_2 < 0.4$)
 Central nervous system depression (disproportionate to hypoxemia)
 Pulmonary edema
Minor
 Tachycardia (>110 beats/min)
 Hyperthermia
 Retinal fat emboli
 Urinary fat globules
 Decreased platelets/hematocrit (unexplained)
 Increased erythrocyte sedimentation rate
 Fat globules in sputum

[a] Criteria for diagnosis of FES requires at least one sign from the major and four signs from the minor criteria categories.
(From Gurd,[98] with permission.)

injury, causing severe hypoxemia, respiratory failure and severe neurologic impairment. Disseminated intravascular coagulation can also occur in conjunction with FES. Not all trauma patients who have demonstrated evidence of fat emboli fit the criteria for diagnosis of FES. Two theories are hypothesized to explain the mechanism of this syndrome: (1) The mechanical theory proposes that long-bone trauma results in release of fat droplets, which enter the vascular system through torn veins. These droplets are transported to the pulmonary vascular bed, where they act as microemboli. (2) The biochemical theory can be divided into two mechanisms, toxic and obstructive. The toxic proposal claims that free fatty acids released at the time of trauma directly affect pneumocytes in the lung and cause adult respiratory distress syndrome. This effect would be enhanced by the trauma-induced release of catecholamines, which would result in further mobilization of free fatty acids. The obstructive theory hypothesizes that an unspecified chemical event at the site of the fracture releases mediators that affect lipid solubility, resulting in coalescence of lipids and consequent embolization. Some or all of these theories may play a role in development of FES. Other predisposing or aggravating factors such as shock, hypovolemia, sepsis, or disseminated intravascular coagulation may be required to trigger the conversion of fat emboli to FES.

Appropriate treatment of FES requires early recognition of the syndrome, reversal of possible aggravating factors such as hypovolemia, early surgical stabilization of fracture sites, and aggressive respiratory support. Corticosteroid therapy is controversial, but may be beneficial. Other pharmacologic interventions, including heparin and dextran, have not been shown to be effective in treating FES.

Summary

Embolic phenomena are a significant cause of morbidity and mortality in the orthopedic surgical patient. Early recognition of these complications and aggressive therapy are critical in ensuring an optimal outcome. The anesthesia care provider can provide invaluable assistance to the orthopedic surgeon in the diagnosis and treatment of these problems.

REFERENCES

1. Modig J: Regional anaesthesia and blood loss. Acta Anaesthesiol Scand 32(98):44, 1988
2. Modig J, Borg T, Karlström G et al: Thromboembolism after total hip replacement: role of epidural and general anesthesia. Anesth Analg 62:174, 1983
3. Lund PC: Peridural anesthesia. A review of 10,000 administrations. Acta Anaesthesiol Scand 6:143, 1962
4. Dawkins CJM: An analysis of the complications of extradural and caudal block. Anaesthesia 24:554, 1969
5. Usubiaga JE: Neurological complications following epidural anesthesia. Int Anesthesiol Clin 13:1, 1975
6. Noble AB, Murray JG: A review of the complications of spinal anaesthesia with experiences in Canadian teaching hospitals from 1959 to 1969. Can Anaesth Soc J 18:5, 1971
7. Phillips OC, Ebner H, Nelson AT: Neurologic complications following spinal anesthesia with lidocaine: a prospective review of 10,440 cases. Anesthesiology 30:284, 1969
8. Kroll DA, Caplan RA, Posner K et al: Nerve injury associated with anesthesia. Anesthesiology 73:202, 1990
9. Selander D, Adshage S, Wolff: Paresthesiae or no paresthesiae? Acta Anaesth Scand 23:27, 1979
10. O'Meara PM, Kaufman EE: Prophylaxis of venous thromboembolism in total hip arthroplasty: a review. Orthopedics 13:173, 1990
11. Horlocker TT, Wedel DJ, Offord KP: Does preoperative antiplatelet therapy increase the risk of hemorrhagic complications associated with regional anesthesia? Anesth Analg 70:631, 1990
12. Scott DL, Ghia JN, Teeple E: Aphasia and hemiparesis following stellate ganglion block. Anesth Analg 62:1038, 1983
13. Moore DC, Crawford RD, Scurlock JE: Severe hypoxia and acidosis following local anesthetic-induced convulsions. Anesthesiology 53:259, 1980
14. Albright GA: Cardiac arrest following regional anesthesia with etidocaine or bupivacaine. Anesthesiology 51:285, 1979
15. Kotelko DM, Schnider SM, Dailey PA et al: Bupivacaine-induced cardiac arrhythmias in sheep. Anesthesiology 60:10, 1984
16. Kasten GW, Martin ST: Successful cardiovascular resuscitation after massive intravenous bupivacaine overdosage in anesthetized dogs. Anesth Analg 64:491, 1985

17. Clarkson C, Hongdeghem L: Mechanism for bupivacaine depression of cardiac conduction: fast block of sodium channels during the action potential with slow recovery from block during diastole. Anesthesiology 62:396, 1985

18. Coyle DE, Sperelakis N: Bupivacaine and lidocaine blockade of calcium-mediated slow action potentials in guinea pig ventricular muscle. J Pharmacol Exp Ther 242:1001, 1978

19. Caplan RA, Ward RJ, Posner K, Cheney FW: Unexpected cardiac arrest during spinal anesthesia: a closed claims analysis of predisposing factors. Anesthesiology 68:5, 1988

20. Selander D, Dhuner KG, Lundborg G: Peripheral nerve injury due to injection needles for regional anaesthesia. An experimental study of acute effects of needle point trauma. Acta Anaesth Scand 21:182, 1977

21. Ott B, Neuberger L, Frey HP: Obliteration of the axillary artery after axillary block. Anaesthesia 44:773, 1989

22. Restelli L, Pincirolli D, Conoscente F, Cammelli F: Insufficient venous drainage following axillary approach to brachial plexus blockade. Br J Anaesth 56:1051, 1984

23. Dhuner K-G: Nerve injuries following operations: a survey of cases occurring during a six-year period. Acta Anaesthesiol Scand 11:289, 1950

24. Nicholson MJ, McAlpine FS: Neural injuries associated with surgical positions and operations. p. 193. In Martin JT (ed): Positioning in Anesthesia and Surgery. WB Saunders, Philadelphia, 1979

25. Marinacci AA: Neurological aspects of complications of spinal anesthesia: without medicolegal implications. LA Neurol Soc J 25:170, 1960

26. Moore DC: Regional Block. 4th Ed. Charles C Thomas, Springfield, IL 1981

27. Urmey WF, Talts KH, Sharrock NE: One hundred percent incidence of hemidiaphragmatic paresis associated with interscalene brachial plexus anesthesia as diagnosed by ultrasonography. Anesth Analg 72:498, 1991

28. Bashein G, Robertson HT, Kennedy WF Jr: Persistent phrenic nerve paresis following interscalene brachial plexus block. Anesthesiology 62:102, 1985

29. Sidhu MS, Asrani RV, Bassell GM: An unusual complication of extradural catheterization in obstetric anaesthesia. Br J Anaesth 55:473, 1983

30. Fischer MMcD, Graham R: Adverse responses to local anaesthetics. Anaesth Intensive Care 12:325, 1984

31. Shanker KB, Palkar NV, Nishkala R: Paraplegia following epidural potassium chloride. Anaesthesia 40:45, 1985

32. Cay DL: Accidental epidural thiopentone. Anaesth Intensive Care 12:61, 1984

33. Cuerden C, Buley R, Downing JW: Delayed recovery after epidural block in labour. Anaesthesia 32:773,1977

34. Pathy GV, Rosen M: Prolonged block with recovery after extradural analgesia for labour. Br J Anaesth 47:520, 1975

35. Abouleish E, Goldstein M: Migration of an extradural catheter into the subdural space: a case report. Br J Anaesth 58:1194, 1986

36. Wanscher M, Riishede L, Krogh B: Fistula formation following epidural catheter: a case report. Acta Anaesthesiol Scand 29:552, 1985

37. Strong WE: Epidural abscess associated with epidural catheterization: a rare event? Report of two cases with markedly delayed presentation. Anesthesiology 74:943, 1991

38. Kennedy TM, Ullman DA, Harte FA et al: Lumbar root compression secondary to epidural air. Anesth Analg 67:1184, 1988

39. Richardson J, Bedder M: Transient anterior spinal cord syndrome with continuous postoperative epidural analgesia. Anesthesiology 72(4):764, 1990

40. Strecker WB, Wood MB, Bieber EJ: Compartment syndrome masked by epidural anesthesia for postoperative pain. J Bone Joint Surg 68:1447, 1986

41. Kane RE: Neurologic deficits following epidural or spinal anesthesia. Anesth Analg 60:151, 1981

42. Palahniuk RJ, Cumming M: Prophylactic blood patch does not prevent post

lumbar puncture headache. Canad Anesth Soc J 26:132, 1979

43. Craft JB, Epstein BS, Coakley CS: Prophylaxis of dural puncture headache with epidural saline. Anesth Analg 52:228, 1973

44. Bart AJ, Wheeler AS: Comparison of epidural saline placement and epidural blood placement in the treatment of post-lumbar-puncture headache. Anesthesiology 48:221, 1978

45. Peterson DO, Borup JL, Chestnut JS: Continuous spinal anesthesia: case review and discussion. Reg Anesth 8:109, 1983

46. Wedel DJ, Mulroy MF: Hemiparesis following dural puncture. Anesthesiology 59:475, 1983

47. Rudehill A, Gordon E, Rahn T: Subdural haematoma. A rare but life-threatening complication after spinal anaesthesia. Acta Anaesthesiol Scand 27:376, 1983

48. Blake DW, Donnan G, Jensen D: Intracranial subdural haematoma after spinal anaesthesia. Anaesth Intensive Care 15:341, 1987

49. Giamundo A, Benvenuti D, Lavano A, D'Andrea F: Chronic subdural haematoma after spinal anaesthesia: a case report. J Neurosurg Sci 29:153, 1985

50. Jonsson LO, Einarsson P, Olsson GL: Subdural haematoma and spinal anaesthesia. Anaesthesia 38:144, 1983

51. King RA, Calhoun JH: Fourth cranial nerve palsy following spinal anesthesia: a case report. J Clin Neurol Ophthalmol 7:20, 1987

52. Abboud TK, Zhu J, Reyes A et al: Efficacy of intravenous caffeine for post dural puncture headache (abstract). Anesthesiology 73:A936, 1990

53. Camann WR, Murray RS, Mushlin PS et al: Effects of oral caffeine on postdural puncture headache: a double-blind, placebo-controlled trial. Anesth Analg 70:181, 1990

54. Winschell SW, Wolfe R: The incidence of neuropathy following upper extremity nerve blocks. Reg Anesth 10:12, 1985

55. De Pablo JS, Diez-Mallo J: Experience with three thousand cases of brachial plexus block; its dangers: report of a fatal case. Ann Surg 128:956, 1948

56. Thompson AM, Newman RJ, Semple JC: Brachial plexus anaesthesia for upper limb surgery: a review of eight years' experience. J Hand Surg 13B:195, 1988

57. Bleyaert A, Soestens M, Vaes L et al: Bupivacaine, 0.125 percent, in obstetric epidural anesthesia. Anesthesiology 51:435, 1979

58. Moore DC, Bridenbaugh LD, Thompson GE et al: Bupivacaine: a review of 11,080 cases. Anesth Analg 57:42, 1978

59. Holdcroft A, Morgan M: Maternal complications of obstetric epidural analgesia. Anaesth Intensive Care 4:108, 1976

60. Moore DC, Bridenbaugh LD, Bagdi PA et al: The present status of spinal (subarachnoid) and epidural (peridural) block: a comparison of two techniques. Anesth Analg 47:40, 1968

61. Eisen SM, Rosen N, Winesanker H et al: The routine use of lumbar epidural anaesthesia in obstetrics: a clinical review of 9,532 cases. Can Anaesth Soc J 7:280, 1960

62. Bonica JJ, Backup PH, Anderson CE et al: Peridural block: analysis of 3,637 cases and a review. Anesthesiology 18:723, 1957

63. Kortum K, Rossler B, Nolte H: Morbidity following spinal anaesthesia. Reg Anaesth 2:5, 1979

64. Bergman H: Spinal anesthesia. Langenbecks Arch Chir 345:515, 1977

65. Moore DC, Bridenbaugh LD. Spinal (subarachnoid) block: a review of 11,574 cases. JAMA 195:907, 1966

66. Sadov MS, Levin MJ, Rant-Sejdina I: Neurological complications of spinal anaesthesia. Can Anaesth Soc J 8:405, 1961

67. Dripps RD, Vandam LD: Long-term follow-up of patients who received 10,098 spinal anaesthetics: failure to discover major neurological sequelae. JAMA 156:1486, 1954

68. Vandam LD, Dripps RD: A long-term follow-up of 10,098 spinal anesthetics. II. Incidence and analysis of minor sensory neurological defects. Surgery 38:463, 1955

69. Vandam LD, Dripps RD: Exacerbation of pre-existing neurologic disease after spinal anesthesia. N Engl J Med 255:843, 1956

70. Vandam LD, Dripps RD: Long-term follow-up of patients who received 10,098 spinal anesthetics. III. Neurological disease incident to traumatic lumbar puncture during spinal anesthesia. JAMA 172:1483, 1960

71. Brown S: Fractional segmental spinal anesthesia in poor-risk surgical patients: report of 600 cases. Anesthesiology 13:416, 1952

72. Garfield JM, Andriole GL, Vetto JT, Richie JP: Prolonged diabetes insipidus subsequent to an episode of chemical meningitis. Anesthesiology 64:253, 1986

73. Kilpatrick ME, Girgis NJ: Meningitis—a complication of spinal anesthesia. Anesth Analg 62:513, 1983

74. Bert AA, Laasberg LH: Aseptic meningitis following spinal anesthesia—a complication of the past? Anesthesiology 62:674, 1985

75. DuPen SL, Peterson DG, Williams A, Bogosian AJ: Infection during chronic epidural catheterization: diagnosis and treatment. Anesthesiology 73:905, 1990

76. Fine PG, Hare BD, Zahniser JC: Epidural abscess following epidural catheterization in a chronic pain patient: a diagnostic dilemma. Anesthesiology 69:422, 1988

77. Rustin MHA, Flynn MD, Coomes EN: Acute sacral epidural abscess following local anaesthetic injection. Postgrad Med J 59:399, 1983

78. Rigler ML, Drasner K, Krejcie TC et al: Cauda equina syndrome after continuous spinal anesthesia. Anesth Analg 72:275, 1991

79. Drasner K, Rigler ML: Repeat injection after a "failed spinal": at times, a potentially unsafe practice. Anesthesiology 75:713, 1991

80. Beck H, Brassow F, Doehn M et al: Epidural catheters of the multi-orifice type: dangers and complications. Acta Anaesthesiol Scand 30:549, 1986

81. Verniquet AJW: Vessel puncture with epidural catheters. Experience in obstetric patients. Anaesthesia 35:660, 1980

82. Srecrama V, Ivan LP, Dennery JM, Richard MT: Neurosurgical complications of anticoagulant therapy. Can Med Assoc J 108:305, 1973

83. Baron HC, LaRaja RD, Rossi G, Atkinson D: Continuous epidural anesthesia in the heparinized vascular surgical patient: a retrospective review of 912 patients. J Vasc Surg 6:144, 1987

84. Rao TLK, El Etr AA: Anticoagulation following placement of epidural and subarachnoid catheters: an evaluation of neurologic sequelae. Anesthesiology 55:618, 1981

85. Kozody R, Palahniuk RJ, Wade JG, Cumming MO: The effect of subarachnoid epinephrine and phenylephrine on spinal cord blood flow. Can Anaesth Soc J 31:503, 1984

86. Modig J, Borg T, Bagge L, Saldeen T: Role of extradural and of general anaesthesia in fibrinolysis and coagulation after total hip replacement. Br J Anaesth 55:625, 1983

87. Thorburn J, Louden JR, Vallance R: Spinal and general anaesthesia in total hip replacement: frequency of deep vein thrombosis. Br J Anaesth 52:1117, 1980

88. Donadoni R, Baele G, Devulder J, Rolly G: Coagulation and fibrinolytic parameters in patients undergoing total hip replacement: influence of the anaesthesia technique. Acta Anaesthesiol Scand 33:588, 1989

89. Davis FM, Laurenson VG, Gillespie WJ et al: Deep vein thrombosis after total hip replacement: a comparison between spinal and general anaesthesia. J Bone Joint Surg 71(2):181, 1989

90. Sharrock NE, Haas SB, Hargett MJ et al: Effects of epidural anesthesia on the incidence of deep-vein thrombosis after total knee arthroplasty. J Bone Joint Surg 73(4):502, 1991

91. Dehring DJ, Arens JF: Pulmonary thromboembolism: disease recognition and patient management. Anesthesiology 73:146, 1990

92. Nielsen PT, Jorgensen LN, Albrecht-Beste E et al: Lower thrombosis risk with epidural blockade in knee arthroplasty. Acta Orthop Scand 61(1):29, 1990

93. Simpson PJ, Radford SG, Forster SJ et al: The fibrinolytic effects of anaesthesia. Anaesthesia 37:3, 1982

94. Carr JB: Fulminant fat embolism. Orthopedics 13:258, 1990

95. Monto RR, Garcia J, Callaghan JJ; Fatal fat embolism following total condylar knee arthroplasty. J Arthroplasty 5:291, 1990

96. Watson JT, Stulberg BN: Fat embolism associated with cementing of femoral stems designed for press-fit application. J Arthroplasty 4:133, 1989

97. Dorr LD, Merkel C, Mellman MF, Klein I: Fat emboli in bilateral total knee arthroplasty. Clin Orthop 248:112, 1989

98. Gurd AR: Fat embolism: an aid to diagnosis. J Bone Joint Surg 52B:732, 1970

99. Vandam LD, Dripps RD: Long-term follow-up of patients who received 10,098 spinal anesthetics. III. Syndrome of decreased intracranial pressure headache and ocular and auditory difficulties. JAMA 161:586, 1956

100. Usubiaga JE: Neurological complications of spinal and epidural analgesia. p. 227. In Saidman LJ, Moya F (eds): Complications of Anesthesia. Charles C Thomas, Springfield, IL, 1970

15

Postoperative Analgesia

Tim J. Lamer

Several studies have documented what many anesthesia care providers and surgeons have known for years: that postoperative pain has been a neglected and often poorly managed aspect of perioperative care.[1-3] Fortunately, clinicians are becoming increasingly familiar with a variety of effective management techniques that can provide excellent analgesia. Furthermore, there is mounting evidence that effective analgesia influences postoperative recovery and morbidity.[4,5] This chapter discusses adverse effects of postoperative pain, modification of these effects by analgesia, and available analgesic techniques relevant to orthopedic surgery. The interested reader is referred to the many excellent reviews of the neuroanatomy and physiology of pain.[6-8]

ADVERSE EFFECTS OF POSTOPERATIVE PAIN

Postoperative pain contributes to a multitude of changes in organ system function, many of which are detrimental to the patient's well-being and recovery (Table 15-1). Some of these changes are related to the type and location of the surgery, while others occur with most operations.

Pulmonary Effects

Postoperative pulmonary dysfunction and pneumonitis are major sources of morbidity and mortality after upper abdominal and thoracic surgery (e.g., anterior spinal fusion). The incidence and severity can be reduced by effective analgesia.[9-11] Fortunately, pulmonary complications (with the exception of pulmonary embolism) are less of a problem after peripheral orthopedic surgery.

Cardiac Effects

Acute pain activates the sympathetic nervous system and the subsequent increase in circulating catecholamines can have adverse effects on patients with coronary artery disease. Increases in heart rate and vascular resistance result in increased myocardial oxygen demand, which can promote myocardial ischemia in vulnerable patients. Effective analgesia can blunt this sympathetic response, and although specific outcome data with respect to cardiovascular morbidity and mortality are lacking, it is tempting to speculate that effective analgesia should have a favorable impact.

363

Table 15-1.   Potential Physiologic
Responses to Pain

Pulmonary
    Reduction in lung volumes (forced vital
        capacity, tidal volume, functional resid-
        ual capacity) and flow parameters (peak
        expiratory flow rate)
    Poor cough
    Secretion retention and atelectasis
Vascular
    Vasoconstriction
    Reduced extremity blood flow
    Enhanced venous thrombosis
Cardiac
    Tachycardia (increased myocardial oxy-
        gen consumption)
    Hypertension (increased myocardial ox-
        ygen consumption)
Endocrine
    Altered protein metabolism (often see
        negative nitrogen balance)
    Fluid and electrolyte changes
    Hyperglycemia
Gastrointestinal/Genitourinary
    Urine retention
    Impaired bowel motility

Effect on Blood Flow

Increased sympathetic tone and other
factors can contribute to reduced limb
blood flow. Neural blockade, especially
continuous brachial plexus and epidural
local anesthetic blockade, can provide a
chemical sympathectomy and improve
blood flow to the involved extremity.[12–15]
This may have a favorable impact on
wound healing, surgical outcome after
vascular reanastomosis procedures, and
thrombotic complications, as discussed
below.

Effect on Coagulation

Surgery creates a situation that is ideal
for the development of venous thrombosis. This (and the potential for pulmonary

embolism) continues to be a major source
of morbidity after hip surgery and certain
other orthopedic procedures. Virchow's
triad of endothelial damage, a hypercoagulable state, and stasis are all present
in the postoperative period. Hypercoagulability may result from the release of
various tissue thromboplastic substances.
Stasis results from immobility and increased sympathetic tone. In addition, fibrinolysis is impaired in most postsurgical patients.[16] Epidural analgesia with
local anesthetics can influence all of
these factors and reduce the incidence of
thromboembolic phenomena. Stasis is reduced as a result of the effect on sympathetic tone, as discussed above. Fibrinolysis may be preserved to a greater
extent with epidural analgesia than with
conventional narcotic analgesia.[17,18] Similarly, some studies suggest an antiplatelet effect of the local anesthetic itself.[19,20]
Several studies have demonstrated a reduction of thromboembolic complications with epidural local analgesia when
compared to systemic narcotic analgesia.[18,21,22]

Chronic Pain and Dysfunction

A certain percentage of patients having
orthopedic surgery will develop chronic
pain syndromes, for example, reflex sympathetic dystrophy, causalgia, chronic
low back pain, and phantom pain after
amputation.[23,24] A small but growing
body of evidence indicates that effective
analgesia utilizing neural blockade may
reduce the incidence and severity of
these unfortunate complications.[25–28] In
addition, pain and guarding after limb
surgery may prompt patients to protect
and immobilize the affected limb, which
can contribute to adhesions and contractures. Effective analgesia can facilitate
mobilization after many orthopedic operations, especially in those patients

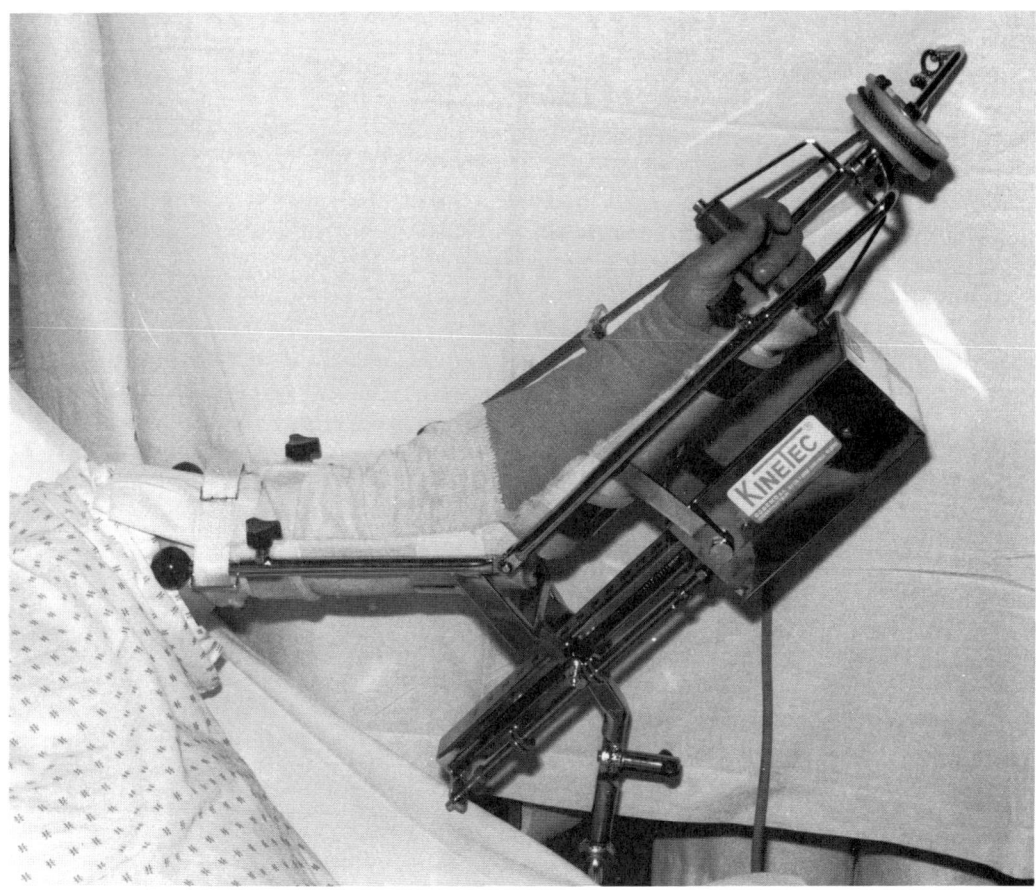

Fig. 15-1. Elbow CPM device for continuous mobilization after reconstructive elbow surgery.

using continuous passive motion (CPM) devices (Fig. 15-1).

Patient Satisfaction

Orthopedic surgery, especially limb surgery, is often performed using regional anesthesia, and it often is convenient and preferable to continue the regional technique into the postoperative period for analgesia. The discussion above outlines the physiologic benefits of aggressively treating postoperative pain. Patient comfort and satisfaction is another important consideration. Several studies have pro-vided overwhelming evidence that epidural narcotic and epidural local analgesia are superior to analgesia with systemic narcotics. These data have been well summarized by Cousins.[29] Effective analgesia may also have a favorable economic impact as several studies have demonstrated a reduction in the duration of hospitalization when epidural analgesia is used instead of conventional systemic narcotic analgesia.[9,25,26,30] The efficacy of intravenous patient-controlled analgesia (PCA) compared to conventional narcotic analgesia (intramuscular or subcutaneous) remains debatable. A number of studies have demonstrated no significant advantage to using PCA; however, the design of these studies is such that the conventionally administered analgesia was closely monitored and truly administered on an as needed basis.[31–34] This does not accurately reflect the usual daily ward situation, in which busy hospital staff are not always able or willing to adequately dose patients, and in this situation, PCA is a significant improvement. New techniques such as transdermal administration of fentanyl[35] and parenteral nonsteroidal anti-inflammatory drugs (NSAIDs) (ketorolac) have some appealing attributes; however, their roles need to be more clearly defined. The next several sections discuss in more detail each of the commonly used analgesic modalities as they apply to orthopedic surgery.

SYSTEMIC ANALGESIA

Although many agents are available for systemic analgesia, opioids and NSAIDs are the most commonly used agents after orthopedic surgery. Systemic opioids may be administered orally or parenterally and parenteral opioids can be administered by intermittent or continuous techniques.

Oral Analgesics

Oral analgesics are often sufficient in alert patients with intact bowel function and pain of mild to moderate intensity. Codeine-, oxycodone-, and hydrocodone-containing preparations are most commonly used; however, morphine, sustained-release morphine, hydromorphone, and levorphanol are occasionally used when stronger analgesics are required (Table 15-2). If antiplatelet effects are not a concern and the patient does not have a history of peptic ulcer disease, oral nonsteroidal analgesics often are effective for mild to moderate pain[36] (Table 15-3. Since a multitude of agents available in this class appear to be equally effective, choice can be based on cost and ease of administration (e.g., bid versus qid dosing).

Many factors make parenteral analgesia necessary or desirable. Clouded sensorium (e.g., early post-general anesthesia), impaired bowel function, and severe pain are all indications for parenteral (or regional) analgesia. As discussed below, we

Table 15-2.   Commonly Used Oral Opioid Analgesics

Drug Name	Usual Dose for Adult (mg)	Commonly Used Trade Names
Propoxyphene HCl[a]	65–130	Darvocet, Darvon
Codeine[a]	30–60	Empirin, Fiorinal, or Tylenol with codeine
Hydrocodone[a]	5–10	Lortab, Vicodin, Co-Gesic
Oxycodone HCl[a]	2.5–10	Percocet, Percodan, Roxicet, Tylox
Hydromorphone[a]	2–4	Dilaudid
Levorphanol	2–4	Levo-Dromeran
Morphine	30–60	
Sustained-release morphine	30–60	M.S. Contin

[a] Often supplied in combination with aspirin or acetaminophen.

Table 15-3. Commonly Used Oral
NSAID Preparations

Drug	Usual Adult Dose
Diflunisal (Dolobid)	500 mg bid
Diclofenac (Voltaren)	75–150 mg tid
Fenoprofen (Nalfon)	300 mg tid
Flurbiprofen (Ansaid)	50–100 mg tid
Ibuprofen (Motrin)	400–600 mg tid
Indomethacin (Indocin)	25–50 mg tid
Ketoprofen (Orudis)	50–100 mg tid
Ketorolac tromethamine (Toradol)	10 mg tid
Meclofenamate (Meclomen)	100 mg tid
Naproxen (Naprosyn)	375–500 mg tid
Naproxen sodium (Anaprox)	275 mg bid
Piroxicam (Feldene)	20 mg qd
Sulindac (Clinoril)	200 mg bid
Tolmetin (Tolectin)	200–400 mg tid
Etodolac (Lodine)	200–400 mg tid

favor regional analgesia when possible. However, some operations do not lend themselves well to regional analgesia, and it may be contraindicated in some patients. In these situations parenteral analgesia is valuable. As mentioned, conventional intermittent narcotic analgesia, by either intramuscular or intravenous administration, has proved to be effective under rigorous study conditions. Because traditional intramuscular administration by nursing staff results in underdosing and inadequate analgesia,[1-3] we favor PCA, continuous narcotic infusions, or a combination.

Continuous Opioid Infusion

Continuous infusions are most appropriate for those patients unable to use PCA devices. These include patients unable to use their hands, those with clouded sensorium (from residual general anesthesia), and patients unable to comprehend equipment instructions (e.g., young children, mentally retarded, or demented patients). Continuous opioid infusion most often is administered intravenously; however, it is important to keep the subcutaneous route in mind in patients with limited intravenous access. Any opioid suitable for injection will work well as long as certain principles are followed. Initially, an adequate loading dose must be used to establish an effective level of analgesia. This is best accomplished by intermittent boluses (or continuous infusion) of the selected narcotic until comfort is obtained, at which time an infusion is started and adjusted based on patient response. If the original infusion dose proves to be inadequate, repeat incremental boluses to re-establish analgesia, followed by a higher infusion dose, will be more effective than simply turning up the infusion. This latter strategy of "catchup" often is ineffective. Lastly, because this technique often is used in patients unable to control their own analgesia, close monitoring of side effects and analgesic efficacy is critical for safe, effective use. We most commonly use morphine or fentanyl (and occasionally hydromorphone) for continuous infusions, using the general dosing guidelines outlined in Table 15-4).

Patient-Controlled Analgesia

PCA has gained acceptance as an effective analgesic technique. Although PCA is more often administered intravenously, subcutaneous and even epidural administration are alternative routes. Many studies have shown intravenous PCA to be safe and effective, and patient satisfaction to be higher with PCA than with conventional systemic analgesia.[37-41] The success of this technique can be undermined by the same attitudes that

Table 15-4. General Dosing Guidelines for Continuous Intravenous or
Subcutaneous Opioid Infusion

	Relative Potency	Loading Dose	Infusion
Morphine	1	0.05–0.20 mg/kg	0.025–0.075 mg/kg/h
Fentanyl	250–500	1.0–3.0 µg/kg	1.0–2.0 µg/kg/h
Hydromorphone	7–10	0.01–0.03 mg/kg	0.005–0.02 mg/kg/h

limit the effectiveness of conventional intramuscular analgesia; that is, the deliberate underdosing by setting unrealistically low bolus doses or long lockout times for fear of overdosing the patient. Therefore, attention to four variables will determine the success of the technique:

1. Effective loading dose
2. Appropriate bolus dose
3. Lockout period
4. Maximum 4-hour dose

It should be pointed out that no single narcotic has been shown to be superior for PCA. Although the ideal narcotic has yet to be discovered, any narcotic when used properly can be effective. In general, drugs with short duration of action (i.e., rapid redistribution) such as fentanyl, sufentanil, and alfentanil are not as desirable for PCA use. As with continuous infusions, an initial effective level of analgesia needs to be established by incremental boluses or continuous infusion. Then the appropriate lockout interval, incremental bolus dose, and maximum dose per unit time need to be determined and programmed into the PCA device (Table 15-5). The appropriate incremental bolus dose delivered when the patient activates the PCA device is crucial to the success of the technique. Since it is well known that significant individual variability exists with respect to narcotic pharmacokinetics and pharmacodynamics, it is unreasonable to expect that all patients can be managed

with the same incremental dose. All too commonly, standard surgical orders prescribe a universal incremental dose for all patients. Early in the treatment, frequent evaluation regarding the efficacy of the chosen dose must be made and adjustments made as necessary. Similarly, programmed lockout intervals should not be set so long that the patient watches the clock in eager anticipation of the next dose. Rather, once the dose has been delivered and the patient experiences the therapeutic effect, the option of administering another bolus dose should exist.

Many modern PCA devices have the capability of providing both the basal level of analgesia using a continuous infusion of narcotic and intermittent patient-activated boluses as needed. Although this is an appealing concept, efficacy studies comparing traditional PCA to PCA plus basal infusion are contradictory.[42–44] Studies currently under-

Table 15-5. Suggested Bolus Dosages and Lockout Periods for the Most Commonly Used PCA Analgesics

Drug	Bolus (mg)[a]	Lockout (min)
Morphine	0.5–3	5–15
Meperidine	10–30	5–15
Hydromorphone	0.1–0.5	5–15

[a] This bolus dosage assumes adequate analgesia has been established by an appropriate loading dose.

way at various institutions will help clarify this issue in the near future.

Transdermal Analgesia

The transdermal application of analgesic agents is an appealing concept because it is noninvasive and does not require normal bowel function (this method also avoids first-pass hepatic metabolism that occurs with oral narcotics). To date, only transdermal fentanyl is available for clinical use. Several studies have shown that transdermal fentanyl provides substantial analgesia.[35,45,46] Currently available patches can be selected to deliver fentanyl at rates of 25, 50, 75, and 100 µg/h, and a single patch will provide continuous analgesia for 3 days.

The technique has two major drawbacks for use in the postoperative period. First, studies have demonstrated a significant delay between initial patch application and peak analgesia. One study examining transdermal fentanyl (75 µg/ml) after major orthopedic surgery demonstrated that is took 2 hours for fentanyl to first appear in the blood and an average of 22 hours to peak blood concentrations.[46] In addition, studies have shown half-lives after removal of the patch ranging from 15 to 25 hours.[46,47] The long time to peak effect and the long half-life make it difficult to titrate or adjust the level of analgesia. Furthermore, the long half-life represents a potential hazard if serious side effects occur. If this method of analgesia is to be useful for acute or postoperative pain, it may be most valuable as a mechanism to provide a basal level of analgesia to which other techniques (e.g., PCA) can be added to fine-tune or optimize pain relief. Since this is a new technique, the role of transdermal analgesia will evolve as more experience is gained.

Parenteral Nonsteroidal Anti-Inflammatory Drugs

Ketorolac is a recently released non-narcotic, nonsteroidal anti-inflammatory, parenteral analgesic. Clinical experience and recent studies have shown this drug to be effective for analgesia for orthopedic surgery without the potential for respiratory depression.[48-50] Although studies indicate efficacy similar to parenteral morphine analgesia, the value of this drug is not necessarily its ability or capacity to replace opioid analgesia, but rather its utility as a supplement or augmentation to opioid analgesia. The combination of an opioid with a NSAID blocks the nociceptive pathway at different levels, thereby improving pain control. Ketorolac can be used to suppress breakthrough pain during epidural opioid analgesia since it is not a respiratory depressant. In addition, ketorolac is often effective in the latter postoperative days and may be used instead of narcotic analgesics, thereby avoiding many of the well-known narcotic side effects. Although gastrointestinal toxicity similar to related (NSAID) oral agents is a theoretical concern, it has not been a significant clinical problem, perhaps because of its limited duration of use in the postoperative setting. The other major concern is the potential for antiplatelet effects. This may be important early in the course of major reconstructive surgery or spine surgery when ongoing blood loss may occur. This drug should be used cautiously or not at all in patients with renal or hepatic dysfunction. Ketorolac may be administered parenterally with an initial loading dose followed by maintenance doses. Recommended dosages are a 30- to 60-mg IM loading dose followed by 15-30 mg IM every 6 hours (note: the manufacturers recommend intramuscular administration; however, this drug has been used effectively intravenously, without apparent complications).

SPINAL OPIOIDS

Several recently published articles and texts provide in-depth information regarding spinal opioid pharmacokinetics.[29,51,52] This section briefly discusses spinal opioid pharmacology and focuses more on practical patient management aspects.

Many studies have demonstrated spinal (epidural, intrathecal) opioid analgesia to be superior to conventional systemic opioid analgesia (including PCA) for a variety of surgical procedures.[53-57] Although morphine is the only drug approved by the Food and Drug Administration for spinal use, all of the currently available narcotics have been used in humans. Morphine and fentanyl have been used most extensively. Reasons for selecting different opioids for spinal use are related primarily to differences in the incidence of side effects, related in large part to the physical properties of the opioid selected.[29]

Physiology

The major advantage of spinal opioid analgesia is the ability to provide intense, selective analgesia without producing the sensory loss, motor loss, and sympathetic blockade that accompanies spinal local analgesia. This is accomplished because spinally applied opioids bind to specific opioid receptors in the dorsal horn of the spinal cord and suppress nociceptive transmission.[29] This antinociceptive effect is likely a pre- and postsynaptic phenomenon. Presynaptic opioid receptor binding may inhibit the release of nociceptive neurotransmitter(s) from C and/or

A-δ fibers as they synapse in the dorsal horn. Postsynaptic opioid receptors also exist and may inhibit neurotransmitter binding or activation of second-order (e.g., spinothalamic tract) neurons. Despite the ability to provide excellent analgesia, spinal opioids do not always provide complete analgesia. Reasons for this are not clear but include the presence of neurotransmitter systems not affected by opioid receptor binding, different opioid receptor subtypes, and also differential sensitivity of afferent fibers to spinal opioid agents.[58] It appears that nociceptive information transmitted via C fibers is more profoundly affected than that transmitted by A-δ fibers.[59] This may explain the observed phenomenon that sharp, well-localized cutaneous and incisional pain is not blocked as well as dull, aching, deep pain. This lack of complete analgesia has led investigators and clinicians to use combinations of spinal local anesthetics plus opioids or opioids plus clonidine to improve analgesia. This concept is discussed later.

Intrathecal Opioid Analgesia

Spinal opioids may be delivered by intrathecal or epidural application. For acute and postoperative pain management, most clinicians use epidural opioids for a number of reasons. The use of epidural catheters allows repeat injections or continuous infusion, thereby allowing more accurate drug dose adjustments and longer periods of analgesia. Most clinicians avoid intrathecal catheters for postoperative analgesia because of the theoretical risk of more serious infection, and because the intrathecal space is more unforgiving (i.e., inadvertent intrathecal injection of drugs intended for intravenous administration is more likely to result in neuronal damage than inadvertent epidural injection.) In addition, intrathecal opioids seem to have a higher incidence of side effects than epidural opioids.[29,60] Intrathecal opioids administered as a single dose are well suited for patients having spinal anesthesia for a surgical procedure, for situations in which indwelling epidural catheters would be undesirable or inadvisable, or for situations in which short-term analgesia is required. When single injections of intrathecal opioids are being considered, morphine may be the best choice because it has the longest duration of action of currently available narcotics and a well-established safety record in terms of lack of neurotoxicity. For most lower extremity operations, 0.125 to 0.25 mg will provide excellent analgesia of *12 to 24 hours* duration. For spine surgery a single dose of 0.25 mg injected directly intrathecally by the surgeon prior to wound closure can provide satisfactory analgesia for 12 to 24 hours. As mentioned above, side effects, particularly vomiting and respiratory depression, are more likely after intrathecal injection than epidural injection.

Epidural Opioid Analgesia

Epidural opioid analgesia is an excellent choice of postoperative analgesia after lower limb surgery. Many of these operations can be performed using epidural anesthesia, and if an epidural catheter is placed for surgery, it can be used for postoperative analgesia. A catheter placed in any of the lumbar interspaces will be sufficient for lower extremity analgesia. For spine surgery, an epidural catheter can be placed under direct vision and externalized during wound closure.[61] Although any narcotic can be used, morphine and fentanyl are used more frequently at our institution and at many others. Either drug can be given by intermittent bolus or continuous infusion

Table 15-6. Doses of Epidural Fentanyl and Morphine for Lower Extremity Surgery

Drug	Loading Dosage	Infusion Dosage
Fentanyl	1.0–1.5 µg/kg	0.075–1.5 µg/kg/h[a]
Morphine	0.03–0.07 mg/kg	0.005–0.0075 mg/kg/h[b]

[a] Usually prepared as a 0.001 percent solution.
[b] Usually prepared as a 0.01 percent solution.

after an appropriate loading dose. Fentanyl's short duration of action makes intermittent-bolus administration an unattractive option. Our preference for either drug is the continuous-infusion technique. This provides more constant drug levels and reliable analgesia without the wide drug level swings and the potential for toxicity that can occur with intermittent boluses. Appropriate doses are outlined in Table 15-6.

The key to successful management of epidural opioid analgesia is careful patient evaluation to allow rapid treatment of inadequate analgesia and minimize side effects. Table 15-7 outlines common management problems and possible responses.

Adverse Effects of Spinal Opioids

Adverse effects of spinal opioids, with the exception of respiratory depression, are usually nuisance problems. From an orthopedic standpoint, perhaps the most troublesome side effect is urinary retention, which occurs in 30 to 60 percent of patients. This appears to be more common with morphine than with fentanyl. In patients with implanted joint hardware, many surgeons are concerned

Table 15-7.   Epidural Opioids: Management Problems and Responses

Inadequate analgesia
    Ensure that the catheter is in the epidural space
        Test dose with 5–10 ml 1.5% lidocaine (chloroprocaine may interfere with fentanyl
            analgesia)
    Bolus and then increase infusion (simply increasing the infusion rate will not produce the
        desired fast response)
        Fentanyl: bolus with 0.5–1.0 μg/kg and increase infusion rate by 10–20 μg/h and reas-
            sess
        Morphine: bolus with 0.025–0.05 mg/kg and then increase infusion by 0.1–0.2 mg/h
    Consider additives: dilute bipuvacaine (or clonidine when it becomes available)
    Add IM ketorolac (30–60-mg load followed by 15–30 mg q6h)
    If analgesia is still inadequate, search for explanation (e.g., psychological issues, neuro-
        pathic pain, tolerance due to previous narcotic use)
    Systemic opioids in conjunction with epidural opioids should be used with extreme cau-
        tion, if at all, because of the increased risk of severe respiratory depression

Side effects
    Excessive somnolence and/or bradypnea (respiratory rate < 8)
        Rule out inadvertent dural puncture; aspirate catheter carefully
        Reduce rate of infusion (with morphine may need to temporarily discontinue infusion)
        Change to a different drug (e.g., if originally using morphine, consider fentanyl)
        Low-dose naloxone infusion[a]
        Naltrexone[b]
    Pruritus
        Try antihistamine first (diphenhydramine 25 mg IM/IV or hydroxyzine 25–50 mg IM
            for average size adult)
        Low-dose naloxone infusion[a]
        Oral naltrexone[b]
    Urine retention
        Intermittent catheter
        Indwelling catheter
        ? Naloxone or naltrexone
    Nausea and vomiting
        Phenothiazine or butyrophenone antiemetic: prochlorperazine 2.5–5.0 IV/IM or dro-
            peridol 0.625–1.25 IV/IM
        Transdermal scopolamine: one disc is designed to be effective for approximately 3
            days
        Diphenhydramine 25 mg q4–6h IV/IM is often very effective
        Low-dose naloxone infusion[a]
        Oral naltrexone[b]

[a] Naloxone infusion: 5–10 μg/kg/h titrated to minimize side effects will maintain analgesia.[83]
[b] Oral naltrexone: 5 mg PO.[84,85]

about the potential need to instrument the urinary tract. The concern is the potential for urinary tract infection with subsequent blood-borne seeding of the implanted joint hardware. Although data on the likelihood of this phenomenon occurring are lacking, the gravity and consequences of this potential complication are sufficient to make many orthopedists wary of the technique. This is an area that requires further study. A recent study has demonstrated that urinary retention may be due to preganglionic sacral parasympathetic inhibition resulting in vesico-sphincter dyssynergy and suggests potential pharmacologic techniques to circumvent this problem (e.g., dopamine agonists).[62] One recent study utilized the addition of droperidol to the epidural opioid mixture. Epidural droperidol significantly reduced the incidence of urinary retention.[63] Further studies will be forthcoming and it is hoped that data will be presented regarding the potential neurotoxicity of epidural droperidol.

Clinically significant nausea and vomiting occurs in 10 to 30 percent of patients receiving epidural opioids. Again, this side effect is more frequent in patients receiving morphine as opposed to fentanyl. Nausea and vomiting presumably are due to narcotic binding to the brain stem vomiting centers which is more likely to occur with the more water-soluble morphine as it remains in the cerebrospinal fluid (CSF) longer, thereby ascending or circulating with the CSF to the brain stem. Management strategies are outlined in Table 15-7.

The mechanism of pruritus has not been elucidated; therefore treatment remains empiric. Antihistamines may be effective; however, if they are not and the pruritus is intense, the decision to begin a low-dose naloxone infusion or to change to an alternate form of analgesia must be made.

As with nausea and vomiting, clinically significant respiratory depression is more common with morphine. This again is due to the ascent of morphine within the CSF to the brain stem respiratory centers. Opioid binding to μ-receptors in the brain stem results in respiratory depression. Although all epidural narcotics have been shown to depress the ventilatory response to carbon dioxide, clinically significant respiratory depression is very

rare with epidural fentanyl.[60] It is more likely with morphine and can be substantially reduced by careful monitoring. Furthermore, once a stable level of analgesia has been established and respiratory depression or excessive somnolence have not occurred within the previous 12 to 24 hours, respiratory depression is extremely rare with epidural morphine. Controversy continues to exist regarding the appropriate monitoring of patients receiving epidural opioids. One issue is whether all patients receiving epidural opioids should be in an intensive care unit. Another is how to monitor for respiratory depression. There are many possible solutions and many institutions have safe epidural opioid practices using different techniques. Ours is perhaps a middle-of-the-road approach. Patients receiving epidural opioids may be transferred directly to general wards in which nurses have been carefully trained and inserviced. For the first 12 hours these patients are monitored with pulse oximetry because it is a noninvasive, continuous monitor that is easy to apply (realizing that significant hypercarbia and somnolence can occur prior to desaturation). Respiratory rate and level of consciousness or arousal are assessed hourly. Hypersomnolence is often a harbinger of respiratory depression and often an indication of excessive epidural opioid administration. Naloxone is available and can be administered immediately in an emergency.

Although Table 15-7 outlines some specific management strategies, it is of special note that most of the side effects due to epidural opioid can be managed with low doses of opioid antagonists (naloxone or naltrexone). Naloxone administered by intermittent injection or as a continuous infusion at rates between 5 and 10 μg/kg/h has been shown to reverse respiratory depression while allowing satisfactory analgesia. Similarly, in patients who can take oral agents, naltrexone administered orally can provide the same result. The use of naloxone or naltrexone is contraindicated in patients chronically exposed to narcotic analgesics as their use in this setting could precipitate a severe opioid withdrawal syndrome.

EPIDURAL LOCAL ANALGESIA

Epidural local anesthesia is particularly well-suited for many lower extremity operations, especially knee operations, which require CPM postoperatively. Epidural local analgesia provides dose-related intense analgesia, prevents muscle spasm, improves lower extremity blood flow by virtue of sympathetic neural blockade, and allows pain-free range of motion to be instituted. Disadvantages are related to the potential for motor and autonomic blockade. Motor fiber block resulting in lower extremity weakness will often prevent early ambulation. Depending on the extent of sympathetic block, hypotension or postural hypotension may be a problem. Sacral parasympathetic block may lead to urinary retention, with the same concerns as mentioned above with spinal opioids.

Epidural local analgesia is chosen instead of epidural narcotic analgesia primarily to obtain sympathetic block and increased lower extremity blood flow when it would be desirable, to avoid the respiratory depressant effects of opioids, and to avoid postoperative skeletal muscle spasm after procedures in which it is a prominent concern. Epidural local anesthetic agents have the potential to provide more intense analgesia than epidural opioids. As mentioned before, epidural opioid analgesia provides very good but not always complete analgesia.

The dose of epidural local analgesia can be adjusted to provide a spectrum of analgesia, from partial sensory block to dense surgical analgesia. This can be a particular advantage in the early postoperative period after notoriously painful operations (e.g., knee replacement or reconstruction followed by immediate CPM).[64,65]

Epidural local analgesia is best obtained by administering an appropriate loading dose followed by continuous infusion. Although intermittent injection can be used, more drug is required with this technique (increasing the likelihood of systemic accumulation), tachyphylaxis (or tolerance) is more likely to occur, and currently available agents all require frequent (i.e., every 2 to 3 hours) administration.[66,67] Continuous infusion provides analgesia with lower anesthetic doses, and minimizes the potential for tachyphylaxis. Although any local anesthetic can be used, bupivacaine is most commonly used because it tends to have more sensorimotor dissociation than other currently available agents. In other words, it is possible to provide sensory block with less motor block. As of 1992, ropivacaine, which may prove to be an excellent infusion agent, is not available.

The key to providing successful analgesia is to establish satisfactory analgesia with a loading dose prior to initiating the infusion. This is best accomplished by beginning the infusion before surgical anesthesia has worn off. We usually start the infusion when the anesthetic level regresses to the T10 level. An infusion of either 0.125 percent or, more commonly, 0.25 percent bupivacaine is administered at a dose of 0.2 to 0.3 mg/kg/h and adjusted to maintain satisfactory analgesia. In order to minimize hypotension, we aim to keep the anesthetic level between T10 and T12. Pharmacokinetic data from *healthy adult patients* receiving prolonged bupivacaine infusions indicate that infusion dosages less than 30 mg/h are safe and do not result in toxic blood levels.[68,69]

Management of epidural local analgesia is similar to management of epidural opioid analgesia. The goals are to optimize analgesia and minimize or treat side effects as best as possible. Table 15-8 outlines the most common management problems. Inadequate analgesia, the most troublesome problem, is managed by ensuring proper catheter position and function and then rebolusing to establish effective analgesia. If analgesia is inadequate despite a seemingly adequate level of anesthesia, a systemic agent such as ketorolac or an opioid (using PCA or transdermal fentanyl) can be added. Another approach would be to consider an epidural opioid and local anesthetic combination.

Side Effects

Hypotension may be a problem and is most likely to occur when fluid or blood replacement is inadequate either intra-

Table 15-8. Epidural Local Analgesia: Management Problems

Inadequate analgesia
 Ensure that catheter is in the epidural space (see Table 15-7)

 Bolus with 5–10 ml of 0.25 percent bupivacaine and then increase infusion rate by 2–4 ml/h

 Increase the concentration of bupivacaine

 Add IM ketorolac or PCA with opioid analgesic

 Narcotic/local anesthetic combination

Side effects
 Urine retention
  Intermittent or indwelling urinary catheter

 Motor block
  Temporarily stop infusion until motor function returns; unfortunately pain often returns as well
  Try narcotic/local combination with reduced local anesthetic combination

 Hypotension
  Ensure adequate intravascular volume and hemoglobin concentration
  Adjust anesthetic level: for most lower extremity surgeries, a T10–T12 level is adequate and should not produce hypotension
  Aspirate catheter to rule out intrathecal migration

 Intravascular toxicity (tinnitus, circumoral paresthesia, dizziness, lightheadedness, visual changes, shivering, or muscle twitching)
  Stop infusion
  Aspirate catheter to confirm
  If intravascular toxicity is suspected (even if aspiration is negative) the infusion should be stopped, the catheter discontinued, and alternate analgesia provided
  Administer oxygen by face mask
  Have resuscitation equipment and anticonvulsant agents (thiopental, midazolam) available

operatively or in the postoperative period. The level of anesthesia needs to be evaluated and adjusted if necessary (either slowing or temporarily stopping the infusion) and intravascular volume status needs to be assessed. Most cases of hypotension will respond to fluid resuscitation. In urgent situations, a vasopressor can be used until the above measures can be instituted.

Motor block often occurs with prolonged infusion, even when a dilute solution is used. As long as ambulation is not required or desired, this is not a problem. When ambulation becomes important for recovery and atelectasis prevention, an alternate analgesic technique must be used.

Despite careful placement into the epidural space, most currently available catheters can puncture the dura or epidural blood vessels. Detection of these potentially serious events can be facilitated by discussing the clinical presentation with the patient and with well-trained, observant nurses. Dural puncture usually presents as a rapid increase in the intensity of the block over a short period of time. Intravascular puncture usually presents with any of the following: tinnitus, circumoral paresthesia, dizziness, lightheadedness, visual disturbance, and muscle twitching. Treatment in either case is to discontinue the infusion and remove the catheter.

One hazard of any local anesthetic technique is its potential to mask a perioperative complication. With complete deafferentation, a compartment syndrome, bladder overdistension, pressure sores, bowel perforation with peritonitis, and other problems could escape early detection. Careful monitoring by nurses and physicians is important to prevent mishaps and detect problems early on.

Epidural Narcotic and Local Anesthetic Combinations

There are many instances when the combination of an epidural opioid plus local anesthetic can be advantageous. The general principle is that the combination of these two agents blocks nociceptive pathways at different sites. Lower doses of each agent can be used than if either agent is used alone. Often this results in improved analgesia with fewer side effects. For example, after reconstructive knee surgery, a combination of epidural 0.0005 percent fentanyl plus 0.075 to 0.100 percent bupivacaine infused at 10 to 14 ml/h often provides excellent analgesia. One recent study did not show any benefit when bupivacaine was added to fentanyl for epidural infusion in patients after knee surgery.[70] Unfortunately, in that study, the epidural infusion was started at 6 ml/h; and we know this is about one-half the required rate to maintain analgesia after knee surgery. Our experience and that of many others indicates that the combination of an epidural opioid plus a local anesthetic is a potentially valuable addition to our analgesic armamentarium.[71–74] Further studies are needed to clarify the role of single-agent versus combination therapy for epidural analgesia. For example, combinations of clonidine plus an opioid or clonidine plus local anesthetic may prove effective in some situations. Further clinical experience with epidural clonidine is necessary to define its place in the postoperative setting.

BRACHIAL PLEXUS ANALGESIA

Many upper extremity surgical procedures result in severe postoperative pain. Shoulder and elbow reconstruction as well as most major hand operations are accompanied by severe pain. Excessive sympathetic tone and vasospasm can lead to poor wound healing and surgical results. Splinting and immobility may lead to excessive scar formation and contractures. Brachial plexus analgesia (BPA) improves pain control, reduces sympathetic tone, improves extremity blood flow, and reduces splinting and muscle spasm to facilitate mobilization of the affected limb. BPA can be accomplished using continuous or intermittent techniques depending on the circumstances of the operation and postoperative recovery period. Interscalene blocks using long-acting agents such as bupivacaine or ropivacaine provide profound analgesia after reconstructive shoulder surgery. Unfortunately, interscalene catheters are notoriously difficult to stabilize and frequently become dislodged with patient movement. Since interscalene blocks are simple to perform, intermittent, daily injections as needed is a reasonable alternative.

For more distal procedures, BPA using a continuous technique is easy to accomplish using the axillary approach or the subclavian perivascular approach.[75–77] The use of a continuous technique allows continuous analgesia, minimizes the potential for tachyphylaxis, allows easy adjustment of anesthetic level depending on the desired degree of sensory or motor block and minimizes the dose of local anesthetic. Both the axillary and subclavian techniques are reliable, effective techniques and selection of one technique over the other is perhaps due to individual familiarity rather than a specific advantage of one technique over the other. A number of commercially prepared kits are available to facilitate catheter placement.

As with other continuous techniques, an effective analgesic level must be obtained with appropriate loading dose before instituting an infusion. This is usually accomplished by beginning an infusion before surgical anesthesia has regressed. If, for some reason, brachial plexus anesthesia was not used for surgery, then a loading dose of approximately 0.75 to 1.0 mg/kg of 0.25 percent bupivacaine can be administered. Bupivacaine is currently the most commonly used infusion agent. Depending on the desired or required intensity of blockade, 0.125 or 0.25 percent bupivacaine at a rate of 8 to 12 ml/h is safe and usually sufficient, and can be adjusted accordingly.[68,77] Management of inadequate analgesia depends on the cause. As with other catheter techniques, it is necessary to ascertain correct catheter position. This can be done by ensuring adequate anesthesia in the desired nerve distribution. If anesthesia is insufficient, a local anesthetic (with epinephrine) test dose is administered (after aspiration) to rule out intravascular placement,[78] after which additional agent is administered to establish anesthesia (for an average adult, we recommend 10 to 20 ml of 2 percent chloroprocaine, as this minimizes the potential for toxicity). Another technique is to inject a small amount of radiopaque dye and note the pattern.[77] If the catheter is within the brachial plexus "sheath," a relatively smooth-contoured, sausage-shaped outline will appear (Fig. 15-2). If the catheter is in a subcutaneous or muscle plane, a "fuzzy blob" of dye or an outline of the muscle will appear. In the absence of anesthesia with a test dose and/or radiologic confirmation of improper placement, the catheter needs to be replaced. (Note: If a previous infusion and test dose have resulted in large doses of local anesthetics, it will be necessary to wait an appropriate amount of time before resuming another infusion.)

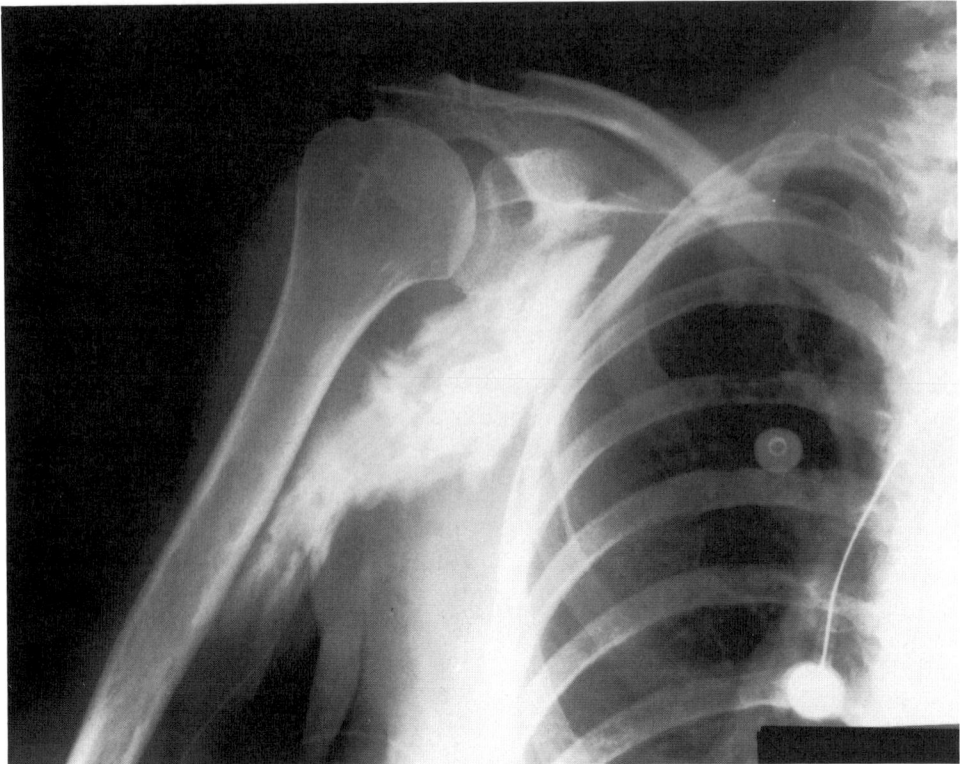

Fig. 15-2. Axillary catheter properly located within the axillary "sheath" outlined by radiopaque dye.

PERIPHERAL NERVE BLOCKS

As with brachial plexus blockade, many other peripheral nerve blocks can be used to provide postoperative analgesia (Table 15-9). Wrist and elbow blocks can provide excellent analgesia for distal upper extremity surgery. Ankle blocks, knee blocks, and sciatic-femoral blocks are excellent analgesic options for lower extremity procedures. Most areas of the body are supplied by nerves that are amenable to peripheral neural blockade. Advantages include the potential for excellent analgesia and minimizing the dose and side effects of systemic analgesics.

Specific nerve block techniques for surgical anesthesia are described elsewhere in this text (see Chs. 12 and 13). The use of long-acting agents such as bupivacaine or ropivacaine can provide 12 to 24 hours of postoperative analgesia.

PSYCHOLOGICAL TECHNIQUES

Clinicians have been made well aware of the significant psychological suffering many chronic pain patients experience. It is easier to forget or ignore psychological factors in patients with acute, postoperative pain for a number of reasons, in-

Table 15-9.   Techniques for Management of Postoperative and Acute Orthopedic Pain Problems

Problem	Techniques[a]
Femur fracture	Femoral nerve block Epidural analgesia
Distal leg fracture	Sciatic nerve block Epidural analgesia
Spine surgery	"Single-shot" intrathecal morphine Epidural opioid analgesia (catheter placed by surgeon)
Hip surgery	"Single-shot" intrathecal morphine Epidural analgesia Lumbar plexus block
Knee surgery	Lumbar plexus block (continuous[86] or single injection) Epidural analgesia
Shoulder surgery	Interscalene block
Elbow or distal upper extremity surgery	Brachial plexus block—continuous or intermittent technique
Arm fracture	Brachial plexus block

[a] Only procedures are listed. Systemic agents can be used to augment the procedures as necessary.

cluding that while postoperative pain is expected but presumed to be of short duration, patients (and physicians) often are not aware that techniques are available to minimize postoperative pain and suffering.

Similar surgical procedures on different patients result in marked differences in pain complaints. For instance, an otherwise healthy individual having elective reconstructive orthopedic surgery to improve function and return to the golf course will have a different pain experience than a patient having palliative surgery because of a metastatic bone neoplasm. In addition, the usual effective analgesic techniques do not always lead to a reduction in pain complaints. Most procedures and medications effectively deal with nociception due to tissue damage but do not always relieve the patient's suffering. The potential reasons are many and complex, and include cultural, social, and psychological factors. Strategies and interventions aimed at relieving both physical and psychological suffering are likely to be more effective than interventions focusing on either one alone.

A simple, effective, and essential step is a thoughtful preoperative visit by the individual(s) who will be responsible for the patient's postoperative analgesia. Since pain is usually the dominant concern and fear of patients, assurance by the anesthesia care provider (and medical and surgical colleagues) that adequate analgesia will be a priority and that many effective options exist will often put patients at ease. For instance, Egbert and others have shown that a preoperative visit has a very favorable effect on postoperative pain and analgesia use.[79]

Many other techniques are available, and perhaps the most important point to make is for clinicians to be aware of these additional techniques and obtain consultation when indicated. Techniques available include but are not limited to the use of various coping strategies, distraction techniques, and relaxation training.[80,81]

In summary, physicians often reflexively prescribe medications and procedures when patients complain of pain. It is important to be aware of and use other available tools and techniques when appropriate.

THE POSTOPERATIVE PAIN SERVICE

The team approach for treating chronic pain patients is well established. Similarly, a team approach may optimize acute and postoperative pain management.[82] The number of individuals required to organize and maintain a postoperative pain service (PPS) depends on many factors, including patient volume, patients' physical status, postoperative monitoring facilities, and availability of trained house staff. A properly trained physician from any discipline could serve as the medical director or as an attending physician on a PPS, although anesthesiologists are uniquely trained and qualified by virtue of their extensive training in regional blockade and opioid pharmacology. In addition to the medical director, the pain service requires a group of interested faculty, a well-trained nursing staff, educated surgical and medical colleagues, pharmacy support, and, in larger practices, assistance from resident physicians or physician extenders (e.g., RN, CRNA, physician assistant) dedicated to the PPS. Twenty-four-hour coverage of the service is essential to optimize patient care and provide personnel to deal quickly with the side effects or complications. Other important duties of the PPS include patient education, education of nurses and physicians, quality assurance, and often research.

In summary, postoperative pain imposes on our patients physical and emotional suffering as well as a wide variety of adverse physiologic changes. We have a variety of pharmacologic, procedural, and psychologic interventions available to prevent or alleviate these undesirable effects. Evidence continues to accumulate that effective analgesia, particularly using regional techniques, positively influences outcome. As physicians and healers, we are obligated to provide our patients with effective analgesia.

REFERENCES

1. Donovan M, Dillon P, McGuire L: Incidence and characteristics of pain in a sample of medical-surgical inpatients. Pain 30:69, 1987
2. Watt-Watson JH: Nurses' knowledge of pain issues: a survey. J Pain Symptom Manage 2:207, 1987
3. Grossman SA, Sheidler VR: Skills of medical students and house officers in prescribing narcotic medications. J Med Educ 60:552, 1985
4. Yeager MP, Glass DD, Neff RK, Brinck-Johnson T: Epidural anesthesia and analgesia in high-risk surgical patients. Anesthesiology 66:729, 1987
5. Lamer TJ: Postoperative pain management with epidural narcotics results in shorter hospital stay than IV or IM narcotics. Reg Anaesth 15:S82, 1990
6. Bonica JJ: Anatomic and physiologic basis of nociception and pain. p. 28. In Bonica JJ (ed): The Management of Pain. 2nd Ed. Lea & Febiger, Philadelphia, 1990
7. Wilson PR, Lamer TJ: Pain mechanisms: anatomy and physiology. p. 65. In Raj PP (ed): Practical Management of Pain. 2nd Ed. Mosby-Year Book, Chicago, 1992
8. Yaksh TL: Neurologic mechanisms of pain. p. 791. In Cousins MJ, Bridenbaugh

PO (eds): Neural Blockade in Clinical Anesthesia and the Management of Pain. 2nd Ed. JB Lippincott, Philadelphia, 1988

9. Lutz LJ, Lamer TJ: Management of postoperative pain: review of current techniques and methods. Mayo Clin Proc 65:584, 1990

10. Cuschieri RJ, Morran CG, Howre JC, McArdle CS: Postoperative pain and pulmonary complications: comparison of three analgesic regimens. Br J Surg 72:495, 1985

11. Shulman M, Sandler AN, Bradley JW et al: Postthoracotomy pain and pulmonary function following epidural and systemic morphine. Anesthesiology 61:569, 1984

12. Bowler GMR, Lamont MC, Scott DB: Effect of extradural bupivacaine or I.V. diamorphine on calf blood flow in patients after surgery. Br J Anaesth 59:1412, 1987

13. Haljamäe H: Effects of anesthesia on leg blood flow in vascular surgical patients. Acta Chir Scan 550(suppl):81, 1988.

14. Haljamäe H, Holm FJ, Akerström G: Epidural versus general anesthesia and leg blood flow in patients with occlusive atherosclerotic disease. Eur J Vasc Surg 2:395, 1988

15. Modig J, Malmberg P, Karlström G: Effect of epidural versus general anesthesia on calf blood flow. Acta Anaesthesiol Scand 24:305, 1980

16. Emeis JJ: The vascular wall and fibrinolysis. Haemostasis 8:332, 1979

17. Henry CP, Odoom JA, Ten Cate H et al: Effects of extradural bupivacaine on the haemostatic system. Br J Anaesth 58:301, 1986

18. Modig J, Borg T, Bagge L, Saldeen T: Role of extradural and of general anaesthesia in fibrinolysis and coagulation after total hip replacement. Br J Anaesth 55:625, 1983

19. Luostarinen L, Evers H, Lyytikäinen MT: Antithrombic effects of lidocaine and related compounds on laser induced microvascular injury. Acta Anaesthesiol Scand 25:9, 1981

20. Borg T, Modig J: Potential antithrombotic effects of local anaesthetics due to their inhibition of platelet aggregation. Acta Anaesthesiol Scand 29:739, 1985

21. Hendolin H, Mattila MAK, Poikolainen: The effect of lumbar epidural analgesia on the development of deep vein thrombosis of the legs after open prostatectomy. Acta Chir Scand 147:425, 1981

22. Modig J, Maripuu E, Sahlstedt B: Thromboembolism following total hip replacement. Reg Anaesth 11:72, 1986

23. Bach S, Noreng M, Tjéllden NU: Phantom limb pain in amputees during the first 12 months following limb amputation, after preoperative lumbar epidural blockade. Pain 33:297, 1988

24. Wall PD: The prevention of postoperative pain. Pain 33:289, 1988

25. Walmsley RHN, Colclough GW, Mazloomdoost M et al: Epidural PCA/infusion for post-nephrectomy pain: shorter hospitalization. Anesthesiology 71:A684, 1989

26. Isaacson IJ, Weitz FI, Berry AJ et al: Intrathecal morphine's effect on the postoperative course of patients underoing abdominal aortic surgery. Anesth Analg 66:S86, 1987

27. McQuay HJ, Carroll D, Moore RA: Postoperative orthopedic pain: the effect of opiate premedication and local anesthetic block. Pain 33:291, 1988

28. Dahl JB, Rosenberg J, Dirkes WE et al: Prevention of postoperative pain by balanced analgesia. Br J Anaesth 64:518, 1990

29. Cousins MJ, Cherry DA, Gourlay GK: Acute and chronic pain: use of spinal opioids. p. 985. In Cousins MJ (ed): Neural Blockade in Clinical Anesthesia and the Management of Pain. 2nd Ed. JB Lippincott, Philadelphia, 1988

30. Bellamy CD, McDonnell FJ, Colclough GW: Postoperative epidural pain management results in shorter hospital stay than IV PCA morphine: a comparison in anterior cruciate ligament repair. Anesthesiology 71:A686, 1989

31. Rogers DA, Dingus D, Stanfield J et al: A prospective study of patient-controlled analgesia. Am Surg 56(2):86, 1990

32. Brewington KC: Patient-controlled analgesia in gynecologic oncology surgery. Ala Med 59(5):15, 1989

33. Welchew EA: On-demand analgesia. A

double bind comparison of on-demand intravenous fentanyl with regular intramuscular morphine. Anaesthesia 38:19, 1983

34. Dahl JB, Daugaard JJ, Larsen HV et al: Patient-controlled analgesia: a controlled trial. Acta Anaesthesiol Scand 31:744, 1987

35. Rowbotham DJ, Wyld R, Peacock JE et al: Transdermal fentanyl for the relief of pain after upper abdominal surgery. Br J Anaesth 63:56, 1989

36. Rigamonti G, Zanella E, Lampugnani R et al: Dose-response study with indoprofen I.V. as an analgesic in postoperative pain. Br J Anaesth 55:513, 1983

37. Ferrante FM, Ostheimer GW, Covino BG: Patient Controlled Analgesia. Blackwell Scientific Publishers, Boston, 1990

38. Egbert A, Parks LH, Short LM, Burnett ML: Randomized trial of postoperative patient-controlled analgesia versus intramuscular narcotics in frail elderly men. Arch Intern Med 150:1897, 1990

39. Eisenach JC, Gore SC, Dewan DM: Patient-controlled analgesia following cesarean section: a comparison with epidural and intramuscular narcotics. Anesthesiology 68:444, 1988

40. Hecker BR, Albert L: Patient-controlled analgesia: a randomized prospective comparison between two commercially available PCA pumps and conventional analgesic therapy for postoperative pain. pain 35:115, 1988

41. Bollish SJ, Collins CL, Kirking DM, Bartlett RH: Efficacy of patient-controlled versus conventional analgesia for postoperative pain. Clin Pharm 4:48, 1985

42. Owen H, Szekely SM, Plummer JL et al: Variables of patient-controlled analgesia. 2. Concurrent infusion. Anaesthesia 44:11, 1989

43. McKenzie R, Rudy T, Tantisira B: Comparison of PCA alone and PCA with continuous infusion on pain relief and quality of sleep. Anesthesiology 73:A787, 1990

44. Vickers AP, Derbyshire DR, Burt DR et al: Comparison of the Leicester Micropalliator and the Cardiff Palliator in the relief of postoperative pain. Br J Anaesth 59:503, 1987

45. Caplan RA, Ready B, Oden RV et al:

46. Plezia PM, Kramer TH, Linford J, Hameroff SR: Transdermal fentanyl: pharmacokinetics and preliminary clinical evaluation. Pharmacotherapy 9:2, 1989

47. Duthie DJR, Rowbotham DJ, Wyld R et al: Plasma fentanyl concentrations during transdermal fentanyl delivery to surgical patients. Br J Anaesth 60:614, 1988

48. O'Hara DA, Fragen RJ, Kinzer M, Pemberton D: Ketorolac tromethamine compared with morphine surfate for treatment of postoperative pain. Clin Pharmacol Ther 41:556, 1987

49. Yee JT, Brown CR, Allbon C, Koshiver J: Analgesia from intramuscular ketorolac tromethamine compared to morphine in severe pain following major surgery. Pharmacotherapy 6:253, 1986

50. Brandon Bravo LJC: The effects on ventilation of ketorolac in comparison with morphine. Eur J Clin Pharmacol 35:491, 1988

51. Cousins MJ, Bridenbaugh PO: Spinal opioids and pain relief in acute care. p. 151. In Cousins MJ, Philips GD (eds): Acute Pain Management. Churchill Livingstone, New York, 1986

52. Cousins MJ, Mather LE: Intrathecal and epidural administration of opioids. Anesthesiology 61:276, 1984

53. Loper KA, Ready LB: Epidural morphine after anterior cruciate ligament repair: a comparison with patient-controlled intravenous morphine. Anesth Analg 68:350, 1989

54. Harrison DM, Sinatra R, Morgese L, Chung JH: Epidural narcotic and patient-controlled analgesia for post cesarean section pain relief. Anesthesiology 68:454, 1988

55. Bengtsson M, Lofstrom JB, Meritz H: Postoperative pain relief with intrathecal morphine after major hip surgery. Reg Anaesth 8:138, 1983

56. Gustafsson LL, Friberg-Niclson S, Garle M: Extradural and parenteral morphine: kinetics and effects in postoperative pain. A controlled clinical study. Br J Anaesth 54:1167, 1982

57. Rechtine GR, Reinert CM, Bohlman HH:

The use of epidural morphine to decrease postoperative pain in patients undergoing lumbar laminectomy. J Bone Joint Surg 66:113, 1984

58. Arner S, Arner B: Differential effects of epidural morphine in the treatment of cancer related pain. Acta Anaesthesiol Scand 29:32, 1985

59. Zieglgansberger W: Opioid actions on mammalian spinal neurons. Int Rev Neurobiol 25:243, 1984

60. Etches RC, Sundler AN, Duley MD: Respiratory depression and spinal opioids. Can J Anaesth 36:165, 1989

61. Ray CD, Bagley R: Indwelling epidural morphine for control of post-lumbar spine surgery pain. Neurosurgery 13:338, 1983

62. Durant PAC, Yaksh TL: Drug effects on urinary bladder tone during spinal morphine induced inhibition of the micturition reflex in unanesthetized rats. Anesthesiology 68:325, 1988

63. Naji P, Farschtschian M, Wilder-Smith O, Wilder-Smith C: Epidural droperidol and morphine for postoperative pain. Anesth Analg 70:583, 1990

64. Pettine KA, Wedel DJ, Cabanela ME, Weeks JL: The use of epidural bupivacaine following total knee arthroplasty. Orthop Rev 18:894, 1989

65. Raj PP, Kinarr DC, Vigdorth E et al: Comparison of continuous epidural infusion of a local anesthetic and administration of systemic narcotics in the management of pain after total knee replacement surgery. Anesth Analg 66:401, 1987

66. Bromage PR, Pettigrew RT, Crowell DE: Tachyphylaxis in epidural analgesia. 1. Augmentation and decay of local anesthesia. J Clin Pharmacol 9:30, 1969

67. Cousins MJ, Mather LE: Clinical pharmacology of local anesthetics. Anaesth Intensive Care 8:257, 1980

68. Denson DD, Raj PP, Saldahna F et al: Continuous perineural infusion of bupivacaine for prolonged analgesia: pharmacokinetic considerations. Int J Clin Pharmacol Ther Toxicol 21:591, 1983

69. Denson DD, Myers JA, Hartwick CT: The relationship between free bupivacaine concentration and central nervous system toxicity. Anesthesiology 61:A211, 1984

70. Badner NH, Reimer EJ, Moote CA, Komar WE: Addition of bupivacaine 0.1% does not improve postoperative epidural fentanyl analgesia after knee joint replacement. Anesthesiology 73:A761, 1990

71. Lee A, Simpson D, Whitfield A, Scott DB: Postoperative analgesia by continuous extradural infusion of bupivacaine and diamorphine. Br J Anaesth 60:845, 1988

72. Hjortsφ NC, Lund C, Mogensen T et al: Epidural morphine improves pain relief and maintains sensory analgesia during continuous epidural bupivacaine after abdominal surgery. Anesth Analg 65:1033, 1986

73. Bisgaard C, Mouridsen P, Dahl JB: Continuous lumbar epidural bupivacaine versus epidural morphine after abdominal surgery. Eur J Anaesthesiol 7:219, 1990

74. Youngstrom P, Eastwood D, Putel H et al: Epidural fentanyl and bupivacaine in labor—double-blind study. Anesthesiology 61:A414, 1984

75. Winnie AP, Collins VJ: The subclavian perivascular technique of brachial plexus anesthesia. Anesthesiology 25:353, 1964

76. Gaumann DM, Lennon RL, Wedel DJ: Continuous axillary block for postoperative pain management. Reg Anesth 13:77, 1988

77. Hall JA, Lennon RL, Wedel JD: Continuous bupivacaine infusion for postoperative pain relief via an axillary catheter. Reg Anesth 15:S58, 1990

78. Lennon RL: The 2-chloroprocaine test for axillary brachial plexus. Anesth Analg 64:646, 1985

79. Egbert LD, Buttel GE, Turndorf H: The value of the preoperative visit by an anesthetist. JAMA 185:553, 1963

80. Van Dulfsen PJ, Syrjula KL: Psychological strategies in acute pain management. Anesth Clin North Am 7:171, 1989

81. Peck C: Psychological factors in acute pain management. p. 251. In Cousins MJ, Phillips GD (eds): Acute Pain Management. Churchill Livingstone, New York, 1986

82. Ready LB, Oden R, Chadwick HS et al: Development of an anesthesiology-based postoperative pain management service. Anesthesiology 68:100, 1988

83. Rawal N, Schott U, Dahlstrom B et al: Influence of naloxone on analgesia and respiratory depression following epidural morphine. Anesthesiology 64:194, 1986

84. Abbound TK, Afrasiabi A, Davidson et al: Prophylactic oral naltrexone with epidural morphine: effect on adverse reactions and ventilating responses to carbon dioxide. Anesthesiology 72:233, 1990

85. Cullen M, Altstatt AH, Kwon NJ et al: Naltrexone reversal of the side effects of epidural morphine. Anesthesiology 69:A336, 1988

86. Schultz P, Anker-Møller E, Dahl JB et al: Postoperative pain treatment after open knee surgery: Continuous lumbar plexus block with bupivacaine vs. epidural morphine. Reg Anesth 16:34, 1991

16

Chronic Pain Management

Peter R. Wilson

This chapter cannot present an encyclopedic overview of pain medicine and management; the reader is referred to standard texts for that purpose.[1,2] However, certain principles of pain medicine are discussed, and certain common orthopedic pain problems illustrated.

Pain is "an unpleasant sensory and emotional experience . . ."[3] that cannot be measured easily, if at all.[4] This problem has been a significant impediment to the development of valid research methodology,[5] and extrapolation of experimental pain models to the clinical situation may not be relevant.[6]

Nociception is the complex sensory response to stimuli that are damaging to normal tissues. It is accompanied by reflex motor (withdrawal) and autonomic ("fight or flight") responses. It is not the same as pain, as it is not necessarily accompanied by the unpleasant experience (for example, nociception still occurs under general anesthesia).

It is clear that many potential nonphysiologic and non-nociceptive factors influence the experience and reporting of pain.[7] They include

Cultural influences (social, religious, ethnic)
Learning, expectation
Cognitive appraisal
Fear and anxiety
Neuroticism, extroversion, introversion
Perceived control
Coping style
Attention/distraction
Depression
Primary, secondary, and tertiary gain
Abnormal illness behavior
Sick role

It is also apparent that the report of pain can be made in the absence of demonstrable pathophysiology. This may imply that there is a psychological basis for the pain.[8] However, it is also possible that there are not adequate diagnostic tools to detect subtle biochemical or pathophysiologic mechanisms responsible for the pain. Therefore, it must always be borne in mind that even apparently simple orthopedic problems might be accompanied by pain with many components. The practitioner must always be alert to the possibility of complicating factors or the presence of multiple pain categories, particularly if there is an unexpected response to injury, surgery, or conservative treatment. Particular care must be taken if the patient is preceded in the pain clinic by letters from attorneys, insurance companies, or worker compensation carriers.

PAIN CATEGORIES

The pathophysiology of nociception and pain has been under intensive scrutiny, and the traditional divisions of pain into "acute," "subacute," and "chronic" categories can no longer be sustained.[9] A more comprehensive description can be justified in the light of new information on pain mechanisms. Several categories, described below, appear to be distinct in terms of pathophysiology, psychology, and therapy.[10] A brief discussion of acute pain management is justified, because chronic pain must arise from acute pain. It is therefore tempting to speculate that prevention or adequate treatment of acute pain will prevent the development of chronic pain.

Acute Pain

Acute (nociceptive) pain (Table 16-1) is probably the most studied and best understood of these proposed pain categories.[11] Activation of appropriate receptors in the peripheral tissues produces activity in A-δ and C nociceptive nerves. This activity is transmitted through well-described pathways in the spinal cord, brain stem, and thalamus to appropriate areas of the cortex where pain is perceived. There are numerous neurotransmitters involved in the transmission and modulation of these impulses (Table 16-2)[12] and generation and transmission of these impulses can be altered at several sites, singly or in combination.

It is not the purpose of this review to discuss in detail the principles of acute pain management, but the principles outlined in Table 16-1 apply: (1) peripheral anti-inflammatory agents reduce nociceptor activation; (2) local anesthetic blockade of peripheral nerves or the central neuraxis is feasible in the short term; (3)

Table 16-1. Acute (Nociceptive) Pain

Pathophysiologic mechanisms
  Biologically useful, warning of impending tissue damage
  Well-defined and well-understood peripheral nociceptive mechanisms, peripheral neural transmission, spinal cord connections, central projections, and descending and local cord modulating mechanisms
  Well-defined neuropharmacology
  Well-defined and useful motor, autonomic, and hormonal reflexes
Psychological factors
  Expectation of occurrence and resolution
  Social, cultural, personal, religious, and domestic factors interact
  Anxiety increases perception
Therapeutic implications
  Peripheral anti-inflammatory agents useful
  Peripheral neural blockade effective
  Central neuraxial blockade effective
  Systemic narcotics useful
  Central (spinal, epidural, intraventricular) narcotics effective
  Anxiolytics possibly useful
  Psychological methods useful

opioid blockade by systemically or spinally administered agents is increasing in application; and (4) other agents such as clonidine and baclofen are being investigated. It is essential to recognize that after it has served its diagnostic function, acute pain has no benefit, and produces many adverse physiologic effects. All efforts must therefore be made to treat and prevent acute pain.[13] It is argued that chronic pain arises from acute pain, and successful treatment of acute pain will therefore prevent chronic pain.

Postoperative Pain

Postoperative pain is discussed in detail in Chapter 15, and summarized in

Table 16-2.   Pain Receptor
Pharmacology

Primary afferent terminals
  Histamine
  Kinins (bradykinin)
  Lipidic acids (leukotrienes, prostanoids)
  Cytokines (interleukins)
  Primary afferent peptides (calcitonin
    gene-related peptide [CGRP]; sub-
    stance P [sP])
Central afferent terminals
  Excitatory amino acids [glutamate, aspar-
    tate]
  Peptides (sP, vasoactive intestinal pep-
    tide [VIP], bombesin, CGRP)
Spinal modulatory systems
  Hyperesthesia (n-methyl-d-aspartate
    [NMDA])
  Allodynia (adenosine)
Spinal analgesic systems
  μ/δ opioid
  α_2-adrenergic
  Serotonin

(From Yaksh[12] with permission.)

Table 16-3. It is again emphasized that
postoperative pain is detrimental to all
physiologic systems. Prevention (or adequate treatment) of postoperative pain is
accompanied by improved outcome and

Table 16-3.   Postoperative Pain

Pathophysiologic mechanisms
  Well-defined surgical tissue damage
  Usually not biologically useful
  Variant of nociceptive pain
  Stress response and reflexes harmful
Psychological factors
  Expectation of occurrence and resolution
  Premorbid psychological factors impor-
    tant
  Sleep deprivation exacerbates adverse ef-
    fects
Therapeutic implications
  Acute pain management principles apply
  Theoretically preventable
  Patient participation in therapy effective
  Cognitive strategies useful

reduced mortality and morbidity (and reduced cost of treatment).

Terminal Pain

Terminal pain may be differentiated
from the other categories because of profound differences in psychological components (Table 16-4). Terminal pain, by
definition, is accompanied by the psychological consequences of the knowledge of impending death. This has become a subspecialty of pain management,
and requires an interdisciplinary approach. It must also be remembered that
several categories of pain can co-exist,
and optimal therapy will require treatment of each component. Again, the
reader is referred to definitive texts for
management of this pain,[14] and is encouraged to evaluate all patients with the
utmost care to define all the pain components.

Table 16-4.   Terminal Pain

Pathophysiologic mechanisms
  Well-defined tissue damage
  Biologically harmful
  Significant nociceptive component
  Stress response and reflexes harmful
  Other pain can co-exist
Psychological factors
  No expectation of resolution of underly-
    ing disease
  Psychological consequences critically im-
    portant
  Anxiety, depression, fear, and anger pres-
    ent
  Significant personal impairment
Therapeutic implications
  Anti-inflammatory agents useful
  Narcotics (systemic and spinal) useful
  Adjuvants (anxiolytic/antidepressant)
    useful
  Neural blockade (temporary or perma-
    nent) useful
  Psychological support essential
  Multidisciplinary approach optimal

Neuropathic Pain

Neuropathic pain (Table 16-5) results from the damage or malfunction of the nervous system.[15,16] Fundamental neurophysiologic mechanisms are unknown, despite much research into the problem.[17] Neuropathic pain syndromes commonly seen in an orthopedic practice include scar pain, reflex sympathetic dystrophy, phantom limb pain, neuroma pain, and radicular and plexus pain (discussed below). Because of the unknown mechanism(s) of neuropathic pain, rational therapy is not possible. Empiric therapy must therefore be used with the utmost caution, and with the intention of avoiding further damage. Objective evidence of successful treatment (such as improvement in function or reduction in

Table 16-5.   Neuropathic Pain

Pathophysiologic mechanisms
    Peripheral and/or central neuraxial damage and/or malfunction
    Neurochemical processes not clearly understood
    Prediction of occurrence/resolution difficult
Psychological factors
    Unknown effect of premorbid personality, co-existing pathology
    Unpredictable psychological consequences
Theraupeutic implications
    Specific, rational therapy impossible at present
    Trials of centrally and peripherally acting agents justified (anticonvulsants, antidepressants, anxiolytics, sympatholytics, corticosteroids, substance P depleters, etc.)
    Prevention difficult (or impossible) at present
    Neural blockade unpredictable
    Neurostimulation and neural ablation unpredictable

medication) must be used in directing therapeutic measures.

Treatment of reflex sympathetic dystrophy and the "failed back" are other examples of conditions for which many treatments have been described. It is the usual in all areas of medicine for initial papers describing a new treatment to report encouraging results. However, subsequent papers often do not confirm the initial optimism. This begs the question: if all new treatments are successful, why are so many described, and why do we keep looking for new ones?

Treatment of neuropathic pain is extremely difficult, and may best be attempted within an interdisciplinary pain clinic, which can address the pain and its adverse physical, physiologic, and psychological effects.

A special situation might pertain to neuromas. The regenerating end of a severed or damaged nerve has been shown to be mechanically sensitive, and to be further activated by norepinephrine. It appears that pain is produced when neuromas are activated mechanically or chemically. This neuroma sensitivity has been shown to be reduced by the application of corticosteroids.[18] It might also be reduced by depletion of the local norepinephrine or by sympathetic blockade. Neuromas may form after any peripheral nerve injury, including surgical incision, and mechanical, chemical (alcohol, phenol, etc.), or thermal (radiofrequency or cryo) trauma. It would therefore seem prudent not to attempt to treat neuromas with techniques that would lead to additional scarring and further neuroma formation.

Chronic Pain

Chronic pain (Table 16-6) does not necessarily relate to the duration of the symptoms, but to the psychosocial factors as-

Table 16-6. Chronic Pain

Pathophysiologic mechanisms
  Poorly defined neurologic mechanisms
  Not biologically useful
  Stress response harmful
Psychological factors
  Premorbid personality important
  Depression common
  Abnormal illness behavior often present
  Secondary gain present
Therapeutic implications
  Pharmacologic agents usually contraindicated
  Neurol blockade usually ineffective
  Cognitive/behavioral strategies often useful

---

sociated with the symptoms.[19] There is significant impairment of physiologic and psychological function, with progressive physical and psychological deconditioning.[20] There is usually secondary gain, and the "sick role" is present. Social functioning in the family and workplace is impaired, and issues of litigation and disability become increasingly important. There might be associated pain of other categories (such as nociceptive or neuropathic pain), but treatment of these has usually been unsuccessful.

This chronic pain syndrome is therefore very resistant to therapy, but the behavioral consequences can sometimes be modified by behavioral programs based on the rehabilitation model. However, the patient has to accept that there is no further treatment available for the underlying pain itself. Outcome measures of such programs include return to work, reduction in medication, and reduction in the utilization of medical services. Third-party payers have begun to evaluate the cost/benefit aspects of such programs, and allow patients to participate in "successful" programs. It should be noted that reduction in pain intensity is not a significant outcome measure.

Psychogenic Pain

The complaint of pain can be a prominent symptom in a number of psychological and psychiatric disorders (Tables 16-7 and 16-8). The incidence and prevalence of these disorders cannot be accurately estimated, and it would seem reasonable to exclude somatic pathology first (especially in an orthopedic clinic). However, such diagnoses should be considered if there is any unusual response to diagnostic or therapeutic maneuvers.

Conversely, chronic somatic pain may be associated with psychiatric disturbances.[21] However, it must be emphasized that the diagnosis of psychogenic pain is made in the absence of pain in the other categories. There are no reliable diagnostic instruments for psychogenic pain, and standard instruments such as the Minnesota Multiphasic Personality Inventory (MMPI) may not be valid in the presence of somatic symptoms.[22] It should also be noted that the diagnosis of psychogenic pain cannot be made on the basis of a placebo response or response to a "differential block." This is a difficult

Table 16-7. Psychogenic Pain

Pathophysiologic mechanisms
  Unknown neuroanatomic, neurophysiologic, neuropathologic, and neuropharmacologic mechanisms
  Interactions with nociceptive and neuropathic pains possible
Psychological factors
  Specific predispositions unknown
  Apparent interactions between premorbid personality and external and internal "stressors" and "hassles"
  Primary, secondary, and tertiary gain variably present
Therapeutic implications
  Specific pharmacological treatment impossible at present
  Behavioral management feasible

Table 16-8. DSM-III-R Diagnoses

Adjustment disorder with physical complaints (309.82)
Body dysmorphic disorder (300.70)
Conversion disorder (300.11)
Delusional disorder, somatic type (297.10)
Dyspareunia (302.76)
Factitious disorder with physical symptoms (301.51)
Generalized anxiety disorder (300.02)
Hypochondriasis (300.70)
Late luteal phase dysphoric disorder (307.90)
Malingering (V65.20)
Opioid withdrawal (292.00)
Overanxious disorder (313.00)
Psychological factors affecting physical condition (316.00)
Separation anxiety disorder (309.21)
Somatization disorder (300.81)
Somatoform pain disorder (307.80)
Undifferentiated somatoform disorder (300.70)
Vaginismus (306.51)

diagnosis of exclusion, and should only be made after exhaustive attempts to define a nociceptive or neuropathic cause.

Sociogenic Pain

Some pain appears to have a primarily sociogenic component (Table 16-9). Examples of this are the pain of litigated injury ("jurisigenic pain": product liability, personal injury, medical malpractice), industrial issues ("repetitive strain"[23,24]), and "compensation neurosis."[25]

In such cases, the physician and medical treatment probably have minimal influence on the outcome.[26] The pain and suffering are removed from the scientific and medical arenas, and managed in the legal arena, which has quite different rules and attitudes.[27] There are few scientific studies of these phenomena.[28]

Table 16-9. Sociogenic Pain

Pathophysiologic mechanisms
  Results from actual or perceived physical or emotional damage
  Medical, personal, work, or product injury
  Intensity of symptoms must be maximized: patient must be as sick as possible for as long as possible to maximize financial return to patient and attorney
Psychological factors
  Conflict between need to recover health and yet retain symptoms until case settled
Therapeutic implications
  Recognize existence of conflicting pressures
  Educate patients and attorneys
  Defense attorney must have the patient as well as possible as soon as possible
  Assume a neutral, helping posture

PAIN MANAGEMENT AND REHABILITATION

Pain causes local muscle spasm, which can itself become painful, thus increasing the "total" pain. This may cause protective disuse of the painful area, which may also lead to pain (e.g., from stiff joints). The inevitable changes associated with any disuse, summarized below, must be reversed by normal use or active physical therapy:

Loss of muscle tone, strength, and endurance
Loss of joint mobility
Contractures of ligaments, tendons, and muscles
Loss of bone calcium
Loss of cardiorespiratory fitness (aerobic power)
Reduction in peripheral blood flow
Changes in motor and sensory function
Changes in autonomic function
Psychological changes (depression, anxiety, anger, etc.)

Successful treatment of any pain must therefore include an assessment of the secondary (deconditioning and disuse) changes, and therapy must be directed toward the reversal of those changes.

Therapeutic Principles

Restoration of normal function, or maximal function within the anatomic and physiologic limitation, is the goal of rehabilitation. These principles apply to all pain therapies. Treatment planning must therefore include realistic functional outcome measures. It is not enough simply to "relieve pain." The goal should be restoration to maximal function, with as much comfort as compatible with that function. Patients should understand at the outset that they might not be completely pain-free, but that their function will be maximized. However, this requires a commitment from the patient and active participation in therapy. This may be difficult to achieve, particularly in the demotivated patient, or the patient in the throes of litigation or other social crisis.

Therapy is therefore directed toward the reversal of the effects of disuse and deconditioning, and includes the following:

Goal-setting with the patient
Restoration of normal function
Specific active and passive exercises
Generalized activity to increase aerobic power
Use of physical modalities to allow mobilization
Use of physical modalities to reduce pain (transcutaneous electrical nerve stimulation [TENS], heat, cold)
Use of appropriate medications (e.g., antiinflammatory drugs)

Again, it is not the purpose of this chapter to describe these principles and modalities in detail, but to reinforce the need for interdisciplinary cooperation.

PAIN MANAGEMENT PRINCIPLES

Pain in orthopedic patients is a complex disorder, and its management is also likely to be complex. There is not likely to be a single modality that will be entirely successful used in isolation. The components of the pain have to be accurately identified and treated. Maximal functional outcome is always the goal.

Pharmacologic Modalities

Pain generation, transmission, and perception can be altered by several mechanisms, summarized in Table 16-10. It must be remembered that some of the

Table 16-10.   Pain Management Principles

Pharmacologic
Peripheral
Anti-inflammatory (steroidal and nonsteroidal) agents
Neural blockade (temporary, local anesthetic)
Central
Opioids (systemic and spinal)
Adjuvants (antidepressants)
Antispasmodics (baclofen, benzodiazepines, etc.)
Physical
Counterirritation
Cold
Heat
Ultrasound, shortwave diathermy, interferential therapy
Gate mechanisms
TENS
Dorsal column stimulation
Manipulation

medications used produce the inevitable biochemical consequences of tolerance, physical dependence, and withdrawal. Other medications (such as the corticosteroids) may have profound metabolic consequences. The place of such therapies in the management of pain syndromes has not yet been clearly defined. No medication should be prescribed without a clear understanding of the indications, goals, and risks, and a full and frank discussion with the patient. It also should be emphasized that the ultimate responsibility for recovery is the patient's.

Diagnostic Blocks

It is sometimes necessary to perform diagnostic local anesthetic nerve blocks. However, there must be a clear understanding of the techniques, goals, and limitations of such procedures. Table 16-11 is a summary of these principles. The information obtained from "diagnostic" blocks may be of significant benefit, but if the results of a block are misinterpreted, the patient may be at an even greater disadvantage than before.[29] For example, it used to be believed that a response to a "placebo" block was indicative of psychogenic pain. It is now clear that any patient, with any mechanism of pain, can respond to a placebo block. The placebo reaction is thought to occur in at least 30 percent of normal individuals. There is no reliable instrument to predict the occurrence of the placebo response in any individual. Similarly, if the position of the needle and spread of injectate are not known (if the injection is done "blind" and not under imaging), then interpretation of the resulting sensations is impossible. Some peripheral (motor) nerves can be located with a nerve stimulator, and some sensory nerves with a paresthesia, but the spread of injectate is unpredictable. It can therefore be seen that significant difficulties may exist in the interpretation of diagnostic blocks.

The question of "differential" blocks is equally difficult. As originally proposed, increasing concentrations of local anesthetic, after a saline "placebo," were injected into the subarachnoid space. This technique purported to differentiate sympathetic pain at low concentrations, somatic pain at moderate concentrations, and psychogenic pain at high concentrations. Unfortunately, there is a fatal flaw in this logic: the response of a particular mixed nerve, either in the periphery or centrally, to a specific concentration of local anesthetic is quite unpredictable. For example, it is possible for 0.125 percent bupivacaine to produce complete motor blockade in some cases, and for 0.5 percent to produce only minimal motor block in others.

As a diagnostic tool, the duration of effect of the block might provide important information. Diagnostic blocks can be planned with short-acting and long-acting local anesthetics (preferably double-

---

Table 16-11.   Diagnostic Nerve Blocks

Objectives
  Define anatomic source(s) of pain (reproduction/relief)
  Define neural pathways of pain
  Define somatic/autonomic components of pain
  Assess referred pain
  Assess non-nociceptive (central neuropathic) components
  Predict psychogenic component
  Determine appropriate duration of effect
Pitfalls
  Placebo response uninterpretable
  Nocebo response uninterpretable
  Nerve supplies overlap
  Referred pain response uninterpretable
  Order of nerve fiber blockade unpredictable
  Unpredictable response to local anesthetic concentration
  Differential nerve block uninterpretable

blind, but at least single-blind). For example, lidocaine can be used in the skin and deeper structures during placement of the needle for a spinal facet block. Bupivacaine can be used for the facet injection itself. If the patient reports 6 to 12 hours of relief, it was probably the bupivacaine in the facet joint. If the patient only reports 2 hours of relief, it was probably the lidocaine in the more superficial structures.

Pain reproduction and referral during diagnostic block are sometimes difficult to interpret (e.g., during lumbar spinal discography[30]). During placement of the needle and injection of the radiographic dye, pain-sensitive structures are stimulated. Patients can often state whether they perceive local pain, with or without referred pain, or their "usual" pain. If they report their "usual" pain in the usual location *and* with the usual radiation, it is reasonable to assume that the structure being stimulated with the needle or contrast medium is the pathologic structure. Further evidence is obtained if the injection of a small amount of local anesthetic abolishes the "usual" pain for the appropriate period. Diagnostic blocks, if carefully planned and executed, and correctly interpreted, can provide invaluable information during the evaluation of orthopedic pain syndromes.

ORTHOPEDIC PAIN SYNDROMES

This section cannot include all orthopedic syndromes, but does include common problems seen in a general orthopedic or pain clinic. A further disclaimer is that there are very few objective outcome data in this field, and therefore many of the following statements are based on clinical impressions, beliefs, institutional traditions, and memories of dramatic cases. However, published support of practices is given where available.

The mainstay of orthopedic pain management is physical therapy (active and passive), often facilitated by anti-inflammatory agents. The biochemical effects of the nonsteroidal anti-inflammatory agents (NSAIDs) has been well defined, and their use is well described. All NSAIDs appear to have similar biochemical effects, but they vary in their pharmacokinetic and adverse effect profiles.

Anti-inflammatory corticosteroids are also widely used in orthopedic pain management. Unfortunately, there are few controlled studies with objective outcome criteria on which to base recommendations. The therapeutic dosage of intra-articular depot steroids has not been evaluated by prospective, dose-ranging, objective studies. Dosages on the package inserts appear to have been derived empirically. No prospective studies of long-term effects of repeated injections are available, but anecdotal evidence suggests that frequent, large doses may damage the joint as well as producing adverse systemic effects. Many practitioners limit the number of injections of a single joint to three per year, but there are no data to guide this practice.

There are few studies of the adverse systemic effects of these drugs on the pituitary–adrenal axis. However, a study of a "traditional" dose of depot methylprednisolone (Depo-Medrol) of 80 mg at 2-week intervals for three doses showed significant depression of adrenal function for at least 3 months.[31]

Degenerative Conditions

Degenerative Joint Disease
The pathophysiology of osteoarthritis is unknown, and there may be little correlation between the radiologic appearance

and symptoms arising from joints or discs.[32,33] Pain arising from this cause should be treated with the rehabilitation principles described above. There is only a limited place for invasive therapy such as intra-articular corticosteroid injection. However, this may be useful for the diagnosis of affected joints, or for specific, temporary treatment of a painful joint that is limiting rehabilitation efforts. However, there may also be associated myofascial pain with trigger points that might respond to local therapy.

Degenerative Disc Disease

Intervertebral discs become dehydrated and desiccated with advancing age. The disc space narrows and becomes less flexible. These changes are readily apparent with radiographs and magnetic imaging. However, there may be little correlation between image appearance and symptoms.[34] Discography may have a limited use in the definition of discs that may be structurally abnormal and symptomatic. However, discs may be structurally abnormal but asymptomatic. Treatment of discogenic pain must be based on rehabilitation methods to reduce stress on any degenerated discs. This is accomplished by improving the tone, strength, and endurance of the postural muscles, and improving ergonomic factors, such as posture. There may be a limited place for anti-inflammatory medication. There are no long-term outcome studies with objective measures that demonstrate efficacy of epidural steroids in degenerative disc disease without acute radiculopathy.

Myofascial Pain/Fibromyalgia

Pain in "soft tissues" is ubiquitous, and many syndromes have been described as a result.[35–37] Table 16-12 reviews current concepts of myofascial pain and fibro-

Table 16-12. Comparison of Fibromyalgia and Myofascial Pain Syndromes

Fibromyalgia
   Widespread (often "total body") pain
   Tenderness of at least 11 of 18 specified points:
      Bilateral nuchal, low cervical, trapezius, supraspinatus, second costochondral junction, lateral epicondyle, gluteal, greater trochanter, medial knee
   Severe fatigue
   Variable autonomic responses (including Raynaud's and sympathetic pain)
   Variable subjective symptoms:
      Chronic headaches, sleep disturbances, anxiety, subjective edema, numbness, irritable bowel, increased symptoms with physical activity, weather changes, stress
   Resistant to treatment: rehabilitation/behavioral principles useful
Myofascial pain syndrome
   Localized tender areas and "trigger points"
   Less impact on overall functioning
   Often good response to physical therapy and trigger point injections
Chronic fatigue syndrome
   Possibly related to chronic viral infection (Epstein–Barr)
   Many of the features of fibromyalgia
   Resistant to treatment: rehabilitation/behavioral principles useful

myalgia. Myofascial pain and "trigger points" are the subjects of entire texts,[38] although other authors ascribe less importance to these conditions,[39] and do not acknowledge the existence of trigger points. The characteristic of these syndromes is the occurrence of localized and referred pain in muscles, muscle attachments and ligaments in the absence of recognizable pathology or significant trauma. There is usually no evidence of degenerative or inflammatory arthritis, inflammatory myalgias, or other systemic disease. Laboratory testing is usually negative. There are no well-defined path-ophysiologic mechanisms in fibromyalgia, the myofascial syndrome, or the chronic fatigue syndrome.[40,41]

Management therefore depends on the application of principles of appropriate ergonomics in the home and workplace and maintenance of a healthy lifestyle, with physical and psychological rehabilitation. In some instances, temporary relief of pain can be obtained by "spray and stretch" techniques, and by localized trigger point injections.[42] Trigger point injections have been carried out with many substances: local anesthetics, corticosteroids, distilled water, and "proliferant" (glucose-phenol-water mixture: "prolotherapy"). Of these possibilities, it would seem rational to use local anesthetic/depot corticosteroid injections to reverse any local inflammatory nociceptive processes. Trigger point injections with local anesthetic and depot corticosteroids are well-established in pain practice. However, there are few data concerning type of local anesthetic or corticosteroid, dosage, number of injections, or frequency. Individual trigger point injections ranging from 0.1 to 20 ml have been reported, lidocaine and bupivacaine are commonly used, and doses of depot methylprednisolone ranging from 1 to 120 mg have also been reported. In the absence of published data, it would seem prudent to use minimal doses of all agents, particularly corticosteroids.

Other modalities, such as acupuncture, massage therapies (e.g., shiatsu), manipulative therapies (e.g., chiropractic), and biobehavioral therapies (e.g., biofeedback), have advocates who claim success. There are few (if any) properly controlled studies of these therapies with objective outcome measures. Studies that are reported are often methodologically flawed, and if not, report "success" at about the placebo rate.

Scar Pain

Surgical, traumatic, and burn scars are painful at the time of the original insult, and may remain painful, or become painful later. Little is known of the mechanisms of persistent scar pain. It is likely that scar pain is a variant of neuropathic pain. Nerves are inevitably damaged in the surgical incision, and may be "trapped" in a suture. The possibility of neuroma formation is therefore always present. A major unanswered question is the reason for the apparent relative rarity of persistent scar pain. Certain scars have the reputation for intransigence, in particular, thoracotomy incisions and bone donor sites (usually iliac crest). In these cases, the neuropathic pain arises from the intercostal and cluneal nerves, respectively. However, any scar has the potential for causing persistent pain. The "failed back" (see below) might be another special case. This type of pain is often reported as continuous and burning, but with intermittent "electric shocks" with movement or minimal trauma.

The treatment of persistent scar pain is difficult in the absence of clearly defined pathological mechanisms. Local counter-irritation (TENS, ice, heat) may assist rehabilitation maneuvers. Injection of local anesthetic/depot corticosteroid into the scar, repeated if necessary, has the reputation of providing increasing relief. The postulated mechanism of this method, if it succeeds in alleviating the pain, is that neuromata in the scar become desensitized and less sensitive to mechanical stimulation. It is hoped that successive injections will lead to progressive improvement. However, the dosages, timing, and frequencies of such injections are not known.

Other therapies have included anticonvulsant and antidepressant medication, opioids, NSAIDs, and benzodiazepines. There are obvious hazards with the long-term use of these groups of medications.

More extreme measures, such as attempts to destroy the putative neuromata with radiofrequency, cryoprobe, surgery, and injections of neurolytic agents, are likely to result in further neural damage and increased pain. There are even reports of dorsal rhizotomy, dorsal column stimulation, implanted peripheral nerve stimulation, and spinal morphine infusion as treatments for scar pain. However, published results of these techniques are more encouraging than actual clinical experience.

Behavioral methods may lead to an increased functional capacity of the patient with severe, incapacitating scar pain. Again, there are few outcome studies.

Low Back Pain

Pathophysiology
Low back pain is a major medical and socioeconomic problem in industrialized societies.[43] Unfortunately, in most cases, the pathophysiologic processes in an individual patient are unknown.[44] Most cases of acute low back pain are *not* caused by intervertebral disc herniation, degenerative disc disease, or degenerative disease of the facet joints. Most cases of chronic low back pain are also *not* caused by these conditions. The diagnosis and management of low back pain is a complex medical, social, and philosophical undertaking.[45,46]

Diagnosis
It may be necessary to undertake a series of diagnostic blocks to determine the anatomic components of back pain. It is often advocated that such injections be carried out under radiologic control (computed tomography or fluoroscopy[47–49]). This practice confirms the anatomic

site of injection, and allows an estimate of the spread of injected solution containing contrast material. It also allows identification of structures that reproduce the pain. In general, two types of pain can be produced during diagnostic blockade. Localized pain indicates irritation of the local tissues. There may also be referred pain from the structure during injection of the contrast material, particularly if the material is hypertonic. The patient may volunteer that this evoked pain is the "usual" pain, or may be asked whether it is the same as usual. If the evoked pain has the same character, location, and radiation as the usual pain, it can generally be assumed that the injected structure is the source of the pain. If injection of local anesthetic then relieves the pain, this provides additional evidence for involvement of that structure. For example, Figure 16-1 shows needles placed in the L4-L5 facet joint and the L5-S1 facet remnant as part of a diagnostic series for mechanical pain after a decompressive laminectomy.

Great care must be used in the interpretation of pain reproduction and relief in the diagnosis of the anatomic structure responsible for the pain. For example, stimulation of the disc during discography is sometimes misleading.[50] On the other hand, injection of the sciatic nerve with local anesthetic has been reported to relieve the pain of lumbar spinal root irritation (proximal to the local anesthetic block).[51] This implies that a distal block can reduce pain arising more centrally by reducing the general neuronal traffic.[52] All available clinical information must be used. For example, if local and referred pain are both reproduced during injection of the contrast medium confirming needle position during facet injection, and a favorable response to local anesthetic and depot corticosteroid occurs, then this might indicate that this particular structure is the likely source of the pain.

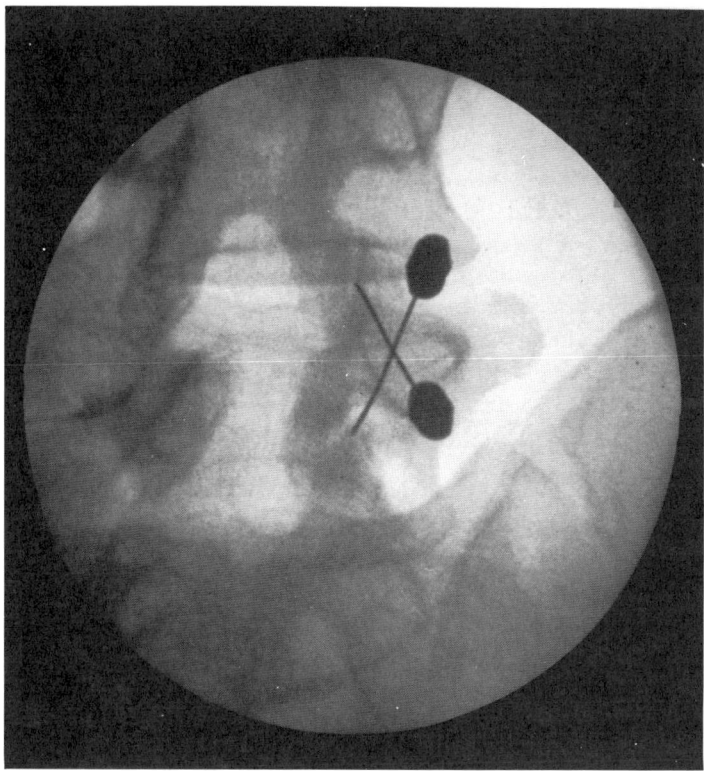

Fig. 16-1. Needles placed through a single skin wheal into the L4-L5 facet joint and the L5-S1 facet remnant for diagnosis of persistent mechanical pain after decompressive laminectomy. Pain was reproduced, then relieved, at the L5-S1 facet remnant, indicating symptomatic instability at that site.

Specific "soft tissue" structures can also be selectively injected. Common sites of pain are the sacroiliac joints, quadratus lumborum and pyriformis muscle attachments, attachments of the thoracolumbar fascia,[53] and the paraspinous muscles themselves. If corticosteroids are included in the injection, and there is local inflammation, the injection might have therapeutic benefit as well.

Diagnostic and Therapeutic Interventions

Epidural Corticosteroid Injection Both subarachnoid[54] and epidural depot corticosteroids have traditionally been used for treatment of low back pain. However, significant questions have been raised about both safety[55] and efficacy.[56] No recommendations can therefore be made on the selection of patients or minimal workup required. In addition, the type or amount of corticosteroid, frequency and technique, and outcome measures have not been clearly defined.

Facet Injection and Denervation Injection of depot corticosteroids into lumbar facet joints has been carried out for more than 15 years, but has only recently been subjected to prospective study.[57] This study was unable to identify clinical facet joint syndromes, and found that only

29 percent of the subjects received pain relief. It also indicated that the facet joint was *not* commonly the single or primary cause of pain in the great majority (more than 90 percent) of low back pain patients.

Other reports indicate that "denervation" of the facet joints in carefully selected patients provides relief of low back pain.[58] However, prospective, long-term, objective data on functional outcome are lacking. I have previously used radiofrequency lysis; cryoneurolysis; and phenol, alcohol, chlorocresol, or ammonium sulfate injections to attempt to improve the outcome of "facet rhizotomy," but has reverted to depot corticosteroid injections combined with aggressive physical rehabilitation. Again, in the absence of prospective, objective functional outcome data, no recommendations can be made.

Discography   Diagnostic discography may provide important information about disc pathology and symptomatology,[59] but this is also disputed.[60]

In rare cases, epidural injections of depot corticosteroids might be warranted as a diagnostic maneuver to determine the presence of a reversible intraspinal process, such as the chemical radiculitis of acute disc herniation or strain of the posterior longitudinal ligament after "whiplash" injury.

It must be stressed that all diagnostic and therapeutic interventions must be carried out with meticulous attention to asepsis, particularly when injecting near implanted hardware.

Treatment Principles

In the absence of acute radiculopathy or myelopathy, which might require surgical intervention, medical treatment of low back pain is based on rehabilitation-sports medicine principles. It should be noted that there is a billion-dollar alternative medicine industry based on the failures of scientific medicine to provide quick and easy "cures" for common complaints: headache, backache, and muscle and joint pains. Most of these interventions have not been "scientifically" tested. However, conventional medical treatment, such as TENS, may be no more effective than placebo.[61]

There must be every effort expended to prevent and reverse the effects of disuse and deconditioning. In the final analysis, it is the patient's own efforts that determine the outcome of any therapy. It follows that there is no quick and easy answer to the complex problem of backache. However, there are certain interventions that may make rehabilitation less painful, and increase compliance with medical advice.

The treatment modalities should be based on the putative pathophysiologic mechanisms of the back pain.[62] An overview of the diagnostic and treatment process is shown in Table 16-13.

Injection of depot corticosteroids into the epidural space is enshrined in the armamentarium of the anesthesia care provider treating back pain. Unfortunately, there are few data demonstrating the efficacy of this practice. There is some evidence of efficacy in the treatment of acute intervertebral disc herniation, but little evidence for efficacy in other back pain syndromes. It appears to be a safe practice, although cases of epidural abscess and arachnoiditis have been reported. Once again, the practice should only be viewed as an ancillary component of the total rehabilitation process.

Other orthopedic pain problems may co-exist with the complaint of low back pain. For example, trochanteric bursitis and pain in the iliotibial tract appear to be more common in back pain patients than in the general population.[63]

Table 16-13. Conservative Low Back Pain Treatment: Phase 1, Dysfunction

Lesion	Manipulation	Injection
Facet joints	Facets	Facet and muscle
Sacroiliac joint	Sacroiliac and muscle	Joint and muscle
Quadratus lumborum	Stretch muscle	Muscle
Pyriformis syndrome	Stretch/relaxation	Muscle
Disc herniation	Rarely	Epidural steroid
Iliac crest syndrome	Stabilize	Muscle attachment

"Failed Back"

The pejorative term, "failed back," is applied to patients who have failed to be "cured" by lumbar laminectomy and/or fusion. It is unclear whether the failure is the fault of the patient or the surgeon(s), or failure of inappropriate surgery. Such patients have invariably had multiple surgical procedures, sometimes with transient benefit, but with an inexorable downhill course. They show the signs and symptoms of chronic pain with deconditioning in all systems, physiological, psychological, and social. The pathophysiology is likely to be complex, with derangements of the structural function of the spine; disc and facet joint damage; damage to muscles and ligaments; and damage to nerve roots and peripheral nerves. There is a limited place for diagnostic injections, as there is little likelihood of corrigible pathology being found. However, there are certain conditions, such as the pseudarthrosis of a failed fusion[64] (Fig. 16-2), painful arthrosis above a fusion, or painful, loose hardware (Fig. 16-3), that might be operable. If such diagnoses are entertained, diagnostic injections of the putative pathologic areas under radiologic control might determine the anatomic pathology.

Rehabilitation of such patients necessarily involves a multidisciplinary team approach. It might be necessary to treat the pain during the process with medications (NSAIDs, opioids, antidepressants, anticonvulsants, antispasmodics), injections of depot corticosteroids, and physical modalities such as TENS. Desperate, last-resort therapies such as implanted dorsal column stimulators or long-term opioid therapy have been used. However, results of such therapies are difficult to evaluate.

Hardware Pain

Internal fixation is a mainstay of orthopedic surgery. In most cases, such hardware becomes incorporated into the callus and causes no problems. However, in a few cases, hardware can loosen and cause pain. This pain is often described as having a deep, toothache quality. It is usually increased by movement and relieved by rest. In the absence of infection, the mechanism is not known. In some cases, a bursa-like structure can be demonstrated radiographically by contrast injection and by aspiration of clear, gelatinous fluid. In such cases, if it is absolutely certain that no infection is present, it is reasonable to inject the hardware with local anesthetic and depot corticosteroid. This may produce transient benefit, and the decision can be made to repeat the injection or remove the hardware. Unfortunately, as in many of the examples

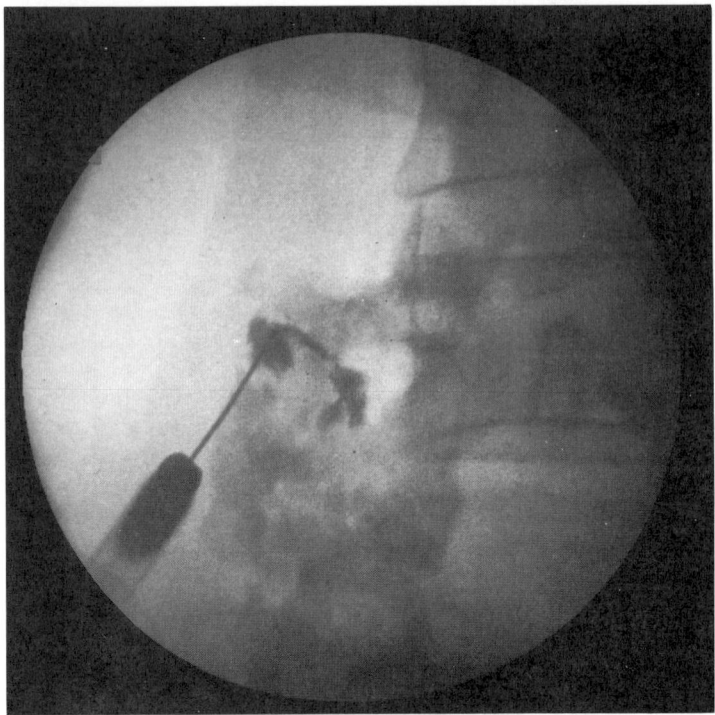

Fig. 16-2. Injection of radio-opaque dye into a lumbar fusion pseudarthrosis reproduced the "usual" pain, which was relieved by the subsequent injection of local anesthetic.

given here, there are no data published, and observations made on the basis of "clinical experience" and anecdotal reports may be misleading or incorrect. Injections in the vicinity of hardware must be carried out under compulsively aseptic conditions, as infection around hardware produces catastrophic complications.

Neck Pain, "Whiplash," and Cervicogenic Headache

Study of the cervical spine is a speciality of its own, and the reader is again referred to the definitive text.[65] The cervical spine is subject to similar pathology as the lumbar spine, and is capable of producing similar symptoms. A summary of the principles of the diagnosis of neck pain is provided in Table 16-14.[66] Chronic neck pain is common in the community, and results in significant disability, impairment, and expense. Local (usually posterior) neck pain is a common predicament in the general population,[67] and referred pain travels into the shoulders, arms, and head.[68] As with the lumbar spine, there may be little correlation between plain radiographic studies and symptoms, although magnetic resonance imaging may prove to be more useful.[69] There is some evidence that neck pain spontaneously resolves with time in the majority of cases, but about one-third continue to experience moderate or severe residual pain.[70] Certain of the cervical pain syndromes may be suitable for treatment in an outpatient pain clinic. However, it must be stressed that serious un-

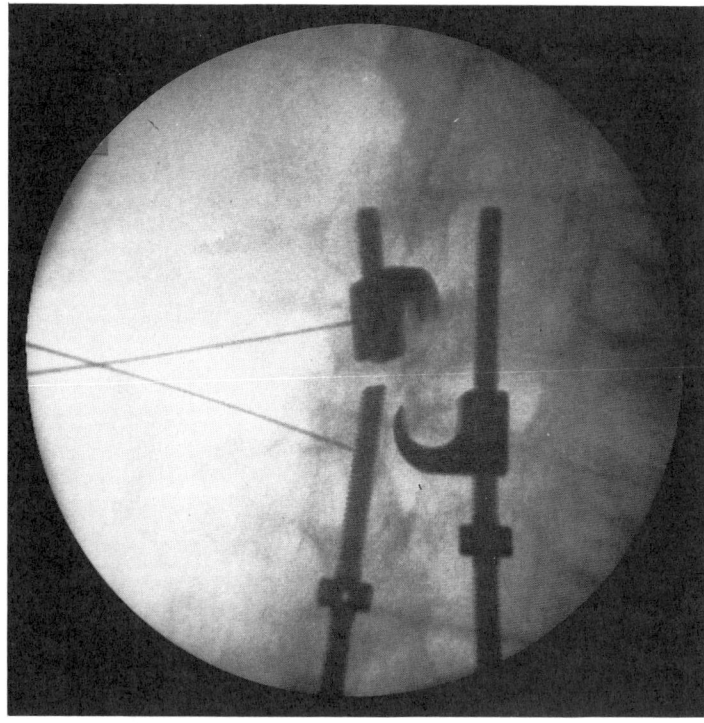

Fig. 16-3. Needles placed through a single skin wheal for diagnostic injection of hardware thought to be loose and causing symptoms. The hook was asymptomatic on injection of dye, but injection of dye around the rod produced the "usual" pain, relieved by the subsequent injection of local anesthetic.

derlying pathology must be excluded before embarking on a symptomatic treatment plan.[71]

Therapy

Cervical Facet Injection   Injection of the cervical facet joints with local anesthetic and depot corticosteroid might produce symptomatic improvement if the joint is painful because of a reversible inflammatory process[72] (Fig. 16-4). However, definitive, prospective studies are required to determine the patients most likely to improve.

Cervical Epidural Steroid Injection Injection of depot corticosteroids into the epidural space would be reasonable if the

inflammatory process is accessible to the steroid. This is probably the case in acute radicular irritation,[73] but is not likely to be the case in whiplash (acceleration–deceleration) injury, where other structures are also likely to be injured. In such cases, it would be appropriate to direct therapy to those. If localized pathology is suspected, trigger point injections, physical modalities, and general rehabilitation may be necessary.

Reflex Sympathetic Dystrophy

Reflex sympathetic dystrophy (RSD), or pain extending beyond the area of injury and persisting beyond the usual heal-

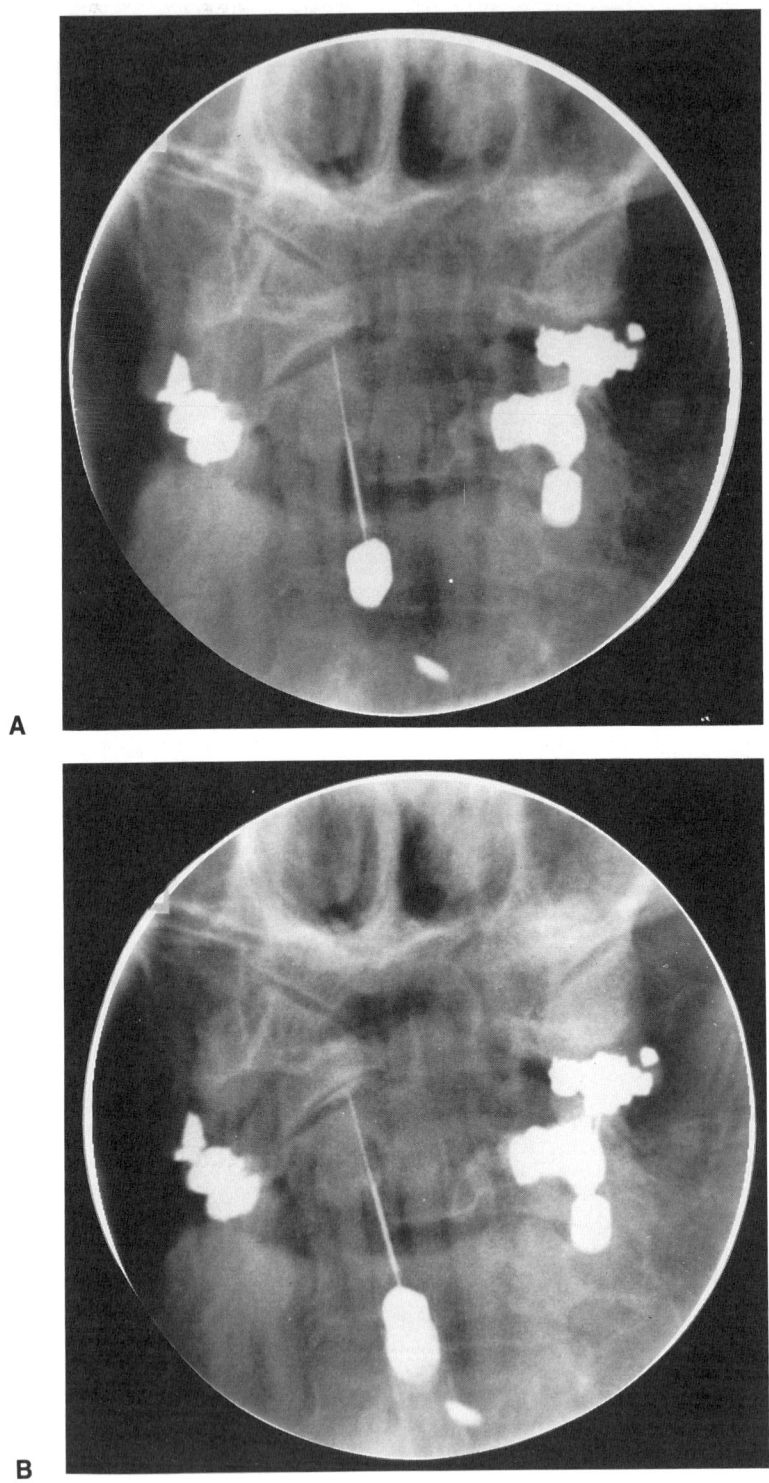

Fig. 16-4. (A) Needle placed in the atlantoaxial joint as part of the investigation of neck pain and headache. (B) Injection of 0.5 ml contrast material reproduced the neck pain and occipital headache, subsequently relieved by injection of 0.5 ml 0.75 percent bupivacaine.

Table 16-14. Differential Diagnosis of Neck Pain

Myelopathy or myeloradiculopathy
  ? Infection
  ? Tumor
  ? Spondylosis with canal stenosis
Acute radicular signs
  ? Infection
  ? Tumor
  ? Disc herniation[a]
  ? "Soft tissue"[a]
Chronic radicular signs
  ? Infection
  ? Tumor
  ? Disc degeneration[a]
  ? Facet arthropathy[a]
Neck pain without referred pain
  ? Infection
  ? Vertebral artery pathology
  ? Facet joint pathology[a]
  ? "Myofascial pain"[a]
  ? Chronic ligamentous strain[a]

[a] Consider treating with physical therapy modalities + corticosteroid injections.
(Adapted from Roberts et al,[66] with permission.)

ing, is a phenomenon recorded since ancient times. It was formalized more than a century ago by scientists such as Weir Mitchell and Claude Bernard, who recognized the importance of the sympathetic nervous system in the maintenance of such pain. There have been innumerable attempts to define the condition (or spectrum of syndromes). The most recent is from the International Association for the Study of Pain Special Interest Group on pain and the sympathetic nervous system.[74]

RSD is a descriptive term referring to a complex disorder or group of disorders that may develop as a consequence of trauma affecting the limbs, with or without obvious nerve lesion. RSD may also develop after visceral diseases and central nervous system lesions or, rarely, without an obvious antecedent event. It consists of pain and related sensory abnormalities, abnormal blood flow and sweating, abnormalities of the motor system and changes in structure of both superficial and deep tissues ("trophic" changes). It is not necessary that all components are present. It is agreed that the name "reflex sympathetic dystrophy" is used in a descriptive sense and does not imply specific underlying mechanisms.

This operational definition is useful, but does not help define the postulated subdivisions or extent of the spectrum of the condition. There are sympathetic components of RSD itself, causalgia, sympathetically maintained pain, phantom limb pain, "pain-dysfunction syndrome" and "reflex orthopedic dystrophy."[75] There have been no validated diagnostic criteria published, which makes evaluation of incidence, treatment, and outcome impossible to determine. There are over 40 therapies published, usually as uncontrolled case studies or anecdotal reports, all with remarkable results. The optimal therapy cannot be determined until the definitive prospective, controlled, double-blind study with objective long-term outcome measures is published. In the interim, an attempt will be made to present a rational approach to the problem. Table 16-15 outlines the clinical assessments necessary in the evaluation of a patient with suspected RSD.

It must be noted that RSD may represent dysfunction in several physiologic systems, and clinical assessment must include all those systems at risk of involvement. It is necessary to examine all components of the nervous system. The sensory, motor, and autonomic components of the peripheral nervous system may all show changes. There may be changes within the central nervous system, and also in psychological functioning. It is difficult to know whether changes are the primary cause or a secondary response to pain, disuse, or the initial injury. Peripheral sensation should

Table 16-15. Clinical Assessment of RSD

Sensory system testing
> The characteristics of the pain and sensory disturbances should be evaluated and recorded
>> Spontaneous pain, often burning in nature, allodynia, hyperpathia, hyperalgesia (mechanical and thermal)
>> Evoked pain from joints, muscles, ligaments, skin
>> Co-existing peripheral nerve damage

Autonomic system testing
> As many functions as possible should be tested as simply and noninvasively as possible
>> Vasomotor function (thermometry [infrared], thermography)
>> Sudomotor function (cobalt blue, starch/iodine, acetylcholine stimulation [QSART])
>> Bone blood flow (three-phase bone scan)
>> Skin capillary microscopy
>> Laser Doppler

Motor system testing
> Muscle strength, joint mobility (active and passive range), presence of tremor

Evaluation of "trophic" changes
> Evaluation of changes in as quantitative manner as possible
>> Bone density (plain radiographs)
>> Edema (measurement of volume compared with the unaffected side)
>> Hair/nail growth

---

be carefully examined clinically. There are few, if any, data to suggest that laboratory testing (such as electromyography, somatosensory evoked potentials, and quantitative sensory thresholds) has any increased sensitivity or specificity in the diagnosis of RSD. However, certain autonomic tests may provide useful quantitative information. Vasomotor function can be measured by infrared thermography simply, accurately, and cheaply with a hand-held infrared thermometer. It can also be measured with thermography, which is complex, accurate, and expensive. Sweating can be quantitated with starch/iodine or cobalt blue powders applied to the skin, or by iontophoresed acetylcholine.[76] This latter test is able to demonstrate an exaggerated response in RSD. Similarly, bone blood flow can be examined with a three-phase bone scan.[77] This scan indicates a delayed periarticular uptake of radioactivity in RSD. Other quantitative tests, such as skin capillary microscopy and laser Doppler skin blood flow measurements, must still be regarded as investigational.

It is also essential to obtain objective measurements, if possible, of the "trophic" changes. Joint movement, active and passive, can be measured directly by goniometer. Strength of convenient actions (e.g., grip strength and pinch apposition and opposition) can be easily measured. Bone density can be estimated by plain radiography (comparing the normal side). Edema of an extremity can be estimated with water displacement.

These measurements can be used to estimate the extent of the trophic changes and disability or impairment, and will enable a quantitative measure of improvement with therapy. One of the most difficult aspects of the diagnosis and therapy of RSD is that many of the changes of RSD are similar to the changes of disuse. It is therefore particularly difficult to ascribe a primary cause. It is not known whether this is important, because the effects of disuse have to be reversed. There is no nerve block, medication, vitamin, dietary supplement, hormone, or other extrinsic maneuver that will reverse the disuse changes. These changes can only be reversed by *use*, and therapy must be directed to that end.

Clinical Criteria

It has been suggested in a preliminary study[78] that there may be 10 easily obtained criteria for the diagnosis of RSD. Five of these are symptoms: burning pain; allodynia or hyperpathia; skin temperature and/or color changes; changes in sweating; and edema, hair, and nail changes. The objective signs are temperature changes (of greater than 1°C), characteristic three-phase bone scan, decrease in bony density, abnormal quantitative sweat test, and appropriate response to diagnostic sympathetic blockade (central or peripheral). It is postulated that any six of these are necessary for the diagnosis of "probable" RSD. However, it must be emphasized that this scoring method has yet to be validated by a prospective study, including treatment and outcome measured by objective criteria. Table 16-16 summarizes proposed diagnostic criteria for RSD. Again, it must be noted that these criteria have not been validated with appropriate prospective studies.

There are potential shortcomings of this method. The signs, symptoms, and investigations may be abnormal in other states, such as simple disuse, the "pain-dysfunction syndrome," and "repetitive strain injury." There is no allowance for tremor or other motor abnormalities. It does not allow for any weighting for importance of a particular symptom or test. It does not take into account the possibilities of different stages and severities. It does not take into account any psychological predispositions or consequences. It does not allow for newer and more precise diagnostic methods.

Pain-Dysfunction Syndromes

Various pain syndromes have been described that may have some or many of the characteristics of RSD, including burning pain, sensory changes, autonomic changes, motor changes, and disuse/dystrophy/atrophy.[79] However, in such cases, sympathetic blockade does not relieve the pain or result in improvement in the condition. There is no comprehensive description of these conditions, which may be reported in the literature as "refractory RSD." The general principles of rehabilitation apply, as there is no specific management.

Therapy

There is not a clear definition of RSD or the other dystrophies, so there cannot be specific therapy. The lack of clear criteria make it impossible to review the literature for optimal therapies. However, of the more than 40 reported, all with similar and good success, some common features pertain (Table 16-17). Again, it should be emphasized that there has not yet been published any good prospective study with objective outcome criteria that indicates optimal therapy for RSD and its variants.

Physical Therapy   Disuse of a limb will cause atrophic changes: loss of muscle tone, strength, and endurance; loss of joint mobility; contractures of ligaments, joints, and muscles; reduction in regional blood flow; changes in kinesthesia; loss of bone calcium; and changes in hair, nails, and sweating. Regardless of the cause, these changes have to be reversed.

Table 16-16.   RSD Diagnostic Criteria

Clinical symptoms and signs of RSD
    Burning pain
    Allodynia/hyperpathia
    Skin temperature/color changes
    Sweating changes
    Edema/hair/nail changes

Laboratory investigations of RSD
    Thermometry/thermography
    Three-phase bone scan
    Bony density
    Quantitative sweat test
    Response to sympathetic blockade (central or peripheral)

Interpretation
    >6   Probable RSD
    3–5   Possible RSD
    <3   Unlikely RSD

Table 16-17. Treatment of RSD:
Combination/Interdisciplinary Therapy

Physical therapy/rehabilitation
  Active and passive range of movement
  Increase strength and endurance
  Desensitize skin and deeper structures
  Proprioceptive retraining
  Encourage normal use
Pain reduction
  NSAIDs
  Peripheral nerve blocks (repeated or continuous)
  Central neuraxial blockade (repeated or continuous)
  Opioids
  TENS
  Heroic, invasive methods (dorsal column stimulation, spinal narcotics)
Sympathetic blockade
  Peripheral end-organ depletion (oral or intravenous regional guanethidine)
  Peripheral blockade (α-blockers)
  Ganglion blockade (stellate, lumbar sympathetic)
  Surgical or chemical sympathectomy (rarely, last resort)
Psychosocial support
  Psychological assessment
  Rehabilitation/vocational counselling
  Medicolegal support

Standard rehabilitation methods usually involve a combination of passive and active exercise, progressing to normal use and work-hardening. In the cases of RSD, pain might be the limiting factor in the rehabilitation process.

Pain Reduction   Pain is prominent in RSD, and reduction in the pain will allow more effective therapy to take place. It might become necessary to coordinate medication or sensory or sympathetic nerve blocks with the therapy to facilitate compliance. There have been reports of both dorsal column stimulation and spinal narcotic administration for relief of pain in RSD.[80]

Sympathetic Blockade   Sympathetic efferent activity can be blocked at the end-organ with guanethidine, bretylium, prazosin, or phentolamine.[81,82] It can be blocked at the sympathetic ganglia temporarily with local anesthetics or for longer periods (in the lumbar region) with neurolytics. Mixed nerves in the periphery or central neuraxis can be blocked temporarily with local anesthetics to provide both somatic pain reduction and sympathetic block.[83] It is not known whether the blood flow changes represent a primary dysfunction, or whether they are related to local reflex changes.[84]

Psychosocial Support   It is not unusual for RSD patients to be depressed and frustrated with their pain and impairment, and to be involved in acrimonious litigation with their employers (or other agencies). Psychosocial support is an essential component in therapy.

It must again be stressed that successful treatment of RSD, including reversal of the dystrophic changes, requires an intensive, dedicated, interdisciplinary team approach, with full cooperation of the patient. It is also necessary to have the full support of the legal, worker compensation, and social welfare systems.

Prevention

It is tempting to speculate that perioperative pain relief and sympatholysis might prevent the development of postoperative RSD. Although there are case reports supporting this theory,[85] there are no prospective controlled studies. It is appealing and rational to suggest that surgery with a high risk of producing RSD (knee arthroscopy, carpal tunnel release) could be performed under intravenous regional anesthesia, including guanethidine or bretylium to produce peripheral sympatholysis. Unfortunately, this hypothesis could only be tested with a very large, controlled prospective study, which is unlikely to be carried out.

"Reflex Orthopedic Dystrophy"

As noted above, there are cases of "sympathetic independent pain." If there is any common feature, it appears to be injury to a minor peripheral sensory nerve. The most common cases seen in my practice are "postarthroscopy knee"[86] and "post-carpal tunnel hand."

In the first type, it is the clinical impression (beware!) that the residual pain and disability is greatly in excess of that expected. Although the knee may have some of the features of RSD, the extent of the sympathetic dysfunction is often restricted. In addition, the usual sympathetic blocks do not provide any relief of pain, and do not allow physical therapy to be carried out. However, injection of the infrapatellar branch of the saphenous nerve where it was damaged by the arthroscope is of diagnostic value. If the knee becomes warm, dry, and comfortable, then the scar and/or nerve can be reinjected with local anesthetic and depot corticosteroid. This injection may need to be repeated on several occasions, presumably to treat the neuroma. The incidence of this condition is not known, although the reported incidence of RSD and neurologic injury both appear to be of the order of 5 percent in a large series (N = 118,590).[87]

In the upper extremity, the hand may have the appearance of RSD, but be unresponsive to sympathetic manipulations. Again, injection of the cutaneous branch of the median (or ulnar, as appropriate) may increase temperature, reduce pain, and allow therapy. Depot corticosteroids may be required around the putative neuroma. The dorsal radial nerve also seems to be vulnerable in fractures of the wrist.

It should again be emphasized that these are clinical impressions awaiting prospective studies for confirmation or refutation.

Phantom Pain

Pain may be experienced in an absent organ or limb, and is assumed to be of central origin.[88,89] The incidence may be as high as 80 percent.[90] There does not appear to be any effective treatment, despite clinical impressions of more than 60 methods.[91] The dangers of relying on clinical impressions have been clearly illustrated by these two surveys by Sherman et al.[90,91] The first survey questioned pain clinics on the modalities in use and the "success rates of each modality." The therapists in the surveyed pain clinics reported success rates of 26 to 73 percent, depending on the modality. Conservative therapies were reported as more effective than surgical ones. There was a reported overall mean success rate of 62 percent, with an average of 52 percent reduction in pain. The same researchers then surveyed a large group of amputees. The respondents reported that they received the same modalities that the pain clinics were using. However, the amputees reported that only 0.4 percent were "cured," and only 0.7 percent received any large permanent change. Overall, only 8.4 percent could be said to have been helped to any real extent. This is a dramatic example of the dangers of misinformation and inappropriate institutional practices arising from inadequate objective follow-up data.[92]

However, a prospective trial of epidural analgesia for 3 days before, during, and after amputation appeared to abolish phantom limb pain for at least a year.[93] This is an encouraging report, and suggests that chronic or neuropathic pain might be preventable with appropriate control of acute pain.

When an amputee complains of pain in the amputated extremity, it is important to determine whether the pain is stump (scar) pain, neuroma pain, phantom pain, or other neuropathic pain (e.g., from nerve root or plexus irritation). It is also important to evaluate the vascular, neurologic, and tumor status, depending on the reason for the amputation.

Other modalities, such as TENS and dorsal column stimulation, have been reported to be useful in the management of phantom pain. However, it must be concluded that there is currently no specific treatment for this variety of neuropathic pain, and general rehabilitation principles will have to be used.

In summary, it has become clear from recent information that several distinct categories of pain can occur, singly or in combination. These categories are defined by their pathophysiology, and the treatment of each depends on that pathophysiology. There can never be a "cookbook" approach to pain management in view of these factors. Orthopedic anesthesia care providers have much to offer in the diagnosis and treatment of acute and chronic orthopedic pain, but the optimal results will be obtained in an interdisciplinary environment.

REFERENCES

1. Bonica JJ (ed): The Management of Pain. 2nd Ed. Lea & Febiger, Philadelphia, 1990
2. Raj PP (ed): Practical Management of Pain. 2nd Ed. Mosby-Year Book, St. Louis, 1992
3. International Association for the Study of Pain, Committee on Taxonomy. Pain (suppl. 3):S1, 1986
4. Chapman CR: The concept of measurement: coexisting theoretical perspectives. p. 1. In Chapman CR, Loeser JD (eds): Advances in Pain Research and Therapy. Vol 12. Issues in Pain Measurement. Raven Press, New York, 1989
5. Lasagna L: Clinical analgesic research: a historical perspective. p. 1. In Max MB, Portenoy RK, Laska EM (eds): Advances in Pain Research and Therapy. Vol. 18. The Design of Analgesic Clinical Trials. Raven Press, New York, 1991
6. Gracely RH: Experimental pain models. p. 33. In Max MB, Portenoy RK, Laska EM (eds): Advances in Pain Research Therapy. Vol. 18. The Design of Analgesic Clinical Trials. Raven Press, New York, 1991
7. Peck CL: Psychological factors in chronic pain management. p. 251. In Cousins MJ, Phillips GD (eds): Acute Pain Management. Churchill Livingstone, New York, 1986
8. American Psychiatric Association. Diagnostic and Statistical Manual of Mental Disorders. 3rd Ed., Revised. American Psychiatric Association, Washington, DC, 1987
9. Wilson PR: Taxonomy again? (editorial). Clin J Pain 7:171, 1991
10. Wilson PR, Lamer TJ: Pain mechanisms: anatomy and physiology. p. 65. In Raj PP (ed): Practical Management of Pain. Mosby-Year Book, St. Louis, 1992
11. Yaksh TL: Neurologic mechanisms of pain. p. 791. In Cousins MJ, Bridenbaugh PO (eds): Neural Blockade. 2nd Ed. JB Lippincott, Philadelphia, 1987
12. Yaksh TL: Pain receptor pharmacology for the clinician. American Society for Regional Anesthesia 1992 Annual Meeting Abstract. p. 255
13. U.S. Department of Health and Human Services, Public Health Service, Agency for Health Care Policy and Research: Acute Pain Management: Operative or Medical Procedures and Trauma. Clinical Practice Guideline, February 1992
14. Foley KM, Bonica JJ, Ventafridda V (eds): Advances in Pain Research and Therapy. Vol. 16. Second International Congress on Cancer Pain. Raven Press, New York, 1990
15. Pain and central nervous system disease. In Casey KL (ed): The Central Pain Syndromes. Raven Press, New York, 1991

16. Levitt M: The theory of chronic deafferentiation dysesthesias. J Neurol Sci 43:71, 1990

17. Yaksh TL, Yamamoto T: Studies on the pharmacology of spinal systems underlying anomalous pain states. p. 197. In Nashold B, Ovelmen-Levitt (eds): Advances in Pain Research and Therapy. Vol. 19. Deafferentiation Pain Syndrome: Pathophysiology and Treatment. Raven Press, New York, 1991

18. Devor M, Govrin-Lippmann R, Raber P: Corticosteroids reduce neuroma hyperexcitability. p. 451. In Fields HL, Dubner R, Cervero F (eds): Advances in Pain Research and Therapy. Vol. 9. Proceedings of the Fourth World Congress on Pain. Raven Press, New York, 1985

19. Large R, Butler M, James F, Peters J: A systems model of chronic musculoskeletal pain. Aust NZ J Psychiatry 24:529, 1990

20. Covington EC: Depression and chronic fatigue in the patient with chronic pain. Prim Care 18:341, 1991

21. Dworkin SF, Von Korff M, LeResche L: Multiple pains and psychiatric disturbance. Arch Gen Psychiatry 47:239, 1990

22. Turk DC: Customizing treatment for chronic pain patients: who, what, and why. Clin J Pain 6:255, 1990

23. Hadler NM: Industrial rheumatology. The Australian and New Zealand experiences with arm pain and backache in the workplace. Med J Aust 144:191, 1986

24. Miller MH, Topliss DJ: Chronic upper limb pain syndrome (repetitive strain injury) in the Australian workforce: a systematic cross-sectional rheumatological study of 229 patients. J Rheumatol 15:1705, 1988

25. Modlin HC: Compensation neurosis. Bull Am Acad Psychiatry Law 14:263, 1986

26. Wiesel SW: Compensation neck pain. p. 823. In The Cervical Spine Research Society Editorial Committee: The Cervical Spine. JB Lippincott, Philadelphia, 1989

27. Rein H: Thermography: medical and legal implications. Leg Med p. 95, 1986

28. Parsons GE, Robinson WT III: Preparation and presentation of medical evidence. p. 947. In Raj PP (ed): Practical Management of Pain. 2nd Ed. Mosby-Year Book, St. Louis, 1992

29. Boas R, Cousins MJ: Diagnostic blockade. p. 885. In Cousins MJ, Bridenbaugh PO (eds): Neural Blockade. 2nd Ed. JB Lippincott, Philadelphia, 1984

30. MacMillan J, Schaffer JL, Kambin P: Routes and incidence of communication of lumbar discs with surrounding neural structures. Spine 16:167, 1991

31. Kay J, Raff H, Findling JW: Epidural triamcinolone causes prolonged and severe suppression of the pituitary-adrenal axis. Anesthesiology 75(3A):A694, 1991

32. Wiesel SW, Tsourmas N, Feffer HL et al. A study of computer-assisted tomography. I. The incidence of positive CAT scans in an asymptomatic group of patients. Spine 9:549, 1984

33. Miller GM, Forbes GS, Onofrio BM. Magnetic imaging of the spine. Mayo Clin Proc 64:986, 1989

34. Gore DR, Sepic SB, Gardner GM: Roentgenographic findings of the cervical spine in asymptomatic people. Spine 11:521, 1986

35. Thompson JM: Tension myalgia as a diagnosis at the Mayo Clinic and its relationship to fibrositis, fibromyalgia, and myofascial pain syndrome. Mayo Clin Proc 65:1237, 1990

36. Yunus MB, Masi AT, Aldag JC: Preliminary criteria for primary fibromyalgia syndrome (PFS): multivariate analysis of a consecutive series of PFS, other pain patients, and normal subjects. Clin Exp Rheumatol 7:63, 1989

37. Bennett RM: Myofascial pain syndromes and the fibromyalgia syndrome: a comparative analysis. p. 43. In Fricton JR, Awad EA (eds): Advances in Pain Research and Therapy. Vol. 17. Myofascial Pain and Fibromyalgia. Raven Press, New York, 1990

38. Travell JG, Simon DG (eds): Myofascial Pain and Dysfunction, The Trigger Point Manual. Vols. 1 & 2. Williams & Wilkins, Baltimore, 1983 and 1992

39. Hadler NM (ed): Clinical Concepts in Regional Muscoloskeletal Illness. Grune & Stratton, Orlando, FL, 1987

40. Holmes GP, Kaplan JE, Gantz NM et al:

Chronic fatigue syndrome: a working case definition. Ann Intern Med 108:387, 1988

41. Goldenberg DL, Simms RW, Geiger A, Komaroff AL: High frequency of fibromyalgia in patients with chronic fatigue seen in a primary care practice. Arthritis Rheum 33:381, 1990

42. Fricton JR: Management of myofascial pain syndrome: p. 325. In Friction JR, Awad EA (eds): Advances in Pain Research and Therapy. Vol. 17. Myofascial Pain and Fibromyalgia. Raven Press, New York, 1990

43. Frymoyer JW, Ducker TB, Hadler NM et al: The future of spinal treatment. p. 43. In Frymoyer JW (ed): The Adult Spine. Vol. 1. Raven Press, New York, 1991

44. Mooney V: Differential diagnosis of low back disorders: principles of classification. p. 1551. In Frymoyer JW (ed): The Adult Spine. Vol. 2. Raven Press, New York, 1991

45. Reesor KA, Craig KD: Medically incongruent chronic back pain: physical limitations, suffering, and ineffective coping. Pain 32:35, 1988

46. Hadler NM: Backache and humanism. p. 55. In Frymoyer JW (ed): The Adult Spine. Vol. 1. Raven Press, New York, 1991

47. Mooney V: Injection: role in pain definition. p. 527. In Frymoyer JW (ed): The Adult Spine. Vol. 1. Raven Press, New York, 1991

48. El-Khoury TY, Ehara S, Weinstein JN, Montgomery WJ et al: Epidural steroid injection: a procedure ideally performed with fluoroscopic control. Radiology 168:554, 1988

49. Walsh TR, Weinstein JN, Spratt KF et al: Lumbar discography in normal subjects. A controlled, prospective study. J Bone Joint Surg 72A:1081, 1990

50. Weinstein J, Claverie W, Gibson S: The pain of discography. Spine 13:1344, 1988

51. Xavier AV, McDanal J, Kissin I: Relief of sciatic radicular pain by sciatic nerve block. Anesth Analg 67:1177, 1988

52. Abram SE: Pain mechanisms in lumbar radiculopathy (editorial). Anesth Analg 67:1135, 1988

53. Collee G, Dijkmans BAC, Vandenbroucke JP, Cats A: Iliac crest pain syndrome in low back pain. A double blind, randomized study of local injection therapy. J Rheumatol 18:1060, 1991

54. Wilkinson HA: Intrathecal Depo-Medrol: a literature review. Clin J Pain 8:49, 1992

55. Johnson A, Ryan MD, Roche J: Depo-Medrol and myelographic arachnoiditis. Med J Aust 155:18, 1991

56. Benzon HT: Epidural steroid injections for low back pain and lumbosacral radiculopathy. Pain 24:277, 1986

57. Jackson RP, Jacobs RR, Montesano PX: Facet joint injection in low-back pain. A prospective statistical study. Spine 13:966, 1988

58. Silvers HR: Lumbar percutaneous facet rhizotomy. Spine 15:36, 1990

59. Executive Committee, North American Spine Society: Position statement on discography. Spine 13:1343, 1988

60. Nachemson A: Lumbar discography—where are we today? Spine 14:555, 1989

61. Deyo RA, Walsh NE, Martin DC et al: A controlled trial of transcutaneous electrical nerve stimulation (TENS) and exercise for chronic low back pain. N Engl J Med 322:1627, 1990

62. Kirkaldy-Willis WH: A comprehensive outline of treatment. p. 247. In Kirkaldy-Willis WH (ed): Managing Low Back Pain. 2nd Ed. Churchill Livingstone, New York, 1983

63. Collee G, Dijkmans BAC, Vandenbroucke JP, Cats A: Greater trochanteric pain syndrome (trochanteric bursitis) in low back pain. Scand J Rheumatol 20:262, 1991

64. Lauerman WC, Bradford DS, Transfeldt EE, Ogilvie JW: Management of pseudarthrosis after arthrodesis of the spine for idiopathic scoliosis. J Bone Joint Surg 73A:222, 1991

65. The Cervical Spine Research Society, Editorial Committee: The Cervical Spine. 2nd Ed. JB Lippincott, Philadelphia, 1989

66. Roberts WA, Garfin SR, White AA: An algorithm for the diagnosis of neck pain. p. 611. In The Cervical Spine Research Society, Editorial Committee: The Cervical Spine. 2nd Ed. JB Lippincott, Philadelphia, 1989

67. Hadler N, Acker JJ: Neck pain. p. 83. In Hadler N (ed): Medical Management of

the Regional Musculoskeletal Diseases. Grune & Stratton, Orlando, FL, 1984

68. Dwyer A, Aprill C, Bogdule N: Cervical zygapophyseal joint pair patterns. I: a study in normal volunteers. Spine 15:453, 1990

69. Ullrich CG: Magnetic resonance imaging of the cervical spine and spinal cord. p. 157. In The Cervical Spine Research Society, Editorial Committee: The Cervical Spine. 2nd Ed. JB Lippincott, Philadelphia, 1989

70. Gore DR, Sepic SB, Gardner GM, Murray MP: Neck pain: a long-term follow-up of 205 patients. Spine 12:1, 1987

71. Wilson PR: Chronic neck pain and cervicogenic headache. Clin J Pain 7:5, 1991

72. Wedel DJ, Wilson PR: Cervical facet arthrography. Reg Anesth 10:/7, 1985

73. Warfield CA, Biber MP, Crews DA, Dwarkanath GK: Epidural steroid injection as a treatment for cervical radiculitis. Clin J Pain 4:201, 1988

74. Jänig W: Experimental approach to reflex sympathetic dystrophy and related syndromes. Pain 46:241, 1991

75. Wilson PR: Sympathetically maintained pain: diagnosis, measurement, and efficacy of treatment. p. 91. In Stanton-Hicks M (ed): Pain and the Sympathetic Nervous System. Kluwer Academic Publishers, Boston, 1990

76. Low PA, Caskey PE, Tuck RR, Fealey RD et al: Quantitative sudomotor axon reflex in normal and neuropathic subjects. Ann Neurol 14:573, 1983

77. Kozin F, Soin JS, Ryan LM et al: Bone scintigraphy in the reflex sympathetic dystrophy syndrome. Radiology 138:443, 1981

78. Gibbons JJ, Wilson PR: "RSD score": criteria for the diagnosis of reflex sympathetic dystrophy and causalgia. Clin J Pain (in press)

79. Amadio PC: Pain dysfunction syndromes. J Bone Joint Surg 70A:944, 1988

80. Barolat G, Schwartzmann R, Woo R: Epidural spinal cord stimulation in the management of reflex sympathetic dystrophy. Appl Neurophysiol 50:442, 1987

81. Bonelli S, Conoscenti F, Movilia PG et al: Regional intravenous guanethidine vs.

stellate ganglion block in re thetic dystrophies: a randor Pain 16:297, 1983

82. Raja SN, Treede R, Davis KD JN: Sympathetic alpha-adrene ade with phentolamine: a dia; for sympathetically maintai Anesthesiology 74:691, 1991

83. Gibbons JJ, Wilson PR, Lamer BA: Interscalene blocks for chr(extremity pain. Clin J Pain (in

84. Wakisaka S, Kajander KC, Be Abnormal skin temperature and sympathetic vasomotor innerva experimental painful periphera athy. Pain 46:299, 1991

85. Hobelman CF Jr, Dellon AL: U longed sympathetic blockade ; junct to surgery in the patient \ pathetic maintained pain. Mic 10:151, 1989

86. Poehling GG, Pollock FE Jr, Kc Reflex sympathetic dystrophy of after sensory nerve injury. Arthr Arthroscopic Related Surg 4:31,

87. Committee on Complications o scopy Association of North . Complications of arthroscopy an scopic surgery: results of a nati(vey. Arthroscopy: J Arthroscopy Surg 1:214, 1985

88. Melzack R: Phantom limbs. Sci . 120, 1992

89. Iacono RP, Linford J, Sadyk R: Pa agement after lower extremity . tion. Neurosurgery 20:496, 1987

90. Sherman RA, Sherman CJ, Pai Chronic phantom and stump pain American veterans: results of a Pain 18:83, 1984

91. Sherman RA, Sherman CJ, Gall survey of current phantom limb pai ments in the United States. Pain 8:8

92. Sherman RA, Ernst JL, Barja RH, GM: Phantom pain: a lesson in t cessity for careful clinical resear chronic pain problems. J Rehab Re 25:7, 1988

93. Bach S, Noreng MF, Tjellden NU: tom limb pain in amputees during th 12 months following limb ampu after preoperative lumbar epidural l ade. Pain 33:297, 1988

Index

Page numbers followed by f *denote figures; those followed by* t *denote tables.*